WILMS vs. Neuroblastoma

hemihypertrophy
aniridia
hematuria
abd mass
mets → LUNG, brain

opsiclonus, myoclonus
calcif's on AXR
mets → bone liver, brain

Chemo phases – induction – consolidation – maintenance

AIDs in kids – mostly b/o drug-abusing parents

- failure to thrive
- lymphadenop.
- hepatomegaly

± diarrhea ⇓ AIDS Clin. complex

ARC – hypergglob.
- anti HTLV 3 AB
- Reversed T_4/T_8

Larry Steven Turtel

Sepsis in Infant < 3 mos

#1 – β strep
#2 – E Coli
#3 – LISTERIA
#4 – Staph
#5 – H Flu

} start AMP/Gent

CP

static encephalop. which affects motor cortex causing fixed motor deficits usually 2° to perinatal inj.

MBD

"Min. brain dysfn" or "learning disability" Has lg spectrum of unrelated phenom. to intellectual impairment

LFTs

Hepatocyte fn { γGTP – most sensitive, SGOT, SGPT

Biliary tree { 5'NT, Alk Phos

Cefuroxane
Cefotriaxone

PED'S ID: RED BOOK
PO Box 1034
Evanston, ILL 60204

Cefuroxime = Zinacef
2nd gen. cephalosp.
crosses BBB

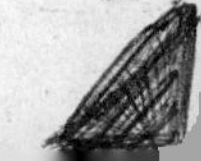

handbook of PEDIATRICS

FOURTEENTH EDITION

handbook of PEDIATRICS

HENRY K. SILVER, MD
Professor of Pediatrics
University of Colorado School of Medicine
Denver, Colorado

C. HENRY KEMPE, MD
Professor of Pediatrics and Microbiology
University of Colorado School of Medicine
Denver, Colorado

HENRY B. BRUYN, MD
Clinical Professor of Medicine and Pediatrics
University of California School of Medicine
San Francisco, California
Consultant in Child Health
City and County of San Francisco

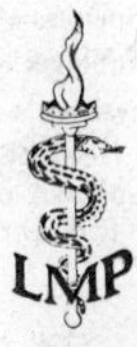

Lange Medical Publications
LOS ALTOS, CALIFORNIA 94022

1983

Lange Medical Publications

Drawer L, Los Altos, California 94022

Spanish Edition: *El Manual Moderno, S.A. de C.V., Av. Sonora 206, 06100-Mexico, D.F.*
Italian Edition: *Piccin Nuova Libraria, S.p.A., Via Altinate, 107, 35121 Padua, Italy*
Portuguese Edition: *Editora Guanabara Koogan, S.A., Travessa do Ouvidor, 11-ZC-00, 20,040 Rio de Janeiro - RJ, Brazil*
Japanese Edition: *Hirokawa Publishing Company, 27-14, Hongo 3, Bunkyo-ku, Tokyo 113, Japan*

International Standard Book Number: *0-87041-066-0*
Library of Congress Catalogue Card Number: *63-10679*

Handbook of Pediatrics, 14th ed. $13.00

A Concise Medical Library for Practitioner and Student

Current Medical Diagnosis & Treatment 1983 (annual revision). Edited by M.A. Krupp and M.J. Chatton. 1130 pp. 1983

Current Pediatric Diagnosis & Treatment, 7th ed. Edited by C.H. Kempe, H.K. Silver, and D. O'Brien. 1106 pp, *illus.* 1982

Current Surgical Diagnosis & Treatment, 6th ed. Edited by J.E. Dunphy and L.W. Way. About 1200 pp, *illus.* 1983

Current Obstetric & Gynecologic Diagnosis & Treatment, 4th ed. Edited by R.C. Benson. 1038 pp, *illus.* 1982

Harper's Review of Biochemistry (formerly **Review of Physiological Chemistry**), 19th ed. D.W. Martin, Jr., P.A. Mayes, and V.W. Rodwell. 638 pp, *illus.* 1983

Review of Medical Physiology, 11th ed. W.F. Ganong. 643 pp, *illus.* 1983

Review of Medical Microbiology, 15th ed. E. Jawetz, J.L. Melnick, and E.A. Adelberg. 553 pp, *illus.* 1982

Basic & Clinical Pharmacology. Edited by B.G. Katzung. 815 pp, *illus.* 1982

Basic & Clinical Immunology, 4th ed. Edited by D.P. Stites, J.D. Stobo, H.H. Fudenberg, and J.V. Wells. 775 pp, *illus.* 1982

Basic Histology, 4th ed. L.C. Junqueira and J. Carneiro. About 510 pp, *illus.* 1983

Clinical Cardiology, 3rd ed. M. Sokolow and M.B. McIlroy. 763 pp, *illus.* 1981

General Urology, 10th ed. D.R. Smith. 598 pp, *illus.* 1981

General Ophthalmology, 10th ed. D. Vaughan and T. Asbury. 407 pp, *illus.* 1983

Correlative Neuroanatomy & Functional Neurology, 18th ed. J.G. Chusid. 476 pp, *illus.* 1982

Principles of Clinical Electrocardiography, 11th ed. M.J. Goldman. 438 pp, *illus.* 1982

Handbook of Obstetrics & Gynecology, 7th ed. R.C. Benson. 808 pp, *illus.* 1980

Physician's Handbook, 20th ed. M.A. Krupp, L.M. Tierney, Jr., E. Jawetz, R.L. Roe, and C.A. Camargo. 774 pp, *illus.* 1982

Handbook of Poisoning: Prevention, Diagnosis & Treatment, 11th ed. R.H. Dreisbach. 632 pp. 1983

Lithographed in USA

Table of Contents

Preface

In the fourteenth edition of this Handbook, the authors have again made extensive revisions and additions, but the format and objectives have remained the same: to present to the medical student, practicing physician, and other health professionals a concise and readily available digest of information pertinent to the diagnosis and management of pediatric disorders. We continue to stress the clinical aspects of the subjects covered—established concepts of pediatric diagnosis and treatment over the purely theoretical or experimental—but have included summaries of physiologic principles as they apply to our knowledge of the various conditions that are discussed.

This Handbook is not intended to be used as a substitute for the more complete pediatric texts and reference works but as a supplement to them; however, recent advances have been included wherever they have seemed to the authors to deserve inclusion in a handbook of this type.

Because of limitations of space, some subjects have been severely condensed or omitted entirely. For the same reason, no attempt has been made to give complete source references.

We have been extremely pleased with the continued success this Handbook has enjoyed among medical students, members of house staffs, practicing physicians, our colleagues in the pediatrics departments at medical schools both here and abroad, and other health professionals. Spanish, Italian, Portuguese, and Japanese editions have been published.

The authors wish to reaffirm their gratitude to all those who assisted in the preparation of the first thirteen editions of the Handbook. During the preparation of this edition, we resubmitted many chapters to our colleagues for comment and criticism. Their names and present affiliations are listed overleaf.

We wish also to take this opportunity to thank our readers throughout the world who have contributed useful suggestions.

Henry K. Silver
C. Henry Kempe
Henry B. Bruyn

Denver, Colorado
San Francisco, California
June, 1983

Acknowledgments

We wish to thank the following individuals from the University of Colorado, Denver:

Roger M. Barkin, MD
Raleigh Bowden, MD
Jane C. Burns, MD
John Burrington, MD
H. Peter Chase, MD
Robert E. Eilert, MD
Philip P. Ellis, MD
Arlene E. Ernest, MA
Donald Ferlic, MD
William Frankenburg, MD
John Githens, MD
Benjamin A. Gitterman, MD
Ronald Gotlin, MD
Keith B. Hammond, MS
William Hathaway, MD
J. Roger Hollister, MD
John R. Lilly, MD
Gary M. Lum, MD
Ida Nakashima, MD
Marianne R. Neifert, MD
Lorrie F. Odom, MD
David Pearlman, MD
Arthur Robinson, MD
Barry H. Rumack, MD
Barton D. Schmitt, MD
John C. Selner, MD
David G. Tubergen, MD

We also wish to thank the following physicians for their generous contributions:

James W. Bass, MD (COL, MC, USA)	Tripler Army Medical Center, Honolulu
Frederic W. Bruhn, MD (COL, MC, USA)	Letterman Army Medical Center, Presidio, San Francisco
Frank Morriss, MD	University of Texas, Houston
Gerhard Nellhaus, MD	University of California, Davis (Sacramento Medical Center)
Robert Peterson, MD	Children's Hospital of Eastern Ontario, Ottawa
Michael A. Simmons, MD	Johns Hopkins University, Baltimore
Charlotte E. Thompson, MD	St. Mary's Medical Center, San Francisco
Anne S. Yeager, MD	Stanford University, Stanford, California

NOTICE

Not all of the drugs mentioned in this book have been approved by FDA for use in infants or in children under age 6 or age 12. Such drugs should not be used if effective alternatives are available; they may be used if no effective alternatives are available or if the known risk of toxicity of alternative drugs or the risk of nontreatment is outweighed by the probable advantages of treatment.

Because of the possibility of an error in the article or book from which a particular drug dosage is obtained, or an error appearing in the text of this book, our readers are urged to consult appropriate references, including the manufacturer's package insert, especially when prescribing new drugs or those with which they are not adequately familiar.

–The Authors

Pediatric History & Physical Examination* | 1

HISTORY

General Considerations

For many pediatric problems, the history is the most important single factor in arriving at a correct diagnosis.

A. Source of History: The history should be obtained from the parent or whoever is responsible for the care of the child. Much valuable information can also be obtained from the child. Adolescents especially should be interviewed alone, since they may deliberately withhold much information in the presence of their parents.

B. Interpretation of History: The presenting complaint as given may be a minor part of the problem. One should be prepared to go on, if necessary, to a more productive phase of the interview, which may have little or no apparent relationship to the complaint as originally presented.

C. Direction of Questioning: After the problem has been presented, fill in with necessary past and family history and other pertinent information. The record should also include whatever may be disclosed concerning the parents' temperaments, attitudes, and methods of rearing children.

Questions should not be prying, especially about subjects likely to be associated with feelings of guilt or shame; however, the parent should be allowed to volunteer information of this nature when prepared to do so. What worried the parents most about the child's illness? What did they expect would happen as a result of the illness? What do they expect will be done? What do they believe caused the illness? What are their basic worries? Hopes?

It is useful and frequently desirable for parents to have some idea of the physician's impressions, of the basic reasoning behind diagnostic and therapeutic considerations, and of the possible course of the child's illness.

D. Recorded History: The history should be a detailed, clear, and chronologic record of significant information. It should include the

*Revised with the assistance of Benjamin A. Gitterman, MD.

parents' interpretation of the present difficulty and indicate the results they expect from consultation.

E. Psychotherapeutic Effects: In many cases, the interview and history-taking is the first stage in the psychotherapeutic management of the patient and the parents. The history-taker should introduce himself or herself. Avoid being hurried or perfunctory. Avoid technical or ambiguous language. Recognize that socioeconomic and cultural background, education, and knowledge influence physician-patient communication.

HISTORY OUTLINE

The following outline should be modified and adapted as appropriate for the age of the child and the reason for consulting the physician:

(1) Name, address, and telephone number; sex; date and place of birth; race, religion, and nationality; referred by whom; father's and mother's names, occupations, and business telephone numbers.

(2) Date of this visit.

(3) Hospital or case number.

(4) Previous entries: Dates, diagnoses, therapy, other data.

(5) Summary of correspondence or other information from physicians, schools, etc.

Presenting Complaint (PC)

Patient's or informant's own brief account of the complaint and its duration.

Present Illness (PI) (or Interval History)

(1) When was the patient last entirely well?

(2) How and when did the disturbance start?

(3) Health immediately before the illness.

(4) Progress of disease; order and date of onset of new symptoms.

(5) Specific symptoms and physical signs that may have developed.

(6) Pertinent negative data obtained by direct questioning.

(7) Aggravating and alleviating factors.

(8) Significant medical attention and medications given and over what period.

(9) In acute infections, statement of type and degree of exposure and interval since exposure.

(10) For the well child, factors of significance and general condition since last visit.

(11) Examiner's opinion about the reliability of the informant.

Previous Health

A. Antenatal: Health of mother during pregnancy. Medical supervision, diet, infections (eg, rubella), other illnesses, vomiting, bleeding, preeclampsia-eclampsia, other complications; Rh typing and serologic tests, pelvimetry, medications, x-ray procedures.

B. Natal: Duration of pregnancy, birth weight, kind and duration of labor, type of delivery, sedation and anesthesia (if known), state of infant at birth, resuscitation required, onset of respiration, first cry.

C. Neonatal: Apgar score, color, cyanosis, pallor, jaundice, cry, twitchings, excessive mucus, paralysis, convulsions, fever, hemorrhage, congenital abnormalities, birth injury. Difficulty in sucking, rashes, excessive weight loss, feeding difficulties. Length of hospital stay.

Development

(1) First raised head, rolled over, sat alone, pulled up, walked with help, walked alone, talked (meaningful words; sentences).

(2) Urinary continence during night; during day.

(3) Control of defecation.

(4) Comparison of development with that of siblings and parents.

(5) Any period of failure to grow or unusual growth.

(6) School grade, quality of work.

Nutrition

A. Breast or Formula Feeding: Type, duration, major formula changes, time of weaning, difficulties.

B. Supplements: Vitamins (type, amount, duration), iron.

C. "Solid" Foods: When introduced, how taken, types, family dietary habits (vegetarian, etc).

D. Appetite: Food likes and dislikes, idiosyncrasies or allergies, reaction of child to eating.

Illnesses

A. Infections: Age, types, number, severity.

B. Contagious Diseases: Age, complications following measles, rubella, chickenpox, mumps, pertussis, diphtheria, scarlet fever.

C. Others.

Immunization & Tests

Indicate type, number, reactions, age of child.

A. Inoculations: Diphtheria, tetanus, pertussis, measles, rubella, typhoid, mumps, others.

B. Oral Immunizations: Poliomyelitis.

C. Recall Immunizations ("Boosters").

D. Serum Injections: Passive immunizations.

E. Tests: Tuberculin, Schick, serology, others.

Operations

Type, age, complications; reasons for operations; apparent response of child.

Accidents & Injuries

Nature, severity, sequelae.

Medications

Chronic use of medications, allergies to medications.

Family History

(1) Father and mother (age and condition of health). What sort of people do the parents characterize themselves as being?

(2) Marital relationships. Little information should be sought at first interview; most information will be obtained indirectly.

(3) Siblings. Age, condition of health, significant previous illnesses and problems.

(4) Stillbirths, miscarriages, abortions; age at death and cause of death of members of immediate family.

(5) Tuberculosis, allergy, blood dyscrasias, mental or nervous diseases, diabetes, cardiovascular diseases, kidney disease, hypertension, rheumatic fever, neoplastic diseases, congenital abnormalities, convulsive disorders, others.

(6) Health of contacts.

Personality History

A. Relations With Other Children: Independent or clinging to mother; negativistic, shy, submissive; separation from parents; hobbies; easy or difficult to get along with. How does child relate to others? Physical deformities affecting personality.

B. School Progress: Class, grades, nursery school, special aptitudes, reaction to school.

Social History

A. Family: Income, home (size, number of rooms, living conditions, sleeping facilities), type of neighborhood, access to playground. Localities in which patient has lived. Who takes care of patient if both parents work outside the home? Who else lives in the home besides immediate family?

B. Family Support Systems: Relatives nearby or close friends to provide support and give parents time away from child.

C. School: Public or private, students per classroom, type of students.

D. Insurance: Blue Cross, Blue Shield, other types of health insurance.

Habits

A. Eating: Appetite, food dislikes, how fed, attitudes of child and parents toward eating.

B. Sleeping: Hours, disturbances, snoring, restlessness, dreaming, nightmares.

C. Recreation: Exercise and play.

D. Elimination: Urinary, bowel.

E. Disturbances: Excessive bed-wetting, masturbation, thumb-sucking, nail-biting, breath-holding, temper tantrums, tics, nervousness, undue thirst, others. Similar disturbances among members of family. School problems (learning, perceptual).

F. Adolescent Habits: Adolescents should be asked about smoking, alcohol or substance abuse, sexual activity, and use of birth control. These questions need not be asked immediately but should be routine if appropriate to the patient's age.

G. Dental Hygiene: Self-care habits (brushing, flossing), most recent preventive check.

H. Safety Habits of Family: Use of infant or child restraining devices in automobiles, careful storage of medicines and toxic substances, covering of electrical outlets, other safety measures.

System Review

A. Ears, Nose, and Throat: Frequent colds, sore throat, sneezing, stuffy nose, discharge, postnasal drip, mouth breathing, snoring, otitis, hearing, adenitis, allergies.

B. Teeth: Age at eruption of deciduous and permanent teeth; number at age 1 year; comparison with siblings.

C. Cardiorespiratory: Frequency and nature of disturbances. Dyspnea, chest pain, cough, sputum, wheeze, expectoration, cyanosis, edema, syncope, tachycardia.

D. Gastrointestinal: Vomiting, diarrhea, constipation, type of stools, abdominal pain or discomfort, jaundice.

E. Genitourinary: Enuresis, dysuria, frequency, polyuria, pyuria, hematuria, character of stream, vaginal discharge, menstrual history, bladder control, abnormalities of penis or testes.

F. Neuromuscular: Headache, nervousness, dizziness, tingling, convulsions, habit spasms, ataxia, muscle or joint pains, postural deformities, exercise tolerance, gait. Screening for scoliosis in adolescents.

G. Endocrine: Disturbances of growth, excessive fluid intake, polyphagia, goiter, thyroid disease.

H. Special Senses.

I. General: Unusual weight gain or loss, fatigue, skin color or texture, other abnormalities of skin, temperature sensitivity, mentality, bleeding tendency, pattern of growth (record previous heights and weights on appropriate graphs). Time and pattern of pubescence. Hyperactivity. Attention span.

The Health Record

Every patient should have a comprehensive medical and health record containing all pertinent information. The parents should be given a summary of this record (including data regarding illnesses, operations, idiosyncrasies, sensitivities, heights, weights, special medications, and immunizations).

PHYSICAL EXAMINATION

Every child should have a complete systematic examination at regular intervals. The examination should not be restricted to those portions of the body considered to be involved on the basis of the presenting complaint.

Approaching the Child

Adequate time should be allowed for the child and the examiner to become acquainted. The child should be treated as an individual whose feelings and sensibilities are well developed, and the examiner's conduct should be appropriate to the age of the child. A friendly manner, quiet voice, and slow and easy approach will help to facilitate the examination. If the examiner is not able to establish a friendly relationship but feels that it is important to proceed with the examination, this should be done in an orderly, systematic manner in the hope that the child will then accept the inevitable.

The examiner's hands should be washed in warm water before the examination begins and should be warm.

Observation of the Patient

Although the very young child may not be able to speak, much information may be obtained by an observant and receptive examiner. The total evaluation of the child should include impressions obtained from the time the child first enters the room; it should not be based solely on the period during which the patient is on the examining table. This is also the best time to assess the interaction of parent and child; the examiner's impressions should be recorded.

In general, more information is obtained by careful inspection than from any other method of examination.

Holding for Examination

A. Before Age 6 Months: The examining table is usually well tolerated.

B. Age 6 Months to 3–4 Years: Most of the examination may be performed while the child is held in the parent's lap or over the parent's shoulder. Certain parts of the examination can sometimes be done more easily with the child prone or held against the parent so that the examiner cannot be seen.

Removal of Clothing

Clothes should be removed gradually to prevent chilling and to avoid resistance from a shy child. In order to save time and to avoid creating unpleasant associations with the doctor in the child's mind, undressing the child and taking the temperature are best performed by the parent. The physician should respect the marked degree of modesty that some children may exhibit.

Sequence of Examination

In most cases, it is best to begin the examination of the young child with an area that is least likely to be associated with pain or discomfort. The ears and throat should usually be examined last. The examiner should develop a regular sequence of examination that can be adapted as required by special circumstances.

Painful Procedures

Before performing a disagreeable, painful, or upsetting examination, the examiner should tell the child (1) what is likely to happen and how the child can assist, (2) that the examination is necessary, and (3) that it will be performed as rapidly and as painlessly as possible.

GENERAL PHYSICAL EXAMINATION

(See also Chapter 8.)

Record temperature, pulse rate, and respiratory rate (TRP); blood pressure (see p 262); weight; and height. The weight should be recorded at each visit; the height should be determined at monthly intervals during the first year, at 3-month intervals in the second year, and twice a year thereafter. The height, weight, and head circumference of the child should be compared with standard charts and the approximate percentiles recorded. Multiple measurements at intervals are of more value than single ones, since they give information regarding the pattern of growth. The blood pressure should also be compared with standard percentiles.

Rectal Temperatures

During the first years of life, the temperature should be taken by rectum (except for routine temperatures of the premature infant and infants under age 1 month, when axillary temperatures are sufficiently accurate). The child should be laid face down across the parent's lap and held firmly with the parent's left forearm placed flat across the child's back; the parent can separate the buttocks with the left thumb and index finger and insert the lubricated thermometer with the right hand. Activity, apprehension, and fear may elevate the temperature.

Rectal temperature may be 1 degree higher than oral temperature. A rectal temperature up to 37.8 °C (100 °F) may be considered normal in a child.

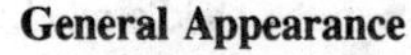

General Appearance

Does the child appear well or ill? Degree of prostration; degree of cooperation; state of comfort, nutrition, and consciousness; abnormalities; gait, posture, and coordination; estimate of intelligence; reaction to parents, physician, and examination; nature of cry and degree of activity; facies and facial expression.

Skin

Color (cyanosis, jaundice, pallor, erythema), texture, eruptions, hydration, edema, hemorrhagic manifestations, scars, dilated vessels and direction of blood flow, hemangiomas, café au lait areas and nevi, Mongolian spots, pigmentation, turgor, elasticity, subcutaneous nodules, sensitivity, hair distribution, character, desquamation.

Practical notes:

(1) Loss of turgor, especially of the calf muscles and skin over the abdomen, is evidence of dehydration.

(2) The soles and palms are often bluish and cold in early infancy; this is of no significance.

(3) The degree of anemia cannot be determined reliably by inspection, since pallor (even in the newborn) may be normal and not due to anemia.

(4) To demonstrate pitting edema in a child, it may be necessary to exert prolonged pressure.

(5) A few small pigmented nevi are commonly found, particularly in older children.

(6) Spider nevi occur in about one-sixth of children under age 5 years and almost half of older children.

(7) Mongolian spots (large, flat, black or blue-black areas) are frequently present over the lower back and buttocks; they have no pathologic significance.

(8) Cyanosis will not be evident unless at least 5 g of reduced hemoglobin is present; therefore, it develops less easily in an anemic child.

(9) Carotenemia is usually most prominent over the palms and soles and around the nose and spares the conjunctiva.

(10) Striae and wrinkling may indicate rapid weight gain or loss.

Lymph Nodes

Location, size, sensitivity, mobility, consistency. One should routinely attempt to palpate suboccipital, preauricular, anterior cervical, posterior cervical, submaxillary, sublingual, axillary, epitrochlear, and inguinal lymph nodes.

Practical notes:

(1) Enlargement of the lymph nodes occurs much more readily in children than in adults.

(2) Small inguinal lymph nodes are palpable in almost all healthy young children. Small, mobile, nontender shotty nodes are commonly found as residua of previous infection.

Head

Size, shape, circumference, asymmetry, cephalhematoma, bossae, craniotabes, control, molding, bruits, fontanelles (size, tension, number, abnormally late or early closure), sutures, dilated veins, scalp, hair (texture, distribution, parasites), face, transillumination.

Practical notes:

(1) The head is measured at its greatest circumference; this is usually at the mid forehead anteriorly and around to the most prominent portion of the occiput posteriorly. The ratio of head circumference to circumference of the chest or abdomen is usually of little value.

(2) Fontanelle tension is best determined with the child quiet and in the sitting position.

(3) Slight pulsations over the anterior fontanelle may occur in normal infants.

(4) Although bruits may be heard over the temporal areas in normal children, the possibility of an existing abnormality should be ruled out.

(5) Craniotabes may be found in normal newborn infants (especially premature infants) and for the first 2–4 months of life.

(6) A positive Macewen sign ("cracked pot" sound when skull is percussed with one finger) may be present normally as long as the fontanelle is open.

(7) Transillumination of the skull can be performed by means of a flashlight with a sponge rubber collar so that it fits tightly when held against the head.

Face

Symmetry, paralysis, distance between nose and mouth, depth of nasolabial folds, bridge of nose, distribution of hair, size of mandible, swellings, hypertelorism, Chvostek's sign, tenderness over sinuses.

Eyes

Photophobia; visual acuity; muscular control and conjugate gaze; nystagmus; Mongolian slant; Brushfield's spots; epicanthic folds; lacrimation; discharge; lids; exophthalmos or enophthalmos; conjunctiva; pupillary size, shape, and reaction to light and accommodation; color of iris; media (corneal opacities, cataracts); fundi; visual fields (in older children).

Practical notes:

(1) Newborn infants usually will open their eyes if placed prone, supported with one hand on the abdomen, and lifted over the examiner's head.

(2) Not infrequently, one pupil is normally larger than the other. This sometimes occurs only in bright or subdued light.

(3) Examination of the fundi should be part of every complete physical examination.

(4) Dilatation of the pupils may be necessary for adequate visualization of the eyes.

(5) A mild degree of strabismus may be present during the first 6 months of life but should be considered abnormal after that time.

(6) To test for strabismus in a very young or uncooperative child, note where a distant source of light is reflected from the surface of the eyes; the reflection should be present on corresponding portions of the 2 eyes.

(7) Small areas of capillary dilatation are commonly seen on the eyelids of normal newborn infants.

(8) Most infants produce visible tears during the first few days of life.

Nose

Exterior, shape, mucosa, patency, discharge, bleeding, pressure over sinuses, flaring of nostrils, septum.

Mouth

Lips (thinness, downturning, fissures, color, cleft), teeth (number, position, caries, mottling, discoloration, notching, malocclusion or malalignment), mucosa (color, redness of Stensen's duct, enanthems, Bohn's nodules, Epstein's pearls), gums, palate, tongue, uvula, mouth breathing, geographic tongue (usually normal).

Practical note: If the tongue can be extended as far as the alveolar ridge, there will be no interference with nursing or speaking. Frenectomy is not a preventive measure for being "tongue-tied."

Throat

Tonsils (size, inflammation, exudate, crypts, inflammation of the anterior pillars), mucosa, hypertrophic lymphoid tissue, postnasal drip, epiglottis, voice (hoarseness, stridor, grunting, type of cry, speech).

Practical notes:

(1) Before examining a child's throat, it is advisable to examine the

mouth. Permit the child to handle the tongue blade, nasal speculum, and flashlight in order to overcome fear of the instruments. Then ask the child to stick out the tongue and say "Ah," louder and louder. In some cases, this may allow an adequate examination. In others, a child who is cooperative enough may be asked to "pant like a puppy"; while this is being done, the tongue blade is applied firmly to the rear of the tongue. Gagging need not be elicited in order to obtain a satisfactory examination. In still other cases, it may be expedient to examine one side of the tongue at a time, pushing the base of the tongue first to one side and then to the other. This may be less unpleasant and is less apt to cause gagging.

(2) Young children may have to be restrained to obtain an adequate examination of the throat. Eliciting a gag reflex may be necessary if the oropharynx is to be adequately seen.

(3) The small child's head may be restrained satisfactorily by the parent's hands placed at the level of the child's elbows while the arms are held firmly against the sides of the child's head.

(4) A child who can sit up can be held on the parent's lap, back against the parent's chest. The child's left hand is held in the parent's left, the right hand in the right, and the hands are placed against the child's groin or lower thighs to prevent slipping. If the throat is to be examined in natural light, the parent faces the light. If artificial light and a head mirror are used, the light should be behind the parent. In either case, the physician uses one hand to hold the head in position and the other to manipulate the tongue blade.

(5) Young children seldom complain of sore throat even in the presence of significant infection of the pharynx and tonsils.

Ears

Pinnas (position, size), canals, tympanic membranes (landmarks, mobility, perforation, inflammation, discharge), mastoid tenderness and swelling, hearing.

Practical notes:

(1) A test for hearing is an important part of the physical examination of every infant and child. If a parent says that the child does not hear well, this must be investigated until disproved.

(2) The ears of all sick children should be examined.

(3) When actually examining the ears, it is often helpful to place the speculum just within the canal, remove it and place it lightly in the other ear, remove it again, and proceed in this way from one ear to the other, gradually going farther and farther, until a satisfactory examination is completed.

(4) In examining the ears, use as large a speculum as possible and insert it no farther than necessary, both to avoid discomfort and to avoid pushing wax in front of the speculum so that it obscures the field. The otoscope should be held balanced in the hand by holding the handle at the

end nearest the speculum. One finger should rest against the child's head to prevent injury resulting from sudden movement.

(5) Pneumatic insufflation to test mobility of the tympanic membrane should always be part of the examination.

(6) The child may be restrained most easily if lying prone.

(7) Low-set ears are present in a number of congenital syndromes, including several associated with mental retardation. The ears may be considered low-set if they are below a line drawn from the lateral angle of the eye to the external occipital protuberance.

(8) Congenital anomalies of the urinary tract are frequently associated with abnormalities of the pinnas.

(9) To examine the ears of an infant, it is usually necessary to pull the auricle backward and downward; in the older child, the external ear is pulled backward and upward.

Neck

Position (torticollis, opisthotonos, inability to support head, mobility), swelling, thyroid (size, contour, bruit, isthmus, nodules, tenderness), lymph nodes, veins, position of trachea, sternocleidomastoid (swelling, shortening), webbing, edema, auscultation, movement, tonic neck reflex.

Practical note: In the older child, the size and shape of the thyroid gland may be more clearly defined if the gland is palpated from behind.

Thorax

Shape and symmetry, veins, retractions and pulsations, beading, Harrison's groove, flaring of ribs, pigeon breast, funnel shape, size and position of nipples, breasts, length of sternum, intercostal and substernal retraction, asymmetry, scapulas, clavicles, scoliosis.

Practical note: At puberty, in normal children, one breast usually begins to develop before the other. Tenderness of the breasts is relatively common in both sexes. Gynecomastia is not uncommon in boys.

Lungs

Type of breathing, dyspnea, prolongation of expiration, cough, expansion, fremitus, flatness or dullness to percussion, resonance, breath and voice sounds, rales, wheezing.

Practical notes:

(1) Breath sounds in infants and children normally are more intense and more bronchial, and expiration is more prolonged, than in adults.

(2) Most of the young child's respiratory movement is produced by abdominal movement; there is very little intercostal motion.

(3) If the stethoscope is placed over the child's mouth and the sounds heard by this route are subtracted from the sounds heard through

the chest wall, the difference usually represents the amount produced intrathoracically.

Heart

Location and intensity of apex beat, precordial bulging, pulsation of vessels, thrills, size, shape, auscultation (rate, rhythm, force, quality of sounds—compare with pulse with respect to rate and rhythm; friction rub—variation with pressure), murmurs (location, position in cycle, intensity, pitch, effect of change of position, transmission, effect of exercise) (see p 261).

Practical notes:

(1) Many children normally have sinus arrhythmia. The child should be asked to take a deep breath to determine its effect on the rhythm.

(2) Extrasystoles are not uncommon in childhood.

(3) The heart should be examined with the child erect, recumbent, and turned to the left.

Abdomen

Size and contour, visible peristalsis, respiratory movements, veins (distention, direction of flow), umbilicus, hernia, musculature, tenderness and rigidity, rebound tenderness, tympany, shifting dullness, pulsation, palpable organs or masses (size, shape, position, mobility), fluid wave, reflexes, femoral pulsations, bowel sounds.

Practical notes:

(1) The abdomen may be examined with the child prone in the parent's lap, held over the shoulder, or seated on the examining table facing away from the doctor. These positions may be particularly helpful where tenderness, rigidity, or a mass must be palpated. In the infant, the examination may be aided by having the child suck at a "sugar tip" or nurse at a bottle.

(2) Light palpation, especially for the spleen, often will give more information than deep palpation.

(3) Umbilical hernias are common during the first 2 years of life. They usually disappear spontaneously.

Male Genitalia

Circumcision, meatal opening, hypospadias, phimosis, adherent foreskin, size of testes, cryptorchidism, scrotum, hydrocele, hernia, pubertal changes.

Practical notes:

(1) In examining a suspected case of cryptorchidism, palpation for the testicles should be done before the child has fully undressed or become chilled or had the cremasteric reflex stimulated. In some cases, examination while the child is in a warm bath may be helpful. The boy

should also be examined while sitting in a chair holding his knees with his heels on the seat; the increased intra-abdominal pressure may push the testes into the scrotum.

(2) To examine for cryptorchidism, one should start above the inguinal canal and work downward to prevent pushing the testes up into the canal or abdomen.

(3) The penis of an obese boy may be so obscured by fat as to appear abnormally small. If this fat is pushed back, a penis of normal size is usually found.

Female Genitalia

Vagina (imperforate, discharge, adhesions), hypertrophy of clitoris, pubertal changes.

Practical note: Digital or speculum examination is rarely done until after puberty.

Rectum & Anus

Irritation, fissures, prolapse, imperforate anus, muscle tone, character of stool, masses, tenderness, sensation.

Practical note: The rectal examination should be performed with the little finger (inserted slowly). Examine the stool on glove finger. Perform gross and microscopic examination, culture, and guaiac test as indicated.

Extremities

A. General: Deformity, hemiatrophy, bowlegs (common in infancy), knock-knee (common after age 2 years), paralysis, edema, coldness, posture, gait, stance, asymmetry.

B. Joints: Swelling, redness, pain, limitation, tenderness, motion, rheumatic nodules, carrying angle of elbows, tibial torsion.

C. Hands and Feet: Extra digits, clubbing, simian lines, curvature of little finger, deformity of nails, splinter hemorrhages, flat feet (feet commonly appear flat during first 2 years of life), abnormalities of feet, dermatoglyphics, width of thumbs and big toes, syndactyly, length of various segments, dimpling of dorsa, temperature.

D. Peripheral Vessels: Presence, absence, or diminution of arterial pulses.

Practical note: Normal femoral arterial pulsations in the newborn period do not definitely exclude coarctation.

Spine & Back

Posture; curvatures; rigidity; webbed neck; spina bifida; pilonidal dimple or cyst; tufts of hair; mobility; Mongolian spots; tenderness over spine, pelvis, and kidneys.

Neurologic Examination (After Vazuka)

A. Cerebral Function: General behavior, level of consciousness, intelligence, emotional status, memory, orientation, illusions, hallucinations, cortical sensory interpretation, cortical motor integration, ability to understand and communicate, auditory-verbal and visual-verbal comprehension, visual recognition of object, speech, ability to write, performance of skilled motor acts.

B. Cranial Nerves:

1. I (olfactory)–Identification of odors, disorders of smell.

2. II (optic)–Visual acuity, visual fields, ophthalmoscopic examination.

3. III (oculomotor), IV (trochlear), and VI (abducens)–Ocular movements, ptosis, dilatation of pupil, nystagmus, pupillary accommodation, pupillary light reflexes.

4. V (trigeminal)–Sensation of face, corneal reflex, masseter and temporal muscle reflexes, maxillary reflex (jaw jerk).

5. VII (facial)–Wrinkling forehead, frowning, smiling, raising eyebrows, asymmetry of face, strength of eyelid muscles, taste on anterior portion of tongue.

6. VIII (acoustic)–

a. Cochlear–Hearing, lateralization, air and bone conduction, tinnitus.

b. Vestibular–Caloric tests.

7. IX (glossopharyngeal) and X (vagus)–Pharyngeal gag reflex; ability to swallow and speak clearly; sensation of mucosa of pharynx, soft palate, and tonsils; movement of pharynx, larynx, and soft palate; autonomic functions.

8. XI (accessory)–Strength of trapezius and sternocleidomastoid muscles.

9. XII (hypoglossal)–Protrusion of tongue, tremor, strength of tongue.

C. Cerebellar Function: Finger to nose; finger to examiner's finger; rapidly alternating pronation and supination of hands; ability to run heel down other shin and to make a requested motion with foot; ability to stand with eyes closed, walk normally, walk heel-to-toe; tremor; ataxia; posture; arm swing when walking; nystagmus; abnormalities of muscle tone and speech.

D. Motor System: Muscle size, consistency, and tone; muscle contours and outlines; muscle strength; myotonic contraction; slow relaxation; symmetry of posture; fasciculations; tremor; resistance to passive movement; involuntary movement.

E. Reflexes:

1. Deep–Bicep, brachioradialis, tricep, patellar, and Achilles reflexes; rapidity and strength of contraction and relaxation.

2. Superficial–Abdominal, cremasteric, plantar, and gluteal reflexes.

3. Pathologic–Babinski's, Chaddock's, Oppenheim's, and Gordon's reflexes.

Development

Both a history for "milestones" and developmental screening tests are part of the routine physical evaluation.

Practical note: Screening devices are not diagnostic of particular problems but merely indicate a need for further developmental evaluation.

Pediatric Management During Illness* | 2

TREATMENT OF CONSTITUTIONAL SYMPTOMS

SHOCK

Shock is a clinical syndrome characterized by prostration and hypotension resulting from profound depression of cell functions associated with or secondary to poor perfusion of vital tissue. If cell function is not improved, shock becomes irreversible and death will ensue even though the initiating cause is corrected.

Clinical Findings

Early signs of shock are agitation, confusion, and thirst. As shock progresses, the patient will become increasingly unresponsive and eventually comatose.

The skin is pale, wet, and cold. The nail beds are cyanotic. Local and peripheral edema may be present. Capillary filling is poor, and skin turgor is decreased. Tachycardia and tachypnea are present.

Newborns in shock appear pale and slightly gray, with poor capillary filling and decreased skin turgor. In late shock, there may be a decrease in skin temperature, particularly of the extremities.

Emergency Treatment of Shock

A. Position Patient: Lay the patient flat. Elevation of the legs is helpful except in respiratory distress, when it is contraindicated. In older children, use of military antishock trousers (MAST suits) may be helpful.

B. Support Life: Establish a patent upper airway, administer oxygen, and support circulation and ventilation. Follow the principles of basic life support outlined in Chapter 30 (see p 715). Prepare to institute advanced life support.

*Revised with the assistance of Roger M. Barkin, MD.

C. Establish Intravenous Access: Establish an intravenous line with a comparatively large-bore catheter.

D. Administer Fluids: Initiate fluid therapy with lactated Ringer's injection or isotonic saline solution given intravenously at a rate of 20 mL/kg over the first 30–60 minutes. Thereafter, administer fluids at a rate sufficient to replace and maintain blood volume.

E. Monitor Central Venous Pressure: Establish a central venous pressure monitor if shock is not easily reversible following initial administration of fluids.

Evaluation of Emergency Treatment

The patient must be observed constantly. The pulse, blood pressure, respiratory rate, and temperature should be taken immediately and monitored every 15 minutes until vital signs stabilize. Determine hematocrit count (this should be done in the emergency department), and send blood for white blood cell count, measurement of electrolytes and glucose level, and typing and cross-matching.

An indwelling catheter should be placed to monitor urine flow. The minimum acceptable urine output is 1 mL/kg/h; the optimal output is 2–3 mL/kg/h.

If response to fluid therapy over the first hour is unsatisfactory, further vigorous antishock therapy should be instituted.

Treatment of Specific Types of Shock

A. Hypovolemic Shock: Hypovolemic shock is characterized by reduction in the effective size of the vascular compartment, with falling blood pressure, poor capillary filling, and a low central venous pressure. Treatment consists of prevention of further fluid loss and replacement of existing volume losses. Vasopressors are not useful. The type of fluid used as a volume expander depends on the cause of the hypovolemia.

1. Blood loss–Whole blood is the replacement fluid of choice for shock due to hemorrhage. Whenever circumstances permit, type-specific blood should be used. Unmatched type O Rh-negative blood may be used but carries an increased risk of reaction.

The rate of blood replacement is determined by the patient's vital signs, the rate of continuing blood loss, the response to the infusion, and the amount of crystalloid solution previously infused.

2. Dehydration–For hypovolemic shock due to dehydration, give lactated Ringer's injection or isotonic saline with 5% dextrose until electrolyte determinations have been obtained. Begin intravenous infusion of fluid at a rate of 20 mL/kg over the first 30–60 minutes; thereafter, administer fluid at a rate calculated to replace the deficit and maintain blood volume.

B. Cardiogenic Shock: This type of shock results from decreased cardiac output, which may be due to cardiac tamponade, myocarditis, abnormal heart rate and rhythm, or biochemical abnormalities.

1. Cardiac tamponade secondary to fluid collection in the pericardial space or constrictive pericarditis is treated by pericardiocentesis or by surgery. Intravenous infusion of crystalloid solution may increase venous pressure enough to allow a delay before more definitive treatment is instituted.

2. Abnormal heart rate and rhythm may cause decreased cardiac output.

a. Marked sinus bradycardia can occur during anesthesia, particularly during surgery of the neck and thorax. Sinus bradycardia can be blocked with atropine, 0.01 mg/kg as a single intravenous dose. The minimum dose of atropine for newborns is 0.15 mg regardless of weight. The maximum dose for older children is 0.6 mg.

b. Atrioventricular block may be secondary to inflammatory disease, surgical trauma, or ischemic injury to the conduction system. If use of atropine is unsuccessful, the ventricular rate may be increased with isoproterenol, the infusion rate being determined by the therapeutic response. A pacemaker may be required temporarily.

c. Ventricular arrhythmias may be secondary to hypoxia, acidosis, or myocarditis. If no specific abnormality can be found, lidocaine, bretylium, or another antiarrhythmia drug may be useful in correcting the arrhythmia.

3. Biochemical disturbances, including acidosis, hypoxia, and hyperkalemia, can result in decreased cardiac output.

C. Bacteremic (Septic) Shock: This is the most common type of vascular shock; it occurs when overwhelming sepsis and circulating bacterial toxins produce peripheral vascular collapse. Clinical recognition is based upon the toxic appearance of the patient, who often has purpura, splinter hemorrhages, hepatosplenomegaly, and jaundice.

Adequate treatment of bacteremic shock depends on supportive care of the patient and proper antibiotic treatment of the primary infection. If sepsis is likely but no specific etiologic agent can be defined immediately, ampicillin, 300–400 mg/kg/d in 6 divided doses, and chloramphenicol, 75–100 mg/kg/d in 4 divided doses, should be started after appropriate specimens for culture have been obtained.

Supportive measures include the following:

1. Fluids–Replace fluids as necessary.

2. Corticosteroids–Corticosteroids may be useful in bacteremic shock (this is controversial); they should be begun early. Give hydrocortisone sodium succinate in doses of 4–5 mg/kg intravenously.

3. Vasopressors–Vasopressor agents may be useful.

4. Heparin–Heparin may be of value when bacterial infections are complicated by disseminated intravascular coagulation.

5. Other drugs–The role of endorphins and naloxone is undefined at present.

D. Anaphylactic Shock: This is an extreme form of allergy or hypersensitivity to a foreign substance and is characterized by very low peripheral resistance. The diagnosis is established by a history of exposure to an antigen followed almost immediately by clinical signs of respiratory distress and circulatory collapse. Urticaria and angioneurotic edema are often present.

1. Tourniquet–If the shock was precipitated by a drug given intramuscularly, apply a tourniquet proximal to the site of injection. The tourniquet should be tight enough to restrict venous return but should not interrupt arterial flow.

2. Epinephrine–Give epinephrine, 1:1000 aqueous solution, 0.01 mL/kg (maximum, 0.35 mL) subcutaneously. This may be repeated in 20 minutes.

3. Corticosteroids–Give hydrocortisone sodium succinate in doses of 4–5 mg/kg intravenously.

4. Aminophylline–For treatment of respiratory distress or wheezing, give aminophylline, 7–8 mg/kg intravenously as a loading dose, followed by a maintenance dose of 16 mg/kg/d.

5. Diphenhydramine–Diphenhydramine, 5 mg/kg/d intravenously in 4 divided doses, is a useful antihistaminic adjunct.

6. Airway–Secretions should be suctioned to maintain a clear airway. Repeated bronchoscopy may be required. Laryngeal edema may necessitate tracheal intubation followed by tracheostomy.

E. Neurogenic Shock: There is usually a history of exposure to anesthetic agents, spinal cord injury, or ingestion of barbiturates, narcotics, or tranquilizers. Examination reveals abnormal reflexes and muscle tone, tachycardia and tachypnea, and low blood pressure. The pathophysiologic mechanism is loss of vessel tone with subsequent expansion of the vascular compartment, resulting in relative hypovolemia. Many anesthetic agents have a direct effect on the myocardium, causing a decreased cardiac output.

1. Underlying problem–Treat the underlying neurologic problem. Head trauma does not produce shock in the absence of involvement of other organ systems unless there is major scalp injury or an open and full fontanelle.

2. Fluids–When head trauma is not present, fluid therapy may stabilize vital signs.

3. Vasopressors–Use of vasopressor drugs (see pp 716–717) may be indicated until definitive treatment has been given.

F. Shock Due to Miscellaneous Causes:

1. Due to pulmonary embolism–Pulmonary embolism may be present if there is a fracture or significant soft tissue injury followed by symptoms of chest pain, dyspnea, cyanosis, and signs of right heart failure. Treatment of shock is supportive, with oxygen and analgesics. If hypotension occurs, isoproterenol is the drug of choice, since it provides a bronchodilator effect. If right heart failure develops, a rapid-acting digitalis preparation such as digoxin should be given.

2. Due to respiratory disease–Respiratory disease due to any cause can result in sufficient hypoxia to cause shock. Shock of this nature is reversible only to the extent that the underlying disease is reversible, and treatment should be directed toward the primary pulmonary disorder. Treatment with oxygen and alkalies will only temporarily improve the patient's condition.

3. Metabolic shock–Shock may be secondary to a number of metabolic conditions, eg, adrenocortical insufficiency and diabetic acidosis.

Prognosis

With prompt and effective emergency care for both the shock and the underlying condition, the immediate prognosis is excellent.

FEVER

In children under age 8 years, the degree of fever may not reflect the severity of the disease process. Extremes of temperature may occur without relation to the significance of the infection. A small infant may have a very serious illness with normal or subnormal temperatures, whereas a 2- to 5-year-old child may have fever above 40 °C (104 °F) with a minor respiratory infection. In children over age 8 years, temperature response is similar to that in adults.

Some children with high temperatures may convulse ("febrile convulsions"), and some of those who convulse will subsequently have an increased risk of epilepsy. Rapid elevation of temperature should therefore receive prompt care in the form of antipyretic therapy. Fever and convulsions may be the presenting findings of a central nervous system infection, and the patient may require a spinal tap for diagnostic evaluation. In general, fever as high as 41 °C (105.8 °F) is not in itself harmful.

Whenever possible, determine the cause of fever (infection, dehydration, reaction to drug, central nervous system disturbance, excessive clothing) and institute specific measures. Nonspecific measures should also be instituted.

Reduction of Fever by Nonspecific Means

The patient with fever above 40 °C (104 °F) may be uncomfortable, dehydrated, and difficult to evaluate. The following measures may be used to reduce fever: Increase fluid intake; bathe with warm or tepid water; and administer antipyretics, ie, acetaminophen, 10–15 mg/kg orally (or rectally if necessary) every 4–6 hours, or aspirin, 10–15 mg/kg orally every 4–6 hours when temperature is above 40 °C (104 °F). Aspirin should not be used in chickenpox or viral influenza because of the suspected increased risk of Reye's syndrome. Administration of both drugs every 6 hours produces a synergistic antipyretic effect.

CARE DURING ILLNESS

REST & ACTIVITY DURING ILLNESS

During most acute illnesses, children may be allowed to establish their own limits of activity, since attempts to enforce bed rest often do more harm than good. When enforced bed rest results in a crying and resentful child, various compromises may be necessary.

The ill child requires a great deal of reassurance and should be spared knowledge of the concern others may feel. It is important to minimize the child's anxiety by discussion and explanation and to avoid the detrimental effects of restlessness and unhappiness that result from overzealous limitations.

In convalescence from a serious illness, consideration should be given to properly controlled occupational and play therapy, a home teaching program for the school-age child, and extra periods of rest until the child is strong enough to do without them.

NUTRITION DURING ILLNESS

Infants

In the severely ill infant, breast feeding may have to be temporarily discontinued. Regular emptying of the mother's breasts, manually or with a pump, may allow prompt reinstitution of breast feeding when the child can again nurse.

When the illness is not severe enough to warrant discontinuing breast feeding altogether, supplemental feedings of water with 5% carbohydrate added will provide the necessary increase in fluid and carbohydrate intake.

Acutely ill infants have a decreased ability to utilize fat and may have increased requirements for carbohydrates, water, and electrolytes to compensate for increased losses. When the acute phase has passed, the formula may be strengthened to overcome deficits of calories, protein, and fat.

Children

Acutely ill children, especially those with pain and fever, are generally anorexic and irritable. One should not attempt to supply optimal food requirements during the acute phase of the illness but should provide the 3 items most needed: water, electrolytes, and sugar, especially to avoid ketosis. It is not unusual to give for several days a diet consisting only of such items as sweetened carbonated beverages, gelatin desserts, ice cream, sherbet, applesauce, and fruit juices as well as an occasional glass of skimmed milk.

Parents should be cautioned to avoid a struggle in feeding the ill child. In general, free choice and frequent small feedings at intervals of 1–2 hours are sufficient to maintain optimal water, electrolyte, and sugar intake during the acute phase of the illness. Requirements for protein should be met in the immediate convalescent period.

When the immediate acute phase has passed, easily digestible solids that the child enjoys may be introduced. Hamburger patty, buttered toast, strained fruits and vegetables, and mashed potatoes with a small amount of butter are successful foods during this period.

Vitamin intake in moderately increased amounts should be continued through the convalescent period.

EMOTIONAL ASPECTS OF HOSPITALIZATION

Hospitalization nearly always involves some degree of psychic trauma, especially in a young child; the need for hospital care must therefore be balanced against the possible emotional consequences. The physician, parents, and hospital staff must try to minimize the psychologic effect of the hospital stay and the procedures involved during the time of the child's hospitalization. Above all, the child must be made to understand the parents' attitude. Candor and reassurance are never more important to a child than at this time. The physician can help by seeing to it that the practical affairs of running a hospital interfere as little as possible with the parents' visits.

Hospital personnel must be brought to a sympathetic awareness of the ill child's emotional needs. The child should be given a reasonable and candid explanation of what is likely to happen. If surgery is to be performed, children should be told how anesthesia will be administered and how they will feel and where they will be after surgery. Explanation and forewarning can make significant modifications in the emotional sequelae of hospitalization, whereas failure to prepare the child may have far-reaching psychologic consequences.

The emotional state of the parents must also be considered. It should be recognized that they may have a sense of guilt for the child's illness and that this reaction may be aggravated when hospitalization is necessary. Their defense mechanisms may be manifested by an inclination to blame others, including the physician.

PREOPERATIVE & POSTOPERATIVE CARE

GENERAL CONSIDERATIONS

Newborn infants withstand surgical procedures better than is usually recognized; this is especially true in the first 72 hours of life. Congenital defects requiring prompt surgery should be repaired as soon as possible after the diagnosis is made.

Psychologic preparation of an older child for anesthesia and surgery is the combined responsibility of all health care providers involved. The parents should be encouraged to discuss surgery with the child, when possible. The child must not be deceived under any circumstances. Simple and honest explanations the day before and on the day of surgery, with a fairly detailed description of what to expect, given in a way that the child can understand, will make for a smoother hospital stay and will significantly decrease untoward psychologic reactions in the postoperative months and years.

Malignant hyperpyrexia may occur as a complication of anesthesia, especially in young boys with undescended testes, lordosis, kyphosis, and muscle disease.

PREOPERATIVE CARE

Preoperative Feeding

Routine stereotyped orders (eg, "nothing by mouth after midnight") must be avoided.

A. Normal Fluid Feeding: Fluid feeding should be administered as follows:

1. Infants–Breast or regular formula feeding may be given up to 4 hours before surgery, or a carbohydrate solution may be substituted.

2. Older children–Five to 6 hours before surgery, give a large glass of strained, sweetened orange juice or carbonated drink. If surgery is scheduled for after 11:00 AM, a liquid breakfast should be given 5–6 hours before surgery.

B. Correction of Fluid and Electrolyte Imbalance: For correction of fluid and electrolyte imbalance, see Chapter 5. It is generally not necessary to correct minor degrees of imbalance, but some attempt should be made to correct major imbalances even if surgery must be delayed. The use of a cutdown for intravenous drip expedites the administration of whole blood and fluids to small children during a major operative procedure and affords a route for the continuous administration of fluids postoperatively. However, the danger of overhydration during surgery must be borne in mind constantly.

Preoperative Medication

See Drug Dosages for Children in Appendix.

Vitamin Therapy

Give vitamin K, 1–3 mg intramuscularly, to all newborn infants and to those who may have a vitamin K deficiency (eg, liver disturbances, chronic gastrointestinal disease, infants in the first 3 months of life).

Antibiotic Therapy

Appropriate chemotherapeutic or antibiotic agents are given depending on the type and site of surgery and possible infecting agent (see Chapter 6).

Reduction of Fever

Children with high fever withstand anesthesia and surgery poorly; attempts should be made to reduce the temperature below 38.9 °C (102 °F) with aspirin orally or rectally, alcohol or tepid water sponges, adequate hydration, and antibiotics if necessary.

Enema

Enemas are generally not necessary unless there is distention or the surgical procedure will involve the bowel.

Sedation

The use of a sedative to allay apprehension and to help relax the child should be considered even though the patient does not complain of these symptoms.

POSTOPERATIVE CARE

The child should be placed in a warm bed, usually on the side or abdomen (to ensure a free airway). Inhalation anesthesia easily produces edema of the upper respiratory tract in children. If inhalation anesthesia has been used, the administration of oxygen in an atmosphere of high humidity diminishes the danger of laryngeal edema and may be instrumental in reducing the need for postoperative tracheostomy. Vaporized detergents containing vasoconstricting agents may also materially aid in decreasing edema of the upper respiratory tract.

Blood & Fluid Replacements

A. Blood: The estimated blood loss should be replaced either during or immediately after surgery.

B. Fluid and Electrolytes: Care should be taken to avoid the administration of excessive amounts of sodium chloride. In most instances, glucose in water should be used.

Sedation

Small doses of phenobarbital for the young child or small doses of morphine for the older child should be given to maintain adequate sedation.

Postoperative Feeding

Oral feedings can usually be resumed 6–12 hours after most surgical procedures. Start with water or clear liquids and advance to the regular diet as rapidly as the child tolerates.

Ambulation

Early ambulation is advisable in the older child. In any case, the hospital stay should be as short as possible. An early return to the home will result in a general improvement in the child's emotional and physical well-being.

Development & Growth | 3

Development and growth are continuous dynamic processes occurring from conception to maturity and taking place in an orderly sequence that is approximately the same for all individuals. At any particular age, however, wide variations are to be found among normal children; these reflect the active response of the growing individual to numberless hereditary and environmental factors.

The body as a whole and the various tissues and organs have characteristic growth patterns that are essentially the same in all individuals.

Development signifies maturation of organs and systems, acquisition of skills, ability to adapt more readily to stress, and ability to assume maximum responsibility and to achieve freedom in creative expression. Growth signifies increase in size.

DEVELOPMENT

The physician should know something about normal development at all ages in order to give comprehensive pediatric care and should be particularly familiar with development during the earliest years, since he or she occupies a unique position as family adviser during this period.

There is no simple practical method of assaying the various behavioral or emotional factors that determine a child's state of development. The following data should merely serve as a screening guide for recognition of marked variations from the average. Overall developmental evaluation is indicated whenever an unexplained persistent retardation is found in any one area.

Various norms of development have been described. Those given below are relatively simple and do not demand specialized testing material.

DEVELOPMENTAL SCREENING*

The Denver Developmental Screening Test (DDST) is a device for detecting developmental delays in infancy and the preschool years. The

*From Frankenburg W: Denver Developmental Screening Test. *J Pediatr* 1967; **71**:181.

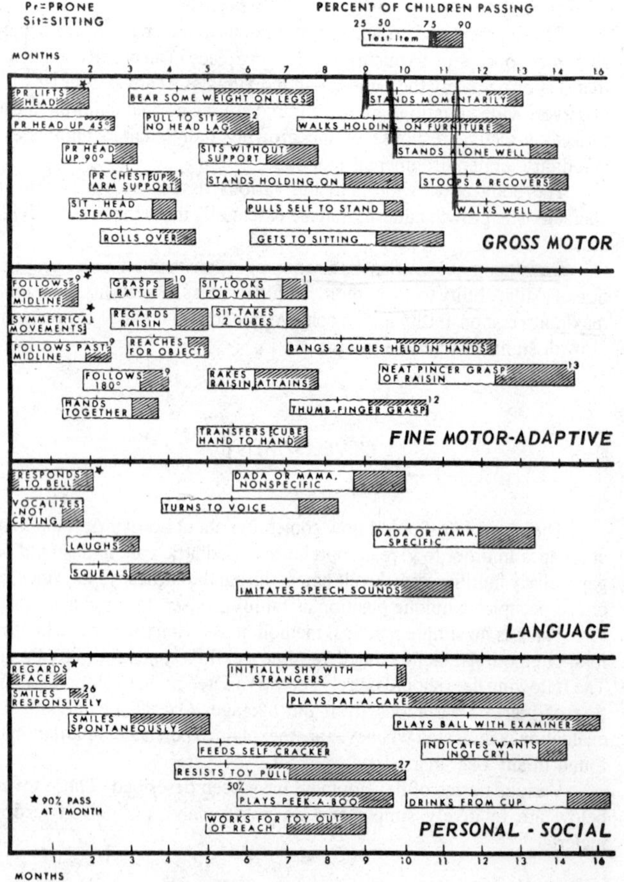

Figure 3–1. Denver Developmental Screening Test.

test is easily and quickly administered and lends itself to serial evaluations on the same test sheet (Fig 3–1).

Test Materials

A skein of red wool, box of raisins, rattle with a narrow handle, small clear bottle with 5/8-inch opening, bell, tennis ball, test form, pencil, and 8 one-inch cubical colored blocks are needed for the test.

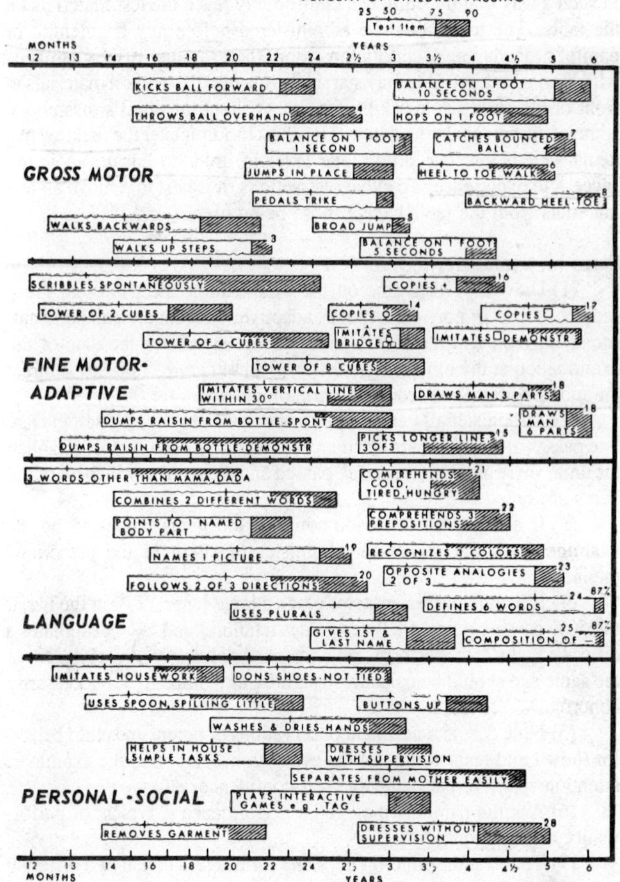

Figure 3–1 (cont'd). Denver Developmental Screening Test.

General Administration Instructions

The parent should be told that this is a developmental screening device to obtain an estimate of the child's level of development and that it is not expected that the child be able to perform each of the test items. This test relies on observations of what the child can do and on reports by a parent who knows the child. Direct observation should be used whenever possible. Since the test requires active participation by the child, every effort should be made to put the child at ease. The younger child may be tested while sitting on the parent's lap. This should be done in such a way that the child can comfortably reach the test materials on the table. The test should be administered before any frightening or painful procedures. A child upon whom the examiner rushes demands will often withdraw. One may start by laying out one or 2 test materials in front of the child while asking the parent about the child's mastery of some of the personal-social items. It is best to administer the first few test items well below the child's age level in order to ensure an initial successful experience. To avoid distractions, it is best to remove all test materials from the table except those being used.

Steps in Administering the Test

(1) Draw a vertical line on the examination sheet through the 4 sectors (gross motor, fine motor-adaptive, language, and personal-social) to represent the child's chronologic age. Place the date of the examination at the top of the age line. For premature children, subtract the months premature from the chronologic age.

(2) Administer all items through which the child's chronologic age line passes unless there are obvious deviations. In each sector, establish the area where all of the items are passed and the point at which all of the items are failed.

(3) If a child refuses to do some of the items requested by the examiner, ask the parent to administer the item in the prescribed manner.

(4) If a child passes an item, place a large letter "P" on the bar at the 50% passing point. "F" designates a failure, and "R" designates a refusal. Failure to perform an item passed by 90% of children of the same age should be considered significant, although not necessarily abnormal.

(5) Note date and pertinent observations of parent and child behavior (how child feels at time of the evaluation, relation to the examiner, attention span, verbal behavior, self-confidence, etc).

(6) Ask the parent if the child's performance is typical of performance at other times.

(7) To retest the child on the same form, use a pencil of a different color for the scoring and age line.

(8) Instructions for administering footnoted items are given below.

Interpretations

The test items are placed into 4 categories: gross motor, fine motor-adaptive, language, and personal-social. Each test item is designated by a bar located under the age scale in such a way as to indicate clearly the ages at which 25%, 50%, 75%, and 90% of the standardization population could perform the particular task. The left end of the bar designates the age at which 25% of the standardization population could perform the item; the point shown at the top of the bar, 50%; the left end of the shaded area, 75%; and the right end, 90%.

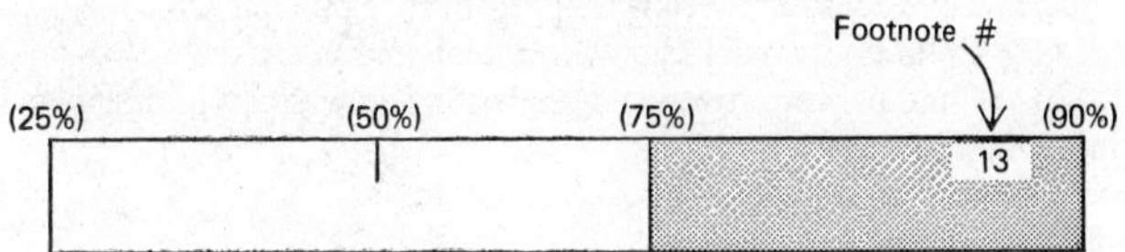

Failure to perform an item passed by 90% of children of the same age should be considered significant. Such a failure may be emphasized by coloring the right end of the bar of the failed item. Several failures in one sector are considered to be developmental delays. These delays may be due either to the unwillingness of the child to perform the task (even though the child is capable) or to an inability to perform the task. General unwillingness may be just as detrimental as an inability to perform. The child's unwillingness may be a temporary phenomenon, such as fatigue, illness, hospitalization, separation from the parent, or fear. Inability to perform the task may be due to general retardation, pathologic factors such as deafness or neurologic impairment, or a familial pattern of slow development in one or more areas.

If unexplained developmental delays are noted and are a valid reflection of a child's abilities, the child should be rescreened a month later. If the delays persist, further evaluation with more detailed diagnostic studies is indicated.

Caution: The DDST is not an intelligence test. It is intended as a screening instrument for use in clinical practice to note whether the development of a particular child is within the normal range.

Directions for Footnoted Items

(1) Child, when prone, lifts chest off table with support of forearms, hands, or both.

(2) Examiner grasps child's hands, pulls child from supine to sitting position; child has no head lag.

(3) Child may use wall or rail only, not person; may not crawl.

(4) Child throws ball overhand 3 feet to within examiner's reach.

(5) Child performs standing broad jump over width of test sheet.

(6) Examiner asks child to walk forward, heel within 1 inch of toe.

(7) Examiner bounces ball to child; child must catch with hands (2–3 trials).

(8) Examiner asks child to walk backwards, toe within 1 inch of heel.

(9) Examiner moves yarn in an arc from side to side, 1 foot above child's head. Note if eyes follow 90 degrees to midline (past midline, 180 degrees).

(10) Child grasps rattle when it is touched to backs or tips of fingers.

(11) Child looks after yarn dropped from sight over table's edge.

(12) Child grasps raisin between thumb and index finger.

(13) Child performs overhand grasp of raisin with tips of thumb and index finger.

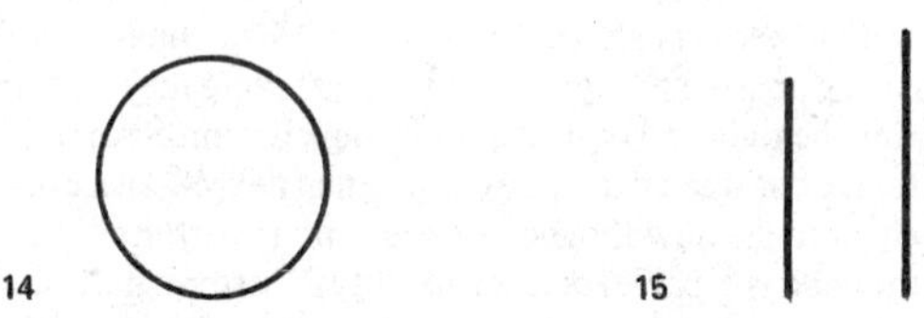

(14) Have child copy. *Do not demonstrate. Do not name form.* Pass any enclosed form.

(15) Ask child, "Which line is *longer*?" (Not *bigger*.) Turn paper upside down and repeat. Pass 3 of 3.

(16) Have child copy. *Do not demonstrate. Do not name form.* Pass crossing lines, any angle.

(17) Have child copy first. If child fails, demonstrate. *Do not name form.* Pass figure with 4 right-angle corners.

(18) When scoring symmetric forms, each pair (2 arms, 2 eyes, etc) counts as one part only.

(19) Point to picture and have child name it.

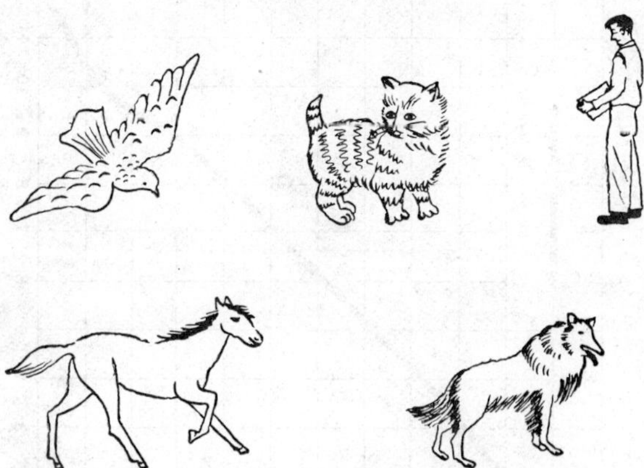

(20) Ask child to "Give block to Mommie (or Daddy)," "Put block on table," and "Put block on floor." *Do not gesture with head or eyes.* Pass 2 of 3.

(21) Ask child, "What do you do when you are cold?" "Hungry?" "Tired?" Pass 2 of 3.

(22) Ask child to "Put clock *on* table, *under* table, *in front of* chair, *behind* chair." *Do not gesture with head or eyes.* Pass 3 of 4.

(23) Ask child to complete the following sentences: "Fire is hot; ice is ________." "Mother is a woman; Dad is a ________." "A horse is big; a mouse is ______." Pass 2 of 3.

(24) Ask child to define 6 of the following: "ball, lake, desk, house, banana, curtain, hedge, pavement." Pass any verbal indication of understanding.

(25) Ask child, "What is a spoon made of?" "What is a shoe made of?" "What is a door made of?" *Do not substitute other objects.* Pass 3 of 3.

(26) Try to get child to smile by smiling, talking, or waving. *Do not touch.* Pass if child smiles responsively in 2 or 3 attempts.

(27) Try to pull toy away when child is playing with toy. Pass if child resists.

(28) Child need not be able to tie shoes or button in the back.

Figure 3–2. Norms of development. (Adapted from Aldrich CA, Norval HA: A developmental graph for the first year of life. *J Pediatr* 1946;29:304.)

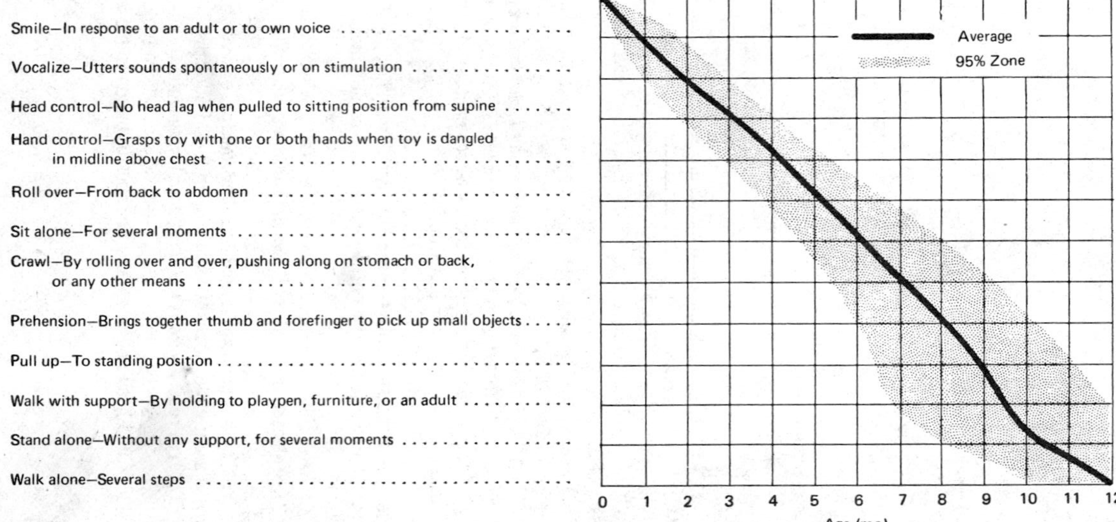

PERSONALITY DEVELOPMENT

Personality development is a dynamic process, and no summary can give a complete picture of what takes place. The goal of the individual, both as a child and as an adult, is to be able to work, to play, to master personal problems, and to love and be loved in a manner that is creative, socially acceptable, and personally gratifying.

The development of personality is a complicated process involving all aspects of the individual and the environment. The process varies from one child to another, but, on the whole, all children pass through various phases of development of which the broad general outlines are essentially the same.

Each successive stage of development is characterized by definite problems the child must solve in order to proceed with confidence to the next. The highest degree of functional harmony will be achieved when the problems of each stage are met and solved at an orderly rate and in a normal sequence. On the other hand, it is important to remember that the successive personality gains the child makes are not rigidly established once and for all but may be reinforced or threatened throughout life. Even in adulthood, a reasonably healthy personality may be achieved in spite of previous misfortunes and defects in the developmental sequence.

It is important to remember that psychologic development takes place within a cultural milieu. Not only the form of large social institutions but the framework of family life, the attitudes of parents, and their practices in child-rearing will be conditioned by the culture of the given period.

Psychologic development in childhood may be roughly divided into 5 stages: infancy (birth–18 months), early childhood (18 months–5 years), late childhood (5–12 years), early adolescence (12–16 years), and late adolescence (16 years–maturity).

Infancy

Perhaps the most striking features of the first year of life are the great physical development that takes place and the infant's growing awareness of *self* as an entity separate from the environment (Fig 3–2).

Much of the psychologic development during the first year is interrelated with physical development, ie, dependent upon the maturation of the body to the extent that the infant can discriminate self from nonself. Knowledge of the environment comes with increasing sharpening of the senses (from indiscriminate mouthing to coordinated eye-hand movements). Beginning of mastery over the environment comes with increasingly adept coordination, the development of locomotion, and the beginnings of speech. The realization of the self as an individual in relation to an environment that includes other individuals is the basis upon which interpersonal relationships are founded.

The newborn infant is at first aware only of bodily needs, ie, of the presence or absence of discomfort (cold, wet, etc). The pleasure of relief from discomfort gradually becomes associated with mothering and later (when perception is sufficient for recognition) with the mother. The infant derives a feeling of security when bodily needs are satisfied and from contact with the mother. The feeding situation provides the first opportunity for development of this feeling of security, and it is therefore important for the physician to ensure that this is a happy event.

The development of the first emotional relationship, then, comes through close contact with the mother. It develops from a meeting of the infant's physical needs into a sustained physical contact and emotional interaction with one person. Prolonged deprivation of this relationship, if no satisfactory substitute is provided, is damaging to the personality. Permanent deprivation leads to restriction of personality development, even to pseudoretardation in all areas. Such behavior may also occur in a home situation, but it is more striking and more common in infants who remain for long periods of time in hospitals or in other institutions where adequate personalized and kindly attention is not given to each infant. The infant who is deprived of the security and affection necessary to produce a sense of trust may respond with listlessness, immobility, unresponsiveness, indifferent appetite, an appearance of unhappiness, and insomnia. In other cases, the continued deprivation of consistent care during infancy may not become apparent until later life, when the individual may feel no reason to trust people and thus lack a sense of responsibility toward others.

No particular techniques are necessary to develop an infant's feeling of security. The infant is not easily discouraged by an inexperienced mother's mistakes; rather, the infant seems to respond to the warmth of her feelings and her eagerness to keep trying. The feeling of security derived from satisfactory relationships during the first year is probably the most important single element in the personality. It makes it possible for the infant to accept restrictions without fearing that each restriction implies total loss of love.

Toward the end of the first year, other personal relationships also are developing, particularly with the father, who is now recognized as comparable in importance with the mother. Relationships perhaps are also forming with siblings.

Early Childhood (18 mos - 5 yrs)

In early childhood, the child's horizon continues to widen. Increased body control makes possible the development of many physical skills. The very important development of speech permits extension of the social environment and increasing ability to understand and perfect social relationships.

Perhaps the central problem of early childhood is still, however, the development of control over the instinctive drives, particularly as they arise in relationship to the parents. The acceptance of limitations on the need for bodily love (the realization that complete infantile dependency is not permitted or desirable) and the control of aggressive feelings are prime examples. This control of primitive feelings is largely accomplished through the psychologic process of "identification" with the parents—the desire in the child to be like the parents and to emulate them. With this desire come the beginnings of conscience as the moral values of the parents are incorporated into the child's own personality.

The child now begins to have a feeling of autonomy—of self-direction and initiative. The child 18 months to 2½ years of age is actively learning to exercise the power of "yes" and "no." The difficulty the 2-year-old has in deciding between the 2 often leads to parental misunderstanding; the child may say "no" but really mean "yes," as if compelled to exercise this new "will" even when it hurts.

At this period, parental "discipline" becomes very important. Discipline is an educative means by which the parent teaches the child how to become a self-respecting, likable, and socially responsible adult. Disciplinary measures have value chiefly as they serve this educative function; if used as an end in themselves, to establish the "authority" of the parent irrespective of the issues at hand, they usually lead only to warfare (open or surreptitious) between parent and child.

The goal is to allow the child to develop the feeling of being a responsible human being without rejecting the help and guidance of others in important matters. The favorable result is self-control without loss of self-esteem. Adults must allow children increasingly wide latitude in undergoing experiences that permit them to make choices they are ready and able to make and yet must also teach them to accept restrictions when necessary.

The parents must be firm and consistent to protect the child against the consequences of immature judgment. Perhaps the most constructive rule a parent can follow is to decide which kinds of conformity are really important and then to clearly and consistently require obedience in these areas. Then "discipline" will have the positive goal of making the child able to live comfortably in society without feeling guilty about basic drives but will not stifle the need for some expression of independence.

Late Childhood

In this period, children achieve a rapid intellectual growth and actively begin to establish themselves as members of society. Psychiatrists call this the latency period, because the force of the primitive drives has been fairly successfully controlled, expressed in a socially acceptable way, or repressed. The energy derived from the instinctive drives whose direct expression society does not permit is diverted into the great

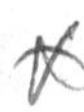
drive for knowledge—a process of "sublimation." At no time in life does the individual learn more avidly and quickly. Reading and writing (the intellectual skills) and a vast body of information are quickly assimilated. The preoccupation with fantasy gradually subsides, and the child wants to be engaged in real tasks that can be carried through to completion. Even in play activities, the emphasis is on developing mental and bodily skills through interest in sports and games.

Late childhood is also a period of conformity to the group. The environment enlarges to include school and, particularly, other children. Much of the emotional satisfaction previously derived from the parents now comes from the child's relationships with peers. The need to become a member of this larger group of equals tends to encourage the qualities of cooperation and obedience to the will of the group (elements of democracy). It also paves the way for questioning parental values where these differ from those of the group—a direct impact of broader cultural values upon the environment of the home.

Early Adolescence (12–16)

After the comparative calm of late childhood, early adolescence is a period of upheaval. With the great changes in body size and configuration comes a new confusion about the physical self (the "body image"). Sexual maturation brings with it a resurgence of the strong instinctual drives that have been successfully repressed for several years. In our culture, in contrast to some primitive cultures, the sexual drive is not permitted direct expression in adolescents in spite of physical readiness.

The calm emotional adjustment is disrupted. Again the child has to learn to control strong feelings: love, hate, and aggression. Again the relationship to the parents is disturbed. The former docile acceptance of them as most important, most powerful, is replaced by rebellion. Yet as strongly as adolescents rebel and insist on independence from their parents, just as strongly do they feel again the old dependence, which is revealed in their unwillingness to accept personal responsibility and their tendency to rely on parental care.

The adolescent's position as an individual must again be realigned, not in relation to the family circle but in relation to society. Adolescents are constantly preoccupied with how they appear in the eyes of others as compared with their own conceptions of themselves. They find comfort in conformity with their own age group, and fads in clothing and manners reach a peak during early adolescence.

Perhaps most helpful to parents is the ability to "ride" with each swing in adolescent behavior and not assume that each change accurately presages the personality of the future adult. Adolescents are inexperienced in their new roles as potential adults, and their behavior tends to be erratic and extreme. Calm and stability provided by the parents can do much to keep them in equilibrium.

Late Adolescence

By age 16 years, most adolescents have again reached comparative equilibrium. Their body growth has slowed somewhat, and they have had time to adapt to the changes. They have acquired sufficient mastery over biologic drives; these drives can now be channeled into more constructive patterns and the beginning of heterosexual social activity, eventually leading to the choice of a companion or marital partner.

The relationship to the parents is now more mature. With the discovery that responsible independence is neither frightening nor overwhelming but a position possible to maintain, the adolescent can cease to rebel and can accept the parents' help in planning constructively for adulthood.

Learning is again rapid, particularly for the intelligent youth, who can absorb much more information than the conventional secondary school education offers.

Active preparation for adulthood characterizes late adolescence in our culture, although, as in more primitive cultures, some adolescents will have already taken on the responsibilities of job and marriage. Biologically, this is certainly feasible; it is the complexity and competition of our modern culture that so greatly prolong the emergence into full adulthood.

GROWTH

General Considerations

A. Fetal Growth: During fetal life, the rate of growth is extremely rapid. During the early months, the fetal rate of gain in length is greater than the rate of gain in weight when expressed as percentage of value at birth. By the eighth month, the fetus has achieved 80% of the birth length and only 50% of the birth weight (Table 3–1).

B. Organs: At birth, the proportion of the weight of the pancreas and the musculature to that of the entire body is less in the infant than in the adult; that of the skeleton, lungs, and stomach is the same; and that of other organs is greater in the infant than in the adult. Major types of postnatal growth of various parts and organs of the body are shown in Fig 3–3.

C. Trunk-Leg Ratio: At birth, the ratio of the lower to the upper segment of the body (as measured from the pubis) is approximately 1:1.7. The legs grow more rapidly than does the trunk; by age 10–12 years, the segments are approximately equal.

D. Height: Rate of growth is generally more important than actual size. For more accurate comparisons, data should be recorded both as

Table 3–1. Fetal and newborn dimensions and weights of the body and its organs.*

Fetal Age (wk)†	Crown-heel (cm)	Crown-rump (cm)	Head Circumference (cm)	Body Weight (g)	Adrenal (g)	Brain (g)	Heart (g)	Kidney (g)	Liver (g)	Lungs (g)	Pancreas (g)	Pituitary (g)	Spleen (g)	Thymus (g)	Thyroid (g)
Prenatal and Newborn															
12	9.0	7.5	7.4	18.6	0.087	2.32	0.098	0.163	0.097	0.69	0.013		0.006	0.010	0.026
16	16.7	12.8	12.6	100	0.417	14.40	0.662	0.962	5.94	3.23	0.095	0.011	0.086	0.122	0.133
20	24.2	17.7	17.6	310	1.07	43	2.08	2.77	16.8	8.18	0.314	0.024	0.41	0.553	0.352
24	31.1	21.9	22.3	670	2.02	91	4.47	5.69	34.5	15.2	0.695	0.040	1.16	1.53	0.684
28	37.1	25.5	26.3	1150	3.16	153	7.70	9.43	57.4	23.7	1.22	0.058	2.43	3.14	1.08
30	39.8	27.1	28.1	1400	3.78	189	9.78	11.5	70.3	28.2	1.53	0.067	3.26	4.18	1.33
32	42.4	28.5	29.9	1700	4.44	228	11.6	13.8	84.3	33.0	1.88	0.076	4.25	5.41	1.54
34	44.8	29.9	31.5	2000	5.11	268	13.7	16.2	100.0	37.8	2.24	0.085	5.36	6.77	1.78
36	47.0	31.2	33.1	2450	5.77	309	15.9	18.6	113.0	42.7	2.61	0.094	6.55	8.22	2.01
38	49.1	32.4	34.4	2900	6.45	352	18.2	21.0	129.0	47.5	3.01	0.103	7.86	9.82	2.26
40	51.0	33.5	35.7	3150	7.10	394	20.6	23.5	143.5	52.5	3.40	0.111	9.22	11.5	2.50
Postnatal															
Age (yr)															
1					4	875	43	62	350	160		0.15	30	23	
5					5	1250	90	110	575	305		0.23	55	28	
10	See Inside Front Cover				6	1325	145	150	825	450		0.33	77	31	
15					8	1340	245	220	1275	675		0.48	125	27	
Adult‡															
Male					6	1375	300	320	1600	1000			165	14	
Female					6	1280	250	280	1500	750			150	14	

*Adapted from Edith Boyd. See also Inside Front Cover. †Time from first day of last menstrual period. ‡Adapted from several sources.

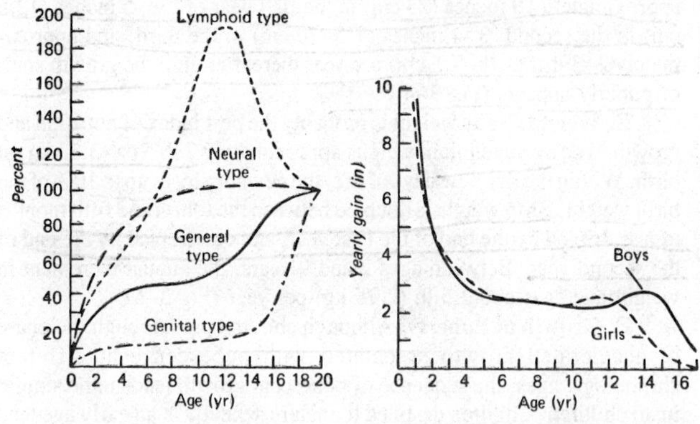

Figure 3–3. Major types of postnatal growth of various parts and organs of the body.

Figure 3–4. Yearly gain in height.

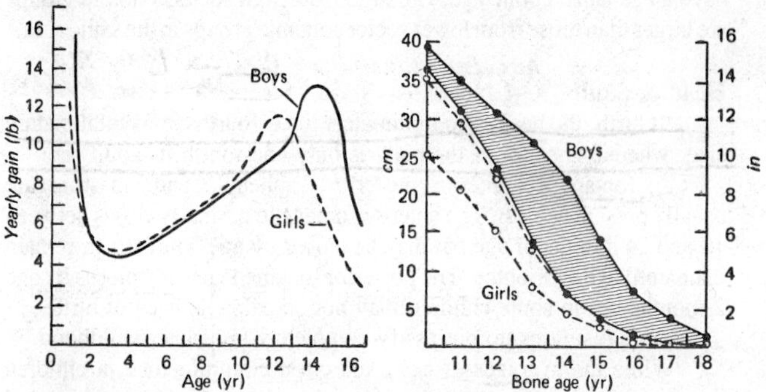

Figure 3–5. Yearly gain in weight.

Figure 3–6. Growth expectancy at bone ages indicated.

Figures 3–3 to 3–6 are redrawn and reproduced, with permission, from Holt LE, McIntosh R, Barnett HL: *Pediatrics,* 13th ed. Appleton-Century-Crofts, 1962, as redrawn from Harris JA et al: *Measurement of Man.* Univ of Minnesota Press, 1930.

absolute figures and as a percentile for that particular age, and the rate of growth should be determined. Birth length is doubled by approximately age 4 years and tripled by age 13 years. The average child grows approximately 10 inches (25 cm) in the first year of life, 5 inches (12.5 cm) in the second, 3–4 inches (7.5–10 cm) in the third, and approximately 2–3 inches (5–7.5 cm) per year thereafter until the growth spurt of puberty appears (Fig 3–4).

E. Weight: Body weight is probably the best index of nutrition and growth. The average infant weighs approximately 7 lb 5 oz (3.33 kg) at birth. Within the first few days of life, the newborn loses up to 10% of the birth weight. Birth weight is doubled between the fourth and fifth months of age, tripled by the end of the first year, and quadrupled by the end of the second year. Between ages 2 and 9 years, the annual increment in weight averages about 5 lb (2.25 kg) per year (Fig 3–5).

F. Growth at Puberty: Although children pass through the phase of accelerated growth associated with pubescence at different chronologic ages, the sequence of pubescent growth tends to be similar in all children. Children destined to mature sexually at an early age tend to be tall and have an advanced bone age (Fig 3–6); late-maturing children are short and show epiphyseal retardation in childhood.

G. Variations in Growth: Obese children are usually taller and have an advanced bone age. Children from high socioeconomic groups are larger than those from lower socioeconomic groups in the same area.

Head & Skull

At birth, the head is approximately three-fourths of its total mature size, whereas the rest of the body is only one-fourth its adult size.

Six fontanelles (anterior, posterior, 2 sphenoid, and 2 mastoid) are usually present at birth. The anterior fontanelle normally closes between 10 and 14 months of age but may be closed by age 3 months or remain open until age 18 months. The posterior fontanelle usually closes by age 2 months but in some children may not be palpable even at birth.

Cranial sutures do not ossify completely until later childhood.

While the averages of head and chest circumference in children during the first 4 years of life are approximately equal, during this period the head circumference may normally be from 5 cm larger to 7 cm smaller than that of the chest. Growth of the skull, as determined by increasing head circumference, is a much more accurate index of brain growth than is the presence or size of the fontanelle.

Sinuses

Maxillary and ethmoid sinuses are present at birth but are usually not aerated for approximately 6 months. The sphenoid sinuses are usually not pneumatized (or visible on x-ray) until after the third year of life.

Frontal sinuses usually become visible by x-ray between 7 and 9 years of age, seldom before age 5.

The mastoid process at birth is relatively large and has a relatively wide communication with the middle ear. Its cellular structure appears gradually between birth and age 3 years.

Eyes

The eyes can follow, even at birth, and the ability to fixate is usually well developed by age 2–3 months. Strabismus normally may be present for the first 6–8 months of life.

Respiration & Heart Rate

The respiratory rate decreases steadily during childhood, averaging approximately 30 breaths per minute during the first year of life, 25 during the second year, 20 during the eighth year, and 18 by the 15th year.

The heart rate falls steadily throughout childhood, averaging about 150 beats per minute in utero, 130 at birth, 105 during the second year of life, 90 during the fourth year, 80 during the sixth year, and 70 during the tenth year.

Abdomen

The abdomen tends to be prominent in infants and toddlers. In the infant, the ascending and descending portions of the colon are short compared with the transverse colon, and the sigmoid extends higher into the abdomen than during later life.

Gas may be visualized roentgenographically almost immediately after birth in the stomach, within 2 hours in the ileum, and, on the average, in 3 or 4 hours in the rectum.

There is a deficiency of the starch-splitting enzyme amylase during early infancy; this prevents optimal handling of long-chain polysaccharides. Amylase is present in significant amounts in the pancreatic juice by age 3 months. Lipase activity is low throughout early childhood. In contrast, trypsin activity is adequate from birth except in the premature infant, in whom low levels are often found.

Muscle

At birth, muscle constitutes 25% of total body weight, as compared with 43% in the adult.

Ossification Centers

At birth, the average full-term infant has 5 ossification centers demonstrable by x-ray: distal end of femur, proximal end of tibia, calcaneus, talus, and cuboid.

The clavicle is the first bone to calcify in utero, calcification beginning during the fifth fetal week.

Epiphyseal development of girls is consistently ahead of that of boys during all of childhood.

Puberty

Sexual maturation is more closely correlated with bone maturation than with chronologic age. The maximal yearly increase in height occurs during the year before menarche in most girls. Climate apparently has little effect on sexual development. Nigerian girls and Eskimo girls have their menarche at approximately the same age. If environmental and nutritional factors are similar, girls of different races tend to have their menarche at approximately the same age.

During the first 1–2 years following menarche, the menstrual periods of most girls are anovulatory and often irregular, and the interval between periods may be longer or shorter than is characteristic during later life.

Girls who mature late are taller (on the average) when final stature is attained.

Some degree of breast hypertrophy (gynecomastia) is relatively common in boys at puberty.

Senses

At birth, the newborn infant has mature sensory receptors for pressure, pain, and temperature over the entire body surface, in the mouth, and in the external genitalia; there are also mature pain receptors in the viscera and proprioceptive receptors in muscles, joints, and tendons.

A. Taste: The ability to taste is present in the newborn infant, who is capable of distinguishing the 4 basic tastes.

B. Olfaction: The human infant is born with fully mature receptors for olfaction.

C. Hearing: Normal infants can hear almost immediately after birth, but they respond to sounds at a subcortical level.

D. Vision: About 80% of newborn infants are hyperopic; the eyeball grows rapidly during the first 8 years of life. Thus, hyperopia should be expected during the preschool and early school years. Strabismus normally may be present for the first 6–8 months of life. Mature adult function of the eye muscles is usually reached by the end of the first year.

At birth, the infant demonstrates an awareness of light and dark, possesses peripheral vision, and is capable of rudimentary fixation on near objects. Other visual functions are deficient. At age 4 months, vision is 20/300–20/200 (6/90–6/60); at age 10 months, 20/200 (6/60); and at age 2 years, 20/40 (6/12). Vision becomes 20/20 (6/6) at age 4 years.

Table 3–2. Dental growth and development.

Primary or Deciduous Teeth

	Calcification		Eruption*		Shedding	
	Begins At	Complete At	Maxillary	Mandibular	Maxillary	Mandibular
Central incisors	4th fetal mo	18–24 mo	6–10 mo	5–8 mo	7–8 yr	6–7 yr
Lateral incisors	5th fetal mo	18–24 mo	8–12 mo	7–10 mo	8–9 yr	7–8 yr
Cuspids	6th fetal mo	30–39 mo	16–20 mo	16–20 mo	11–12 yr	9–11 yr
First molars	5th fetal mo	24–30 mo	11–18 mo	11–18 mo	9–11 yr	10–12 yr
Second molars	6th fetal mo	36 mo	20–30 mo	20–30 mo	9–12 yr	11–13 yr

Secondary or Permanent Teeth

	Calcification		Eruption*	
	Begins At	Complete At	Maxillary	Mandibular
Central incisors	3–4 mo	9–10 yr	7–8 yr (3)	6–7 yr (2)
Lateral incisors	Maxilla 10–12 mo Mandible 3–4 mo	10–11 yr	8–9 yr (5)	7–8 yr (4)
Cuspids	4–5 mo	12–15 yr	11–12 yr (11)	9–11 yr (6)
First premolars	18–24 mo	12–13 yr	10–11 yr (7)	10–12 yr (8)
Second premolars	24–30 mo	12–14 yr	10–12 yr (9)	11–13 yr (10)
First molars	Birth	9–10 yr	5½–7 yr (1)	5½–7 yr (1a)
Second molars	30–36 mo	14–16 yr	12–14 yr (12)	12–13 yr (12a)
Third molars	Maxilla 7–9 yr Mandible 8–10 yr	18–25 yr	17–30 yr (13)	17–30 yr (13a)

*Figures in parentheses indicate order of eruption. Many otherwise normal infants do not conform strictly to the stated schedule.

Water Content

The water content of the body is approximately 95% of weight during early fetal life, 65–75% at birth, and 55–60% at maturity.

Blood

If the umbilical cord is not clamped for 2–3 minutes after delivery of the infant, 75–135 mL of blood will be transferred from the placenta to the infant. Late clamping will produce a red blood cell count approximately 1 million/μL higher, a hemoglobin level approximately 2.5 g/dL higher, and a hematocrit count 7% higher than if early clamping were carried out.

At birth, 5% of all red blood cells may be reticulocytes; they drop to less than 1% after the second week of life. Nucleated red cells (up to 5% as a percentage of the total number of nucleated cells) and immature lymphocytes may be present in the newborn but disappear within the first week of life. Fetal hemoglobin accounts for 80% of total hemoglobin at birth (cord blood), 75% of the total at age 2 weeks, and 55% at age 5 weeks; it falls to 5% by age 20 weeks.

The leukocyte count is high at birth, rises slightly during the first 48 hours after birth, falls for the next 2 or 3 weeks, and then rises again. In some infants, it reaches its highest level in life sometime before the seventh month. The lymphocyte count is highest during the first year of life and then falls progressively during the remainder of childhood.

Children have a higher sedimentation rate than do adults.

Urine

The average infant secretes 15–50 mL of urine per 24 hours during the first 2 days of life, 50–300 mL/d during the next week, and 400–500 mL/d by the latter half of the first year. There is subsequently a gradual increase in urinary output; 700–1500 mL/d is secreted between ages 8 and 14 years.

Tears

Tears can be produced during the early weeks of life.

Teeth

Stages of dental growth and development are shown in Table 3–2.

Nutrition & Feeding* | 4

The act of feeding is important to the young child not only because of the nutritive substances obtained from the food but also because of the emotional and psychologic benefits derived. Drinking and eating are intense experiences to an infant and can and should be sources of great satisfaction. From these experiences, and from the persons who feed them, infants obtain many of their early ideas about the nature of life and people.

Parents must be made to understand that there is much individual variation in the nutritional needs and desires of infants and that differences occur in the same child at various times.

The feeding of children is constantly being made more flexible and simple as knowledge of their nutritional requirements increases; however, certain basic information and data are necessary for a practical understanding of the subject.

Neither strict adherence to a time schedule nor feeding when the infant cries is necessary for successful and satisfactory feeding. For most parents and infants, a flexible schedule with reasonable regularity is most satisfactory, but in some cases either a strict routine or complete ''demand'' feeding gives better results.

BREAST FEEDING

Advantages & Disadvantages

A. Advantages: Apart from considerations of economy and convenience (temperature, asepsis, automatic adjustment in most instances to infant's needs), breast feeding is superior to bottle feeding because the composition of breast milk is ideal for nearly all infants (Table 4–1); because breast milk contains specific antibacterial and antiviral activity that protects infants from gastrointestinal and respiratory disease; because breast feeding produces less infantile allergy; and because breast feeding can be psychologically beneficial to both mother and infant. Breast feeding should be encouraged whenever feasible, although suc-

*Revised with the assistance of Marianne R. Neifert, MD.

Table 4–1. Composition of milk and commercial formula (per 100 mL).*

Component	Unit	Human Milk	Typical Commercial Formula	Whole Cow's Milk
Osmolality	mosm/kg water	282	290	275
Energy	kcal	72	68	61
Carbohydrate (lactose)	g	7.3	7.2	4.7
Fat	g	4.2	3.6	3.3
Minerals				
Calcium	mg	25	51	119
Chloride	mg (mEq)	40 (1.1)	53 (1.5)	102 (2.9)
Copper	μg	35	41	30
Fluorine	μg	7	20	15
Iodine	μg	7	10	5
Iron	μg	40	150 (1200 w/Fe)	50
Magnesium	mg	3	41	13
Manganese	μg	0.4	3	2–4
Phosphorus	mg	15	39	93
Potassium	mg (mEq)	58 (1.5)	78 (2)	152 (3.9)
Sodium	mg (mEq)	15 (0.8)	25 (1.1)	49 (2.1)
Zinc	μg	166	500	380
Proteins				
Casein	mg	187	1185	2700
Lactalbumin	mg	161	52	400
Total proteins	g	0.9	1.5	3.3
Vitamins				
A (retinol equivalents)	μg (IU)	47 (155)	75 (250)	31 (126)
B_6 (pyridoxine)	μg	28	40	42
B_{12} (cyanocobalamin)	ng	26	150	357
C (ascorbic acid)	mg	4	5.5	0.9
D	μg (IU)	0.04 (1.6)	1 (40)	1 (42)
E (total tocopherols)	μg (IU)	315 (0.32)	1700 (1.7)	80 (0.08)
K	μg	0.21	3	6
Folic acid	μg	5.2	5	5
Niacin	μg	200	790	84
Pantothenic acid	μg	225	300	314
Riboflavin	μg	35	100	162
Thiamine	μg	16	65	30

*Adapted from various sources.

cess will be influenced by the mother's attitude toward nursing, emotional status, home conditions and support systems, breast anatomy, and general health; the father's interest; and the infant's maturity, weight, vigor, appetite, and feeding characteristics.

Breast milk alone is sufficient to ensure adequate growth for the first several months, and, in fact, an early diet of breast milk alone provides optimal infant nutrition. The iron in breast milk is readily available to the child, providing the term infant with an adequate source of iron for the first 4–6 months of life. Iron deficiency anemia among breast-fed infants is uncommon.

B. Disadvantages and Contraindications: Breast feeding may be temporarily impossible for a weak, ill, or premature infant or one with a cleft palate, although in such cases breast milk may be expressed and fed in another way.

Hormones used in oral contraceptives may interfere with optimal milk production.

Breast milk may need to be supplemented with formula if the mother's supply remains inadequate, as evidenced by the infant's poor weight gain, after 3 weeks of trial. Bottle feeding may be substituted for breast feeding if the mother is severely ill or decides not to continue nursing. Menstruation is not a contraindication to breast feeding. An unidentified inhibitor of glucuronyl transferase present in some mothers' milk may be responsible for prolonged unconjugated hyperbilirubinemia in some healthy, thriving breast-fed infants. Permanent weaning is not indicated, although a short trial off breast milk will result in a sharp fall in the bilirubin level. Galactosemia remains a rare absolute contraindication to breast feeding.

Colostrum

Colostrum is an alkaline, yellow breast secretion that may be produced during the last few months of pregnancy and for the first 2–4 days after delivery. It has a higher specific gravity (1.040–1.060); a higher content of protein, fat-soluble vitamins, and minerals; and a lower carbohydrate and fat content than does breast milk.

Colostrum contains secretory IgA, leukocytes, and other immune substances that play a part in the immune defenses of the newborn. Colostrum has a natural laxative action and is an ideal starter food.

Transmission of Drugs & Toxins in Breast Milk

A. Factors Affecting Drug Excretion in Milk: Virtually all drugs consumed by the mother will appear in her milk to some degree, usually in homeopathic amounts. Drug excretion into milk is affected by the drug's ionization, lipid solubility, protein binding, molecular size, and other factors, so generalizations are difficult to make. Effects on the infant also depend upon the route of administration, the dosage, and the mother's timing in taking the drug as well as the drug's metabolites and whether it is absorbed in the gastrointestinal tract. It is thought that the amount of drugs in breast milk is least when the infant is nursed just before the mother takes medications.

B. Drugs Hazardous to the Infant: While it is wise to carefully observe a nursing infant whose mother is being medicated, very few drugs are actually contraindicated. These include radioactive compounds, antimetabolites, lithium, valium, chloramphenicol, and tetracycline. When a course of therapy of a potentially hazardous drug will be brief, the mother can temporarily interrupt breast feeding and maintain her supply by expressing and discarding her milk.

Prelactation (Colostrum) Phase

Although the milk may not "come in" until 2–4 days after delivery, prelactation nursing is very important because of the value of colostrum, the effect of the nursing stimulus to increase milk supply and lessen engorgement, and the opportunity nursing provides for the mother and infant to become accustomed to one another. While some infants nurse irregularly the first few days, others demand feeding as often as every 2 hours. Nursing is commonly limited to 5 minutes per breast per feeding the first day, 10 minutes per breast per feeding the second day, and 15 minutes or longer per breast per feeding thereafter.

There is no need for routine supplementation for the full-term, healthy infant who appears satisfied, but when the infant is persistently hungry or has an underlying condition (ie, hypoglycemia) requiring increased caloric intake, then glucose water or formula may be offered after nursing until the milk comes in. Once milk is in, there is no need for further supplementation if feedings are frequent enough.

Lactation Phase

Forty-eight to 96 hours postpartum, the mother's breasts change from soft to firm and full as engorgement (lactogenesis) occurs. The infant may be fed at each hungry period, day and night, and should be allowed to nurse at the first breast for approximately 10 minutes, then put to the other breast and allowed to suckle as long as required (unless the nipples are sore). At the next feeding, the last breast nursed should be offered first. During the early weeks of lactation, the milk supply seems to be more sensitive to negative stimuli such as maternal fatigue, anxiety, and lack of suckling. The infant will usually have frequent, somewhat loose bowel movements (often with each feeding) during this period.

The let-down reflex, by which milk is actively ejected through the duct system for easy access to the infant, is usually conditioned and evident by 2 weeks. The mother feels "tightening," "stinging," "tingling," or "burning" circumferentially in both breasts shortly after the infant begins nursing. The nursing mother should eat a well-balanced diet with additional intake of protein, calcium, and fluids. Drinking a glass of liquid with each nursing is helpful. Additional rest, with several naps each day, should be encouraged.

"Frequency days," or "appetite spurts," when infants desire to nurse more often than their established routine, typically occur for several days at approximately 3 weeks, 6 weeks, 3 months, and 6 months of age. Increased frequency of nursing increases the milk supply and allows resumption of the former nursing schedule. Supplemental feedings should not be used during the first month, but an occasional bottle may be offered thereafter if the mother's milk supply is well established. The infant should remain familiar with the bottle nipple if the mother has a commitment to return to work, and bottle feedings will need to be instituted. "Solid" food should not be necessary until well after 3 months of age. A woman with activities outside the home should feel free to take her nursing infant with her and breast-feed discreetly when the infant is hungry.

Weaning

There is no "best time" for weaning, which depends on the needs and desires of both infant and mother. Gradual weaning is preferred. Cup or bottle feedings are increased progressively over a period of several weeks as breast feedings are omitted. Older infants may be weaned directly to the cup.

ARTIFICIAL FEEDING
(Bottle Feeding)

Several types of commercially prepared infant formulas are available: milk-based or soy-based; with or without iron; in ready-to-feed, concentrated, or powdered form; as well as numerous preparations for special indications (Table 4–2). Various bottles, including plastic, glass, and disposable, and a multitude of rubber nipples, long, short, and orthodontically shaped, are available. In general, the mother's preference for standard milk-based formula and bottle and nipple should be respected. The infant who is fed an adequate amount of accurately mixed formula (Table 4–3) and held while being fed will gain the physical and emotional satisfaction that accompanies breast feeding.

Evaporated milk formula is still a suitable alternative to proprietary infant formulas and is prepared as follows: To make 32 oz of formula, mix 1 can (13 oz) of whole evaporated milk, 1½ cans (19 oz) of water, and 2 tablespoons of corn syrup. To make 5 oz, mix 2 oz of evaporated milk, 3 oz of water, and 1 teaspoon of corn syrup.

Infants should be fed formula for a minimum of 6 months, or, ideally, for the entire first year of life. Low-fat and skimmed milk are inappropriate for use in the first year of life.

Preparation of the Formula

(1) The formula should be mixed correctly. *No* water is added to ready-to-feed preparations. Most concentrated formulas are mixed 1:1

Table 4–2. Normal and special infant formulas.*

Product	Protein Source	CHO Source	Fat Source	*Indications for Use*	Comments (Nutritional Adequacy)
Milk and milk-based formulas					
Cow's milk Evaporated milk (several brands)	Milk protein.	Lactose, sucrose.	Butterfat.	For full-term and premature infants with no special nutritional requirements.	*If not fortified,* supplement with iron and vitamins C and D.
Commercial formulas for infants					
Enfamil (Mead Johnson)†	Nonfat cow's milk.	Lactose.	Coconut, soy.	For full-term and premature infants with no special nutritional requirements.	Available fortified with iron, 12 mg/L.
Similac (Ross)†	Nonfat cow's milk.	Lactose.	Coconut, corn.	For full-term and premature infants with no special nutritional requirements.	Available fortified with iron, 12 mg/L.
SMA (Wyeth)†	Milk protein, demineralized whey.	Lactose.	Oleo, coconut, safflower, soy.	For full-term and premature infants with no special nutritional requirements.	Supplemented with iron, 12 mg/L.
Products for milk protein–sensitive infants ("milk allergy")					
Isomil (Ross)	Soy.	Sucrose, corn sugar.‡	Coconut, soy.		Soy protein isolate.
Meat base (Gerber)	Beef hearts.	Sucrose, modified tapioca starch.	Sesame.		
Prosobee (Mead Johnson)	Soy protein isolate.	Sucrose, corn syrup solids.	Soy.	For infants with milk protein allergy or lactose intolerance.	Hypoallergenic. Zero band antigen.
Products for premature infants					
Enfamil premature formula (Mead Johnson)	Demineralized whey, nonfat cow's milk.	Lactose, corn syrup solids.	MCT§ (coconut source), corn, coconut oils.	For rapidly growing low-birth-weight infants and infants with special nutritional requirements.	Protein, 3 g/100 kcal. Ca/P ratio 2:1. E/PUFA ratio 1.7:1. Supplemental vitamin E is recommended.

Ensure, Osmolite (Ross)	Sodium and calcium caseinates, soy protein isolate.	Hydrolyzed corn syrup.	MCT (coconut source), corn, soy oils.	For infants intolerant to hypertonic liquid diet (pre- or postoperative feedings).	Osmolality 300 mosm/kg water.
Similac 24 LBW (Ross)	Nonfat cow's milk.	Lactose, corn syrup solids.	MCT, coconut, soy oils.		Protein, 2.7 g/100 kcal. E/PUFA ratio 1.7:1. Osmolality 290 mosm/kg water.
Elemental diets for tube feeding and products for oral supplements					
Ensure (Ross)	Sodium and calcium caseinates, soy protein isolate.	Sucrose, corn syrup solids.	Corn oil.	Used for low-residue liquid diet.	Osmolality 450 mosm/kg water at 1 kcal/mL.
Flexical (Mead Johnson)	Casein hydrolysate.	Corn syrup solids, modified tapioca starch.	20% MCT, 80% soy.	For infants with fat malabsorption.	Osmolality 723 mosm/kg water at 1 kcal/mL.
Hycal (Beecham)		Glucose.			A flavored product for calorie supplementation only.
Polycose (Ross)		Glucose polymers.			A powdered or liquid calorie supplement.
Vital (Ross)	Partial hydrolyzed proteins.	Glucose oligo- and polysaccharides, sucrose.	Safflower, MCT.	Nutritionally complete, hydrolyzed diet from soy, whey, and meat protein with free amino acids. Osmolality 450 mosm/kg water at 1 kcal/mL.	
Vivonex (Eaton)	L-Amino acids.	Glucose, glucose oligosaccharides.	Safflower oil.	Used as general dietary supplement or as sole nutritional source in malabsorption.	Pure amino acid base. Also high in nitrogen. Osmolality 800 mosm/kg water at 1 kcal/mL.

*Committee on Nutrition, American Academy of Pediatrics: Commentary on breast feeding and infant formulas including proposed standards for formulas. *Pediatrics* 1976;57:278. Committee on Nutrition, American Academy of Pediatrics: Nutritional needs of low-birth-weight infants. *Pediatrics* 1977;60:519.

†Ready-to-use, concentrated liquid, and powder forms.

‡Composed of glucose, maltose, and dextrins.

§Medium-chain triglycerides (MCT).

//Powder form.

Table 4–2 (cont'd). Normal and special infant formulas.*

Product	Protein Source	CHO Source	Fat Source	Indications for Use	Comments (Nutritional Adequacy)
Low-sodium formulas					
Lonalac (Mead Johnson)‖	Casein.	Lactose.	Coconut.	For children with congestive cardiac failure.	For long-term management, additional sodium must be given. Supplement with vitamins C and D and iron. Na = 1 mEq/L.
Partially demineralized whey formulas					
Similac PM 60/40 (Ross)‖	Whey, casein.	Lactose.	Coconut, corn.	For newborns predisposed to hypocalcemia.	Low phosphorus. Relatively low solute load. Na = 7 mEq/L.
Products for infants with malabsorption syndromes					
Alacta (Mead Johnson) (available internationally but not in USA)		Lactose.	Butterfat.	For infants with poor fat tolerance or poor fat absorption.	Supplement with vitamins A, D, and C and iron. To increase calories, supplement with carbohydrates. Renal solute load is high if powder only is used to increase calories to 67 kcal/dL.
Nutramigen (Mead Johnson)	Casein hydrolysate.	Sucrose, modified tapioca starch.	Corn.	For infants and children intolerant to food proteins and for galactosemic patients.	Enzymatic hydrolysate of casein.
Portagen (Mead Johnson)	Sodium caseinate.	Sucrose, corn syrup solids.	MCT (coconut source), corn.	For management of chyluria, intestinal lymphangiectasia, various forms of steatorrhea, biliary atresia.	Fat in MCT and corn oil.

Pregestimil (Mead Johnson)	Casein hydrolysate, L-amino acids.	Corn syrup solids, modified tapioca starch.	MCT, corn oil.	For infants with malabsorption syndromes, especially after diarrhea and in malnutrition.	Contains added iron and vitamins. Protein is enzymatically hydrolyzed milk protein.
RCF (Ross)	Soy.		Sucrose, corn sugar.‡	For infants with CHO intolerance.	CHO is added according to amount infant will tolerate.
Products for infants with inborn errors					
Lofenalac (Mead Johnson)	Casein hydrolysate, L-amino acids.	Corn syrup solids, modified tapioca starch.	Corn.	For infants and children with phenylketonuria.	Must be supplemented with other foods to provide minimal phenylalanine.
MSUD Diet (Mead Johnson)//	L-Amino acids.	Corn syrup solids, modified tapioca starch.	Corn oil.	For children with branched-chain ketoaciduria.	Leucine-, isoleucine-, and valine-free; must be supplemented.
Phenyl-free (Mead Johnson)	L-Amino acids.	Sucrose, corn syrup solids, modified tapioca starch.	Corn oil.	For children over 1 year of age with phenylketonuria.	Phenylalanine-free. Permits increased supplementation with normal foods.
Product 80056 (Mead Johnson)		Corn syrup solids, modified tapioca starch.	Corn oil.	Used for formulation of special diets.	Protein-free; carbohydrate, fat, vitamin, and mineral mix.

*Committee on Nutrition, American Academy of Pediatrics: Commentary on breast feeding and infant formulas including proposed standards for formulas. *Pediatrics* 1976;**57**:278. Committee on Nutrition, American Academy of Pediatrics: Nutritional needs of low-birth-weight infants. *Pediatrics* 1977;**60**:519.

†Ready-to-use, concentrated liquid, and powder forms.

‡Composed of glucose, maltose, and dextrins.

§Medium-chain triglycerides (MCT).

//Powder form.

Table 4–3. Composition and schedule of formula feedings for infants up to 1 year of age.*

Age (mo)†	0	1	2	3	4	5	6	7	8	9	10	11	12
Calories‡	100–130 kcal/kg/d (45–60 kcal/lb/d)					100–110 kcal/kg/d (45–50 kcal/lb/d)				90–100 kcal/kg/d (40–45 kcal/lb/d)			
Fluid	130–200 mL/kg/d (2–3 oz/lb/d)			130–165 mL/kg/d (2–2.5 oz/lb/d)						130 mL/kg/d (2 oz/lb/d)			
Number of feedings§	6–7/d		4–5/d				3–4/d					3/d	
Amount (oz) per feeding	2.5–4	3.5–5	4–6	5–7	6–8	7–9//							

*Some prepared milk formulas may be deficient in vitamins C and D and need to be supplemented with vitamins (25–50 mg of vitamin C and 400 units of vitamin D daily). Iron supplementation of formulas has been recommended.

†Underweight or overweight infants generally have the same food requirements as do infants of the same age with a normal weight. Undiluted whole milk or formulas of equal parts of evaporated milk and water should not be used for young infants, since their kidneys do not have a range of safety in the event of high environmental or body temperature.

‡The larger amounts should be used for younger infants.

§Will vary somewhat with individual infants.

//Decrease sugar in individually mixed formulas by ½ oz (15 g) every 2 wk starting at age 5 mo. Whole milk may be substituted for evaporated milk when sugar is no longer added to formula, but evaporated milk may be continued indefinitely.

with water. Most powdered formulas are mixed in proportions of 1 scoop (which comes in the can) to 2 oz of water.

(2) Most infants do not require more than 1 quart of formula per day.

(3) Sterilization of formula, water, bottles, and nipples is not required if the equipment is washed well with hot soapy water and a hygienic water supply is available. It is best to prepare only one bottle of formula at a time. If bottles of formula must be stored before being used, they must be sterilized.

(4) If the nipple holes are the right size, a drop of milk will form on the end of the nipple when the cool bottle is turned upside down and will drop off with little shaking of the bottle.

(5) One pint of whole milk per day is adequate for the child age 1–5 years who otherwise is receiving a reasonable diet.

Feeding the Infant

(1) The bottle should be held, not propped.

(2) More water may be added to the formula if the infant consistently finishes each bottle and caloric intake is adequate.

(3) The infant need not empty every bottle.

(4) The infant should be "burped" during and at the end of feeding.

(5) After feeding, the infant should be placed on the side (preferably the right side) or prone.

(6) A few ounces of water (which may be sweetened) should be offered between feedings once or twice a day, especially during excessively hot weather or during febrile illnesses.

Vitamins

Infants who are fed one of the complete proprietary infant formulas do not require additional vitamin supplements. Those fed evaporated milk formula should have daily supplements of vitamins C and D. Supplemental vitamin D, generally recommended for breast-fed infants, is most conveniently given as a multivitamin liquid preparation.

Supplemental vitamins are usually unnecessary for the older child who is eating a relatively well balanced diet. Ingestion of more than the daily dietary requirement of vitamins is unnecessary and potentially harmful.

Night Feedings

Infants will "sleep through the night" (8-hour interval between feedings) at an average age of approximately 6 weeks (range, newborn to 15 months). There is no correlation between the interval between feedings at night and such things as the infant's age when solids are added to the diet, type of milk offered, or caloric intake.

Weaning

Small amounts of fluid may be offered from a cup when the infant is about age 6 months. The infant should not be allowed to nurse from the bottle throughout the night because this is associated with "bottle mouth caries." Weaning from the bottle is best done gradually and may not be completed until the child is over 1 year old.

"SOLID" FOODS

Common Solid Foods & Time of Adding to Diet

Breast-fed infants may not need solid foods during the first 6 months of life or longer. Even for formula-fed infants, solid foods need not be added earlier than as follows: single-grain cereal (preferably rice), 3–4 months; puréed vegetables, 4–5 months; fruits and juices, 5–6 months; strained meat and egg yolk, 6–7 months; junior type foods, 7–8 months; finely chopped table foods, 9 months; and egg white, 12 months.

(1) There is no exact time or order for starting solid foods. The first physiologic requirement for foods other than milk occurs about age 4–6 months, when a need for iron develops. When solid foods are started, they should initially be given in small amounts for several consecutive days to determine the infant's reaction and any adverse response. The amount should be gradually increased if the food is well tolerated. If the infant continues to refuse a food, another food may be tried; if that is also rejected, discontinue the attempt for 1–2 weeks before trying again. Foods prepared commercially have no nutritional advantage over those prepared at home, provided that the foods prepared at home are not seasoned.

(2) Many infants can learn to take semisolid food from a small spoon by age 4 months. If the infant cannot master spoon feeding, postpone the attempt for a few weeks; otherwise, undesirable behavior may result and may make spoon feeding difficult for months.

Table 4–4. Approximate daily expenditure of calories during the first year of life.

Use	Amount (kcal/kg/d)
Basal metabolism	55
Specific dynamic action of foods	9
Caloric loss in the excreta	8–11
Allowance for bodily activity	22
Growth	15–20
Total	110–120

(3) The transition from strained to chopped foods should be gradual and may be started when the infant begins to make chewing motions.

(4) Egg, wheat, orange juice, corn, and other allergenic foods should not be given (especially when there is a family predisposition to allergy) until the child is in the latter part of the first year of life.

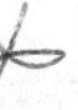

(5) Infants should be allowed to feed themselves with fingers or a spoon when they wish to do so.

(6) Avoid feeding nuts, popcorn, and other foods that are easily aspirated to all children under age 4 years.

The approximate daily expenditure of calories for the first year of life and the recommended dietary allowances for the maintenance of good nutrition are shown in Tables 4–4 and 4–5.

DIGESTION DURING INFANCY

Protein digestion and absorption are excellent during infancy. Amylase is present only in small quantities. The gastric glands are functionally active at birth and secrete hydrochloric acid (small quantities), pepsin, and rennin. Salivary digestion is relatively unimportant during early infancy.

Breast-fed infants usually empty the stomach in 2–3 hours; bottle-fed infants require 3–4 hours or longer; newborns may empty the stomach even more slowly.

VITAMIN DEFICIENCIES & HYPERVITAMINOSES

VITAMIN A DEFICIENCY & EXCESS

Deficiency

Deficiency of vitamin A, which is fat-soluble, is uncommon and occurs in children only when the diet is deficient or absorption or storage of the vitamin is impaired (chronic use of unfortified skimmed milk, chronic intestinal disorders, celiac syndrome, hepatic and pancreatic diseases, or prolonged use of mineral oil). Vitamin A deficiency is characterized by failure to gain weight or to grow, xerophthalmia or extreme conjunctival dryness progressing to keratomalacia, and dryness, scaliness, and follicular hyperkeratosis of the skin. Eye adaptation to the dark is impaired (night blindness) when serum vitamin A levels are less than 20 μg/dL.

Vitamin A deficiency should be treated by use of daily doses of

Table 4–5. Recommended dietary allowances of the Food and Nutrition Board, National Academy of Sciences–National Research Council (revised 1980).*
Designed for the maintenance of good nutrition of practically all healthy people in the USA.

	Age (yr)	Weight (kg)	Weight (lb)	Height (cm)	Height (in)	Protein (g)	Fat-Soluble Vitamins: Vitamin A (μg RE)†	Vitamin D (μg)‡	Vitamin E (mg α-TE)§
Infants	0–0.5	6	13	60	24	kg X 2.2	420	10	3
	0.5–1	9	20	71	28	kg X 2	400	10	4
Children	1–3	13	29	90	35	23	400	10	5
	4–6	20	44	112	44	30	500	10	6
	7–10	28	62	132	52	34	700	10	7
Males	11–14	45	99	157	62	45	1000	10	8
	15–18	66	145	176	69	56	1000	10	10
	19–22	70	154	177	70	56	1000	7.5	10
	23–50	70	154	178	70	56	1000	5	10
	51+	70	154	178	70	56	1000	5	10
Females	11–14	46	101	157	62	46	800	10	8
	15–18	55	120	163	64	46	800	10	8
	19–22	55	120	163	64	44	800	7.5	8
	23–50	55	120	163	64	44	800	5	8
	51+	55	120	163	64	44	800	5	8
Pregnant//						+30	+200	+5	+2
Lactating//						+20	+400	+5	+3

	Age (yr)	Water-Soluble Vitamins: Vitamin B_6 (mg)	Vitamin B_{12} (μg)	Vitamin C (mg)	Folacin¶ (μg)	Niacin (mg NE)#	Riboflavin (mg)	Thiamine (mg)
Infants	0–0.5	0.3	0.5**	35	30	6	0.4	0.3
	0.5–1	0.6	1.5	35	45	8	0.6	0.5
Children	1–3	0.9	2	45	100	9	0.8	0.7
	4–6	1.3	2.5	45	200	11	1	0.9
	7–10	1.6	3	45	300	16	1.4	1.2
Males	11–14	1.8	3	50	400	18	1.6	1.4
	15–18	2	3	60	400	18	1.7	1.4
	19–22	2.2	3	60	400	19	1.7	1.5
	23–50	2.2	3	60	400	18	1.6	1.4
	51+	2.2	3	60	400	16	1.4	1.2
Females	11–14	1.8	3	50	400	15	1.3	1.1
	15–18	2	3	60	400	14	1.3	1.1
	19–22	2	3	60	400	14	1.3	1.1
	23–50	2	3	60	400	13	1.2	1
	51+	2	3	60	400	13	1.2	1
Pregnant//		+0.6	+1	+20	+400	+2	+0.3	+0.4
Lactating//		+0.5	+1	+40	+100	+5	+0.5	+0.5

*See footnotes on last page of table.

Table 4–5 (cont'd). Recommended dietary allowances.*

	Age (yr)	Minerals: Calcium (mg)	Iodine (μg)	Iron (mg)	Magnesium (mg)	Phosphorus (mg)	Zinc (mg)
Infants	0–0.5	360	40	10	50	240	3
	0.5–1	540	50	15	70	360	5
Children	1–3	800	70	15	150	800	10
	4–6	800	90	10	200	800	10
	7–10	800	120	10	250	800	10
Males	11–14	1200	150	18	350	1200	15
	15–18	1200	150	18	400	1200	15
	19–22	800	150	10	350	800	15
	23–50	800	150	10	350	800	15
	51+	800	150	10	350	800	15
Females	11–14	1200	150	18	300	1200	15
	15–18	1200	150	18	300	1200	15
	19–22	800	150	18	300	800	15
	23–50	800	150	18	300	800	15
	51+	800	150	10	300	800	15
Pregnant//		+400	+25		+150	+400	+5
Lactating//		+400	+50		+150	+400	+10

*The allowances are intended to provide for individual variations among most normal persons as they live in the USA under usual environmental stresses. Diets should be based on a variety of common foods in order to provide other nutrients for which human requirements have been less well defined.

†Retinol equivalents: 1 RE = 1 μg retinol or 6 μg β-carotene.

‡As cholecalciferol: 10 μg cholecalciferol = 400 IU vitamin D.

§α-Tocopherol equivalents: 1 mg D-α-tocopherol = 1 α-TE.

//The increased iron requirement during pregnancy cannot be met by the iron content of habitual American diets or by the existing iron stores of many women; therefore, the use of 30–60 mg supplemental iron is recommended. Iron needs during lactation are not substantially different from those of nonpregnant women, but continued supplementation of the mother for 2–3 months after parturition is advisable in order to replenish stores depleted by pregnancy.

¶The folacin allowances refer to dietary sources as determined by *Lactobacillus casei* assay after treatment with enzymes ("conjugases") to make polyglutamyl forms of the vitamin available to the test organism.

#Niacin equivalents: 1 NE = 1 mg niacin or 60 mg dietary tryptophan.

**The RDA for vitamin B_{12} in infants is based on average concentration of the vitamin in human milk. The allowances after weaning are based on energy intake (as recommended by the American Academy of Pediatrics) and consideration of other factors such as intestinal absorption.

vitamin A, 25,000 IU for 1–2 weeks, together with a high-protein diet. It is usually necessary to replenish liver stores of vitamin A for several weeks before the serum levels increase. In cases of malabsorption, a water-miscible vitamin A preparation can be given. When xerophthalmia is present, vitamin A may be injected intramuscularly in daily doses of up to 25,000 IU for several days.

Excess

Vitamin A toxicity in infants is characterized by irritability, anorexia, tense fontanelles, craniotabes, bone pain, and skin desquamation, especially of the palms and soles. In older children, cortical hyperostosis may occur (see Chapter 20). Clinical improvement begins within a few days after discontinuing excessive intake of vitamin A.

VITAMIN B_1 (THIAMINE) DEFICIENCY (Beriberi)

Thiamine is water-soluble. Thiamine deficiency results from inadequate intake of the vitamin, which in developed countries is usually due to idiosyncrasies of diet or excessive cooking or processing of foods. It is characterized by anorexia, listlessness, irritability, vomiting, constipation, and edema. Cardiac manifestations include dyspnea, tachycardia, cyanosis, and heart failure. Central nervous system signs include apathy, drowsiness, peripheral neuritis (including neuritis of the cranial nerves), loss of deep tendon reflexes, paresthesias, convulsions, and coma.

The condition can be prevented by instituting a normal diet containing at least 0.4 mg of thiamine daily. In acute deficiency states, give thiamine, 10 mg intravenously, followed by 10 mg intramuscularly twice daily for 3 days, and an additional 10 mg/d orally for 6 weeks.

VITAMIN B_2 (RIBOFLAVIN) DEFICIENCY

Riboflavin is water-soluble. Riboflavin deficiency may be due to decreased intake or malabsorption. It is characterized by thinness, maceration, and superficial fissuring of the skin at the angles of the mouth; smoothness, loss of papillary structure, and redness of the tongue; and fissures and seborrheic dermatitis, especially in the nasolabial folds. Ocular manifestations may also occur, with vascularization and infiltration of the cornea, itching, excessive tearing, photophobia, and ultimately interstitial keratitis.

Treatment consists of correcting dietary deficiencies and giving riboflavin, 0.5–1 mg orally 3 times daily for several weeks. If oral administration is not possible, riboflavin may be given in doses of 2 mg/d intramuscularly for several weeks. A diet containing 0.6 mg of riboflavin per 1000 kcal must be maintained.

NIACIN (NICOTINIC ACID) DEFICIENCY (Pellagra)

Niacin is water-soluble. Niacin deficiency is the principal but not the only dietary defect in pellagra. Pellagra usually occurs in low-income groups or in patients with anorexia or with gastrointestinal disease associated with severe malabsorption. Early symptoms may include burning sensations, numbness, dizziness, anorexia, and weakness. Cutaneous manifestations include sharply demarcated, symmetric areas of erythema appearing on the exposed portions of the body. These may become dark red and are followed by scaling and residual pigmentation. Superficial vesicles may develop and ulcerate or become infected. Gastrointestinal symptoms include swelling and redness of the tongue, stomatitis, and vomiting and diarrhea. Effects upon the central nervous system include depression, insomnia, disorientation, and delirium.

Treatment consists of giving nicotinamide, 10–25 mg 3 times daily for 2 weeks, and ensuring an adequate diet containing sufficient B complex vitamins. Nicotinic acid (niacin) is less frequently used because of its vasodilating effects.

VITAMIN B_6 (PYRIDOXINE) DEFICIENCY

Pyridoxine is water-soluble. Pyridoxine deficiency usually occurs in conjunction with inadequate intake of other B vitamins due to poor diet or malabsorption states. Isolated pyridoxine deficiency can occur when heat processing of formulas reduces the amount of pyridoxine to insufficient levels or during treatment with isoniazid, which is a pyridoxine antagonist. Pyridoxine requirements are increased in the presence of other drugs, including penicillamine, contraceptive steroids, and hydralazine. Clinical features of deficiency in young infants include abnormal central nervous system activity (irritability, aggravated startle responses, and seizures) and gastrointestinal distress (abdominal distention, vomiting, and diarrhea). Other manifestations include anemia, peripheral neuropathy, and dermatitis, including chelosis, glossitis, and seborrhea around the eyes, nose, and mouth.

Pyridoxine deficiency is treated by giving pyridoxine, 5 mg intramuscularly followed by 0.5 mg/d orally for 2 weeks. The diet should be corrected. Children receiving penicillamine or isoniazid should receive supplementary pyridoxine, 2 mg/kg/d. Pyridoxine deficiency should be considered in the differential diagnosis of neonatal seizures when other more common causes have been eliminated, and pyridoxine, 100 mg intramuscularly, should be tried.

Infants are occasionally "pyridoxine-dependent" and develop manifestations of pyridoxine deficiency unless they are given large amounts of this vitamin (10–100 mg/d orally).

VITAMIN C (ASCORBIC ACID) DEFICIENCY
(Scurvy)

Vitamin C is water-soluble. Prolonged vitamin C deficiency, as can occur with food faddism, famine, or use of a diet consisting solely of unsupplemented cow's milk during infancy, causes scurvy. Scurvy most commonly appears in children between 7 months and 2 years of age; it is rare in newborns. It is characterized by progressive irritability, especially when the child is handled. The legs are held in the typical "frog-leg position." The extremities are very tender when handled, are moved very little (pseudoparalysis), may be edematous, and may have palpable subperiosteal hemorrhages.

There may be hemorrhages into the skin and into or from mucous membranes. Gums are bluish-purple and swollen, especially around erupted teeth. The costochondral junction shows marked angular mushrooming, and the sternum is depressed. Serum and white blood cell ascorbic acid levels are reduced. X-rays show thinning of bone cortices, loss of trabecular pattern ("ground glass" appearance), and thickening and irregularity at the epiphyseal line, with a subepiphyseal zone of rarefaction. Lateral spurring from the line of increased density and epiphyseal separation may occur. Shadows of subperiosteal hemorrhages become visible during healing when the elevated periosteum calcifies.

The therapeutic dose of vitamin C is 100 mg 3 times daily. (Citrus juices sufficient to give an equivalent amount of vitamin C are also satisfactory.) With treatment, clinical improvement is rapid (within 48 hours), but x-ray evidence of healing may not appear for a week or more. Recovery is usually complete.

VITAMIN D (CALCIFEROL) DEFICIENCY
(Rickets)

Vitamin D is fat-soluble. Vitamin D deficiency may occur with inadequate intake of vitamin D and insufficient exposure to ultraviolet rays. It is more likely to occur, however, during periods of rapid growth and produces the most marked changes in the bones that are growing most rapidly. It is uncommon in infants during the first 2–3 months of life, except in small premature infants with immaturity of the mechanism responsible for the normal postnatal rise of 1,25-dihydroxycholecalciferol levels.

Rickets may also occur as a result of malabsorption of calcium in children with steatorrhea, inadequate dietary calcium intake with vegan diets, malabsorption of vitamin D in children with hepatobiliary disease, inability to form the active metabolite (1,25-dihydroxycholecalciferol) in children with renal disease, or vitamin D resistance in children with X-linked disease.

Clinical Findings

A. Head: Craniotabes (early), asymmetry, bossing ("hot cross bun" skull), increased size of fontanelles and skull, and delayed closure of fontanelles may be present.

B. Teeth: Delayed dentition, defects of tooth enamel, and a tendency to develop caries may occur. The permanent teeth may be affected.

C. Thorax: Costochondral prominence ("rachitic rosary"), "pigeon-breast" deformity, flaring of the chest, and a depression along the insertion of the diaphragm (Harrison's groove) may be present.

D. Extremities: Widening of the epiphyses and bending of the shafts of the long bones may be seen. Greenstick fractures may occur.

E. Other Bones: There may be scoliosis or kyphosis and deformity of the pelvis.

F. Other Findings: Other findings include relaxation of ligaments and poor development and tone of the muscles, with resultant deformities at the joints, protrusion of the abdomen, weakness, and constipation. Shortness of stature may be an end result. Infantile tetany may occur.

Laboratory Findings

Serum calcium levels are usually normal except in children with tetany. Serum phosphorus levels are decreased, and alkaline phosphatase levels are increased.

X-Ray Findings

Cupping, fraying, and flaring are seen at the ends of the bones. The shafts are denser than normal, and the trabeculae are prominent. The distance between the calcified portion of the shaft and the epiphyseal center is increased. Periosteal reaction may occur.

Treatment & Prognosis

In cases of inadequate intake of vitamin D and insufficient exposure to ultraviolet rays, rickets is cured by vitamin D (oleovitamin D, ergocalciferol, or cholecalciferol), 5000 IU/d orally for 4–5 weeks. Radiologic and biochemical signs of improvement appear after the first week of therapy. Some cases of rickets are exceedingly resistant and require huge doses of vitamin D (25,000–150,000 IU/d). Recently, in patients with hepatobiliary, renal, and vitamin D-resistant rickets, good biochemical, radiologic, and growth responses have occurred with the use of 1,25-dihydroxycholecalciferol in doses of 20–80 ng/kg/d. Biochemical signs of improvement occur promptly and should be monitored during treatment. The need for supplemental calcium, phosphorus, or both must be individually determined. Healing of rickets may be complete, but in severe cases some deformity usually remains.

VITAMIN E (α-TOCOPHEROL) DEFICIENCY

Vitamin E is fat-soluble. Vitamin E deficiency can occur in children with chronic malabsorption syndromes (eg, hepatobiliary, small intestinal, and pancreatic diseases) and in premature infants with limited tissue stores of vitamin E, with intestinal malabsorption, and during rapid growth. Vitamin E deficiency has occurred as a hemolytic anemia in infants consuming a diet high in polyunsaturated fats and also receiving oxidant compounds such as iron. The anemia is associated with dependent edema.

Treatment with α-tocopherol acetate, 30 mg (30 IU) daily, has been recommended for premature infants.

DISORDERS OF NUTRITION

INFANTILE CALORIC UNDERNUTRITION
(Marasmus)

Marasmus is a syndrome of generalized undernutrition in infants. It is due to insufficient caloric intake, most often secondary to extreme poverty but occasionally caused by improper feeding technique, neglect, or organic disease. Initially, there is failure to gain weight, followed by loss of weight and ultimately emaciation. Loss of subcutaneous fat, muscle wasting, fretfulness or listlessness, sunken cheeks, and a wide-eyed appearance are typical. The abdomen may be flat or distended, the pulse and temperature are decreased, and edema is typically absent. Total serum protein, albumin, hemoglobin, and blood urea nitrogen levels are low.

Treatment consists of providing an adequate diet and treating the underlying disorder if there is one. Intravenous restoration of adequate blood volume may be required initially. Because children with marasmus may have secondary disaccharide intolerance, a lactose-free formula should be provided initially. Vitamin supplements should be given. Exposure to infectious diseases must be avoided. The prognosis depends on the severity, duration, and timing of the malnutrition.

PROTEIN DEPRIVATION (Kwashiorkor)

Kwashiorkor is the most prevalent serious form of malnutrition worldwide. It is caused by severe protein deficiency, usually in the presence of adequate caloric intake. Kwashiorkor typically occurs in children between 1 and 5 years of age, following weaning from the breast. It is characterized by retarded growth and development, apathy, anorexia, edema, abdominal distention, skin and hair depigmentation and other cutaneous lesions, diarrhea, and anemia. Levels of serum enzymes, cholesterol, total lipids, and albumin are low. Hypoglycemia is common, and fatty infiltration of the liver is typical.

Children with protein deprivation should be given *gradually* increasing amounts of protein and placed on a balanced diet containing all the essential amino acids and adequate vitamin supplements. An elemental formula may be used initially. Concomitant infections should be treated appropriately. Long-term sequelae depend on the severity of the malnutrition.

ZINC DEFICIENCY

Severe acquired zinc deficiency has been most commonly observed in association with the use of total parenteral nutrition and is a particular problem in infants with very low birth weights. Symptoms include acro-orificial skin rash, diarrhea, cessation of weight gain, and depressed mood. Mild to moderate deficiencies may result from disease states in which either intestinal absorption of zinc is decreased or urinary excretion of zinc is increased. Inadequate dietary zinc intake, poor bioavailability of dietary zinc, or both may cause a chronic mild zinc deficiency. Mild to moderate deficiencies are characterized by poor growth, lethargy, anorexia, impaired taste perception, and delayed sexual maturation. Acrodermatitis enteropathica, an autosomal recessive disorder of intestinal zinc absorption, results in the clinical features of severe acquired zinc deficiency during early infancy or following weaning in breast-fed infants.

Infants with mild to moderate zinc deficiencies are treated with Zn^{2+}, 0.5–1 mg/kg/d orally; zinc sulfate or other zinc salts are used. For treatment of infants with severe zinc deficiency associated with intravenous nutrition, give Zn^{2+}, 100 μg/kg/d intravenously; a higher dosage may be required if gastrointestinal fluid losses are great. Premature infants being fed intravenously should receive Zn^{2+}, 300 μg/kg/d. Acrodermatitis enteropathica rapidly improves with use of Zn^{2+}, 30–50 mg/d orally.

Fluid & Electrolyte Disorders | 5

*Robert W. Winters, MD**

FUNDAMENTAL CONSIDERATIONS

Fluid and electrolyte therapy should be divided into 3 phases: (1) repair of preexisting deficits, (2) provision of maintenance requirements, and (3) correction of ongoing losses.

Repair of Preexisting Deficits

Water, sodium, chloride, and potassium deficits occur via renal or extrarenal routes. The aim of therapy is to estimate and correct these deficits as soon and as safely as possible. These losses are best expressed in terms of body weight (milliliter or milliequivalent per kilogram of body weight).

Provision of Maintenance Requirements

Normal expenditures of water and electrolytes through the usual channels as the result of normal metabolism must be replaced. These replacements are called maintenance requirements; they bear a close relationship to metabolic rate and are ideally formulated in terms of caloric expenditure. However, it is easier to calculate maintenance requirements in terms of body weight, although factors that alter metabolic rate must be given consideration.

Correction of Ongoing Losses

Extrarenal losses may occur during therapy, usually via the gastrointestinal tract through loss (vomiting or diarrhea) or removal (suction) of secretions. Replacement of such losses should be made contemporaneously with losses and should be similar in type and amount to the fluid being lost. Hence, such a replacement is best formulated as milliliter of fluid and milliequivalent of electrolyte replaced per milliliter of fluid and milliequivalent of electrolyte lost.

*Medical Director, Home Nutrition Support, Inc., Fairfield, NJ; formerly Professor of Pediatrics, College of Physicians and Surgeons, Columbia University, New York, NY.

CALCULATION & CORRECTION OF FLUID & ELECTROLYTE LOSSES

DEFICIT THERAPY

History

A detailed analysis of the history should be undertaken in order to determine (1) the magnitude of the deficit of water and electrolytes; (2) whether an acid-base disturbance is present and, if so, what type; and (3) whether a significant potassium deficit is present.

The history should include information pertinent to the following: (1) type, severity, and duration of the loss; (2) an estimate of the weight loss (a recent pre-illness weight is often available, especially in infants); (3) estimates of the type and amount of the loss and of the intake (a balance sheet should be prepared); (4) frequency and approximate quantity of urine voided during illness; and (5) presence of fever or sweating.

Physical Examination

A. Signs of Dehydration: Skin and subcutaneous tissue signs include dryness of the skin and mucous membranes, depression of the anterior fontanelle, and poor skin turgor. (Chronically malnourished infants may exhibit poor skin turgor without significant dehydration, whereas obese infants may become quite dehydrated without developing poor turgor.) Sclerematous changes of skin suggest hypertonic dehydration. Cardiovascular system signs include poor peripheral circulation, tachycardia, oliguria, and hypotension. Fever, especially in the absence of infection, is a sign of dehydration. In the average infant, when these signs are marked the total water deficit will be about 10–15% of body weight; in children, about 5–10% of body weight.

B. Signs Suggesting Specific Abnormalities: (For clinical signs of specific electrolyte disturbances, see pp 86 ff.)

1. Hyperpnea is seen in metabolic acidosis, respiratory alkalosis, and sometimes advanced pulmonary disease with respiratory acidosis.
2. Hypoventilation is present in respiratory acidosis due to central respiratory depression.
3. Cyanosis often occurs with respiratory acidosis.
4. Positive Chvostek and Trousseau signs and tetany may indicate respiratory or metabolic alkalosis.
5. Generalized seizures may be seen in alkalosis, water intoxication, and respiratory acidosis.

Laboratory Examination

Laboratory examination gives information about abnormalities in (1) volume of body fluids and (2) concentration of specific components of the extracellular fluid.

A. Abnormalities in Volume of Body Fluids: An increase in the packed cell volume, hemoglobin, and serum proteins indicates hemoconcentration and (except in burns) diminished volume of the extracellular fluid. Intelligent interpretation of these indices requires an estimate of the pre-illness values.

The specific gravity of the urine in dehydration is usually above 1.010 unless diabetes insipidus or renal disease is present. However, a number of factors (solute excretion, potassium depletion) exert marked influences upon renal concentrating ability. Therefore, the specific gravity may not be very high in spite of severe dehydration. Significant glycosuria and proteinuria will elevate the specific gravity.

Slight proteinuria, hyaline casts, and a few formed elements are often found in the urine of dehydrated patients and under these circumstances are not indicative of intrinsic renal disease. Ketonuria may be present. Nitroprusside and ferric chloride tests for ketones in urine should be performed. Confirmation of the presence of ketones may be obtained by retesting the urine after volatilization of the ketones by acidification and boiling. A freshly voided urine specimen should be tested for pH, using indicator papers.

Elevated blood urea nitrogen or serum creatinine levels in the absence of preexisting renal disease nearly always indicate a significant reduction in functional extracellular volume. Therefore, measurement of either of these substances is valuable in aiding interpretation of serum electrolyte determinations and in management of dehydrated patients.

B. Abnormalities in Concentration of Specific Components: Abnormalities of serum sodium, potassium, and bicarbonate are discussed in subsequent sections. Initial study of the serum electrolytes is highly desirable in any patient presenting with a serious disturbance of hydration or acid-base balance. In evaluating these studies, it is important to exclude an obvious laboratory error by subtracting the sum of bicarbonate and chloride (both in mEq/L) from the value for sodium (in mEq/L). The difference is normally 10 mEq/L and may be even greater, depending upon the normal values of any given laboratory; when the difference is less than 5 mEq/L, or when it is negative, a laboratory error has been made. This relationship can also be used to predict the serum sodium level from data on bicarbonate and chloride (serum Na^+ = bicarbonate + Cl^- + 10), but this calculation is accurate only in the absence of excesses of other serum anions (phosphate, keto acids, etc).

Determination of the initial level of serum sodium is most important, since dehydration can then be classified on this basis as isotonic (normal serum Na^+), hypotonic (low serum Na^+), or hypertonic (high serum Na^+). Recognition of the hypertonic state is particularly important, since hypertonic dehydration requires specific therapeutic measures (see p 79). With hyperglycemia, serum sodium may be low even with hypertonic or isotonic dehydration; this is because glucose contrib-

Table 5–1. Magnitude of deficits of water and sodium.*

	Water (mL/kg)	Sodium (mEq/kg)
Isotonic	100–120	8–10
Hypertonic	100–120	2–4
Hypotonic	100–120	10–12

*Values shown are those usually found in infants with severe dehydration.

utes to the effective osmotic pressure of extracellular fluid and draws water out of cells, thus diluting extracellular constituents. Hyperlipemia can produce artifactual hyponatremia owing to displacement of plasma water by lipids.

General Comments About Deficits

A. Magnitude of Deficits: The usual magnitude of deficits of sodium and water encountered in severe dehydration in infants is shown in Table 5–1.

Chloride deficits tend to parallel sodium deficits but are also affected by the type of acid-base disturbance that develops. Potassium depletion usually complicates most instances of dehydration except those associated with adrenocortical insufficiency or advanced renal insufficiency. These deficits are usually about 8–10 mEq/kg in severe cases; they may be higher in patients with alkalosis.

All of the above figures apply to severe dehydration in an infant. Less severe cases of dehydration require proportionally less replacement. In children with severe dehydration, the deficits are only about three-fourths of those encountered in infants.

B. General Outline of Treatment:

1. Initial therapy should be aimed at restoring blood and extracellular fluid volume in order to relieve or prevent shock and to restore renal function. The fluids should always be given intravenously. While awaiting the results of the initial laboratory determinations, initiate treatment with isotonic sodium solution (10–20 mL/kg), either sodium chloride, balanced sodium solution (Table 5–2), or lactated Ringer's

Table 5–2. Isotonic "balanced" sodium solution.

	Volume (mL)	mEq		
		Na^+	Cl^-	HCO_3^-
$NaHCO_3$ (1 mEq/mL)	30	30		30
0.9% NaCl	682	105	105	
Pyrogen-free water or 5% glucose	qs ad 1000			
Totals	1000	135	105	30

injection. If the circulatory status does not improve following this infusion (1–2 hours), a colloid solution (10–20 mL/kg) should be given over the next 1–2 hours.

2. The next phase of treatment—repair of the remaining deficits of sodium, chloride, and water—should be started as soon as the circulatory status is improved. Replacement during this phase depends upon the relationship between water and sodium losses as these are reflected in the initial serum sodium.

a. Isotonic dehydration–Additional isotonic sodium solution, 40–60 mL/kg, should be given over the next 12–18 hours for infants; 20–40 mL/kg is more appropriate for children.

b. Hypotonic dehydration–In severe hyponatremia, particularly when it is associated with symptoms suggesting cellular overhydration or persistently poor circulatory status, an infusion of hypertonic sodium solution calculated according to the formula given on p 90 should be given. Lesser degrees of hypotonicity may be managed adequately by providing isotonic sodium solution in amounts 10–20 mL/kg greater than those given above for isotonic dehydration.

c. Hypertonic dehydration–In severe hypernatremic states, convulsions often accompany rapid reduction of serum sodium to normal levels. Since circulatory collapse does not often accompany this type of dehydration, it is wise to reduce serum sodium to normal over a longer period (48–72 hours).

3. Repair of potassium deficits may be started after deficits of sodium, water, and chloride have been largely repaired (generally 18–24 hours after admission); since potassium must be administered slowly (see p 87), significant deficits require several days for repletion.

4. Restoration of protein and caloric deficits may be started as soon as the patient can tolerate full oral feedings. Several weeks may be required for complete repair of these deficits.

In treating deficits, body weight and serum electrolytes and blood urea nitrogen or serum creatinine should be closely monitored. Satisfactory treatment of the dehydration will be accompanied by an acute gain of about 10% of body weight and a prompt fall in the level of blood urea nitrogen or serum creatinine.

Use of Solutions for Fluid Therapy

Many fluids of highly complex composition have been recommended for treating dehydration. However, such specialized fluids are expensive and unnecessary. Virtually every problem encountered can be effectively managed with the use of combinations of the following simple, commonly available fluids: (1) 0.9% saline solution (155 mEq of Na^+ and Cl^- per liter), (2) 5% saline (855 mEq of Na^+ and Cl^- per liter), and (3) 5 or 10% glucose in water. Appropriate additions of the following (available in ampules) may be made: potassium chloride (1 or 2 mEq of K^+ and Cl^- per milliliter) and sodium bicarbonate (1 mEq of Na^+ and HCO_3^- per milliliter). These additives should never be given undiluted.

An example of an isotonic "balanced" sodium solution (135 mEq of Na^+, 105 mEq of Cl^-, and 30 mEq of HCO_3^- per liter) is given in Table 5–2.

MAINTENANCE REQUIREMENTS FOR FLUID & ELECTROLYTES

Maintenance therapy attempts to provide adequate water, sodium, chloride, and potassium to meet normal requirements. It is virtually impossible to satisfy protein, carbohydrate, and fat requirements by giving presently available solutions by a peripheral venous route, but fortunately this is seldom necessary. When total parenteral nutrition is necessary, a central venous catheter should be used. Sufficient carbohydrate should be provided to prevent ketosis and to minimize protein breakdown but not so much that severe glycosuria is produced. In general, these aims can be met by giving an amount of carbohydrate that provides about 25% of the total caloric expenditure (ie, 25 kcal from carbohydrate, or 6.5 g of glucose, per 100 kcal expended). To be effective, the carbohydrate should be given either continuously over the entire 24-hour period for which it is intended or in multiple small doses during that period. It will not be effective and may produce glycosuria if given over only a few hours. Average maintenance requirements are shown in Table 5–3.

The maintenance requirements as given do not include allowances for such complicating factors as fever, excessive sweating, excessive insensible loss through hyperventilation, or impaired renal function. Appropriate adjustments for these circumstances are best determined by close observation of the patient and serial measurements of serum electrolytes and blood urea nitrogen or serum creatinine.

Table 5–3. Average maintenance requirements for fluid and electrolyte therapy.

	H_2O (mL/kg)	Na^+ (mEq/kg)	K^+ (mEq/kg)	Carbohydrate (g/kg)
Premature	50–70	1.5–2.0	1.5–2.0	2–3
Newborn	40–60	0.8–1.0	0.8–1.0	2–3
4–10 kg	100–120	2.0–2.5	2.0–2.5	5–6
10–20 kg	80–100	1.6–2.0	1.6–2.0	4–5
20–40 kg	60–80	1.2–1.6	1.2–1.6	3–4
Adult total	2500–3000	50	50	100–150

Composition of Maintenance Solutions

The solutions shown in Table 5–4 will meet the requirements listed in Table 5–3. An alternative solution similar in sodium, potassium, and carbohydrate composition may be made by mixing 160 mL of a balanced isotonic sodium solution (see Table 5–2) or lactated Ringer's injection with 840 mL of 5% glucose in water and adding 20 mL of potassium chloride (concentration 1 mEq/mL) to ensure a final potassium chloride concentration of 20 mmol/L.

Maintenance Therapy in Newborns

Maintenance requirements for newborn and low-birth-weight infants are not well understood. They are certainly more variable than in older infants and children. The figures in Table 5–4 represent rough but probably safe approximations for the first few days of life. In general, in this period of life, the safest policy is to give too little rather than too much unless there are unexpectedly large extrarenal losses (eg, due to phototherapy). Older premature infants will require more liberal amounts of water and electrolytes.

Table 5–4. Maintenance solutions.

	Volume (mL)	mEq				Carbohydrate (g)
		Na^+	K^+	Cl^-	HCO_3^-	
$NaHCO_3$ (1 mEq/mL)	20	20			20	
KCl (1 mEq/mL)	20		20	20		
5% glucose in water	qs ad 1000					43.5
Total	1000	20	20	20	20	43.5

Time Plan for Administration of Maintenance Requirements

Each day's maintenance requirements should be administered intravenously throughout the 24 hours if possible. They should never be administered rapidly in a single continuous dose. Hypodermoclysis has no role in modern fluid therapy.

REPLACEMENT OF ONGOING LOSSES OF FLUID & ELECTROLYTES

Replacement of ongoing extrarenal losses should proceed as the losses are incurred, and the composition of the solution being administered should approximate that of the fluid lost.

Determination of Ongoing Losses

A. Losses of Gastrointestinal Secretions: Gastrointestinal secretions may be lost as a result of vomiting or suction. The approximate composition of most gastrointestinal secretions is shown in Table 5–5. Although pure gastrointestinal juices are isotonic, in practice they are often hypotonic owing to dilution from ingestion of water or ice, flushing of the suction tube with water, or swallowing of saliva. When this occurs, appropriate downward adjustments of the concentration of the various ions may be necessary. Volumes of losses incurred must be accurately measured; their electrolyte composition may be determined either by direct measurement or by reference to Table 5–5.

Table 5–5. Composition of gastrointestinal secretions.

	mEq/L				
	H^+	Na^+	K^+	Cl^-	HCO_3^-
Gastric	40–60	20–80	5–20	100–150	
Biliary		120–140	5–15	80–120	30–50
Pancreatic		120–140	5–15	40–80	70–110
Small bowel		100–140	5–15	90–130	20–40

B. Losses Due to Diarrhea: The electrolyte composition of diarrheal stools is quite variable (see Table 5–6). Estimation of stool volume is difficult. The infant with diarrhea who is receiving full oral feedings may have a stool volume of 50 mL/kg/d or more; with limited oral feedings, 10–25 mL/kg/d is a more reasonable estimate. In difficult cases, measurement of both stool volume and electrolyte composition may be necessary for accurate replacement of losses.

Table 5–6. Composition of diarrheal stools.

	mEq/L of Stool Water		
	Na^+	K^+	Cl^-
Average	50	35	45
Range	(40–65)	(25–50)	(25–55)

Replacement Solutions for Major Ongoing Losses

A. Losses of Gastric Juices: Losses of gastric juice may be replaced with a solution similar to that shown in Table 5–7, preferably given intravenously.

B. Losses of Small Bowel Juices: These losses may be replaced by a balanced isotonic sodium solution (Table 5–2) to which is added 15 mL of potassium chloride (concentration 1 mEq/mL) in order to give a final potassium chloride concentration of 15 mmol/L.

Table 5–7. Replacement of gastric juice.

	Volume (mL)	mEq		
		Na^+	K^+	Cl^-
0.9% NaCl	580	90		90
KCl (1 mEq/mL)	40		40	40
Pyrogen-free water or 5% glucose	qs ad 1000			
Total	1000	90	40	130

C. Losses Due to Diarrhea: See Table 5–8. An alternative fluid consists of 2 parts of isotonic balanced sodium solution (see Table 5–2) or lactated Ringer's injection and 1 part of 5% glucose in water to which is added potassium chloride, 20–40 mEq/mL, to give a final potassium chloride concentration of 20–40 mmol/L.

In any situation involving ongoing large losses, replacement therapy must be guided by serial blood chemistry studies and, if possible, direct analysis of the fluid being lost. The solutions recommended above represent only approximations and should be altered according to results of laboratory tests and the response of the patient.

Replacement of Ongoing Losses

In small children with extensive ongoing losses, it is especially important that replacement not be allowed to fall behind contemporary

Table 5–8. Replacement of losses caused by diarrhea.

	Volume (mL)	mEq			
		Na^+	K^+	Cl^-	HCO_3^-
KCl (1 mEq/mL)	40		40	40	
$NaHCO_3$ (1 mEq/mL)	60	60			60
5% glucose	300				
Pyrogen-free water or 5% glucose	qs ad 1000				
Total	1000	60	40	40	60

losses. Contemporary losses should be estimated and replacement given every 6–8 hours in amounts sufficient to cover the previous 6- to 8-hour period. Waiting for a period of 24 hours is not recommended. It is frequently possible and desirable to anticipate losses and replace them as they occur.

Solutions for replacement of any 1 day's contemporary losses should be given by slow intravenous drip. The precautions outlined on p 87 should be followed.

FLUID & ELECTROLYTE MANAGEMENT IN COMMON PEDIATRIC DISORDERS

INFANTILE DIARRHEA

Principal Clinical & Laboratory Manifestations

The principal manifestations of infantile diarrhea are dehydration and shock, metabolic acidosis with compensatory hyperventilation, and potassium depletion. Hypernatremia, when present, constitutes a special complicating factor that must be recognized on admission and managed with the aid of frequent laboratory determinations of serum sodium levels. A chronic nutritional problem frequently underlies diarrhea and requires continuing attention during convalescence.

Treatment

A. Moderately Severe Diarrhea Without Hypernatremia: The usual deficits found in balance studies in diarrheal disease are H_2O, 100–150 mL/kg; Na^+, 8–12 mEq/kg; Cl^-, 7–10 mEq/kg; and K^+, 8–12 mEq/kg.

1. Omit all oral feedings initially.

2. Rapid rehydration must be carried out intravenously. The first infusion should consist of isotonic balanced sodium solution (see p 72) or lactated Ringer's injection, 10–20 mL/kg. In severe cases, this may be followed by an infusion of Plasmanate. This should be completed by 2–4 hours after admission, by which time the patient's circulatory status and renal function should be improved.

3. Further hydration at a slower rate, by the methods outlined on p 72, should be completed by 12–24 hours after admission.

4. In marked hyponatremia, it may be advisable to use hypertonic sodium solutions instead of isotonic solutions; if the former are used, a total of 3 mEq/kg of potassium should be distributed throughout all subsequent fluids for the first day (see p 73).

5. Maintenance requirements as well as replacement of losses from

continuing diarrhea should be administered parenterally as previously described until oral fluids can be tolerated.

6. Fluids may be given orally only after the stools are no longer watery or voluminous, fever or dehydration (or both) is overcome, abdominal distention and anorexia have been relieved, and vomiting has stopped. At this time, oral feedings may be started as outlined in Chapter 16.

B. Milder Diarrhea: Milder diarrhea without vomiting may be managed as outlined in Chapter 16.

C. Diarrhea With Hypernatremia: Hypernatremia should be suspected in young infants with diarrheal disease and sclerematous changes, especially over the buttocks and thighs. Such infants often display prominent central nervous system disturbances (lethargy, coma, muscular rigidity, exaggerated reflexes, convulsions, and elevated levels of cerebrospinal fluid protein). Intracranial bleeding and subdural effusions have been reported in such infants; permanent central nervous system damage may occur.

The rapid return of serum sodium to normal levels should be avoided, since it is frequently associated with severe convulsions. Careful laboratory guidance of treatment is essential. In general, it is preferable to rehydrate these patients with a fluid containing sodium, 15–30 mEq/L, rather than to use completely sodium-free fluids. The exact amounts given are dictated by the individual case; generally no more than 150 mL/kg (including maintenance requirements) should be given on the first day. Potassium deficits are variable in hypernatremia; in most instances, no potassium need be added to the fluid therapy for the first day. It may be added subsequently if hypokalemia develops.

Even with a slow rate of reduction of serum sodium to normal, convulsions and twitchings may appear. In some instances, definite hypocalcemia may be found; if present, it may be treated by the addition of 10% calcium gluconate to the daily infusion in amounts calculated to supply calcium at a rate of 1–2 mg/kg/h. This represents 10–20 mg/kg/h of calcium gluconate. Symptomatic treatment of convulsions may be necessary; phenobarbital or diazepam may be used.

PYLORIC STENOSIS & VOMITING

Principal Clinical & Laboratory Manifestations

The principal problems encountered in pyloric stenosis are dehydration, metabolic alkalosis, and potassium depletion. In older children, vomitus is generally bile-stained, which reflects the loss of small bowel juices and is more likely to be associated with a hyperchloremic acidosis with superimposed starvation ketosis.

Treatment

A. Replacement of Losses Due to Vomiting: After the diagnosis is established, give nothing by mouth (see Chapter 16). Rehydration should be carried out initially with isotonic sodium solution, 10–20 mL/kg. (Sodium chloride should be used when alkalosis is present; a balanced sodium solution [see p 72] is more appropriate for patients with acidosis.) Following this, a transfusion of Plasmanate (10–20 mL/kg) may be needed to combat shock.

Further hydration should then be carried out according to the method outlined on p 72. In cases of pyloric stenosis, it is of particular importance to begin potassium repletion as soon as this is safe; give potassium, 3 mEq/kg/d for at least 3 days. The potassium should be distributed throughout the daily fluids so that its concentration does not exceed 40 mEq/L.

Maintenance fluid and electrolyte requirements (see Table 5–3) should also be given parenterally.

In cases of vomiting not due to pyloric stenosis, the same general regimen should be followed. However, because the acid-base disturbance is usually a metabolic acidosis, balanced sodium solutions incorporating some bicarbonate or lactate are preferred over sodium chloride solutions. Large amounts of bicarbonate are not necessary. If present, ketosis is managed by providing adequate carbohydrate.

B. Pre- and Postoperative Replacement of Losses in Pyloric Stenosis: After the deficit has been completely restored and a start has been made on potassium repletion, surgery may be performed (usually after 36–48 hours). After surgery, no special precautions are needed with respect to electrolytes. Give full maintenance requirements of water and electrolytes.

1. On the first day, offer 50% of the maintenance fluid and electrolytes orally in multiple small feedings (15–30 mL). Give the balance parenterally.

2. On subsequent days, give full or partial maintenance requirements orally as tolerated. Start milk feedings with small amounts of half-skimmed milk, proceeding to dilute evaporated milk and then full formula as tolerated.

3. Combined oral and parenteral intake should provide additional potassium, 3 mEq/kg/d, for the first 3 postoperative days.

4. If vomiting occurs, ascertain the cause; discontinue all oral feedings for 8–12 hours and give maintenance requirements parenterally (see p 74).

PREOPERATIVE PREPARATION FOR MAJOR SURGERY

(See also Chapter 2.)

Adequate preparation for surgery must include attention to the fluid, electrolyte, and nutritional status of the child.

Treatment

A. Preparation for Surgery: Dehydrated infants and young children are poor surgical risks. The fluid, electrolyte, and blood losses during a long operation predispose to shock and its complications. Replacement of fluid and electrolyte deficits should therefore be completed before surgery, and at the time of surgery the volume and composition of the body fluids should, if possible, be normal. Even in emergencies, sodium and water deficits should be repaired before surgery is undertaken.

B. Preoperative Fluids: If preoperative orders call for no oral intake after midnight, it is wise to give 50% of the calculated 24-hour maintenance fluid and electrolyte requirements intravenously from midnight to the time of operation.

C. Fluids During Surgery: During surgery, fluids should be administered intravenously. In the small child and infant, a surgical cutdown is best if an intravenous site is not secure. A slow drip of 5% glucose in water can be used to keep the intravenous route open until surgery, but care should be taken not to administer excessive amounts of this solution.

D. Whole Blood: Whole blood should be immediately available during any surgical procedure. Blood should be administered as it is lost.

POSTOPERATIVE PERIOD AFTER MAJOR SURGERY

(See also Chapter 2.)

The principal problems in the postoperative period differ depending on whether there has or has not been extrarenal loss of fluid and electrolytes. Little is known of the metabolic response to surgery in the infant, and the assistance of a consultant may be advisable in unusual cases.

Treatment

A. Patients Without Extrarenal Losses or Preexisting Deficits:

1. Water–Requirements are the same as for any maintenance program except in those few patients who, for incompletely understood reasons, show acute (usually transient) oliguria postoperatively. This complication must be carefully watched for to avoid water intoxication.

2. Glucose–Requirements are the same as for any maintenance program.

3. Sodium and chloride–Maintenance requirements of sodium (see Table 5–3) may be given with safety, although some physicians prefer moderate sodium restriction for 1–2 days after surgery.

4. Potassium–Maintenance requirements of potassium may be given as soon as renal function and circulation are adequate. It must be reemphasized that a large preexisting potassium deficit should be corrected before surgery. When this is not possible, potassium repletion should be instituted on the first postoperative day. It is imperative, however, that precautions regarding potassium administration be applied (see p 87). Potassium-containing juices and other fluids given orally usually can meet the need during this period. If potassium intake remains inadequate after 1–2 days, potassium should be included in the parenteral fluids in amounts of 2–3 mEq/kg/d and should be given with the precautions outlined. Postoperative alkalosis due to potassium depletion is a syndrome that usually appears after the second or third postoperative day unless there has been a previous uncorrected deficit. Preparations suitable for parenteral potassium administration are outlined in the section on hypokalemia.

5. Nitrogen–Nitrogen intake need not be encouraged during the immediate postoperative period. With minimal water intake, dehydration may actually be precipitated as a result of the large urinary losses of water incurred in clearing the urea produced by catabolism of dietary protein. Parenteral administration of whole protein (plasma) is of little value to protein nutrition, since considerable time is required for breakdown of plasma into amino acids.

B. Patients With Extrarenal Losses: In these patients, ongoing losses must be replaced at the same time as maintenance requirements are being provided. Replacement should proceed as the loss is being incurred and with solutions of similar composition, usually by parenteral routes. Serial serum electrolyte determinations may be useful in complicated cases for checking adequacy of replacement.

C. Oral Feedings: Oral feedings of liquid or soft diets should be started as soon as tolerated.

D. Nutritional Deficits: Patients having severe nutritional deficits secondary to incompetent gastrointestinal function should be considered for total parenteral nutrition delivered by central venous catheter.

INTESTINAL OBSTRUCTION

(See also Chapter 16.)

In intestinal obstruction, there is continuing gastrointestinal secretory activity while absorptive function is depressed, resulting in either the accumulation or loss through vomiting of large quantities of gastrointestinal fluids. This produces abdominal distention, vomiting, dehydration, and shock; depletion of potassium, sodium, and chloride in varying combinations; and associated gross disturbances in acid-base balance.

Nothing should be given orally or by tube to the obstructed patient, since food or fluid often stimulates increased secretion. If it is judged necessary to offer fluids orally, give only isotonic solutions.

Treatment

A. Immediate Measures: Relieve distention by continuous suction from the small intestine and give nothing by mouth.

B. Replacement of Deficits: Replacement of deficits should follow the principles already outlined. The anion composition of the sodium solutions used for rehydration should be adjusted according to the prevailing disturbance of acid-base equilibrium—sodium chloride for alkalosis and a balanced sodium solution for acidosis.

Significant potassium deficits complicate virtually every case of intestinal obstruction; these should be managed according to the methods outlined on p 87.

If warranted, surgery should be delayed until the water, sodium, and chloride deficits have been corrected (in 36–48 hours) and some progress has been made on repair of the potassium deficit.

C. Maintenance Requirements: Fluid and electrolyte requirements must be met as needed. On the first postoperative day, give the maintenance requirement of sodium and chloride. If there is evidence of hypokalemia, the full potassium requirement (2.5–3 mEq/kg) should be given. (Observe precautions in potassium therapy as noted on p 87).

D. Replacement of Losses: Ongoing losses incurred through suction must be continuously replaced (volume for volume) with an appropriate solution. Blood losses must also be replaced.

E. Oral Feedings: Oral feedings may be begun only in the absence of abdominal distention and nausea or vomiting and after bowel sounds have returned. On the first day of oral feedings, give 25% of the total water and electrolyte requirements in the form of clear fluids in small, frequent feedings. The balance must be given parenterally. Increase oral feeding with clear fluids or diluted formula gradually until full maintenance requirements are tolerated.

SALICYLISM

Salicylate intoxication occurs frequently and usually results from cumulative effects of prolonged administration of presumed safe doses of aspirin to ill infants and children, accidental ingestion of large quantities of aspirin, or accidental ingestion of methyl salicylate (oil of wintergreen). Severity of toxicity does not necessarily relate to dosage.

Pathologic Physiology & Clinical Findings

Three basic effects of toxic amounts of salicylate account for the various metabolic disorders encountered in salicylism: (1) central respiratory stimulation; (2) abnormal metabolism of carbohydrate and lipid, resulting in ketosis; and (3) increase in metabolic rate. The first of these leads to marked hyperventilation, which is the most prominent and important clinical sign in salicylism. When this is the only major disturbance, respiratory alkalosis results. In infants and young children, ketosis often occurs simultaneously with respiratory stimulation, and this leads to a mixed disturbance of acid-base equilibrium in which plasma bicarbonate is reduced but blood pH may be normal, acid, or alkaline.

In moderate or severe cases, hyperventilation may be accompanied by vomiting, sweating, flushed appearance, stupor, convulsions, and fever. A disturbance in blood coagulation (hypoprothrombinemia or thrombocytopenia) may lead to internal or external bleeding. Moderate degrees of dehydration occur as a result of polyuria, sweating, vomiting, and increased insensible water loss. The dehydration is usually isotonic, although it may be hypertonic in infants.

Exact diagnosis of the acid-base disturbance in any given patient is important in the design of therapy. Of greatest importance is the differentiation of patients with alkalosis from those with acidosis, since large amounts of bicarbonate administered to the former may precipitate tetany and convulsions.

Determination of the pH of arterial or arterialized venous blood is the only absolute method for confident diagnosis. Lacking this, the following may be helpful:

A. pH of Urine: Alkalosis is likely when the urine is alkaline, but "paradoxic aciduria" may occur (see p 94).

B. Age Factor: Younger children and infants are more apt to be acidotic, especially if there has been an interval of several hours since ingestion of salicylate.

C. Dietary History: If the child's oral intake has been poor as a result of a febrile illness for which aspirin was given, acidosis is more likely.

D. Other Urinary Findings: Additional urinary findings may include reducing substance levels of 1+ to 2+, proteinuria of 1+ to 2+, small numbers of formed elements, and a positive result in the ferric chloride (Gerhardt) test after boiling the urine. The latter, however, does not necessarily indicate toxic levels of salicylates; positive results are also obtained when there are coal tar derivatives and phenols in the urine. In the presence of acidosis, a nitroprusside (Rothera) test for acetone may yield positive results. (Salicylates per se do not give a positive reaction in the test.) Salicylism may mimic diabetic coma in producing not only acidosis but also reducing substances and acetone in the urine.

Treatment

A. General Measures:

1. Induce emesis if possible; otherwise, perform gastric lavage with a balanced sodium solution (see Table 5–2).

2. Treat dehydration and peripheral vascular collapse, if present, as outlined on p 72.

3. Vitamins K and C should be given, particularly if there is a disturbance of blood coagulation.

4. If hyperpyrexia is present, reduce body temperature by sponging with cool (not cold) water.

5. Maintenance fluids should be generous because of the increased metabolic rate; in a moderately severe case of salicylism, maintenance requirements may be 50% above the usual range. Generous amounts of carbohydrate should be given; use 10% glucose.

6. Potassium depletion complicates nearly every case and should be managed as outlined on p 86.

B. Treatment of Acid-Base Disturbances:

1. Alkaline pH–All sodium and potassium should be in the form of chlorides. Do not give respiratory depressants (eg, morphine); rebreathing or breathing CO_2-enriched mixtures is ineffective, since it provokes intolerable dyspnea.

2. Normal or acid pH–Patients presenting with these types of disturbances show a marked tendency to recover through an alkalotic phase even when no large amounts of alkalinizing salts are given. Therefore, most of the sodium and potassium administered to such patients should be in the form of the chloride, with only moderate amounts in the form of bicarbonate.

C. Treatment of Severe Cases:

1. Acute pulmonary edema may occur in severe salicylism. It should be treated vigorously with positive-pressure oxygen, tourniquets, and aminophylline. Morphine should be avoided.

2. Respiratory depression usually occurs as an accompaniment of acute pulmonary edema. It may be severe enough to warrant artificial ventilation.

3. Severe cases may require one or more of the following measures designed to remove salicylate from the body at a rate faster than can usually be accomplished by conservative management alone:

a. Measures designed to accelerate salicylate through the renal route–These measures all are designed to alkalinize the urine (preferably to a pH above 7.5), since alkaline urine markedly enhances the rate of clearance of salicylate. Large loads of sodium bicarbonate (up to 10 mmol/kg) have been advocated by some workers but may produce severe systemic alkalosis. Such large amounts are not recommended. Administration of acetazolamide (Diamox), 5 mg/kg intramuscularly and repeated twice at 4-hour intervals (if necessary), may produce an alkaline urine. One report states that unexpected death followed administration of acetazolamide, whereas other reports, generally discussing less severe cases, mention no such complications.

b. Measures designed to remove salicylate via the extrarenal route–Exchange transfusion has been used successfully but is inefficient and only applicable to the small infant. Intermittent peritoneal dialysis, using a fluid with the composition of normal extracellular fluid plus human serum albumin in a final concentration of 5 g/dL, has also been used successfully. Hemodialysis is unquestionably the most efficient method for removal of salicylate, but it presents formidable technical difficulties in infants and small children.

SPECIFIC ELECTROLYTE DISTURBANCES

HYPOKALEMIA & POTASSIUM DEPLETION

Predisposing Factors

A. Extrarenal Losses: Losses without commensurate intake, eg, vomiting, diarrhea, intestinal suction.

B. Renal Losses:

1. Acid-base disturbances, including metabolic acidosis and metabolic and respiratory alkalosis.
2. Adrenocortical factors, including excessive endogenous (stress) adrenocortical secretion, exogenous adrenal steroid or corticotropin (ACTH) therapy (particularly in the presence of a large sodium intake), primary aldosteronism, and Bartter's syndrome.
3. Use of diuretics.
4. Polyuric phase of acute tubular necrosis or in primary renal or adrenal disease ("potassium-losing nephritis").

C. Diabetes: Recovery phase of diabetic acidosis.

Clinical Findings

Potassium depletion of considerable proportions may exist with little clinical evidence.

A. Symptoms and Signs: Deep tendon reflexes are depressed. Muscle weakness and hypotonia are usually vague and are not helpful signs in most pediatric patients. Frank paralysis is rare. Abdominal distention with diminished or absent peristalsis is sometimes seen. A fall in diastolic blood pressure may be seen when careful serial blood pressure records are available. Cardiac failure may occur.

B. Laboratory Findings: Serum potassium levels may be less than 3 mEq/L, particularly in the presence of alkalosis. Levels may be normal in acidosis even though a significant deficit of total body potassium is present. Likewise in dehydration with prerenal azotemia, the initial serum potassium level may be normal or even elevated but will drop sharply with rehydration.

C. Electrocardiographic Findings: When the serum potassium concentration drops to (or below) 3 mEq/L, the electrocardiographic changes described below may be observed. However, they are not specific for potassium depletion. The final diagnosis depends on the serum potassium level. The reversal of an altered electrocardiographic pattern following administration of potassium is also helpful.

1. Frequently, an associated slight prolongation of the Q–T interval that is not due to a lengthening of the ST segment as is the case in hypocalcemia.

2. A decrease in height and inversion of the T wave. T waves are also influenced by the pH and the bicarbonate, sodium, and calcium concentrations of the blood.

3. Rounding and prolongation of the T wave, so that it may run into the following P wave.

4. Depression of the ST segment.

5. Possible inversion of the P wave; extrasystoles (especially ventricular) and atrioventricular block.

Precautions & Treatment

Because of the dangers of potassium intoxication, do not give more than 3 mEq/kg during a 24-hour period for the replacement of potassium deficits except in unusually severe cases. This limiting factor makes potassium replacement a prolonged procedure. The total amount of potassium to be administered varies with the deficit present and the ongoing losses. At the first observation, estimate the deficit as closely as possible and determine the maintenance needs (see p 74). Keep an accurate account of the ongoing losses (see p 76). On the basis of this information, recalculate the **total potassium needs** daily and give potassium, up to 5 mEq/kg/d, as long as required. With good renal function, extra potassium will be excreted and will not be toxic as long as the rate of administration is slow (see precautions given in ¶ B2, below).

A. Oral Administration: If the patient has no gastrointestinal obstruction and can tolerate oral feedings without nausea or vomiting, adequate potassium is present in the ordinary full diet. With any dietary restriction, the patient's potassium intake may be inadequate and should be checked. Potassium added to milk, orange juice, or ginger ale up to a level of 60–80 mEq/L (total) may be offered. Potassium chloride (KCl) is the preferred salt. However, potassium sometimes produces pylorospasm with nausea, vomiting, and anorexia; this is especially likely when potassium levels exceed 80 mEq/L. Potassium given without fluid (eg, capsules) may exert a local damaging effect on gastrointestinal mucosa. A common—but false—assumption is that the potassium deficit will cease once the patient is able to resume full oral feedings. To be sure potassium replacement is adequate, the electrolyte composition of orally ingested fluids and foods should be determined by calculation.

B. Parenteral Administration: Potassium salts may be given intravenously. The following precautions should be observed when potassium is given by parenteral routes:

1. Solutions containing potassium, 20–40 mEq/L, are usually satisfactory. Avoid solutions containing more than 40 mEq of potassium per liter.
2. Before giving potassium, review and analyze the patient's history, calculate preceding intake and probable need, look for physical signs of hypokalemia, determine serum potassium levels, and check the ECG.
3. Do not start potassium administration until the patient is excreting adequate amounts of urine.
4. Do not give potassium to a patient who may still be in shock, to patients with oliguria or anuria, or to those suspected of having chronic nephritis with potassium retention.
5. Do not give more than a *total* of 5 mEq of potassium per kilogram per day, but give it continuously over the entire 24-hour period for which it is intended. It ordinarily takes several days to completely correct a marked potassium deficiency.
6. If any symptoms of hyperkalemia appear during therapy, stop the infusion, again determine the serum potassium concentration, and take another ECG.

C. Control of Potassium Therapy:

1. Serial determinations of serum potassium and bicarbonate concentrations are desirable.
2. If analysis of serum is impossible, take serial ECGs.
3. Potassium therapy is indicated as long as the serum potassium level remains below 3.5 mEq/L.

D. Preparations Commonly Used in Parenteral Potassium Therapy:

1. Potassium chloride, 1 mEq/mL or 2 mEq/mL.
2. Potassium phosphate salts–
   a. KH_2PO_4 0.3 g, K_2HPO_4 1.55 g } in 10 mL of water
   A 10-mL vial contains 20 mEq of K^+ and 10 mmol of P.
   b. KH_2PO_4 1 g, K_2HPO_4 4.59 g } in 20 mL of water
   A 20-mL vial contains 120 mEq of K^+ and 60 mmol of P.

These potassium phosphate solutions should be added to other solutions. They are of value in diabetic acidosis, where hypokalemia may be accompanied by hypophosphatemia.

HYPERKALEMIA & POTASSIUM INTOXICATION

Predisposing Factors

Predisposing factors include shock and oliguria, particularly in the presence of continuing intake of potassium or the release of large amounts of potassium from the cells, and chronic renal disease with nitrogen retention.

Clinical Findings

A. Symptoms and Signs: Symptoms are frequently absent, but listlessness, mental confusion, and paresthesias may be present. Bradycardia, peripheral vascular collapse, and cardiac arrest may occur.

B. Laboratory Findings: Serum potassium concentration is above 6 mEq/L.

C. Electrocardiographic Findings: The following correlate roughly with increasing potassium concentration: peaked T waves, an increase in QRS duration, an increase in P–R interval, and a totally irregular rhythm and heart block.

Treatment

Severe hyperkalemia should be considered a metabolic emergency, and treatment should be carefully monitored by serial measurements of serum potassium levels and serial ECGs.

(1) Withhold potassium by all routes.

(2) Give insulin and glucose.

(3) Give 10% calcium gluconate (1–2 mg of calcium per kilogram per hour [see p 79]) cautiously intravenously; additional calcium salts should be added to intravenous infusions as needed. (Amounts and rates of administration of calcium should be guided by electrocardiographic changes.) Special attention must be paid to monitoring the infusion site whenever calcium is given, since infiltration will be accompanied by a skin slough.

(4) Some authorities recommend digitalization.

(5) Utilize measures designed to rid the body of excess potassium. Give potassium-free resin such as sodium polystyrene sulfonate (Kayexalate), 1 g/kg, either by retention enema or as multiple divided doses by mouth. The oral route is preferred in the absence of vomiting, since results with oral usage are more predictable. If enemas are used, they should be given several times a day with a volume of 250 mL each time. Peritoneal dialysis or hemodialysis may be indicated.

HYPONATREMIA & SODIUM DEPLETION

Hyponatremia may be classified as acute salt depletion, acute dilutional hyponatremia, chronic dilutional hyponatremia, or inappropriate secretion of antidiuretic hormone (ADH).

Acute Salt Depletion

A. Predisposing Factors:

1. Untreated adrenal insufficiency (adrenal crisis).

2. Repeated administration of diuretics to patients with restricted sodium intake.

3. Removal of a large ascitic fluid collection, as in a cirrhotic (or occasionally a nephrotic) patient on a low salt intake.

4. Excessive sweating without salt replacement, especially in children with mucoviscidosis.

5. Administration of a large non-salt-containing clysis (isotonic glucose) to a salt-depleted individual.

6. Chronic renal disease.

B. Symptoms and Signs: Symptoms and signs are essentially those of a combination of water intoxication and peripheral vascular collapse. They include cool, clammy skin; low blood pressure; weakness; central nervous system stimulation and sometimes convulsions; and thirst.

C. Treatment: Prompt intravenous administration of hypertonic salt solution (5% sodium chloride containing 855 mEq of Na^+ and Cl^- per liter) is indicated. Dosage is calculated as follows:

$$\begin{bmatrix}\text{mEq of Na}^+\\ \text{needed}\end{bmatrix} = \begin{bmatrix}140 - \text{Patient's serum Na}^+\text{ level}\\ \text{(in mEq)}\end{bmatrix} \times \begin{bmatrix}\text{60\% body weight}\\ \text{(in kg)}\end{bmatrix}$$

To avoid a large chloride excess, it may be desirable to give some of the sodium as sodium bicarbonate (usually one-third) and the rest as sodium chloride.

It is advisable to attempt only about 50% of the total correction initially over a period of 4–6 hours. Then recheck the plasma Na^+ concentration to ascertain the degree of correction achieved—further hypertonic infusion may be unnecessary. In general, hypertonic sodium therapy should be reserved for serious, symptomatic hyponatremia.

Acute Dilutional Hyponatremia (Water Intoxication)

A. Predisposing Factors:

1. Excessive administration of salt-free fluids.

2. Failure to excrete water due to endogenous factors (excessive ADH secretion, as seen in some postoperative patients and secondary to morphine administration) or excessive administration of vasopressin.

B. Symptoms and Signs: These include gain in weight, vomiting, convulsions, and oliguria (in severe instances). Urine osmolality (specific gravity) is significantly higher than plasma osmolality. Blood urea nitrogen or serum creatinine level is nearly always normal.

C. Treatment: In the presence of severe symptoms, treatment should consist of rapid infusion of hypertonic salt solution calculated and carried out as described above.

Chronic Dilutional Hyponatremia

Chronic dilutional hyponatremia is seen in chronic edematous states of various types. It is generally refractory to treatment with hypertonic salt solution unless there is a superimposed acute salt depletion. In general, chronic dilutional hyponatremia should not be treated, although fluid restriction may be tried. Its occurrence indicates a poor prognosis. Patients with chronic dilutional hyponatremia are prone to develop a superimposed acute salt depletion, since they are frequently on a low sodium intake because of their edema and are subjected to diuretic measures.

Inappropriate Secretion of ADH

Inappropriate secretion of ADH occurs in patients with tuberculous and other types of meningitis, bilateral far-advanced pulmonary disease, and many other types of serious systemic disease. These patients are well hydrated and have normal blood urea nitrogen and serum creatinine levels but produce small volumes of concentrated urine. They become hyponatremic when water intake continues at usual levels (see Acute Dilutional Hyponatremia, above). Treatment of hyponatremia requires water restriction; the water balance should be negative, ie, water intake should be less than measured urine output plus estimated insensible and other losses.

HYPERNATREMIA

Since hypernatremia is a potent stimulus for thirst, it occurs only in patients who do not have free access to water (infants and unconscious persons). It may be seen in any situation where loss of water exceeds loss of salt and special circumstances limiting water intake are present, eg, infantile diarrhea, excessive administration of table salt to infants with mild diarrhea, and solute diuresis secondary to tube feeding of unconscious patients with large amounts of protein.

The treatment of infants with hypernatremia has been outlined earlier. In other instances, adequate water should be provided. In patients with diabetes insipidus, vasopressin should be given.

Table 5–9. Composition of parenteral and oral solutions. (All values per liter.)

Solution and Route	Na^+ (mEq)	K^+ (mEq)	Cl^- (mEq)	Other (mEq or as noted)
5% and 10% glucose in water (IV, subcut)*				CHO, 50 and 100 g
Isotonic (0.9%) NaCl (IV, subcut)	154		154	
Hypertonic (3%) NaCl (IV)	515		515	
Hypertonic (5%) NaCl (IV)	855		855	
Normosol-R (or Normosol-R in D5-W) (IV)	140	5	98	Mg^{2+}, 3; Ac, 27; gluconate, 23; CHO, 50 g
Polysal (IV, subcut)	140	10	103	Ca^{2+}, 5; Mg^{2+}, 3; Ac, 47; citrate, 8
Polysal elixir (oral)	5†	1.5†	4.3†	Ca^{2+}, 0.2; Mg^{2+}, 0.1; lactate, 2.4†
Lytren‡ (oral)	50	20	30	Ca^{2+}, 4; Mg^{2+}, 4; citrate, 35; P, 10 mmol; lactate, 4
Ringer's injection (IV, subcut)	145	4	155	Ca^{2+}, 6
Lactated Ringer's injection (IV)	129	4	109.5	Ca^{2+}, 3.5; lactate, 27
1 M sodium lactate (11.2%) (for dilution)	1000			Lactate, 1000
0.167 M sodium lactate (1.97%) (IV, subcut)	167			Lactate, 167
Normosol-M in D5-W (IV)	40	13	40	Mg^{2+}, 3; Ac, 16; CHO, 50 g
Darrow's solution (K lactate) (IV, subcut)	123	35	105	Lactate, 53
Gastric replacement with 10% dextrose (Baxter)§ (IV, subcut)	63	17	150	NH_4^+, 70
Intestinal replacement with 10% dextrose (Baxter)§ (IV, subcut)	138	12	100	Lactate, 50
Potassium chloride (1 or 2 mEq/mL) (ampules; to be added to other fluids)		1000 2000	1000 2000	
Sodium bicarbonate (1 mEq/mL) (ampules; to be added to other fluids)	1000			HCO_3^-, 1000
Whole blood, citrated// (IV)				
Plasma (275 mL)	40	1.4¶	25	Protein, 18 g
Cells (225 mL)		23		Protein, 75 g
ACD diluting solution (125 mL)	5			CHO, 3.75 g

*Contains 50 or 100 g CHO and 200 or 400 kcal/L.
†Per undiluted teaspoon (5 mL).
‡Available as solution.
§Contains 100 g CHO and 400 kcal/L.
//Values per unit of whole blood (625 ml).
¶Bank blood potassium levels may rise to as much as 30 mEq/L of plasma.

DISTURBANCES OF ACID-BASE EQUILIBRIUM

Disturbances of acid-base equilibrium may be calculated by use of the Henderson-Hasselbalch equation, which expresses the bicarbonate-carbonic acid system as follows:

$$pH = 6.10 + \log \frac{(HCO_3^-)}{(H_2CO_3 + \text{Dissolved } CO_2)}$$

In healthy adults, the ratio of HCO_3^- to (H_2CO_3 + dissolved CO_2) is about 24:1.2 or 20:1, representing a normal pH of 7.40 with a plasma bicarbonate content of 25.2 mmol/L (ie, plasma bicarbonate = 24.0 + 1.2 = 25.2). In infants, the normal value for the ratio is 20:1 at pH 7.40, and the normal plasma bicarbonate is 21 mmol/L.

The denominator term is a function of the partial pressure of carbon dioxide (P_{CO_2}) in the alveolar air and can therefore be readily adjusted by changes in pulmonary ventilation. The plasma bicarbonate content includes both HCO_3^- and (H_2CO_3 + dissolved CO_2), and determination of the pH is necessary to ascertain the value of each. In practice, this is desirable but not absolutely necessary, since an analysis of the clinical findings will nearly always clarify the diagnostic issue unless one is dealing with a complex acid-base problem.

Classification of Acid-Base Disturbances

Disturbances of acid-base equilibrium can be classified as either metabolic or respiratory, depending upon whether the primary distortion affects the numerator (HCO_3^-) or the denominator (H_2CO_3) of the Henderson-Hasselbalch equation. Compensatory adjustments occur in the metabolic disorders primarily through alterations in the alveolar partial pressure of CO_2, which adjust the denominator, as well as through renal adjustment, which tends to restore the numerator. Compensatory adjustments in respiratory disorders are principally renal and therefore affect the numerator in a direction that tends to restore the absolute value of the ratio towards normal (20:1).

A. Metabolic Acidosis: Metabolic acidosis results from an abnormal retention or production of fixed (nonvolatile) acids—as in diabetes, excessive ammonium chloride ingestion, diarrhea, starvation ketosis, salicylate intoxication, or renal insufficiency—which leads to a reduction in the numerator (HCO_3^-). Compensation occurs through hyperventilation, reducing the denominator. The kidney responds by increasing excretion of titratable acid and ammonium. In addition, there may be some buffering of hydrogen ions by cellular or bone exchanges. Therapy should include attempts to control acid production as well to rehydrate the patient and should provide adequate amounts of sodium and potassium. *Large* amounts of sodium bicarbonate should not be given acutely, since they tend to produce an alkalosis during recovery phases. No sodium bicarbonate is necessary if the plasma bicarbonate level is above 15 mmol/L in acute acidosis and renal function is potentially normal.

B. Metabolic Alkalosis: A primary loss of hydrogen ions, as in loss of hydrochloric acid by vomiting or the ingestion of excessive amounts of sodium bicarbonate, leads to an increase in the numerator of the equation. Any circumstances leading to chloride depletion coupled with sodium depletion also tend to be associated with metabolic alkalosis. In theory, hypoventilation should provide respiratory compensation, but this may be limited by oxygen demands. It is quite unpredictable for unknown reasons. Renal compensation initially leads to an alkaline urine with loss of potassium and sodium, but when chloride or potassium depletion (or both) supervenes, the urine pH becomes acid ("paradoxic aciduria" with alkalosis). Some buffering occurs when hydrogen ions from cellular and bone sites are exchanged for sodium or potassium (or both) from the blood. Therapy should treat the primary loss as well as provide adequate sodium, water, and potassium.

Chloride depletion has been found to occupy a special role in states where bicarbonate concentration is elevated. An adequate chloride intake must be provided to correct metabolic alkalosis.

C. Respiratory Acidosis: Primary retention of CO_2 due to hypoventilation resulting from pulmonary disease or central factors raises the denominator. Compensation is renal; titratable acid and ammonium are excreted, while serum bicarbonate is increased. Buffering through extrarenal ion exchange is similar to that in metabolic acidosis. Treatment should be for the primary disease. High concentrations of oxygen should be avoided unless the patient can be artificially ventilated. If the P_{CO_2} can be brought to normal by therapy, the patient will become alkalotic unless the bicarbonate concentration is readjusted to normal; this requires an adequate chloride intake.

D. Respiratory Alkalosis: A primary loss of CO_2 due to hyperventilation caused by emotional factors or salicylate intoxication or, rarely, primary central nervous system disease leads to a reduction in the denominator of the equation. Renal and extrarenal compensation is similar to that in metabolic alkalosis. Therapeutic measures should include rebreathing in emotional hyperventilation, rehydration with adequate potassium supplements, and calcium infusions for tetany.

Anti-infective Chemotherapeutic Agents & Antibiotic Drugs* | 6

Antimicrobial therapy is the use of chemotherapeutic agents (eg, sulfonamides and antibiotics) for the treatment of infectious disease by attack upon the etiologic agent. Maximum success in the use of these substances depends upon (1) identification of the pathogens to be eliminated, (2) selection of the therapeutic agent or agents most active against the pathogen, (3) administration of an adequate amount of drug to destroy the pathogen, and (4) selection of the appropriate route for the appropriate duration of time to achieve maximal contact of the agent with the pathogen.

Methicillin, oxacillin, and nafcillin are resistant to staphylococcal penicillinase and are used in the treatment of infections due to penicillin-resistant staphylococci. Cloxacillin and dicloxacillin are oral drugs effective against penicillin-resistant staphylococci. Ampicillin (a broad-spectrum antibiotic), cephalexin, and trimethoprim-sulfamethoxazole are useful in treating chronic urinary tract infections. Gentamicin, tobramycin, and amikacin may be used for systemic therapy of *Pseudomonas* or otherwise resistant gram-negative infections. Carbenicillin, ticarcillin, piperacillin, and mezlocillin are penicillins given intravenously for treatment of *Pseudomonas* infections. Oral carbenicillin is useful only for treatment of urinary tract infections. Clindamycin is a semisynthetic antibiotic derived from lincomycin; it is active against staphylococci, most streptococci, and many anaerobes. Moxalactam and cefotaxime, which are newer "third-generation" cephalosporins, are used for treatment of *Haemophilus influenzae* infections and offer the advantage of effectively penetrating the cerebrospinal fluid. It should be noted also that meningitis of unknown cause in premature infants and infants under 1 month of age should be treated with ampicillin plus erythromycin but that infants over 1 month of age should be given ampicillin plus chloramphenicol, since half of these cases are due to *H influenzae*, against which chloramphenicol is effective. Chloramphenicol blood levels should be monitored.

The antibacterial spectrum of antimicrobial agents and the choice of anti-infective agents are shown in Tables 6–1 and 6–2.

*Revised with the assistance of Frederic W. Bruhn, MD (COL, MC, USA).

Table 6–1. Antibacterial spectrum of antimicrobial agents.

Mode of Action	Activity Principally Against		
	Gram-Positives	Broad-Spectrum	Gram-Negatives
Bactericidal	Penicillins, bacitracin, vancomycin	Carbenicillin, cephalosporins, ampicillin, penicillin*	Streptomycin, gentamicin, kanamycin, moxalactam
Bacteriostatic	Erythromycin, clindamycin	Tetracyclines, sulfonamides, chloramphenicol	Nalidixic acid

*In very large doses, penicillin may be bactericidal against a number of gram-negatives.

General Indications

Antibiotic and chemotherapeutic agents are indicated (1) for diseases in which a specific microbial etiologic agent has been identified by culture or serology, (2) for diseases in which the clinical picture implies a definite etiologic diagnosis, and (3) as a possible lifesaving measure for a desperately ill patient when an exact or complete etiologic diagnosis has not yet been made.

Development of Resistance

Resistance develops (1) if strains that are already genetically resistant to the agent being used gain dominance by selection or (2) if "spontaneous" mutation to a state of resistance occurs.

Adequate dosage and combined therapy prevent or slow down the development of resistant strains. Topical therapy should often supplement systemic therapy in chronic infections.

Precautions in Newborns & Premature Infants

Great caution is necessary in preventing overdosage in order to avoid serious and permanent damage (especially in premature infants, newborn infants, and oliguric children).

Precautions in Oliguric Children

Regular drug dosages are too high for children with reduced renal function. Dosage and time schedules must be adjusted to renal output in the case of the more toxic agents (bacitracin, cephalothin, chloramphenicol, colistin, flucytosine, gentamicin, kanamycin, neomycin, novobiocin, polymyxin, streptomycin, tetracyclines, trimethoprim with sulfamethoxazole, and vancomycin).

PEDIATRIC ANTIMICROBIAL THERAPEUTIC AGENTS

Amikacin Sulfate (Amikin)

Use: Bactericidal for some gram-positive enteric bacteria, including

Table 6–2. Choice of anti-infective agents.

Organism (and Gram Reaction)	Drug(s) of First Choice	Drug(s) of Second Choice
Actinomyces (+)	Penicillin	Tetracyclines, erythromycin
Bacillus anthracis (+)	Penicillin	Tetracyclines, erythromycin
Bacteroides (–)*	Chloramphenicol, clindamycin	Penicillin, metronidazole, carbenicillin
Bordetella pertussis (–)	Erythromycin	Tetracyclines
Brucella (–)	Tetracyclines + streptomycin	Chloramphenicol
Campylobacter (–)	Erythromycin	Gentamicin
Candida albicans	Amphotericin B	5-Flucytosine, ketoconazole
Chlamydiae (agents of lymphogranuloma venereum, psittacosis, and trachoma)	Tetracyclines, erythromycin	Chloramphenicol, sulfonamides
Clostridia other than *Clostridium difficile* (+)	Antitoxin + penicillin	Chloramphenicol, metronidazole
Clostridium difficile	Vancomycin	
Corynebacterium diphtheriae (+)	Antitoxin + penicillin	Erythromycin, clindamycin
Enterobacter (–)*	Gentamicin	Cephalothin, mezlocillin, tetracyclines + streptomycin
Erysipelothrix (+)	Penicillin	Tetracyclines, erythromycin
Escherichia coli (–)*	Ampicillin, gentamicin	Tetracyclines, cephalothin, sulfonamides, cephalexin
Francisella tularensis (–)	Streptomycin + tetracyclines	
Haemophilus influenzae (–)*	Ampicillin, chloramphenicol	Streptomycin, moxalactam, trimethoprim-sulfamethoxazole
Klebsiella pneumoniae (–)*	Kanamycin, cephalothin	Gentamicin, tetracyclines + streptomycin
Leptospira icterohaemorrhagiae	Tetracyclines	Penicillin
Listeria monocytogenes (+)	Ampicillin, tetracyclines	Penicillin
Mycobacterium leprae (+)	Sulfones (eg, dapsone)	Clofazimine, rifampin
Mycobacterium tuberculosis (+)*	Isoniazid + rifampin **or** Isoniazid + ethambutol†	Ethionamide, streptomycin, PAS
Mycoplasma pneumoniae	Tetracyclines, erythromycin	
Neisseria gonorrhoeae (–)	Penicillin + probenecid	Ampicillin + probenecid, spectinomycin, tetracyclines, cefoxitin

*Sensitivity tests usually indicated.

†Ethambutol should be used with caution in children too young to complain of or be tested for changes in visual acuity.

Table 6–2 (cont'd). Choice of anti-infective agents.

Organism (and Gram Reaction)	Drug(s) of First Choice	Drug(s) of Second Choice
Neisseria meningitidis (–)	Penicillin	Ampicillin, chloramphenicol
Nocardia (+)*	Trimethoprim-sulfamethoxazole	Sulfonamides + agent chosen by sensitivity tests
Proteus mirabilis (–)*	Ampicillin, penicillin	Kanamycin, cefoxitin
Proteus vulgaris, Proteus morganii, *Proteus rettgeri* (–)*	Gentamicin	Chloramphenicol, cefoxitin
Pseudomonas aeruginosa (–)*	Gentamicin, carbenicillin, mezlocillin	Tobramycin
Rickettsiae (–)	Chloramphenicol (+ corticosteroids for Rocky Mountain spotted fever)	Tetracyclines
Salmonella other than *Salmonella typhi* (–)*	Ampicillin, trimethoprim-sulfamethoxazole	Chloramphenicol, cephalothin, tetracyclines, kanamycin
Salmonella typhi (–)*	Ampicillin	Chloramphenicol, trimethoprim-sulfamethoxazole
Shigella (–)*	Trimethoprim-sulfamethoxazole	Ampicillin
Spirillum minor (–)	Penicillin	Tetracyclines
Staphylococcus (+)* if sensitive	Penicillin	Erythromycin, lincomycin, cephalothin
Staphylococcus (+)* if resistant to penicillin	Methicillin, nafcillin, dicloxacillin, cloxacillin	Cephalothin, erythromycin, lincomycin, clindamycin, vancomycin
Streptococcus (+) (group A, B, and nonenterococcal group D)	Penicillin	Erythromycin, cephalothin, ampicillin
Streptococcus faecalis (+)* (group D enterococci)	Penicillin + streptomycin **or** Ampicillin + gentamicin	Cephalothin
Streptococcus (Diplococcus) pneumoniae	Penicillin	Ampicillin, erythromycin, clindamycin
Treponema pallidum	Penicillin	Cephalothin, erythromycin, tetracyclines
Yersinia pestis (–)	Streptomycin + tetracyclines	

*Sensitivity tests usually indicated.

†Ethambutol should be used with caution in children too young to complain of or be tested for changes in visual acuity.

Escherichia coli, Klebsiella, Enterobacter, indole-negative and indole-positive *Proteus, Pseudomonas,* and *Serratia.*

Dosage: 15 mg/kg/d intramuscularly or intravenously in 2 or 3 divided doses; and reduced in the presence of impaired renal function.

Toxicity: Similar to other aminoglycosides.

Comment: Semisynthetic aminoglycoside with pharmacologic characteristics of kanamycin and spectrum of activity similar to gentamicin and tobramycin.

Aminosalicylic Acid (PAS, PAS-C)

Use: Tuberculosis.

Dosage: (For PAS.) 250–300 mg/kg/d orally in divided doses every 6 hours; 12 g/d for adolescents.

Toxicity: Gastrointestinal symptoms, hypersensitivity (skin, genital, drug fever), renal irritation, hematologic or hepatic damage, hypokalemia, goiter.

Comment: Avoid or reduce dosage by half when renal function is impaired. Stop drug at first sign of skin rash. PAS-C is more soluble and causes less gastrointestinal irritation than does PAS. Use of rifampin or ethambutol has replaced use of PAS as the second drug in initial treatment regimens.

Amphotericin B (Fungizone)

Use: Active against a variety of fungi (*Candida, Cryptococcus, Blastomyces, Sporotrichum, Coccidioides, Histoplasma, Aspergillus* species, and others).

Dosage:

Intravenous: 0.5–1 mg/kg/d or every other day, given over 4–6 hours.

Intrathecal: 0.5–1 mg in 10 mL of spinal fluid every other day.

Incompatibility: Do not mix with other drugs except heparin. Must only be administered in 5% dextrose.

Toxicity: Chills, fever, malaise. Significant renal, hepatic, and bone marrow damage. Thrombophlebitis, calcifications, hypokalemia.

Comment: Indicated only in severe systemic fungal infections. Administration of corticosteroids before the daily dose is given may ameliorate side effects. Blood levels should be followed. No initial reduction for renal failure. Uninfluenced by dialysis.

Bacitracin

Use: Effective against gram-positive organisms; ineffective against gram-negatives.

Dosage:

Intrathecal or intraventricular: 500–5000 units/d (1000 units/mL).

Topical: 500 units/mL for eye or skin infection.

Toxicity: Transient nephrotoxicity, nausea and vomiting. Topical or oral use harmless except for large denuded areas.

Comment: Largely superseded by penicillinase-resistant penicillins. Relatively safe for children under 1 year of age.

Cefaclor (Ceclor)

Use: Active against essentially the same spectrum as most cephalosporins but with the distinct advantage of activity against *Haemophilus influenzae* including β-lactamase-producing strains.

Dosage: 20–40 mg/kg/d orally in 3–4 divided doses for children.

Toxicity: See Cephalexin.

Comment: Used primarily in treatment of milder infections due to potentially ampicillin-resistant strains of *H influenzae*.

Cefamandole (Mandol)

Use: Essentially the parenteral equivalent of cefaclor.

Dosage: 50–150 mg/kg/d intramuscularly or intravenously in divided doses every 4–6 hours for children.

Toxicity: See Cephalothin.

Comment: Do not use for the treatment of bacterial meningitis.

Cefazolin (Ancef, Kefzol)

Use: Like cephalothin, with certain differences. Activity against gram-positives is about 2-fold less, but that against gram-negatives is about twice as high.

Dosage: 25–100 mg/kg/d intramuscularly or intravenously in divided doses every 6 hours to a maximum of 4 g. Dosage in neonates and premature infants not well established.

Toxicity: Less renal toxicity than cephaloridine; SGOT rises, allergy (see Cephalothin), positive Coombs test.

Comment: Because it is slowly excreted, this drug achieves substantially higher serum levels than does cephalothin after intravenous or intramuscular administration. It is well tolerated intramuscularly. Never use in the treatment of meningitis.

Cefotaxime (Claforan)

Use: Central nervous system infections (eg, meningitis, ventriculitis) when use of a broad-spectrum agent is necessary. Active against the same spectrum of organisms as cephalothin.

Dosage: 50 mg/kg intravenously every 12 hours for premature infants and neonates 0–1 week of age or every 8 hours for neonates 1–4 weeks of age. For infants and children 1–12 years of age, use 50–180 mg/kg intramuscularly or intravenously in 4–6 divided doses; the higher dosages are used in more severe infections (eg, meningitis). For an older child or adolescent whose body weight is 50 kg or more, use the adult dose of 1 g every 6–8 hours; do not exceed 12 g.

Toxicity: See Cephalothin. Local reaction at the injection site is common.

Comment: Indications for this drug are the same as for cephalothin and include treatment for infections due to susceptible organisms in all organ systems.

Cefoxitin (Mefoxin)

Use: Structurally similar to the cephalosporins, with certain differences in spectrum: less active against gram-positive cocci; more active against gram-negative bacilli primarily owing to resistance to β-lactamases; also active against penicillinase-producing *Neisseria gonorrhoeae;* and has a good anaerobic spectrum.

Dosage: 50–200 mg/kg/d intravenously in 4–6 divided doses.

Toxicity: See Cephalothin.

Comment: Useful addition to therapeutic regimen in selected patients but should not be used alone when resistant gram-negative bacilli may be etiologic.

Cephalexin (Keflex)

Use: Cee Cephalothin.

Dosage: 50–100 mg/kg/d orally (not well established); 1–2 g/d for adults.

Toxicity: Nausea, vomiting, diarrhea. Occasional SGOT rise, rash, pruritus.

Comment: The same precautions apply to the use of this drug in persons who are sensitive to penicillin as apply to cephalothin, cephaloridine, and cephaloglycin. The peak blood and urine levels are delayed when the drug is administered with food, but the absorption is still good. Bactericidal activity against sensitive organisms is not as rapid as with cephalothin and cephaloridine. Unit for unit, this drug is not quite as active as the latter 2 drugs against sensitive organisms. Blood levels, in general, are adequate for sensitive gram-positive organisms and for many gram-negative organisms, but the peak blood level achieved on a standard dose varies considerably from individual to individual. The drug should not be relied on for initial therapy in seriously ill persons. In the first 6 hours following a single dose, 80–90% of the drug is excreted. Because of rapid excretion, frequent doses of probenecid may be necessary if high blood levels must be maintained.

Cephalothin (Keflin)

Use: Equivalent to penicillin against gram-positive organisms except enterococci *(Streptococcus faecalis),* which are relatively insensitive. Highly resistant to staphylococcal penicillinase. Effective against most *Escherichia coli,* indole-negative *Proteus,* and most *Klebsiella.* Ineffective against *Pseudomonas,* most *Serratia,* and most *Enterobacter.* When used for gram-negative infections, individual sensitivities should be determined. This drug should definitely not be used in the treatment of meningitis.

Dosage:

Oral: Not absorbed.

Intramuscular: 60–150 mg/kg/d in divided doses every 4–6 hours, given in a large muscle.

Intravenous: 60–150 mg/kg/d in divided doses every 4–6 hours. For newborns, 50–150 mg/kg/d in divided doses every 4–6 hours. For adolescents, up to 12 g/d in the usual case. In severe infections, may be used in doses of 150–200 mg/kg/d, with up to 24 g being used in adults. Should not be used in bacterial meningitis.

Incompatibility: Do not mix with polymyxin B, tetracyclines, erythromycin, calcium chloride, or calcium gluconate.

Toxicity: Pain at injection site, thrombophlebitis, sterile abscesses, drug fever, positive direct Coombs test, anemia, thrombocytopenic purpura; brown-black precipitate in Benedict's test or Clinitest for glucose (when glucose is normal).

Comment: Cephalothin was of special use as a penicillin substitute in penicillin-sensitive persons. It is currently less desirable for this purpose than cefazolin, because it achieves lower serum levels, causes more pain on injection, and increases the risk for nephrotoxicity. Anaphylaxis has been reported but is rare clinically, although the incidence of "sensitivity" to cephalothin as demonstrated by in vitro tests in penicillin-sensitive persons is high. The reason for this discrepancy is not known at present. Cephalothin causes a positive direct Coombs response in normal persons and, because of difficulty in cross-matching blood, should be avoided in persons who may require transfusion.

Chloramphenicol (Chloromycetin)

Use: Bacteriostatic for a wide range of gram-positive and gram-negative organisms, rickettsiae, and chlamydiae. Beginning in 1972, strains of *Salmonella typhi* isolated from Mexico and the southern USA were found to be resistant. Effective against most *Bacteroides* species and anaerobic streptococci.

Dosage:

Oral: 50–100 mg/kg/d (crystalline) in divided doses every 6 hours. Palmitate is unpredictably absorbed.

Intramuscular: Should not be used since absorption is poor.

Intravenous: 100–150 mg/kg/d in divided doses every 12 hours (microcrystalline); 100 mg/kg/d in divided doses every 6–8 hours (succinate). For full-term newborns, 25–50 mg/kg/d in divided doses every 6–12 hours. For premature infants, 25 mg/kg/d in divided doses every 6–12 hours. This drug should be avoided in premature infants. If used, serum levels should be followed to avoid toxicity initially and to avoid inadequate dosage as renal and liver functions mature. An adequate blood level is 10–12 μg/dL. For adolescents, 100 mg/kg/d.

Incompatibility: Do not mix with polymyxin B, tetracyclines, vancomycin, hydrocortisone, B complex vitamins.

Toxicity: In newborns up to 5 months of age, "gray syndrome" with vasomotor collapse; usually with dosage over 80 mg/kg/d. Aplastic anemia and other hematopoietic toxicity. Gastrointestinal symptoms, stomatitis, candidal infections. Allergy, hepatitis, and neurologic abnormalities occur rarely.

Comment: Should not be used when an equally effective drug is available. Diffuses well into most body spaces. Current indications include (1) *Haemophilus influenzae* meningitis when an ampicillin-resistant organism is a possibility; (2) purulent meningitis when true penicillin allergy exists and a causative organism is sensitive; (3) certain anaerobic infections (eg, brain abscess); (4) typhoid fever due to sensitive strains; and (5) Rocky Mountain spotted fever.

Clindamycin (Cleocin)

Use: Gram-positive organisms except *Streptococcus faecalis;* anaerobic organisms including *Bacteroides fragilis*. Some activity against methicillin-resistant staphylococci.

Dosage: 8–16 mg/kg/d for mild to moderate infections; 16–20 mg/kg/d for severe infections. Divide dosage into 3 or 4 equal doses. For adolescents, give 600–1200 mg/d in divided doses every 6 hours; for severe infections in adolescents, give 1200–1800 mg/d in divided doses every 6 hours. ***Caution:*** Do not use in infants under 1 month of age.

Incompatibility: Erythromycin, B complex vitamins.

Toxicity: Generally well tolerated. Toxic reactions include nausea, vomiting, diarrhea, and occasionally pseudomembranous colitis. Irreversible hematopoietic toxicity has been rarely reported. Skin rash appears to be relatively common. Transient elevations in alkaline phosphatase and serum transaminase levels usually return to normal during therapy.

Comment: This drug is structurally similar to lincomycin, with somewhat better and more rapid absorption after oral dosage and greater activity in vitro against staphylococci and pneumococci. It is active against α- and β-hemolytic streptococci but is only slightly more effective than erythromycin. It is not indicated for infections due to enterococci, gonococci, meningococci, or *Haemophilus influenzae* and is inactive against gram-negative rods.

Erythromycin

Use: Gram-positive cocci, clostridia, *Bordetella pertussis, Corynebacterium diphtheriae,* rickettsiae, *Brucella,* some *Bacteroides,* chlamydiae, *Legionella pneumophila.* Resistance of some group A streptococci and some pneumococci has been reported, although this is rare at present. May be of use in chronic bronchitis, cystic fibrosis, and some urinary tract infections because of action against L forms. Probably as effective as tetracycline for symptomatic relief of mycoplasmal infections, although the organisms continue to be shed.

Dosage:

Oral: 30–50 mg/kg/d in divided doses every 6 hours. For full-term newborns and premature infants, 20–40 mg/kg/d in divided doses every 6 hours.

Intramuscular or intravenous: 10–20 mg/kg/d intramuscularly in divided doses every 6 hours; 40–70 mg/kg/d intravenously in divided doses every 6 hours given over a period of 20–60 minutes. For full-term newborns and premature infants, 10 mg/kg/d intramuscularly or intravenously in divided doses every 12 hours. For adolescents, up to 2 g/d intramuscularly or intravenously; higher doses could be used in severe infections.

Incompatibility: Many other antibiotics, B complex vitamins.

Toxicity: Painful injection, gastrointestinal symptoms, candidiasis, drug fever. Estolate (Ilosone) is associated with intrahepatic cholestatic jaundice when treatment is for more than 10 days.

Comment: Do not use concomitantly with lincomycin. Peak serum levels from the estolate salt are higher than levels from other salts. Cerebrospinal fluid penetration is poor.

Ethambutol (Myambutol)

Use: Tuberculosis.

Dosage: 15 mg/kg/d; retreatment, 25 mg/kg/d for 60 days, then 15 mg/kg/d given in a single dose.

Toxicity: Retrobulbar neuritis (3%). Examine visual acuity and color discrimination each month. Anaphylactoid reactions. Peripheral neuritis. May cause hyperuricemia.

Comment: Experience in the pediatric age range is limited; ethambutol probably should not be given to children under age 3 years because it may cause eye damage. There is frequent development of resistance if the drug is used alone.

Ethionamide (Trecator)

Use: Effective in the treatment of tuberculosis and atypical mycobacterial infections.

Dosage: 15–20 mg/kg/d orally up to 0.75–1 g daily.

Toxicity: Anorexia, nausea, vomiting, diarrhea, mental depression, headache, asthenia, convulsions, peripheral neuropathy, acne, allergic skin reactions, purpura, sialorrhea, metallic taste, stomatitis, gynecomastia, impotence, menorrhagia, hepatitis, hair loss, goiter, and hypothyroidism.

Comment: To prevent serious hepatotoxicity, serum SGOT levels should be determined every month or more frequently and the drug stopped if the SGOT level exceeds 100 IU/L. Strongly encouraged patients must often endure unpleasant but nonserious side effects.

Flucytosine (Ancobon)

Use: Antifungal agent active against some strains of *Candida, Cryptococcus neoformans, Torulopsis glabrata.*

Dosage: 150 mg/kg/d orally in divided doses every 6 hours.

Comment: Ninety percent of the drug is excreted in the urine. Drug resistance has been reported during therapy. Sensitivity studies are indicated. Currently, it is suggested that patients on therapy be followed with blood creatinine, blood urea nitrogen, SGOT, serum alkaline phosphatase, hematocrit, and white blood count determinations. A synergistic effect between flucytosine and amphotericin B may be achieved if flucytosine is combined with small doses of amphotericin B.

Gentamicin (Garamycin)

Use: Most gram-negatives, including *Pseudomonas* and *Proteus*. Of particular use in *Serratia marcescens* infections. Some activity against gram-positives, including coagulase-positive staphylococci. Relatively inactive against pneumococci and streptococci.

Dosage:

Oral: 10–15 mg/kg/d (about 0.2% of a single dose is absorbed). May be of use in nursery outbreaks of diarrhea due to enteropathogenic *Escherichia coli* but is not recommended for routine use.

Topical: Cream, 0.1%, and ointment, 0.1%.

Intramuscular or intravenous: 5 mg/kg/d for newborn infants under 1 week of age; 7.5 mg/kg/d for those over 1 week of age. Intravenous administration should extend over a 30-minute period. In neonates and patients with renal failure, obtain serum levels during therapy, since individual variations occur. For urinary tract infections, 2–3 mg/kg/d in 2–3 divided doses is adequate.

Intraventricular: Unproved value.

Toxicity: Irreversible vestibular damage has occurred, most often in uremic patients, and is related to excessive plasma levels. There is considerable variability in the serum level achieved at the same dose per kilogram in different patients. Serum levels should be measured in any patient requiring long-term therapy. Transient proteinuria, elevated blood urea nitrogen levels, oliguria, azotemia, macular skin eruption, and elevated SGOT levels have been reported. If used in uremic patients, the dosage schedule should be modified. Should be used with caution in patients receiving ototoxic drugs. Overall toxicity is probably the same as or less than that of kanamycin.

Comment: Parenteral therapy with this drug should be reserved for serious *Pseudomonas* infections, hospital-acquired infections, and life-threatening infections of unknown but suspected gram-negative origin. If cultures later are positive for an organism sensitive to less toxic drugs, therapy should be changed to one of these drugs. Every effort should be made to use this drug selectively so that drug resistance will not develop. Relative resistance has developed during therapy. Topical therapy with gentamicin for superficial infections of the skin or mucous membranes due to *Pseudomonas* has been effective. To achieve synergy, gentamicin can be used in combination with a penicillin that is active against *Pseudomonas*.

Griseofulvin

Use: Determatophytosis due to *Epidermophyton*, *Microsporum*, *Trichophyton*.

Dosage: (For griseofulvin.) 20 mg/kg/d orally in divided doses every 6–12 hours. For microcrystalline (Grisactin), 10 mg/kg/d in divided doses every 6–12 hours. For adolescents, 1 g/d (griseofulvin); 0.5 g/d (Grisactin).

Toxicity: Leukopenia and other blood dyscrasias, headache, incoordination and confusion, gastrointestinal disturbances, rash (allergic and photosensitivity), renal damage, lupuslike syndrome.

Comment: Do not use in patients with hepatocellular failure or porphyria. Used primarily in scalp and nail infections when topical therapy is unsuccessful.

Isoniazid (INH, Nydrazid)

Use: Tuberculosis.

Dosage:

Oral: 15–20 mg/kg/d in divided doses every 6–12 hours. Give no more than 300 mg/d.

Intramuscular: 10 mg/kg/d in divided doses every 12 hours. For newborns up to 1 month of age, give 5–10 mg/kg/d. BCG vaccination may offer a better alternative than INH prophylaxis for the child of an infected mother.

Toxicity: Neurotoxic, owing to pyridoxine deficiency (rare in children). Gastrointestinal symptoms, seizures, hypersensitivity. Reactions are rare, but more common in the elderly and the malnourished.

Comment: Although it is generally stated that addition of pyridoxine to the treatment regimen is unnecessary in children, exceptions to this rule occur, and some authorities recommend routine supplementation with pyridoxine. Isoniazid may inhibit metabolism of phenytoin, thereby causing high serum levels.

Kanamycin (Kantrex)

Use: Bactericidal for staphylococci, coliforms, *Proteus,* some *Pseudomonas,* mycobacteria. Of use in special circumstances in some *Vibrio, Salmonella,* and *Shigella* infections. Inactive against streptococci, anaerobic bacteria, and *Pseudomonas aeruginosa.*

Dosage:

Oral: Not absorbed.

Intramuscular: 15 mg/kg/d in divided doses every 12 hours. For full-term newborns, 15 mg/kg/d. For premature infants, 10 mg/kg/d; avoid using intravenously. For adolescents, 1 g/d in divided doses every 12 hours.

Intravenous: 15–20 mg/kg/d in divided doses every 6–8 hours. (For serious infections only.) For adolescents with serious infections, 2 g/d intravenously for a short time.

Toxicity: Limit use to 10 days. Irreversible deafness occurs after prolonged administration of high doses. (Cumulative ototoxicity with other ototoxic drugs occurs.) Nephrotoxicity is transient unless prior renal impairment was present. The safe total dose is 0.5 g/kg.

Comment: Modify dosage and use with caution in oliguric patients.

Ketoconazole (Nizoral)

Use: An imidazole antifungal agent with a broad spectrum of activity against various superficial and deep fungal pathogens. Approved for use in patients with selected forms of candidiasis, coccidioidomycosis, histoplasmosis, chromomycosis.

Dosage: 200–400 mg orally every day for adults. For children weighing under 20 kg, 20–40 kg, or over 40 kg, dosage is 50 mg, 100 mg, or 200 mg, respectively, given orally every day.

Toxicity: Nausea, vomiting, and anorexia are relatively common. Rash, hepatocellular dysfunction, and thrombocytopenia have been reported.

Comment: Ketoconazole is an attractive alternative to amphotericin

B because it is administered orally and is less toxic. However, current studies have not shown ketoconazole to be superior to amphotericin B in the treatment of patients with severe, life-threatening systemic mycoses.

Lincomycin (Lincocin)

This drug is similar but inferior to clindamycin and has been supplanted by clindamycin for clinical use.

Mebendazole (Vermox)

Use: Drug of choice for trichuriasis; also active against hookworm, pinworm, ascaris.

Dosage: 100 mg orally twice daily for 3 days.

Toxicity: Transient abdominal pain, diarrhea.

Comment: The drug has not been studied well in children under age 2 years.

Methacycline (Rondomycin)

See Tetracyclines.

Methenamine Mandelate (Mandelamine)

Use: Genitourinary infections. Not effective against *Proteus*.

Dosage: 100 mg/kg orally immediately and then 50 mg/kg/d in divided doses every 8 hours.

Comment: Urine *must* be kept acid for the drug to be effective. Primarily used for suppression of chronic urinary tract infection.

Metronidazole (Flagyl)

Use: *Trichomonas, Giardia, Entamoeba histolytica,* anaerobic bacteria including *Bacteroides fragilis*.

Dosage: 250 mg orally every 8 hours for adults; 30 mg/kg/d in 3 divided doses for children.

Toxicity: Nausea, anorexia, and other gastrointestinal intolerance. Glossitis and stomatitis. Leukopenia, dizziness, vertigo, ataxia, urticaria, and pruritus.

Comment: Recent studies indicate an increase in malignant tumors and genetic mutations in animals treated with metronidazole. It should be used with caution and only when clearly indicated. When taken with alcohol, the so-called disulfiram reaction may occur.

Moxalactam (Moxam)

Use: Active against many enteric β-lactamases. Relatively inactive against gram-positive and anaerobic organisms. Primary use is in neonatal meningitis due to susceptible gram-negative organisms. May become a suitable alternative to chloramphenicol in ampicillin-resistant severe *Haemophilus influenzae* infections.

Dosage: 50 mg/kg intravenously every 12 hours for newborns 1 week or less of age, every 8 hours for neonates, or every 4–6 hours for infants and children.

Toxicity: Similar to that of cephalosporins. In patients with bleeding diathesis secondary to vitamin K deficiencies, prothrombin time should be monitored regularly.

Comment: Patients with gram-positive infection, particularly group B streptococcal meningitis, should *not* be treated with this agent.

Nalidixic Acid (NegGram)

Use: Useful only in gram-negative urinary tract infections with *Escherichia coli, Enterobacter, Klebsiella,* and *Proteus. Pseudomonas* is generally resistant.

Dosage: 40–50 mg/kg orally in divided doses 4 times daily for initial therapy. For prolonged therapy, reduce dosage to 15 mg/kg/d. For adolescents, give 4 g/d; in prolonged therapy, reduce to 2 g/d.

Toxicity: Gastrointestinal symptoms, hypersensitivity (pruritus, rash, urticaria, eosinophilia), seizures, pneumonitis.

Comment: Resistance may develop rapidly. Use cautiously in patients with liver disease or impaired renal function. Do not use in children under 1 month of age. Use *only* for urinary tract infections.

Neomycin (Mycifradin, Neobiotic)

Parenteral use is superseded by penicillinase-resistant penicillins. Since neomycin oral therapy has been reported to cause malabsorption states, its use is no longer recommended.

Nitrofurantoin (Furadantin)

Use: Many gram-negative organisms are susceptible to concentrations achieved in urine.

Dosage: 5–7 mg/kg/d orally. Reduce after 10–14 days to 2–4 mg/kg/d. For infants, 1.5 mg/kg/d. For adolescents, 300 mg every day in divided doses every 6 hours.

Toxicity: Primaquine-sensitive hemolytic anemia, peripheral neuropathy, rash, chills, fever, myalgialike syndrome, cholestatic jaundice.

Comment: Should only be used for urinary tract infections. Dosage should be reduced in patients with impaired renal function.

Nystatin (Mycostatin)

Use: *Candida albicans* and other yeasts.

Dosage:

Oral: Not absorbed. For children under 2 years of age, 400–800 thousand units/d; for those over 2 years of age, 1–2 million units/d in divided doses every 6–8 hours. For full-term newborns and premature infants, 200–400 thousand units/d.

Topical: 100 thousand units/g for eye or skin infection.

Toxicity: None.

Comment: Use orally *after* meals.

Oleandomycin

See Erythromycin.

The Penicillins

Because of protein binding, serum killing power is the preferred test of bacterial sensitivity and efficacy of therapy. All penicillins are cross-allergenic. The mechanism of action of tetracyclines and chloramphenicol is antagonistic to that of the penicillins. In serious infections, all penicillins should be given in divided doses so that a dose is given at least every 4 hours.

A. **Penicillins Rendered Ineffective by Staphylococcal Penicillinase:** (Ampicillin, carbenicillin, amoxicillin, penicillin G, procaine penicillin G, benzathine penicillin G, phenoxymethyl penicillin.)

1. Ampicillin–

Use: 50–80% of *Escherichia coli,* some salmonellae, shigellae, *Proteus*. *Enterobacter* and *Klebsiella* are usually resistant. Gram-positive cocci, nonpenicillinase-producing staphylococci, and *Haemophilus influenzae* are sensitive. *H influenzae* resistance is well documented and is increasing.

Dosage:

Oral: 50–150 mg/kg/d in divided doses every 6 hours.

Intramuscular or intravenous: 150–400 mg/kg/d in divided doses every 4 hours. Not stable in intravenous bottle. For meningitis, begin with at least 200 mg/kg/d in divided doses every 4 hours. For newborns, 100 mg/kg/d in divided doses every 6–8 hours. (For meningitis, a higher dose may be required.)

Toxicity: Low toxicity. Diarrhea, skin rash, drug fever. Superinfection.

Comment: Useful for genitourinary infections, chronic *Salmonella* carriers, and *H influenzae* meningitis. A loading dose of 50 mg/kg is desirable in serious infections. Contains about 1.7 mEq of sodium per 500 mg of drug. Ampicillin levels in the cerebrospinal fluid drop after the third day in meningitis as the pleocytosis decreases. Although ampicillin is usually effective, causes of resistance of *H influenzae* meningitis to intravenous therapy have been well documented. The drug must be given parenterally for the entire course. Patients with suspected *H influenzae* meningitis should be treated with chloramphenicol in addition until sensitivity is established.

2. Carbenicillin–

Use: Active against *Pseudomonas,* indole-positive *Proteus,* and *Serratia*. In general, its spectrum against gram-negative bacteria is comparable to that of ampicillin but is less active.

Dosage:

Oral: (For carbenicillin indanyl sodium [Geocillin].) 50–100 mg/kg/d in divided doses every 6 hours, up to 4 g/d, for urinary tract infection only.

Intravenous: 600 mg/kg/d in divided doses every 2–4 hours (not well established). For newborns, 400 mg/kg/d (not well established). For adolescents, up to 30 g/d.

Comment: Relatively high doses of this drug are required. Its main use is in *Pseudomonas* infections in patients with compromised renal function. SGOT level rises have been reported. This may be due to muscle necrosis after intramuscular injection. Carbenicillin is probably synergistic with gentamicin. Contains 6 mEq of Na^+ per gram.

3. Amoxicillin–

Use: Spectrum similar to ampicillin.

Dosage: 20–50 mg/kg/d orally in divided doses every 8 hours up to 1.5 g/d.

Comment: Better absorbed than ampicillin. Diarrhea less common than with ampicillin.

4. Penicillin G, potassium or sodium salt–

Use: Gram-positive and gram-negative cocci, gram-positive bacilli. In high doses, some gram-negative organisms.

Dosage:

Oral: 100–400 thousand units one-half hour before meals, 4 times daily.

Intramuscular: 20–50 thousand units/kg/d in divided doses every 4–6 hours.

Intravenous: 20–500 thousand units/kg/d in divided doses every 4 hours. For newborns, 50 thousand units/kg in divided doses every 8–12 hours.

Intrapleural or intraperitoneal: 10–20 thousand units mL.

Intrathecal or intraventricular: (Rare indications.) 5–10 mL/24 h (1000 units/mL).

Incompatibility: Do not mix with amphotericin B, metaraminol, phenylephrine, tetracyclines, vancomycin, vitamin C.

Toxicity: Hypersensitivity (anaphylaxis, urticaria, rash, drug fever). Change in bowel flora, candidiasis, diarrhea, hemolytic anemia. Neurotoxic in very large doses.

Comment: High concentration in the urine makes this agent useful in treatment of some urinary tract infections with gram-negative rods. One million units of potassium penicillin G contain 1.7 mEq of potassium. Avoid pushing large doses of potassium salt, as in initiating therapy for meningitis; use sodium salt instead.

5. **Procaine penicillin G–**

Dosage: 25–100 thousand units intramuscularly in divided doses every 12–24 hours up to 4.8 million units.

Toxicity: May cause sterile abscesses, particularly in newborns. Contains 120 mg of procaine per 300,000 units of penicillin G, which may be toxic.

6. **Benzathine penicillin G–**

Dosage: 0.6–1.2 million units intramuscularly every month.

Comment: The preferred drug for rheumatic fever prophylaxis. Increasing the dose gives a more sustained rather than a higher blood level.

7. **Phenoxymethyl penicillin–**

Dosage: 50–100 thousand units/kg/d orally every 6 hours up to 6 g/d. (125 mg = 200 thousand units.)

Comment: Stable in acid and therefore better absorbed than oral penicillin G. Not as effective as penicillin G against some *Neisseria*.

B. Penicillins Resistant to Staphylococcal Penicillinase: (Methicillin, nafcillin, oxacillin, cloxacillin, dicloxacillin.)

1. **Methicillin–**

Use: Penicillinase-producing staphylococci. Less effective than penicillin G for other gram-positive cocci.

Dosage: 200–300 mg/kg/d intravenously or intramuscularly in divided doses every 4 hours. Not stable in intravenous bottle. Deterioration in dextrose in water or normal saline solution is rapid and is prevented by adding $NaHCO_3$, 6 mEq/L. For full-term newborns, 200–250 mg/kg in divided doses every 6–8 hours for the first 10 days and then every 4–6 hours. For premature infants, 100 mg/kg in divided doses every 6–8 hours for the first 10 days and then every 6 hours.

Incompatibility: Do not mix with tetracyclines, kanamycin, neomycin.

Toxicity: Hypersensitivity, kidney damage, hematuria (thought to be a hypersensitivity phenomenon). Reversible bone marrow depression. Painful when given intramuscularly.

Comment: If therapy is initiated with methicillin because of suspected penicillin resistance, change to penicillin G when sensitivity to this agent is shown. One gram contains 2.5 mEq of sodium.

2. **Nafcillin–**

   Use: Staphylococci (penicillin-resistant and penicillin-sensitive), pneumococci, streptococci.

   Dosage: 50–250 mg/kg/d intramuscularly or intravenously in divided doses every 4 hours. For adolescents, up to 18 g/d. Oral doses are not recommended because absorption is unreliable.

   Incompatibility: Do not mix with B complex vitamins.

   Toxicity: Similar to that of methicillin. Thrombophlebitis with intravenous use.

   Comment: Good choice for coverage of gram-positive cocci before culture and sensitivity results are available.

3. **Oxacillin–**Cloxacillin and dicloxacillin are preferred.

4. **Cloxacillin–**

   Use: Penicillinase-producing staphylococci.

   Dosage: 50–100 mg/kg/d orally in divided doses every 6 hours given 1–2 hours before meals.

   Toxicity: Probably similar to that of other penicillins.

   Comment: Penicillinase-resistant. Dicloxacillin in equivalent dose is probably more active and better absorbed. For osteomyelitis, use a dosage of 100 mg/kg/d.

5. **Dicloxacillin–**

   Use: Penicillinase-producing staphylococci.

   Dosage: 25–50 mg/kg/d. In serious infections, begin with 50 mg/kg/d and reduce dosage if serum killing power indicates this is possible.

   Toxicity: Gastrointestinal irritation, which appears to be dose-related.

C. Penicillins Active Against *Pseudomonas*: (Carbenicillin, ticarcillin, mezlocillin, piperacillin, azlocillin.)

Use: Used primarily in patients at risk of acquiring severe *Pseudomonas* infections (eg, infection in an immunocompromised host, infection in a patient with severe burns or cystic fibrosis).

Dosage: For carbenicillin, see above. For mezlocillin and ticarcillin, 75 mg/kg intravenously every 12 hours in newborns less than 1 week of age, every 8 hours in neonates, or every 6 hours in infants and children. Dosages of piperacillin and azlocillin have not been established for use in pediatric patients.

Toxicity: Allergy (cross-reactive with other penicillins), thrombophlebitis, thrombasthenia. Sodium content of mezlocillin is less than that of the other drugs in this class.

Comment: Limited usefulness in most pediatric patients. Cost may be a factor in determining which drug to use.

Polymyxin B (Aerosporin)

Parenteral use of polymyxin B has been supplanted by use of aminoglycosides and penicillins effective against *Pseudomonas,* since these drugs are less toxic.

Rifampin

Use: *Neisseria, Haemophilus influenzae, Mycobacterium,* gram-positive cocci.

Dosage: Not available in solution owing to instability. For oral use, place contents of 300-mg capsule in tablespoon of applesauce or pudding; each teaspoon equals 100 mg. Dose is 15 mg/kg/d. For adults, 600 mg/d.

Toxicity: Occasionally rashes, cholestatic hepatitis. The drug imparts a harmless orange color to urine, sweat, tears, and contact lenses.

Comment: This drug's most striking contribution has been to the care of patients infected with multiple-resistant strains of *M tuberculosis.* Although the results have been remarkably good, when used alone the development of resistance is rapid; therefore, the drug should always be used in combination with one or 2 drugs to which the organisms are sensitive. It has also been found to be of value in the treatment of atypical mycobacterial infections. It may have a place in the therapy of the carrier of *N meningitidis* or *H influenzae* who poses a hazard. The drug has also been used with success in the treatment of infections with *N gonorrhoeae* and staphylococci but offers no advantage over other drugs.

Spectinomycin (Trobicin)

Use: *Neisseria gonorrhoeae.*

Dosage: 2 g intramuscularly as a single dose for adults; 35 mg/kg intramuscularly as a single dose for children.

Comment: Spectinomycin is in the same class of drugs as streptomycin and kanamycin. Toxicity reported after a single dose includes urticaria, dizziness, nausea, chills, fever, and insomnia. It is likely that the drug has some renal toxicity on prolonged use. Spectinomycin is not effective in eradicating concomitant incubating syphilis.

Streptomycin Sulfate

Use: *Mycobacterium tuberculosis, Haemophilus influenzae,* some gram-negatives. Synergistic with penicillin against enterococci. Resistance develops quickly.

Dosage:

Oral: Not absorbed. 40 mg/kg/d in divided doses every 6 hours.

Intramuscular: 20–40 mg/kg/d in divided doses every 12–24 hours. For newborns, 10–20 mg/kg/d. Use with caution.

Aerosol: 2 mL every 6 hours (150 mg/mL).

Toxicity: Damage to vestibular apparatus. Fatal central nervous system and respiratory depression. Bone marrow depression, renal toxicity, hypersensitivity, superinfection.

Comment: Should never be used as the only drug. Dihydrostreptomycin is toxic to the eighth nerve and should not be used. May be used in *H influenzae* meningitis if other drugs cannot be given.

Sulfonamides: Sulfadiazine, Sulfisoxazole (Gantrisin), Sulfamethoxazole (Gantanol), Trisulfapyrimidines, Trimethoprim With Sulfamethoxazole (Co-trimoxazole, Bactrim, Septra)

Use: Bacteriostatic against gram-negative organisms. Approximately 80% of shigellae are resistant. Trimethoprim-sulfamethoxazole (Bactrim, Septra) has a wide range of antibacterial activities but is primarily used for resistant *Salmonella typhi* and chronic urinary tract infections. It is also effective in prophylaxis and treatment of *Pneumocystis carinii* infections (trimethoprim, 20 mg/kg/d, with sulfamethoxazole, 100 mg/kg/d).

Dosage: (For sulfadiazine, triple sulfas, and sulfisoxazole.)

Oral: 120–150 mg/kg/d in divided doses every 6 hours.

Intravenous: 120 mg/kg/d in divided doses every 6–12 hours; alkalinize urine. For newborns, do not use (risk of kernicterus).

Dosage: (For sulfamethoxazole.) 50 mg/kg/d orally in divided doses every 12 hours.

Dosage: (For trimethoprim-sulfamethoxazole.) Capsule contains 80 mg of trimethoprim and 400 mg of sulfamethoxazole; pediatric suspension contains 20 or 40 mg of trimethoprim and 100 or 200 mg of sulfamethoxazole per 5 mL. Oral dosage is 150 mg/m^2/d of trimethoprim and 750 mg/m^2/d of sulfamethoxazole.

Toxicity: Crystalluria (mechanical urinary obstruction); keep fluid intake high. Hypersensitivity (fever, rash, hepatitis, lupuslike state, vasculitis). Neutropenia, agranulocytosis, aplastic anemia, thrombocytopenia. Hemolytic anemia in individuals deficient in glucose-6-phosphate dehydrogenase. (There is a high correlation between G6PD deficiency and sickle cell anemia, so do not use in these patients.) Trimethoprim-sulfamethoxazole may produce rashes and gastrointestinal or hematologic symptoms.

Comment: Useful in infections of the urinary tract and for rheumatic fever prophylaxis. (Should not be relied upon for treatment of group A streptococcal infections.) Sulfadiazine is preferred for central nervous system infections since diffusion into the cerebrospinal fluid is better. Sulfamethoxazole is intermediate-acting and causes a slightly higher incidence of urinary sediment abnormalities.

Tetracyclines

Use: Gram-positive and gram-negative bacteria, rickettsiae, chlamydiae, *Mycoplasma pneumoniae, Brucella,* some *Bacteroides.*

Dosage: (For tetracycline, chlortetracycline, and oxytetracycline.)

Oral: 20–40 mg/kg/d in divided doses every 6 hours. Do not give with milk.

Intramuscular: 12 mg/kg/d in divided doses every 12 hours; achieves poor levels; painful.

Intravenous: 12 mg/kg/d in divided doses every 12 hours.

Aerosol: 1 mL every 12 hours (50 mg/mL in 75% propylene glycol).

Dosage: (For demeclocycline [Declomycin] and methacycline [Rondomycin].) 12 mg/kg/d orally in divided doses every 6 hours. For newborns, do not use.

Incompatibility: Do not mix with amphotericin B, cephalothin, chloramphenicol, heparin, hydrocortisone, methicillin, penicillin G, polymyxin B.

Toxicity: In children under 7 years of age, tetracyclines cause damage to teeth and bone. Deposition in teeth and bone of premature and newborn infants can result in enamel dysplasia and growth retardation. Outdated tetracyclines can produce Fanconi's syndrome. Pseudotumor cerebri, bulging fontanelles. Nausea, vomiting, diarrhea, stomatitis, glossitis, proctitis, candidiasis. Overgrowth of staphylococci in bowel. Disturbed hepatic and renal functon. Drug fever, rash, photosensitivity.

Comment: Cross-resistance among the tetracyclines is complete.

Tobramycin (Nebcin)

Use: Semisynthetic aminoglycoside nearly identical to gentamicin in spectrum; is probably more active against *Pseudomonas aeruginosa* and less nephrotoxic than gentamicin.

Dosage:

Oral: Not well absorbed.

Intramuscular or intravenous: 3–5 mg/kg/d in divided doses every 8 hours.

Toxicity: Similar to that of gentamicin, although less nephrotoxic.

Vancomycin (Vancocin)

Use: Staphylococci, other gram-positive cocci, *Clostridium, Corynebacterium.* Main use is in treatment of pseudomembranous enterocolitis, methicillin-resistant staphylococcal infection, susceptible shunt infections, and penicillin-resistant pneumococcal infections.

Dosage:

Oral: Not absorbed. 2–4 g/d in divided doses every 6 hours.

Intravenous: 40 mg/kg/d. For adolescents, 2–3 g/d in divided doses every 4–6 hours.

Incompatibility: Do not mix with chloramphenicol, heparin, hydrocortisone, penicillin G.

Toxicity: Painful when given intramuscularly; do not use. Troublesome symptoms during intravenous administration include rash, chills, thrombophlebitis, and fever. Hypotension may result from infusion given too rapidly. Nephrotoxicity and irreversible ototoxicity have occurred. Does not interfere with the action of any known antibiotic.

Comment: Before the advent of the penicillinase-resistant antibiotics, vancomycin was used successfully in the treatment of subacute bacterial endocarditis, osteomyelitis, and serious soft tissue infections. It is effective orally in staphylococcal enterocolitis.

MODIFICATIONS OF ANTIBIOTIC DOSES FOR OLIGURIC PATIENTS

If creatinine clearance is less than 10 mL/min, the patient should receive a full loading dose and then half that dose at the intervals recommended in Table 6–3.

If creatinine clearance is greater than 10 mL/min but less than 40 mL/min, the intervals between doses should be half as long as those suggested below.

When possible, serum killing power or other means of measuring circulating antibioticlike activity should be used, as the recommendations below are based on the serum half-life after a single injection, and accumulation of partially degraded active metabolites may occur with some drugs in the uremic individual.

Patients with lowered creatinine clearance but with normal blood urea nitrogen or serum creatinine concentrations should be given ordinary therapeutic doses unless severe liver disease is present.

ANTIVIRAL CHEMOTHERAPY

Some therapeutic agents are available for viral infections. The following drugs have limited usefulness.

Table 6–3. Modifications of antibiotic doses for oliguric patients.*

Antibiotic	Modification of Dose Required in Uremia (Creatinine Clearance < 10 mL/min) Extent	Interval Between Doses
Ampicillin	Minor	8–10 h
Cephalothin	Minor	24 h
Chloramphenicol	None, except newborn and liver disease	8 h
Erythromycin	None	8 h
Gentamicin	Major	2–3 d
Isoniazid	Minor	8 h
Kanamycin	Major	3–4 d
Methicillin	Minor	8–10 h
Nafcillin	Minor	8–12 d
Nitrofurantoin	Avoid	
Penicillin G	Minor	8–10 h
Polymyxin B	Major	3–4 d
Streptomycin	Major	3–4 d
Sulfisoxazole	Minor	12–24 h
Tetracycline	Major	3–4 d
Vancomycin	Major	9 d

*Modified from Kunin CM: A guide to use of antibiotics in patients with renal disease. *Ann Intern Med* 1967;**67**:151.

Acyclovir (Zovirax)

Use: Selective antiviral activity against herpes simplex virus. For use in immunocompromised hosts or neonates with severe or systemic herpes simplex infections.

Dosage:

Intravenous: 5 mg/kg infused over 1 hour, every 8 hours, not to exceed 15 mg/kg/d.

Topical: Dermatologic ointment, 5% concentration.

Toxicity: Thrombophlebitis, rash, elevated creatinine, and encephalopathic changes characterized by lethargy, confusion, hallucinations, and seizures. Because acyclovir is preferentially taken up and selectively converted to the active form by herpesvirus-infected cells (and not by normal uninfected host cells), it has a lower potential for toxicity.

Comment: Best results are obtained with early diagnosis and treatment. The frequent application of topical ointment decreases viral shedding and may speed healing.

Amantadine (Symmetrel)

Use: Limited to prophylactic administration during identified A_2 influenza virus epidemics. Of questionable therapeutic value if given within 48 hours of onset of symptoms. Does not appear to interfere with immunity induced by vaccination.

Dosage: 3 mg/kg/d orally (do not exceed 150 mg/d) in 2 or 3 doses for children 1–9 years of age; 200 mg/d orally in 2 doses (total dose) for children 9–12 years of age; 200 mg/d orally in 1 or 2 doses for adults.

Toxicity: Central nervous system irritability (nervousness, insomnia, dizziness, lightheadedness, drunken feelings, slurred speech, ataxia, inability to concentrate). Occasional depression and feelings of detachment; blurred vision (heightened with higher dosage, 300–400 mg/d, in elderly); less commonly, dry mouth, gastrointestinal upset, skin rash. Rarely, tremors, anorexia, pollakiuria, nocturia.

Idoxuridine (Stoxil)

Use: At present, limited to acute superficial herpes simplex or vaccinia virus keratitis. Should be administered under an ophthalmologist's supervision. Some prefer concomitant local corticosteroid administration.

Dosage: Supplied as an 0.1% ophthalmic solution or an 0.5% ophthalmic ointment. Solution should be used initially; place 1 drop in each infected eye every hour while awake and every 2 hours at night; with definite improvement, decrease to every 2 hours around the clock and continue treatment for 3–5 days after healing appears to be complete. Ointment: Instill 5 times a day (every 4 hours), with last dose at midnight.

Toxicity: Too frequent administration leads to small punctate defects in the cornea. Ingestion of 15 mL of solution or 20 mg of ointment is not known to be associated with poisoning. Idoxuridine is no longer used systemically.

Vidarabine (Adenine Arabinoside)

Use: Active against a number of poxviruses and herpesviruses. Clinically useful in the treatment of varicella-zoster infection and herpes simplex encephalitis if treatment is begun early.

Dosage:

Intravenous: 15 mg/kg/d in a single dose infused over 12 hours.

Topical: Ophthalmic cream, 3% concentration.

Toxicity: Gastrointestinal disturbance, tremors, weakness. Thrombophlebitis is common, and slow infusions of dilute solutions are recommended.

Comment: Best results are obtained with early diagnosis and treatment. The institution of parenteral therapy after 72 hours of illness in a patient with systemic disease will result in limited clinical effect.

7 | Immunization Procedures, Vaccines, Antisera, & Skin Tests*

Active immunity may be conferred by the administration of immunizing products, antigens, or vaccines that stimulate the production of antibodies and induce cell-mediated reactions. It is often possible to combine these materials for administration; the use of a mixture of different antigens need not inhibit the response. When live virus vaccines are used, the original virus inoculum must replicate in order to stimulate active immunity.

Passive immunity is conferred by the administration of serum from animals, from human donors who have been actively immunized against the disease, or from human donors who have recovered from the disease. This immunity is transient and is used only when antibodies must be made available immediately and for a short time.

Useful general information for pediatricians is provided in the American Academy of Pediatrician's *Red Book,* 1982 (PO Box 1034, Evanston, IL 60204).

AGENTS CONFERRING ACTIVE IMMUNITY

PRECAUTIONS & CONTRAINDICATIONS

Precautions

A. Consent: Parents, guardians, and patients should be informed of the nature of the proposed immunization and should provide consent (ideally, written informed consent).

B. Storage and Dosage: Biologic products are susceptible to inactivation by heat and light, and proper storage is therefore essential. Directions regarding storage and dosage schedules are provided by the manufacturer in the package insert and must be followed carefully. Expiration dates should be observed. Complete records should be kept.

C. Method of Administration: Rigorous aseptic technique must be used. Any material containing adjuvant, alum, aluminum hydroxide, or phosphate must *only* be injected intramuscularly. A "sterile abscess"

*Revised with the assistance of Anne S. Yeager, MD.

is less likely to occur if the material is injected deeply into the tissue and the site of injection is massaged after the needle is withdrawn.

D. Adverse Reactions: Parents should be urged to report any adverse reactions (ie, reactions other than simple local tenderness). If a mild febrile response occurs, aspirin may be recommended. Any child with a severe reaction, especially high fever or central nervous system disturbance, must be carefully evaluated before further immunization is undertaken. Any child who develops a severe febrile reaction or central nervous system disturbance after receiving pertussis vaccine must *not* be given further pertussis vaccine injections; if such a reaction occurs after administration of diphtheria-tetanus-pertussis (DTP) vaccine, future immunization is limited to use of diphtheria-tetanus (DT) toxoid.

Contraindications

A. General: Always consult the manufacturer's package insert regarding contraindications.

B. Infection or Disease: Immunization should be deferred in an infant with a febrile respiratory infection or other infection or an apparent major disease. However, the presence of simple rhinorrhea or a "cold" need not interfere with routine immunization in infants.

C. Immune Deficiency: A child with suspected or established immune deficiency should be carefully evaluated. If there is a defect in cell-mediated immunity, live virus vaccines must *not* be administered.

D. Seizures or Convulsions: While children with developmental retardation can receive routine immunization, those subject to seizure disorders or to febrile convulsions must *not* receive pertussis vaccine. Children with central nervous system disorders that appear stable must be individually evaluated before immunization.

PRIMARY IMMUNIZATION OF CHILDREN NOT IMMUNIZED IN INFANCY

The recommended schedule for active immunization of children is shown in Table 7–1.

In a child under 7 years of age, live diphtheria-tetanus-pertussis vaccine (DTP) and live trivalent oral poliovaccine (TOPV) are given 3 times at intervals of 2 months. Combined measles, mumps, and rubella vaccine is administered at the same visit or midway between injections. Boosters of DTP and TOPV are desirable 1 year after the start of immunization (Table 7–1). Children over 7 years of age receive diphtheria-tetanus toxoid (Td) instead of DTP in an otherwise similar schedule. Those over 18 years of age should probably receive inactivated trivalent vaccine (Salk type) instead of TOPV for primary immunization, with booster injections as recommended by the manufacturer. The

Table 7–1. Recommended schedule for active immunization of children.*

Normal Infants and Children		Persons Not Immunized in Infancy (7–18 yr)	
Age	Product Administered or Test Recommended†	Schedule	Product Administered†
2 mo	DTP,‡ TOPV§	Initial	Td,// TOPV
4 mo	DTP, TOPV	1 mo later	Measles vaccine, mumps vaccine, rubella vaccine
6 mo	DTP, TOPV¶	2 mo later	Td, TOPV
15–19 mo	DTP, TOPV, measles vaccine, mumps vaccine, rubella vaccine,# tuberculin test**	6–12 mo later	Td, TOPV
4–6 yr (school entry)	DTP, TOPV, tuberculin test	14–16 yr of age	Td
Every 10 yr thereafter	Td//	Every 10 yr thereafter	Td

*Reproduced, with permission, from Jawetz E, Grossman M: Introduction to infectious diseases. Chap 21, pp 797–813, in: *Current Medical Diagnosis & Treatment 1983.* Krupp MA, Chatton MJ (editors). Lange, 1983.

†Follow manufacturer's directions for dose and precautions. A physician may choose to obtain informed consent for immunizations.

‡**DTP**: Toxoids of diphtheria and tetanus, aluminum-precipitated or aluminum hydroxide-adsorbed, combined with pertussis bacterial antigen. Three doses IM at 4- to 8-wk intervals. Fourth dose IM about 1 yr later. Not suitable for children over age 7 yr. A child who experiences any type of seizure after immunization should receive only diphtheria-tetanus (DT) vaccine subsequently. (Excerpt from: *Report,* 19th ed. Committee on Infectious Diseases, American Academy of Pediatrics, 1982.)

§**TOPV**: Trivalent (types I, II, and III) oral live poliomyelitis virus vaccine. Inactivated trivalent vaccine (Salk type) preferred for immunodeficient children, for children with immunodeficient members of the household, and for those initially immunized after age 18 yr, but not recommended for others.

//**Td**: Tetanus toxoid and diphtheria toxoid, purified, suitable for adults. This should be given every 7–10 yr.

¶Optional dose, if exposure to wild poliomyelitis virus is anticipated.

#Measles, mumps, and rubella vaccines are live vaccines of attenuated viruses grown in cell culture. They may be administered as a mixture or singly at 1-mo intervals. Persons who received measles vaccine (inactivated) before 1968 or before age 15 mo should be reimmunized with measles vaccine. Some physicians prefer to give rubella vaccine to prepubertal females (age 10–14 yr). These live vaccines are not recommended for severely immunodeficient children.

**It is desirable to give a tuberculin test prior to measles vaccination and at intervals thereafter, depending on probable risk of exposure.

References:

Cody CL et al: Adverse reactions associated with DTP and DT administration. *Pediatrics* 1981;**68**:650.

Committee on Control of Infectious Diseases: *Report,* 19th ed. American Academy of Pediatrics, 1982.

Immunization Practices Advisory Committee, Centers for Disease Control: Diphtheria, tetanus and pertussis. *Ann Intern Med* 1981;**95**:723.

rationale for use of different toxoids is based on the following factors: (1) Older children have a higher risk of febrile reactions to pertussis vaccine and a lower risk of severe pertussis; (2) in older children, a reduced dose of highly purified diphtheria toxoid will ensure a low rate of hypersensitivity reactions while still providing effective immunization; and (3) live poliovaccine strains may carry a slightly higher risk of disease if they are administered to adults not previously immunized.

IMMUNIZATION OF INSTITUTIONALIZED CHILDREN

Institutionalized children should receive the immunizations recommended in Table 7–1. In addition, influenza virus vaccine, repeated annually, may be desirable (see below). Immune globulin for hepatitis A may be desirable (Table 7–2). No definitive recommendations exist regarding hepatitis B vaccine for patients at present. Pneumococcal polyvalent polysaccharide vaccine and meningococcal A and C vaccine may be considered for use in some children under special circumstances (see below).

IMMUNIZATIONS FOR ALL CHILDREN

Diphtheria

Immunization against diphtheria is effected by administration of toxoid to stimulate antitoxin production. Levels of antitoxin are related to immunity against disease, but they do not protect against the carrier state.

A. Diphtheria (D): This toxoid is used only when combined preparations are contraindicated.

B. Diphtheria-Tetanus (DT) (Pediatric): This preparation is adsorbed for delayed absorption. It contains the same materials as DTP (below) and is used in children who cannot receive pertussis vaccine. Three doses of 0.5 mL are given intramuscularly at 4–8 week intervals, with a booster injection 6–12 months later. DT toxoid should not be given to adults.

C. Diphtheria-Tetanus (Td) (Adult): This preparation contains less diphtheria toxoid than does DT and rarely produces reactions in older children and adults. The dose is 0.5 mL intramuscularly, given at intervals shown in Table 7–1.

D. Diphtheria-Tetanus-Pertussis (DTP): This vaccine is used routinely in infants and children. It combines diphtheria and tetanus toxoids with a suspension of *Bordetella pertussis* organisms. Three doses of 0.5 mL are given intramuscularly at 2-month intervals; the first

Table 7–2. Materials available for passive immunization.*

Indication	Product	Dosage	Comments
Black widow spider bite	Black widow spider antivenin, equine.	One vial (6000 units) IM or IV.	Use should be limited to children < 15 kg, the only group with significant morbidity or mortality. Available from Merck Sharp & Dohme.
Botulism	ABE polyvalent antitoxin, equine. (Hexavalent ABCDEF, bivalent AB, and monovalent E antitoxins are also available.)	One vial IV and 1 vial IM; repeat after 2–4 h if symptoms worsen, and after 12–24 h.	For treatment of botulism. Available from CDC.† Twenty percent incidence of serum reactions. Prophylaxis is not routinely recommended but may be given to asymptomatic persons with unequivocal exposure.
Diphtheria	Diphtheria antitoxin, equine.	20,000 (1 vial)–120,000 units depending on severity and duration of illness; may be given IM or ½ IM and ½ IV.	For treatment of diphtheria. Active immunization and (perhaps) erythromycin prophylaxis should be given to nonimmune contacts of active cases. Contacts should be observed for signs of illness so that antitoxin may be administered if needed. Also available from CDC.†
Gas gangrene	Gas gangrene antitoxin, polyvalent, equine.		Clinically ineffective; no longer manufactured. Not recommended for use.
Hepatitis A ("infectious")	Immune globulin.	0.02 mL/kg IM as soon as possible after exposure up to 6 wk. A protective effect lasts about 2 mo. For chronic exposure, a dose of 0.1 mL/kg is recommended every 6 mo.	Modifies but does not prevent infection. Recommended for household contacts and other contacts of similar intensity. Not office or school contacts unless an epidemic appears to be in progress. Also recommended for travel to endemic areas. Personnel of mental institutions, facilities for retarded children, and prisons are at risk of acquiring hepatitis A, as are those who work with nonhuman primates.

Hepatitis B ("serum")	Hepatitis B immune globulin (regular immune globulin may be effective as well).	0.06 mL/kg IM as soon as possible after exposure, preferably within 7 d. A second injection should be given 25–30 d after exposure. (Dose of immune globulin uncertain; 0.1–0.2 mL/kg suggested.)	Administer to nonimmune individuals as postexposure prophylaxis following either parenteral exposure to or direct mucous membrane contact with HBsAg-positive materials. Should not be given to persons already demonstrating anti-HBsAg antibody. Administration of various live virus vaccines should be delayed for at least 2 mo. A single dose of 0.13 mL/kg is given to newborns of mothers who develop hepatitis B in the third trimester and who are seropositive at time of delivery.
Hepatitis non-A non-B	Immune globulin.	0.02–0.04 mL/kg IM as soon as possible after exposure.	Give to individuals with parenteral exposure to sera from patients with hepatitis, or other close contacts.
Hypogammaglobulinemia	Immune globulin.	0.6 mL/kg IM every 3–4 wk.	Give double dose at onset of therapy. Immune globulin is of no value in prevention of frequent infections in the absence of demonstrable hypogammaglobulinemia.
Measles	Immune globulin (measles immune globulin no longer available).	0.25 mL/kg IM as soon as possible after exposure. Immunoincompetent patients should receive 20–30 mL.	Live measles vaccine will usually prevent natural infection if given within 48 h following exposure. If immune globulin is administered, delay immunization with live virus for 3 mo.
Mumps	Mumps immune globulin, human.	1.5 mL IM for child; 4.5 mL for > 12 yr of age.	Efficacy doubtful; no longer available.
Pertussis	Pertussis immune globulin.	1.5 mL IM (child).	Efficacy doubtful, both for treatment as well as prophylaxis. Available from Cutter Laboratories.

*Modified and reproduced, with permission, from Cohen SN: Immunization. Chapter 39 in: *Basic & Clinical Immunology,* 4th ed. Stites DP et al (editors). Lange, 1982.

†Centers for Disease Control, (404) 329–3670 during the day, (404) 329–2888 nights, weekends, and holidays.

Note: Passive immunotherapy or immunoprophylaxis should always be administered as soon as possible after exposure to the offending agent. Immune antisera and globulin are always given IM unless otherwise noted. Always question carefully and test for hypersensitivity before administering animal sera (see text).

Table 7–2 (cont'd). Materials available for passive immunization.*

Indication	Product	Dosage	Comments
Poliomyelitis	Immune globulin.	0.15 mL/kg IM.	Indicated only for exposed, unimmunized subjects. Immunize with live or inactivated vaccine after 2–3 mo, with subsequent boosters.
Rabies	Rabies immune globulin. (Equine antirabies serum is available but is much less desirable and requires a higher dose.)	20 IU/kg, up to half of which is infiltrated locally at the wound site, and the remainder given IM.	Give as soon as possible after exposure. Recommended for all bite or scratch exposures to bat, skunk, fox, coyote, or raccoon, despite animal's apparent health, if the brain cannot be immediately examined and found rabies-free. Not recommended for individuals with demonstrated antibody response from preexposure prophylaxis. Must be combined with rabies immunization. Also available through CDC.†
Rh isoimmunization (erythroblastosis fetalis)	Rh_0 (D) immune globulin.	One dose IM within 72 h of abortion, amniocentesis, obstetric delivery of an Rh-positive infant, or transfusion of Rh-positive blood in an Rh_0 (D)-negative woman.	For nonimmune females only. May be effective even if more than 72 h have elapsed. One vial contains 300 μg antibody and can reliably inhibit the immune response to a fetomaternal bleed of 7.5–8 mL as estimated by the Betke-Kleihauer smear technique.
Rubella	Immune globulin.	20–40 mL IM at time of exposure.	Prevents disease in recipient but ***not*** in fetus of exposed mother—hence not recommended.
Snakebite	Coral snake antivenin, equine. Crotalid (pit viper) antivenin, polyvalent, equine.	At least 3–5 vials IV (preferred) or IM.	Dose should be sufficient to reverse symptoms of envenomation. Consider antitetanus measures as well. Available from Wyeth Laboratories ([215] 688–4400) or CDC.†

Tetanus	Tetanus immune globulin. (Bovine and equine antitoxins are available but are not recommended. They are used at 10 times the dose of tetanus immune globulin.)	Prophylaxis: 250–500 units IM. Therapy: 3000–6000 units IM.	Give in separate syringe at separate site from simultaneously administered toxoid. Recommended only for major or contaminated wounds in individuals who have had fewer than 2 doses of toxoid at any time in the past (fewer than 3 doses if wound is more than 24 h old or otherwise highly tetanus-prone).
Vaccinia	Vaccinia immune globulin.	Prophylaxis: 0.3 mL/kg IM. Therapy: 0.6 mL/kg IM. May be repeated as necessary for treatment and at intervals of 1 wk for prophylaxis.	May be useful in treatment of vaccinia of the eye, eczema vaccinatum, generalized vaccinia, and vaccinia necrosum and in the prevention of such complications in exposed patients with skin disorders. Available from CDC.†
Varicella	Varicella-zoster immune globulin or zoster immune globulin.	3–5 mL IM within 96 h of exposure.	Available for nonimmune immunosuppressed or immunoincompetent children under 15 yr of age who have household, hospital (same 2- or 4-bed room or adjacent beds in large ward), or playmate (> 1 h play indoors) contact with a known case of varicella-zoster, and for neonates whose mothers have developed varicella within 4 d before or 48 h after delivery. The products modify natural disease. Immune globulin, 0.6–1.2 mL/kg IM, also may modify the illness. Available from local American Red Cross chapters. For information, contact main office, (617) 731–2130.

*Modified and reproduced, with permission, from Cohen SN: Immunization. Chapter 39 in: *Basic & Clinical Immunology*, 4th ed. Stites DP et al (editors). Lange, 1982.

†Centers for Disease Control, (404) 329–3670 during the day, (404) 329–2888 nights, weekends, and holidays.

Note: Passive immunotherapy or immunoprophylaxis should always be administered as soon as possible after exposure to the offending agent. Immune antisera and globulin are always given IM unless otherwise noted. Always question carefully and test for hypersensitivity before administering animal sera (see text).

dose is usually given when the infant is 2 months of age (Table 7–1). Booster doses are given at 15–19 months and 4–6 years of age. Thereafter, the pertussis component of the vaccine is eliminated. DTP and live virus vaccines can be given during the same office visit but at different sites of injection.

Measles

Live attenuated measles virus vaccine is grown in cell culture. The vaccine is given as a single dose in a child 15–19 months of age and generally provides permanent immunity. The manufacturer's directions should be followed.

The "further attenuated" measles virus vaccine (Moraten strain) is the only vaccine currently available in the USA. It produces negligible side effects and does not require simultaneous administration of measles immune globulin. Infants under 15 months of age should *not* receive vaccine. Those who received vaccine before 15 months of age in the past or who received inactivated vaccine in the past should be reimmunized with live vaccine, particularly when there is known risk of exposure to measles. In epidemic situations, children 6–15 months of age should also be immunized; they should be given a second dose of live vaccine after 15 months of age.

Contraindications to measles vaccine include pregnancy, immunodeficiency, immunosuppression, recent administration of immune globulin, and known hypersensitivity to materials in the vaccine (ie, those listed in the manufacturer's package insert).

Inactivated measles virus vaccine alters immunologic reactivity and should *not* be used. This vaccine is not available in the USA.

Mumps

Mumps is usually benign but can be accompanied by aseptic meningitis, pancreatitis, orchitis, or oophoritis. Live vaccine confers immunity.

Live attenuated mumps vaccine is a chick embryo-adapted virus. It is dispensed as a freeze-dried powder that must be reconstituted before administration. (Follow manufacturer's directions.) Mumps vaccine is usually combined with live measles and rubella vaccines (mumps-measles-rubella vaccine [MMR]) for administration to infants.

Contraindications are listed in the manufacturer's package insert and include immunodeficiency, hypersensitivity to eggs, and all contraindications (listed above) for measles vaccine.

Pertussis

Immunization with suspensions of phase I *Bordetella pertussis* prepared as vaccine can effectively reduce the risk of clinical pertussis. Usually, infants are immunized with DTP, and children over 6 years of age do not receive pertussis vaccine. Any child who develops a severe febrile reaction or central nervous system involvement after receiving pertussis vaccine must *not* be given pertussis vaccine again and should subsequently receive DT or Td.

Poliomyelitis

Live trivalent oral poliovaccines (TOPV) provide effective immunity and are the choice for immunization of infants in most countries. Some countries (eg, Sweden) utilize repeated injections of inactivated poliovaccines (IPV).

A. Live Poliovaccine (Sabin): Attenuated strains of virus types I, II, and III are grown in cell culture. Standardized suspensions of virus are stored frozen until they are administered orally (oral poliovaccine [OPV]). TOPV is commonly administered to infants 3 times at 2-month intervals. This usually assures development of antibodies and immunity to all 3 types of viruses. Boosters are frequently given at 15–19 months and at 4–6 years of age; they may be given later in life under special circumstances (eg, travel to endemic regions, an outbreak of poliomyelitis).

Live monovalent vaccines are not available in the USA but can be obtained from the Centers for Disease Control and public health departments for use in epidemic situations.

B. Inactivated Poliovaccine (Salk): Mixtures of all 3 types of viruses grown in cell culture and inactivated by formaldehyde (IPV) are available. Although IPV is not generally recommended, it is the preparation of choice for immunization of immunodeficient children, for primary vaccination of persons over 18 years of age, and for immunocompromised adults. The manufacturer's directions regarding dosage schedule should be followed.

Rubella

Rubella is a benign disease in children, but infection in pregnant women and the resulting fetal infection can have catastrophic consequences. Maternal antibodies can fully protect the fetus.

It is urged that all infants be given live attenuated rubella vaccine (strain RA 27/3 grown in diploid cells), usually in combination with live measles vaccine (see above). The manufacturer's directions should be followed.

Rubella vaccine is sometimes given to prepubertal girls. It is sometimes given to nonpregnant, susceptible women (ie, those with negative serologic test results) who are using effective methods of contraception. The vaccine strain occasionally has been isolated from placental tissues of women inadvertently vaccinated during pregnancy, but no fetal abnormalities have been definitely associated with such an occurrence.

Tetanus

Tetanus toxoid is an excellent immunizing agent. Every child should receive adsorbed tetanus toxoid during infancy, usually administered in the form of DTP vaccine (see under Diphtheria, above, and Table 7–1). Older children and adults receive Td or booster injections of purified tetanus toxoid (T) every 7–10 years. More frequent boosters may be accompanied by local hypersensitivity reactions.

IMMUNIZATIONS FOR CHILDREN WITH SPECIAL INDICATIONS

Cholera

For children traveling to or residing in areas where cholera is endemic (or for travel to countries that require a certificate of cholera vaccination), suspensions of killed *Vibrio cholerae* can be given in doses recommended by the manufacturer. The vaccine gives only partial resistance and must be repeated at 6-month intervals. Control of sanitation and use of chemoprophylaxis are also necessary. The vaccine is not recommended in the control of cholera outbreaks.

Influenza

Epidemic influenza A or B may cause serious respiratory disease in infants or children with cardiac, pulmonary, metabolic, renal, or neurologic disease. Children at increased risk also include those with chronic cardiovascular and respiratory diseases, immunodeficiency, and immunosuppression. Institutionalized children or those in child-care centers are at special risk. For these individuals, influenza vaccines may reduce the risk of serious illness or complications. *Only* children at increased risk should receive the vaccine. Routine immunization is not recommended for normal healthy infants and children.

The subtypes of influenza A and B to be incorporated into vaccines are selected every year, based on the strains expected to circulate during the next season. Viruses are grown in embryonated chicken eggs, purified, chemically inactivated, and made into ''split'' virus products. To avoid severe febrile reactions, only the split virus form of vaccine should be given to children. More than one injection is usually required for primary immunization. Boosters are indicated every year. The manufacturer's directions for dosage regimen and precautions should be followed. Hypersensitivity to eggs is a contraindication.

Meningococcal Meningitis

Polysaccharide preparations derived from meningococcus groups A and C are available. They can provide resistance against infection in children over 2 years of age but are not employed for routine immunization. They are given principally when an outbreak of meningococcal meningitis is imminent or if an individual plans to visit or reside in a country with epidemic meningococcal disease. The manufacturer's directions for dosage regimens should be followed.

Plague

For children traveling to or residing in areas where plague is highly endemic, suspensions of killed *Yersinia pestis* can be given in doses recommended by the manufacturer. Control of exposure to vectors and use of chemoprophylaxis are necessary.

Pneumococcal Pneumonia

A mixture of capsular polysaccharides from 14 types of pneumococci, including those that account for about 80% of bacteremic infections, is available. This preparation is not recommended for routine immunization. It should be considered for use in children at high risk of death from pneumococcal infection and in children over 2 years of age who suffer from sicklemia, asplenia, nephrosis, and B-cell immunodeficiencies. While the vaccine is well tolerated in children, those under 2 years of age often fail to develop adequate antibody responses; these children in high-risk groups must receive penicillin prophylaxis against life-threatening pneumococcal infections. A few children between 2 and 6 years of age may also require additional penicillin prophylaxis. The manufacturer's directions for dosage regimen, limitations, and side effects should be followed.

Rabies*

Rabies develops following bites by rabid animals. It is almost always fatal. Because the disease is so feared, many persons receive rabies treatment after contact with an animal even when the chance may be very small that the animal was rabid.

A. Human Diploid Cell (HDC) Vaccine:

1. Postexposure immunization–Before HDC vaccine was developed, decisions about whom to immunize were more difficult to make. They are made easier now because the vaccine is prepared from human diploid cells, requires only 5 injections, regularly stimulates a good antibody response, and is virtually free from significant neurologic side effects.

Rabies vaccine (HDC, killed virus) is given to the patient on days 0, 3, 7, 14, and 28 after "significant exposure." A wild animal bite or scratch is considered a "significant exposure," but other exposures must

*Consultation regarding rabies is available from the Centers for Disease Control; telephone (404) 329-3696 or (404) 329-3670 during the day or (404) 329-2888 during nights, weekends, and holidays.

be evaluated on the basis of individual circumstances and epidemiologic considerations. The manufacturer's directions for use of the vaccine must be followed. The bite wound must always be cleansed and flushed, and when use of rabies immune globulin is indicated, part of the immune globulin must be injected around the bite wound (Table 7–2).

2. Preexposure prophylaxis–HDC vaccine is indicated when there is a substantial risk of exposure to rabid animals (eg, in persons residing in areas of high endemicity). Prophylaxis involves 3 injections in 3–4 weeks.

B. Duck Embryo Vaccine: Inactivated vaccine prepared from rabies virus grown in duck embryo tissue is no longer manufactured in the USA. That preparation, as well as vaccines derived from other animal tissues, may be available in other countries. Manufacturer's directions must be followed, and the risk of allergic encephalomyelitis from the vaccine must be considered. Numerous and frequent injections (eg, 23 injections) are often required, and the efficacy of vaccines such as these is not well established.

Rickettsiae (Typhus & Rocky Mountain Spotted Fever)

Inactivated suspensions of the rickettsiae of typhus and of Rocky Mountain spotted fever have been used for immunization against these infections in individuals at special risk. At present, such vaccines are not available; new, more immunogenic preparations are being developed.

Smallpox

Live vaccinia virus was long used and was highly effective for the prevention of smallpox. It was a major factor in the eradication of that disease from the world in 1980. At present, no indication exists for the use of this vaccine in civilians. However, since military personnel are still being immunized with the vaccine, it is important to be aware of complications of vaccinia. The vaccine should never be given to persons with eczema, other forms of dermatitis, or impaired cell-mediated immunity, because it may produce eczema vaccinatum, vaccinia necrosum, or postvaccinial encephalitis.

Tuberculosis

Bacille Calmette-Guérin (BCG) is an attenuated strain of *Mycobacterium bovis;* different substrains of the organism are produced as vaccine in different countries. These substrains exhibit marked differences in invasiveness or immunogenicity. Administration of BCG is limited to individuals who have negative results in the tuberculin skin test and who are at very high risk of infection (eg, persons exposed to infective tuberculosis in the family). The manufacturer's directions must be followed. Use of BCG varies widely in different countries, depending on socioeconomic conditions and on available measures for medical and public health control of active tuberculosis. Any form of immune deficiency is an absolute contraindication to the administration of BCG. The proposed effect of BCG is the substitution of an attenuated strain, which can give partial resistance during primary infection, for a wild virulent strain. The tuberculin skin test in a child injected with BCG will yield positive results, at least temporarily. Therefore, the skin test cannot be used as a means for the early detection of infection. BCG organisms resistant to isoniazid (INH) have been produced. Thus, children with continued heavy exposure to tuberculosis can be treated with INH after BCG vaccination.

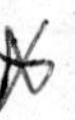

Typhoid

For children traveling to areas where exposure to typhoid is likely, suspensions of killed *Salmonella typhi* can be given as immunization, as recommended by the manufacturer. The most effective vaccines can transform a serious infection into a mild or subclinical one. To maintain resistance, booster injections are required at intervals.

Varicella

A vaccine of live attenuated varicella-zoster, Towne 125 strain, has been proposed for use in susceptible immunosuppressed children receiving chemotherapy for neoplasia. This vaccine is currently under evaluation and appears to be protective and relatively safe.

Yellow Fever

For children residing in or visiting areas where yellow fever is endemic, a single injection of live attenuated vaccine (consisting of the 17D strain of yellow fever virus) is indicated. The vaccine is administered only by certain public health officials and may be repeated 6–8 years later. A valid certificate for yellow fever vaccination is required for travel to some countries.

MATERIALS USED FOR PASSIVE IMMUNIZATION

ADMINISTRATION OF ANIMAL SERA

Precautions

A. History: Before the administration of animal sera to a patient, routine inquiry should be made regarding the history of allergy in the patient or the patient's family and whether such sera have been administered previously. Reactions due to horse serum sensitivity, while not frequent, may be severe, especially in an allergic patient who is known to be sensitive to horse dander.

B. Testing for Sensitivity: Intradermal and conjunctival sensitivity tests should be performed routinely. They must be done if the history suggests or indicates allergy.

1. Procedure–Give 0.05 mL of 1:10 dilution of serum in normal saline intradermally and 2 drops into the conjunctival sac of one eye. Readings are made at 20 minutes.

2. Results–A positive eye reaction consists of a marked reddening of the conjunctiva. Local corticosteroid therapy is indicated. A positive skin reaction consists of pseudopod formation with erythema larger than 1.5 cm. If a reaction is positive, serum must be administered cautiously, or (preferably) the patient must first be desensitized (hyposensitized). In general, the conjunctival test is more sensitive than the skin test.

Desensitization (Hyposensitization)

The salient feature in the production of desensitization (hyposensitization) is the administration of a series of divided doses of the serum. In the presence of sensitivity, proceed as follows: Initially, give no more than 0.1 mL of the serum subcutaneously. Double the dose every 20 minutes until a total of 1.6 mL has been given. Absorption may be delayed by the use of a tourniquet if the local reaction is too severe. Twenty minutes after the last dose, give 0.1 mL of serum diluted 1:20 in a saline solution intramuscularly or very slowly intravenously. Double the dose after 20 minutes, and repeat the procedure at 20-minute intervals until the full dose has been administered.

If a reaction occurs, the previous dosage is repeated but not until all signs and symptoms have disappeared.

If untoward symptoms become severe, inject epinephrine hydrochloride, 1:1000, 0.2–0.5 mL subcutaneously. Desensitization should be discontinued altogether if severe reactions follow each successive dose. The temporary use of parenteral hydrocortisone should be considered in the presence of any sensitivity.

Reduction of Serum Reactions

A. Dilution: Unpleasant serum reactions may be reduced by diluting the serum 10–20 times with 5 or 10% glucose in physiologic saline or by injecting the serum slowly into the tubing of the infusion apparatus during administration of intravenous fluids.

B. Retarding Absorption: The intramuscular administration of animal serum is best made into the anterior thigh in order to allow tourniquet application to retard absorption if a reaction occurs.

C. Drugs: Antihistaminic substances may be given prophylactically 1 hour before administration and repeated as required. The following may also be given intravenously with antiserum when diluted:

chlorpheniramine, 2–10 mg intravenously; diphenhydramine, 2–10 mg intravenously; and tripelennamine, 5–25 mg intravenously. (Intramuscular or subcutaneous administration requires no dilution.)

Treatment of Reactions

Epinephrine hydrochloride, 1:1000, should always be on hand for immediate use. Give 0.2–0.5 mL intramuscularly.

Hydrocortisone orally or intravenously is of no immediate use but may minimize late reactions. (For children with a history of previous reactions, hydrocortisone may be given prophylactically at the time of administration.)

SKIN TESTS

Blastomycin Skin Test

This test is no longer used. Diagnosis is by culture.

***Brucella* Skin Test**

This test is of little use. Diagnosis is by culture and serology.

Chancroid Skin Test (Ducrey Test)

This test is no longer used. Diagnosis is by smear and culture.

Coccidioidin Skin Test

A. Test Material: A 1:100 dilution of the filtrate obtained from a culture of *Coccidioides immitis* grown in a synthetic medium. Spherulin (derived from spherules of *Coccidioides* in culture) is more sensitive but less specific than coccidioidin as a skin testing material.

B. Indications: For detecting sensitivity to *C immitis*. The test does not evoke humoral antibodies.

C. Dosage and Administration: The 1:100 material is injected intradermally and read at 24 and 48 hours. Patients with coccidioidal erythema nodosum are likely to be very sensitive; therefore, an initial testing with 1:10,000 dilution is advisable. If this is negative, 1:100 can be used.

D. Results and Interpretation: Induration over 5 mm in diameter at either 24 or 48 hours is considered positive. Positive reactions may be obtained 2–3 weeks after infection and remain positive for many years.

Histoplasmin Skin Test

A. Test Material: Culture filtrate of *Histoplasma capsulatum*.

B. Indications: For epidemiologic studies. The histoplasmin skin test stimulates a rise in antibodies and is therefore rarely employed in diagnosis. There are probably cross-reactions with other fungi. Serologic tests have taken the place of the histoplasmin skin test.

C. Dosage and Administration: 0.1 mL of a 1:100 dilution is injected intradermally and read at 48 and 72 hours.

D. Results and Interpretation: The reaction is positive if at either reading the area of induration is more than 5 mm in diameter.

Toxoplasma Skin Test

A. Test Material: Extract of killed *Toxoplasma* organisms.

B. Indications: For detecting past or present *Toxoplasma* infection in epidemiologic surveys. The test is not used clinically and has been replaced by serologic tests for diagnosis.

C. Dosage and Administration: 0.1 mL of a 1:500 dilution is injected intradermally and read in 24–48 hours.

D. Results and Interpretation: Present or past infection is indicated by redness and swelling more than 5 mm in diameter. False-positive results do occur.

Tuberculin Skin Test (Mantoux Test)

A. Test Material: Purified protein derivative of tuberculin (PPD). PPD is a highly purified protein fraction isolated from culture filtrates of human type strains of *Mycobacterium tuberculosis*. It is supplied in first, intermediate, and second test strengths.

B. Indications: For determination of tuberculin sensitivity.

C. Dosage and Administration: Injections should be made intradermally on the flexor surface of the forearm so as to raise a small bleb. Care should be taken to avoid injecting tuberculin subcutaneously. If this occurs, no local reaction develops and a general febrile reaction may result.

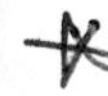

The recommended method for Mantoux testing with PPD is as follows: (1) When tuberculous illness is suspected, inject 0.1 mL of first strength PPD intradermally. If the result is negative, the test is repeated with intermediate strength PPD (a strength representing a 5-fold increase in PPD concentration, or equal to 5 "tuberculin units" [5 TU]). If old tuberculin (OT) is used, begin with a 1:1000 dilution. (2) For survey purposes, in the absence of illness suggestive of tuberculosis, begin with intermediate strength PPD (5 TU). Young children rarely develop severe cutaneous reactions, and thus it is appropriate to start with intermediate strength.

D. Results and Interpretation: A definite palpable induration of 10 mm or more is considered positive. Erythema alone must be disregarded, and readings are best made at 72 hours. Young children may have indurations of less than 10 mm. Such smaller indurations cannot be disregarded in children in the USA, where only 0.5% of children entering kindergarten have positive reactions. Children with findings compatible with tuberculosis should be treated even when the Mantoux test results in an induration smaller than 10 mm. Once a child has exhibited a positive result in the tuberculin skin test, the test should not be repeated.

Negative results in the Mantoux test occur in patients with measles and other viral illnesses, persons who have received live virus vaccines, and patients who are immunosuppressed or immunocompromised. False-positive results in the Mantoux test (often indurations of small diameter) occur in patients with infections due to nontuberculous mycobacteria.

Tuberculin Skin Test (Tine Test)

A. Test Material: Dried purified protein derivative of tuberculin (PPD) or old tuberculin (OT) on disposable metal tines.

B. Indications: For screening apparently healthy groups. This test should not be used for diagnosis of tuberculosis. It is less sensitive and less specific than the intradermal Mantoux test with PPD.

C. Dosage and Administration: The volar surface of the mid forearm is cleansed, and the tines are firmly but briefly pressed into the skin. The metal tines deliver an approximate dose of intermediate strength when pressed into the skin. The results are read in 48 hours.

D. Results and Interpretation: Size of induration is compared with the pattern provided by the manufacturer. If significant induration is found in a healthy child, results are usually confirmed by intradermal Mantoux test before chemoprophylaxis is considered.

Tularemia Skin Test

The tularemia skin test employs a suspension of killed *Francisella tularensis* and is used for epidemiologic purposes in suspected outbreaks of tularemia. The material is not generally available, and the test is not used for diagnosis. Diagnosis is by clinical findings and results of cultures.

8 | The Newborn Infant: Assessment & General Care*

CLINICAL ASSESSMENT

Clinical evaluation of a newborn infant should include consideration of (1) aspects of the maternal and obstetric history, including labor, delivery, and medications; (2) the need for resuscitation and its effectiveness; (3) the physical examination, including gestational age assessment and search for possible birth injuries and congenital anomalies; and (4) assessment of the level of care required by the neonate.

High-Risk Factors in Obstetric History

The risk of neonatal mortality or morbidity is increased in pregnancies associated with previous neonatal death or complications, multiple gestation, incompetent cervix, antepartum hemorrhage (placenta previa, abruptio placentae), premature rupture of membranes, Rh sensitization, maternal infection (especially rubella, cytomegalovirus, herpesvirus hominis infection, and amnionitis), chronic maternal disease (cardiac; renal; endocrine, especially diabetes), hypertension, failure to obtain prenatal care, maternal age less than 15 years or greater than 40 years, antepartum trauma, or major surgery. Complications during labor or delivery (prolapsed cord, abnormal presentation [face, brow, breech; shoulder dystocia], fetal distress, prolonged labor, mid- or high-forceps delivery), complications of analgesia and anesthesia, and prolonged rupture of membranes may also cause increased neonatal mortality.

In recognized high-risk pregnancies, the condition of the fetus during labor should be continuously monitored. Fetal distress is often accompanied by meconium passage and is diagnosed by abnormal fetal heart rate pattern (bradycardia, late decelerations, loss of beat-to-beat variability) or fetal acidosis ($\text{pH} < 7.25$).

IMMEDIATE CARE OF THE NEWBORN

In the Delivery Room

(1) Aspirate mucus gently from infant's nose and throat with a

*Revised with the assistance of Michael A. Simmons, MD.

rubber-bulbed syringe (preferable) or a catheter attached to a glass trap. This should be done, if possible, with infant's head down before the first breath is taken and is conveniently carried out before delivering the infant's shoulders.

(2) Neither immediate nor delayed clamping of the cord appears to be clearly superior in the healthy full-term infant.

(3) Dry infant thoroughly, keep infant warm (preferably under a radiant heater), and wrap infant in warm blankets for transfer to nursery.

(4) Administer naloxone (Narcan) to reverse respiratory depression due to morphine, codeine, or other opiates, or use mechanical ventilation.

(5) Assign Apgar score at 1 and 5 minutes (Table 8–1).

(6) Carry out brief initial screening examination, checking for gross abnormalities, adequate chest expansion and air exchange, abdominal masses, torsion of testes, signs of adequate perfusion, and number of umbilical arteries.

(7) Identify infant with bracelet and footprinting or necklace.

(8) For resuscitation, avoid vigorous chest pressing, alternate hot and cold baths, jackknifing, holding the infant upside down for more than a few seconds, spanking, and rubbing the spine. Do not weigh or bathe infant until the infant's condition is stabilized.

(9) Encourage parental contact if the infant's condition permits.

In the Nursery

(1) Place infant in heated crib. Prevent contamination. Assess gestational age. Administer vitamin K_1 (phytonadione [AquaMephyton, Konakion]), 1 mg intramuscularly. Perform eye care if not done in delivery room. Instill 1% silver nitrate or suitable antibiotic into the eyes. A mild chemical conjunctivitis may result. Do not weigh or bathe infant until infant is stabilized and temperature is normal. Wipe away

Table 8–1. Apgar score of newborn infant.

	Sign	Score 0	Score 1	Score 2
A	Appearance (color)	Blue; pale	Body pink; extremities blue	Completely pink
P	Pulse (heart rate)	Absent	< 100	> 100
G	Grimace (reflex irritability in response to stimulation of sole of foot)	No response	Grimace	Cry
A	Activity (muscle tone)	Limp	Some flexion of extremities	Active motion
R	Respiration (respiratory effort)	Absent	Slow; irregular	Good strong cry

excess vernix and debris around infant's face. After infant has stabilized, bathe infant with water and bland soap. Do not use hexachlorophene for routine bathing. (In presence of skin infection, use hexachlorophene according to instructions.) After initial bath, cleanse infant's skin daily (and when soiling occurs) with water.

(2) Keep infant under close observation for at least 4–8 hours. If there is a great deal of mucus, elevate the foot of the crib and aspirate mucus with a suction tube. Examine the umbilical cord for bleeding. Check axillary temperature every hour until it is stabilized and above 36 °C (96.8 °F). Check to see that voiding of urine and passage of meconium stools occur.

(3) Routine rubs with chemotherapeutic or antibiotic ointments are not needed and are not recommended for use because of the danger of sensitization. Talcum and oils generally are not necessary and (especially if perfumed) may lead to sensitization. Cord care with triple dye (brilliant green, proflavine, and crystal violet) significantly reduces colonization with staphylococci.

(4) For prevention of infections, see discussion in Chapter 9.

RESUSCITATION

During Delivery of the Potentially Asphyxiated Newborn

(1) Give mother 100% oxygen continuously by mask.

(2) Deliver infant slowly, keeping the head down.

(3) In the presence of meconium, aspirate infant's upper airway thoroughly with a suction catheter prior to delivery of the shoulders.

Immediately After Delivery

(1) Place infant in 30-degree Trendelenburg position. Permit adequate delivery of placental blood to the infant unless hemolytic disease of the newborn (erythroblastosis fetalis) is suspected or the term infant is small for gestational age (SGA).

(2) Clear infant's airway again with gentle bulb suction.

(3) Stimulate infant by flicking soles of feet or gently flexing and extending extremities. ***Caution:*** Do not spank or swing the infant or immerse the infant alternately in cold and hot water.

(4) Dry infant to reduce heat loss and keep warm. An overhead radiant warmer may be of value.

After Clamping & Cutting the Cord

A. Immediate Measures: Place infant in 15- to 30-degree Trendelenburg position and keep infant warm.

B. Oxygen: Administer oxygen by means of a head box or mask if required.

C. Apgar Score: Check Apgar score (Table 8–1).

1. Resuscitation of the vigorous newborn (1-minute Apgar score > 7)–

a. If the infant is breathing well, briefly and gently suction the mouth, nose, and pharynx with bulb syringe or soft rubber catheter; pass catheter through mouth into stomach to check patency of esophagus, and aspirate stomach contents, noting volume.

b. If the infant is dusky but the respiratory effort is adequate, gently suction the mouth, nose, and pharynx and administer oxygen by face mask. Keep warm. Stimulate gently.

2. Resuscitation of the moderately depressed newborn (1-minute Apgar score 4–7)–

a. Suction the nose and throat briefly while administering oxygen by face mask.

b. If initial heart rate of less than 100 accelerates promptly and good muscle tone is developing, infant may not need more than oxygen by face mask.

c. If bradycardia or weak respiratory efforts persist, administer intermittent positive pressure ventilation (IPPV) with bag and mask and 100% oxygen at 30–40 breaths per minute and 25–35 cm of water pressure. Listen to both sides of chest for adequate ventilation, and listen for heart rate. If heart rate does not accelerate after 1 minute, proceed to intubation.*

3. Resuscitation of the severely depressed newborn (1-minute Apgar score 0–3)–

a. Suction briefly, intubate, and administer IPPV with 100% oxygen via bag to tube at a rate of 30–40 respirations per minute and a pressure of 25–35 cm of water. Auscultate over both lungs and withdraw endotracheal tube slightly if breath sounds on left are poor.

b. If heart rate is less than 50 or decelerating after 60 seconds of IPPV, begin external cardiac massage at a rate of 60 compressions per minute. Measure umbilical artery pH and P_{CO_2}, and determine base excess. Correct acidosis, if present, by adequate ventilation. Consider administration of diluted sodium bicarbonate, based on observed base deficit. In the presence of hypotension or known blood loss, administer whole blood (which may be obtained from placenta) or plasma volume expander.

c. If there is no sustained heart rate response after 5 minutes of cardiac massage, continue IPPV and therapy for acidosis; obtain chest x-ray to look for diaphragmatic hernia, pneumothorax, etc; and consider needle and syringe aspiration of pleural spaces as indicated. Consider intracardiac epinephrine, 0.5 mL of 1:10,000 solution.

*Intubation should be performed by experienced persons.

GENERAL CARE

The infant should be wrapped in a blanket or placed in an incubator in a recovery area of the nursery and carefully observed for abnormal appearance, vital signs, or symptoms. The newborn infant in satisfactory condition after the recovery period should be evaluated (taking into account the gestational age and possible factors of risk), weighed, and bathed with a bland soap and plain water. Bathing with a solution of 1% hexachlorophene *followed by thorough rinsing* should be reserved for infants with a significantly increased risk of skin infections. (Avoid excessive use.) Routine umbilical care with triple dye has been recommended for these infants. Bacitracin ointment may be used to reduce staphylococcal colonization.

Routine Care of the Term Appropriate-for-Gestational-Age (AGA) Newborn (See Fig 8–1.)

Feeding can be started as early as age 2–6 hours in vigorous term infants. Sterile water or 5% glucose in water should be offered initially. When the infant has demonstrated an ability to suck and swallow adequately and has taken one of these liquids well, breast milk or full-strength milk formula (20 kcal/oz), 2–4 oz per feeding, can be offered every 4 hours or more often on demand. Avoid high-protein formulas.

Urination and passage of meconium stools should be documented in the first 24 hours. Circumcision has not been proved to be necessary or beneficial; however, if performed, it should be delayed until at least the second day of life.

In most states, screening for phenylketonuria is mandatory. Samples of blood or urine for screening tests should be taken only after adequate intake of milk for 24 hours.

Routine Care of the Preterm Newborn

A. Incubator: Prematurely born neonates should be cared for in incubators designed to keep them warm, to protect them from infection, to provide an atmosphere with increased humidity and oxygen if required, and still to allow them to be carefully observed with minimal handling.

Infants may be placed in a neutral thermal environment (ie, environment with temperature at which oxygen consumption is minimal) appropriate for their weight and postnatal age, or they may be servocontrolled to maintain a skin temperature of 36–36.5 °C (96.8–98 °F). Humidity is maintained at about 50%. Preterm infants who weigh 1800–2000 g or more can often maintain their body temperature out of an incubator.

B. Monitoring: Infants of less than 36 weeks' gestational age have

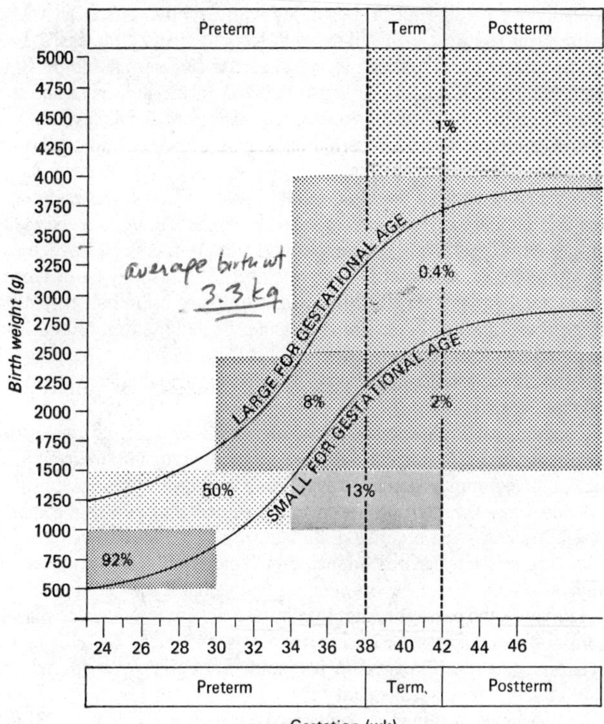

Figure 8–1. Neonatal mortality risk based on weight and gestational age. (Colorado data.)

an increased risk of apnea and bradycardia. When available, the use of apnea (or heart rate) monitors is advised with these infants.

C. Feeding: Preterm newborns weighing less than 1700 g should be given 10% dextrose solutions intravenously to supplement the inadequate oral intake that occurs during the first few days after birth. If glycosuria occurs in a markedly preterm infant, the concentration of dextrose should be reduced. Intravenous supplementation should be continued until the infant is receiving a combined intravenous and oral intake of at least 100 mL/kg/d.

Infants of less than 34–36 weeks' postconceptual age usually do not suck and swallow well enough to take nipple feedings. These infants can be gavage-fed via intermittent (or in some cases continuous) nasogastric polyethylene feeding tubes, beginning with 2–5 mL of sterile water. Subsequent feedings with full-strength formula may be increased 1–5 mL in volume every 3 hours. Residual gastric contents should be aspirated before each feeding to assess delayed gastric emptying and the infant's ability to tolerate an increased volume of formula. Residual gastric contents of greater than 2 mL should lead to caution during further feeding advancements.

When gavage-fed infants are about 34–36 weeks old postconceptually and demonstrate good sucking ability, nipple feedings may be tried. In premature infants in whom conventional feedings have been poorly tolerated, nasogastric or nasojejunal feedings may be of value.

Preterm infants (< 36 weeks) should be given iron supplementation in the form of either commercial formulas containing iron or oral iron preparations. The recommended intake of elemental iron from age 2 months is 2 mg/kg/d. Vitamin A, C, D, and folic acid supplementation is also indicated.

Peripheral intravenous hyperalimentation with amino acid, glucose, and lipid solutions has been used in very premature infants when oral alimentation is impossible or difficult to achieve. Neutral nitrogen balance can be achieved with intravenous alimentation containing amino acids, 2 g/kg/d, and 60 kcal/kg/d.

D. Oxygen: Preterm infants should not routinely be placed in oxygen-supplemented environments. Hypoxemia is the only indication for augmented oxygen therapy. Infants who are cyanotic may be placed temporarily in oxygen-rich environments sufficient to relieve the cyanosis, but it is essential to determine arterial P_{O_2} or arterialized capillary P_{O_2} for management of more prolonged oxygen exposure. Therapy should be aimed at maintaining the arterial P_{O_2} between 50 and 80 mm Hg to avoid retrolental fibroplasia.

E. Special Nursery for High-Risk Newborns: In general, infants with an 8% or greater chance of dying (Fig 8–1) and those with significant morbidity factors should be cared for in a special nursery for high-risk newborns.

F. Transportation of High-Risk Newborns: The transportation of ill or high-risk infants to a referral nursery should be done swiftly, with a nurse or physician accompanying the infant if possible. Portable incubators with adequate means for temperature and oxygen support are essential.

G. Hyperglycemia: Avoid excessive hyperglycemia when administering glucose solutions intravenously. Glucose concentrations greater than 10% are rarely indicated for intravenous infusion.

Special Care of the Small-for-Gestational-Age (SGA) Newborn (See Fig 8–1.)

Approximately two-thirds of preterm SGA infants and one-third of term SGA infants develop neonatal hypoglycemia (blood glucose < 30 mg/dL). These infants are optimally managed by the prophylactic administration of intravenous dextrose solutions and frequent blood glucose determinations during the first few days of life.

Special Care of the Large-for-Gestational-Age (LGA) Newborn (See Fig 8–1.)

Particular attention must be given to LGA newborns because their large size may fail to stimulate an adequate level of concern in those caring for them even though they actually have a much higher risk of morbidity for a given gestational age than do AGA infants.

LGA infants should be observed carefully for hypoglycemia, transient tachypnea, and birth injuries (intracranial hemorrhage, phrenic nerve paralysis, Erb's palsy).

PHYSICAL EXAMINATION

Current management of the newborn infant is based in part on gestational age and the adequacy of intrauterine growth for that gestational age. A clinical assessment of gestational age made within the first 6 hours is based on historical data and the presence or absence of certain physical features.

A complete physical examination of the newborn who is vigorous at birth may be postponed until the infant has been observed to progress uneventfully through the recovery and transitional period of the first 6–12 hours of life. An infant who is obviously ill at birth deserves a thorough examination as soon as a relatively stable state is reached following any required resuscitative measures.

Characteristics of the Term Newborn

A term newborn has the following characteristics at birth and shortly thereafter:

A. Resting Posture: Extremities are flexed and somewhat hypertonic (determined to some extent by intrauterine position [eg, following frank breech presentation, the neonate's thighs may be flexed onto the abdomen]). Fists are clenched. Asymmetries of skull, face, jaw, or extremities may result from intrauterine pressures.

B. Skin: Skin is usually ruddy and often mottled. Localized cyanosis of hands and feet (acrocyanosis) normally disappears after several days except when the infant is cool. Subcutaneous tissues may feel full and slightly edematous in the term newborn; skin may appear dry and peeling in the postterm newborn.

1. Lanugo (fine downy growth of hair) may be present over the shoulders and back.

2. Vernix caseosa (whitish or clay-colored, cheesy, greasy material) may cover the body but is usually on the back and scalp and in the creases of the term infant.

3. Milia of the face (distended sebaceous glands producing tiny whitish papules) are especially prominent over the nose, chin, or cheeks.

4. Mongolian spots (benign bluish pigmentation over the lower back, buttocks, or extensor surfaces) may be found in infants of dark-skinned races.

5. Capillary hemangiomas ("flame nevi") are common on the eyelids, forehead, and neck.

6. Petechiae are sometimes present over the head, neck, and back, especially in association with nuchal cord; if generalized, thrombocytopenia should be suspected.

7. Newborns of 32 weeks' or more gestational age may perspire when too warm. The forehead is usually the first site noted.

C. Head: The head is large in relation to the rest of the body; it may exhibit considerable molding with overriding of the cranial bones.

1. Caput succedaneum (localized or fairly extensive ill-defined soft tissue swelling) may be present over the scalp or other presenting parts. It usually extends over a suture line.

2. Cephalhematoma (see Chapter 9).

3. Anterior and posterior fontanelles may measure 0.6–3.6 cm in any direction and are soft. They may be small initially. A third fontanelle between these 2 is present in approximately 6% of infants and is more likely to occur in children with various abnormalities.

4. Transillumination normally produces a circle of light no greater than 1.5 cm beyond the light source in term infants.

5. Craniotabes (slight indentation and recoil of parietal bones elicited by lightly pressing with thumb) is normal in newborns.

D. Face:

1. Eyes–The irises are slate-gray except in dark-skinned races. Tears may or may not be present. Most term infants look toward a light source and transiently focus on a face. Subconjunctival, scleral, and retinal hemorrhages are abnormal. The pupillary light reflex is present. Lens opacities are abnormal. A red reflex can be seen on ophthalmoscopic examination. The infant will turn to follow a face more than other stimuli.

2. Mouth–Small, pearllike retention cysts at the gum margins and the midline of the palate (Bohn's and Epstein's pearls) are common and insignificant. The tonsils are usually quite small.

3. Nose–The newborn, a preferential nose-breather, experiences respiratory distress in bilateral choanal atresia. Patency should be confirmed by passage of a nasogastric tube if obstruction is suspected.

4. Ears–Eardrums may be difficult to visualize but have a characteristic opaque appearance and decreased mobility. Severe malformation of pinnas may be associated with abnormalities of the genitourinary tract. Normal newborns respond to sounds with a startle, blink, head turning, or cry.

5. Cheeks–The cheeks are full because of the sucking pads.

E. Chest:

1. Breasts–Breasts are palpable in most mature males and females; size is determined by gestational age and adequacy of nutrition.

2. Lungs–Breathing is abdominal and may be shallow and irregular; rate is usually 40–60 breaths per minute, with a range of 30–100 breaths per minute. Breath sounds are harsh and bronchial. Faint rales may be heard immediately following birth and normally clear in several hours.

3. Heart–Rate averages 130 beats per minute, but rates from 90 to 180 may be present for brief periods in normal infants. Sinus arrhythmia may be present. The apex of the heart is usually lateral to the midclavicular line in the third or fourth interspace. Transient murmurs are common. During the first day, systolic blood pressure taken in the arm by the flush, palpation, or auscultation method is 45–55 mm Hg and by the Doppler method is 55–65 mm Hg.

F. Abdomen: The abdomen is normally flat at birth but soon becomes more protuberant; a markedly scaphoid abdomen suggests diaphragmatic hernia. Two arteries and one vein are usually present in the umbilical cord. The liver is palpable; the tip of the spleen can be felt in 10% of newborns. Both kidneys can and should be palpated. Bowel sounds are audible shortly after birth. Between 5 and 25 mL of cloudy white gastric fluid can be aspirated from the stomach.

G. Genitalia: Appearance in both sexes is dependent on gestational age. Edema is common, particularly after breech delivery.

1. Females–The labia minora and clitoris are covered by labia majora in term neonates. A mucoid secretion exudes from the vaginal orifice.

2. Males–Testes are in the scrotum; rugae cover the scrotum. The prepuce is adherent to the glans of the penis. White epithelial pearls 1–2 mm in diameter may be present at the tip of the prepuce.

H. Anus: Patency should be checked. An anteriorly displaced anus may be associated with stenosis.

I. Hips: Dislocation is suspected if abduction of the thighs is limited. Test for dislocation as follows: (1) Place the middle fingers over the greater trochanters and the thumbs over the region of the lesser trochanters. Apply pressure against the greater trochanters and bring the thighs into abduction. A snap felt in abduction (Ortolani's sign) is suggestive of dislocation, although a faint click is not uncommon during the first 24 hours after birth or even longer in breech presentations. (2) With one hand, fix the pelvis, with the thighs abducted. Apply pressure with the thumb against the inner thigh, and feel for a snap as the head of the femur slips over the acetabular rim. (3) Attempt to telescope the femur by pulling forward and pushing backward. Reexamine at 1 week and periodically thereafter.

J. Feet: Many apparent abnormalities may be only the transient results of intrauterine position. Clubfoot requires prompt orthopedic attention.

K. Neurologic Examination:

1. Neurologic development is dependent on gestational age.
2. Most reflexes, including the Moro, tonic neck, grasp, sucking, rooting, stepping, Babinski, deep tendon, abdominal, cremasteric, and Chvostek reflexes, are normally present at birth.

L. Weight: As a rule, male infants weigh more than female; white infants more than nonwhite; and second-born infants more than first-born.

Characteristics of the Preterm Newborn

The preterm or premature infant is comparatively inactive, with a feeble cry and irregular respirations (periodic breathing). The infant has a relatively large head, prominent eyes, and a protruding abdomen. The skin is relatively translucent, often wrinkled, red, and deficient in subcutaneous fat. The nails are soft, lanugo is prominent, and vernix is thick. The musculature is poorly developed, the thorax less rigid, and breast engorgement usually absent. Testes may be undescended.

In general, preterm infants weigh less than 2500 g and have a crown-heel length of less than 47 cm, a head circumference of less than 33 cm, and a thoracic circumference of less than 30 cm.

The preterm infant has physiologic handicaps due to functional and anatomic immaturity of various organs.

A. Body Temperature: Body temperature is more difficult to maintain owing to decreased insulation by subcutaneous fat and large surface area/body weight ratio. Consequently, body temperature falls unless the environment is thermally supported.

B. Respiration: Respiratory difficulties are common because of weak gag and cough reflexes (increased risk of aspiration); pliable thorax and weak respiratory musculature (results in less efficient ventilation); deficiency of surfactant (allowing alveoli to collapse on exhaling and contributing to the respiratory distress syndrome); and defects in central nervous system control (apnea).

C. Renal Function: Because of immature renal function, iatrogenic disturbances of water or electrolyte balance may occur. Large solute or water loads may not be adequately excreted.

D. Resistance to Infection: Ability to combat infection is decreased owing to inadequate placental transmission of 19S immunoglobulins; relative inability to produce antibodies; and impaired phagocytosis, leukocyte bactericidal capacity, and inflammatory response. Epidermal and mucosal barriers in preterm infants are not as effective as those in term infants.

E. Hyperbilirubinemia: Because of impaired conjugation and excretion of bilirubin, hyperbilirubinemia is more common and more severe in preterm infants.

F. Hemorrhage: Hemorrhagic diathesis is more common owing to clotting factor deficiencies and increased permeability of vessels.

G. Anemia: Deficient antenatal accumulation of iron and vitamin E and rapid body growth and blood volume expansion contribute to a more pronounced anemia in the first months of life.

H. Nutritional Disturbances: Disturbances of nutrition may be a consequence of the faulty absorption of fat, fat-soluble vitamins, and certain minerals as well as reduced stores of calcium, phosphorus, proteins, ascorbic acid, and vitamin A.

Characteristics of the Small-for-Gestational-Age (SGA) Newborn

Regardless of gestational age, the SGA infant's weight is less than the tenth percentile for that age, and the infant often appears malnourished. With increasingly severe intrauterine growth retardation, the infant's length as well as weight are compromised. In severe SGA neonates, the weight, length, and head circumference are all below the tenth percentile for gestational age.

SGA infants have higher morbidity and mortality rates than do AGA infants. SGA infants should be carefully examined for congenital anomalies, evaluated for intrauterine infection, and watched for the possible development of hypoglycemia, hyperviscosity, and feeding difficulties.

SGA infants may not require as warm an incubator as do preterm AGA infants of the same weight.

Characteristics of the Large-for-Gestational-Age (LGA) Newborn

An LGA neonate is one whose birth weight is greater than the 90th percentile for gestational age. Only a portion of LGA neonates are infants of diabetic mothers, but all LGA infants have higher morbidity and mortality rates than do AGA infants of the same gestational age. Birth injuries—especially brachial plexus injuries and fractures of the clavicle—and hypoglycemia are more common in LGA infants. Transient tachypnea (not progressing to respiratory distress syndrome) and developmental retardation subsequent to the neonatal period are also more common.

Infants of diabetic mothers have a characteristic macrosomic appearance. They are obese and plethoric and have round, full faces. In addition to the above problems they share with other LGA infants, they have an increased incidence of renal vein thrombosis (manifested by flank mass and hematuria) and congenital anomalies (especially skeletal and frequently below the waist) as well as an increased incidence of respiratory distress syndrome, hypocalcemia, and hyperbilirubinemia.

LABORATORY DATA

Blood (See also Normal Blood Chemistry Values in Appendix.)

Red cell counts and hemoglobin may be as much as 20% higher in capillary blood than in venous blood at birth. Nucleated red blood cells up to 500/μL may be found normally. Pyknocytes ("burr cells") may be present (< 2% in full-term and up to 6% in premature infants). The sedimentation rate is greatly accelerated. Plasma proteins and blood glucose are reduced. The reticulocyte count is elevated (2–6%). Fetal hemoglobin is 44–95% of total hemoglobin. Red cell instability is higher, and the half-life of red cells is shorter. Extracellular water content and total body water are high. Asymptomatic hypertyrosinemia often occurs, especially in low-birth-weight infants; its significance is not yet clear. The level of thyrotropin (thyroid-stimulating hormone, TSH) may be temporarily elevated in stressed infants. Serum calcium is depressed in preterm and stressed term infants.

Prothrombin, plasma thromboplastin component, proconvertin, and Stuart-Prower factor are reduced. Proaccelerin may be normal or elevated. Plasminogen level is reduced.

Gastrointestinal Tract

Gastrointestinal enzymes are adequate except for digestion of starches. Lactose malabsorption is common, especially in premature infants. Pancreatic amylase remains low for months.

Electrocardiography

Right ventricular preponderance may continue for a few months. Ectopic beats are relatively common during the first week.

Cerebrospinal Fluid

Spinal fluid is xanthochromic and frequently contains increased numbers of leukocytes and elevated protein (mean > 100 mg/dL). Red blood cells may be present.

ASSESSMENT OF RISK & LEVEL OF CARE REQUIRED

A newborn's risk of dying in the neonatal period can be estimated on the basis of birth weight and gestational age by referring to Fig 8–1. The mortality risk increases with decreasing gestational age and with inappropriately grown neonates.

Factors that affect the mortality rate include the following: (1) gestational age, (2) weight, (3) high-risk obstetric history, (4) low Apgar score at 5 minutes, (5) difficult or prolonged resuscitation, (6) severe birth injury, and (7) abnormal physical findings at birth (eg, congenital anomalies).

NORMAL PHYSIOLOGIC EVENTS DURING THE NEONATAL PERIOD

Transition From Fetus to Newborn

A. Cardiovascular System:

1. A remarkable transition from the fetal parallel pulmonary and systemic circulations to the adult arrangement of these circulations in series occurs at birth. This transition is not complete, however, for several days to weeks, when the ductus arteriosus and foramen ovale are closed and the pulmonary vascular resistance has diminished. Table 8–2 describes the changes that occur during this transition.

Table 8–2. Changes in the circulatory mechanism at birth.*

Structure	Prenatal Function	Postnatal Function
Aorta	Receives mixed blood from heart and pulmonary arteries.	Carries oxygenated blood from left ventricle.
Ductus arteriosus	Shunts mixed blood from pulmonary artery to aorta.	Generally occluded by 4 mo and becomes ligamentum arteriosum.
Ductus venosus	Carries oxygenated blood from umbilical vein to inferior vena cava.	Obliterated to become ligamentum venosum.
Foramen ovale	Connects right and left atria.	Functional closure by 3 mo, although probe patency without symptoms may be retained by some adults.
Inferior vena cava	Carries oxygenated blood from umbilical vein and ductus venosus and mixed blood from body and liver.	Carries only unoxygenated blood from body.
Pulmonary arteries	Carry some mixed blood to lungs.	Carry unoxygenated blood to lungs.
Umbilical arteries	Carry oxygenated and unoxygenated blood to placenta.	Obliterated to become vesical ligaments on anterior abdominal wall.
Umbilical vein	Carries oxygenated blood from placenta to liver and heart.	Obliterated to become ligamentum teres (round ligament of liver).

*Adapted from Scammon.

2. The fetus pumps almost half of the cardiac output to the placenta and only a small percentage to the lungs and kidneys. After the umbilical cord is clamped, the cardiac output is redistributed so that the lungs and kidneys receive a much greater proportion.

3. The mean systemic arterial blood pressure is about the same in the fetus and the newborn but increases during the neonatal period and subsequently.

B. Respiratory System:

1. The factors causing the infant to take the first breath are thought to be low Pa_{O_2}, high Pa_{CO_2}, low pH, evaporative cooling, and gasp reflex due to recoil of thorax after delivery.

2. Intrathoracic negative pressures as great as 60–70 cm of water are required to expand the lungs during the first few breaths. In the normal newborn, succeeding breaths require 5–15 cm of water pressure.

3. The liquid present in the lungs of the newborn prior to the first breath is normally absorbed within a few hours.

C. Blood Gases and pH:

1. The pH of fetal blood is only slightly lower (0.05 pH unit) than the adult value. During labor, the pH falls slightly, and the vigorous newborn attains a relatively normal acid-base state within 1–3 hours of birth. By 24 hours of age, the healthy neonate has a blood pH of 7.4.

2. Fetal P_{CO_2} is slightly higher than the maternal P_{CO_2}. During labor, P_{CO_2} rises somewhat, but following recovery from birth the normal neonate has a lower P_{CO_2} (approximately 32 mm Hg) than does the adult.

3. The fetal hemoglobin oxygen saturation is relatively high, but the fetal Pa_{O_2} (about 30–40 mm Hg) is much lower than adult values. During the first 24 hours of neonatal life, the Pa_{O_2} increases from about 55 mm Hg shortly after birth to about 90 mm Hg.

Changes Occurring After Birth

A. Metabolic:

1. The principal metabolic substrate for the human fetus is glucose. Following birth, the neonate develops the metabolic capacity to utilize fats and amino acids absorbed from the diet.

2. The metabolic rate increases gradually during the neonatal period. At birth, term infants have a higher metabolic rate than do preterm infants.

3. One-third of healthy term infants and about one-half of preterm neonates develop clinically apparent "physiologic jaundice" during the first week of life. Clinical jaundice is not manifest until the second or third day of life, with peak bilirubin levels on days 5–7. Term infants rarely exceed indirect bilirubin levels of 12 mg/dL, and preterm infants rarely exceed 15 mg/dL. The etiologic factors are not completely understood, but an important cause is the delayed maturation of hepatic

glucuronyl transferase, which is necessary for bilirubin conjugation.

B. Renal: In late gestation, the fetal urine flow rate is high and the urine osmolality low. The newborn initially also excretes a dilute urine (between 100 and 400 mosm/L) the osmolality of which varies inversely with the urine flow rate (5–0.5 mL/kg/h for well-hydrated neonates). With increasing age, the neonatal kidney excretes a more concentrated urine with a greater urea content. The ability to excrete many drugs is altered.

C. Immunologic: Passive immunity against diphtheria, tetanus, pneumococcal infection, the rash-producing toxins of streptococci that cause scarlet fever, and the viruses of measles, rubella, herpes simplex, infectious hepatitis, mumps, and poliomyelitis is present in most infants at birth if the mother is immune.

At birth, the term infant's serum concentration of IgG (derived from the mother) is similar to that of adults, and there are low or undetectable amounts of IgA, IgM, IgD, and IgE. The greater the gestational age, the higher the IgG level. The lack of IgM antibodies, which are especially effective in killing gram-negative bacteria, predisposes neonates to gram-negative infections. However, in fetal infections with syphilis, toxoplasmosis, rubella, cytomegalovirus, and herpesvirus hominis, the IgM levels may be increased in serum from cord blood and venous blood.

IgG concentrations decrease until about age 2 or 3 months, then rise again as the neonate responds to antigenic stimuli in the environment. Infants begin to synthesize IgM globulins in the first days of life. Breast-fed neonates receive secretory IgA antibodies in colostrum and human milk.

D. Clinical:

1. Birth recovery period–For about 30 minutes, the infant is active and alert, the heart rate is rapid, and there may be nasal flaring, mild grunting and retracting, auscultatory rales, irregular respiratory movements, and mucus present in the mouth. Bowel sounds are absent. Body temperature falls. During the subsequent 0.5–2 hours, the infant falls asleep and has decreased heart and respiratory rates, and bowel sounds are present. Then the neonate arouses and again is active, with labile heart rate and swift color changes due to vasomotor instability and a period of hemoconcentration at about 6 hours of age that contributes to a plethoric appearance. Meconium is usually passed during this period but may be delayed (in about 6% of newborns) for over 24 hours. Urination usually occurs soon after birth but may be delayed until the second day in about 8% of newborns. Body temperature returns to normal.

2. Weight–Both term and preterm newborns lose weight initially. Term infants lose 5–10% of their birth weight by the third to fifth day (> 12% may be excessive) and regain their birth weight by the second week of life. Preterm neonates may experience a greater relative weight loss and require longer to regain their birth weight, primarily because of the difficulty in providing them with an adequate caloric intake. Healthy term neonates subsequently gain about 30 g/d.

3. Position–Relaxation from the intrauterine to the infantile position occurs. The head may be lifted from prone position. Asymmetries diminish.

4. Skin–Skin change is from ruddy to paler pink. Desquamation of trunk and extremities is usually mild but may be extensive, especially in postmature infants. Fissures may develop at ankles and wrists. Lanugo begins to fall out. Petechiae disappear. Rashes (erythema neonatorum toxicum) are common during the first few days. Harlequin color change (midline demarcation of body into pale and plethoric halves) may occur.

5. Head and face–Molding and caput disappear. Eyes may show muscular imbalance. Intracranial pressure increases on the first day and then drops. Head size may decrease during the first days of life.

6. Chest–Breast engorgement may increase, and secretion may be present. (This is not likely to occur in premature infants.)

7. Abdomen–Vomiting is common, usually caused by irritation of gastric mucosa by foreign material (eg, blood, amniotic fluid) ingested at or after birth. The umbilical cord dries up and falls off during the first or second week.

8. Genitalia–Pseudomenstruation may occur in females.

9. Urinary tract–The urine is pale, acid, of low specific gravity, and may contain reducing substance, acetone, and casts but less than 10 red and 10 white cells per microliter. Rarely, ingested sugars may be present in urine. Galactosuria with a peak at 3 days may be present. Urates may cause pink staining of the diaper and a false-positive reaction for protein. Urinary 17-ketosteroid excretion level is elevated for the first week of life.

10. Blood–Hemoglobin and erythrocytes increase during the first day, and then both fetal and adult fractions of hemoglobin fall. A relative hypoglycemia often develops; infants may remain asymptomatic in spite of blood glucose levels below 30 mg/dL. If glucose concentration is below 30 mg/dL, treatment is necessary. Levels of L-thyroxine (T_4), protein-bound iodine (PBI), and uptake of tagged triiodothyronine (T_3) by red blood cells are elevated, with highest levels being reached on the second to fifth day of life. Less elevation occurs in infants who are kept warm. Plasma 17-hydroxycorticosteroid levels are maintained at near-adult levels.

11. Gastrointestinal tract–Gas is visible by x-ray in the gastrointestinal tract within a few minutes after birth. Swallowed air reaches the cecum in 3–5 hours and the descending colon in 10 hours. Hydrolysis of lactose in the intestines may be relatively impaired during the first few days of life. Stools frequently contain many eosinophils

Stools may contain blood that was previously swallowed. Ninety percent of infants pass their first stools with 24 hours. Meconium stools may be passed for 1–3 days; these are followed by rather frequent transitional stools (loose, slimy, brown to green) for 2–3 days and subsequently by milk stools.

DISTURBANCES DUE TO ANTENATAL FACTORS*

Maternal Factors Affecting the Newborn

A. Infection: Infants born of mothers who have had rubella during pregnancy may be small for gestational age; may have brain lesions (microcephaly, hydrocephalus, meningoencephalitis), eye lesions (cataracts, glaucoma, microphthalmia, retinitis), deafness, cardiac defects (especially pulmonary valve or artery stenosis or both, patent ductus arteriosus, and ventricular septal defect), pulmonary complications, thrombocytopenic purpura ("blueberry muffin" lesions), hepatosplenomegaly, hepatitis, jaundice, bone lesions, peculiar dimples of the skin, areas of skin pigmentation, retardation of somatic growth, chromosomal abnormalities, abnormal fingerprints and palmar creases; and may shed virus for many months (with or without clinical abnormalities) and have psychomotor retardation. Cord IgM levels may be elevated.

Syphilis may produce abortions, stillbirths, or congenital syphilis. Influenza during the first trimester may cause congenital anomalies. Maternal urinary tract disease may increase the incidence of prematurity. Toxoplasmosis, cytomegalovirus, and live virus vaccines may produce disease in the infant. A number of other viruses (mumps, varicella, herpesvirus hominis, rubeola, coxsackieviruses and other picornaviruses, poxvirus, serum and infectious hepatitis virus, and arboviruses), bacteria (including *Mycobacterium tuberculosis*), and other infectious agents (malaria parasites, *Histoplasma*) may be transplacentally transmitted to the fetus and produce disease.

B. Noninfectious Maternal Factors:

1. Diabetes mellitus.

2. Congenital thrombocytopenic purpura may occur if the mother has had thrombocytopenia or platelet isoimmunization or received quinine.

*Amniocentesis has been recommended for (1) pregnancy in a woman age 35 years or older; (2) pregnancy in a woman who has previously had a child with Down's syndrome or any other genetic disorder or who is a carrier of an X-linked disease; and (3) pregnancy in which one parent is a translocation carrier, in which both parents are carriers of an autosomal recessive trait (for a disease or defect), or in which the parents previously had a child with a neural tube defect.

3. Iodine deficiency, an enzymatic defect of thyroid metabolism, or excessive therapy of maternal hyperthyroidism may result in cretinism in the child.

4. Severe iron deficiency predisposes to anemia in the infant.

5. Rh and ABO factor sensitization.

6. Severe anoxia during pregnancy may predispose to congenital abnormalities.

7. Acetonuria during pregnancy, possibly due to malnutrition, may be associated with lowered intelligence quotient in the offspring.

8. Use of drugs or other substances by the mother may affect the newborn. **Progestins, testosterone, and other hormones** may cause virilization and advanced bone age of the female fetus. **Thalidomide** may cause phocomelia. **Nitrofurantoin** may cause hemolysis; **sulfonamides, novobiocin, oxacillin, cephalothin, sodium benzoate, and salicylates** may cause competitive binding with albumin in serum with resultant hyperbilirubinemia due to displacement of bilirubin; and **chloramphenicol** can lead to cardiovascular collapse and the "gray syndrome." **Aminopterin, methotrexate, and chlorambucil** may cause anomalies and abortions. **Dicumarol** may cause hemorrhage and fetal death. **Heroin, morphine, and other narcotics** may cause tremors, neonatal death, and neonatal withdrawal symptoms in maternal addiction. **Smoking** may cause infants to be small for gestational age. **Streptomycin** may cause deafness. Certain **cancer chemotherapeutic agents and phenothiazines** may cause a parkinsonismlike syndrome. **Mepivacaine and lidocaine** may cause central nervous system depression or seizures and irritability. **Thiazides** may cause electrolyte imbalance, thrombocytopenia, and leukopenia. **Inorganic mercury** may cause brain damage with cerebral palsy. **Reserpine** may cause nasal congestion, bradycardia, hypothermia, and drowsiness in the newborn. **Tetracyclines** may produce retarded bone growth and mottled and stained teeth. **Magnesium sulfate** may cause depression or convulsions in the newborn. **General anesthetics** may cause respiratory depression; **spinal anesthetics,** maternal hypotension with fetal distress; and **paracervical block,** fetal bradycardia. **Oxytocin induction** may lead to water intoxication in the mother and hyponatremia, hypotension, and hypotonia in the infant. **Vitamin K_3** may cause hyperbilirubinemia; **salicylates,** coagulation defects with neonatal bleeding; **quinine,** thrombocytopenia and deafness; and **ganglionic blocking agents,** paralytic ileus. **Phenobarbital** may increase the rate of neonatal drug metabolism; a large dose may depress the infant. **Hexamethonium** may produce ileus; **atropine,** tachycardia; **prochlorperazine,** depression; **chloroquine,** retinal damage; **corticosteroids,** adrenal insufficiency; and **oral hypoglycemic agents,** hypoglycemia. **Radioiodine** may produce fetal thyroid destruction. **Thiouracil derivatives, potassium iodide, and potassium perchlorate** may produce congenital goiter.

9. Certain iodine-containing dyes for cholecystograms cause a prolonged increase in protein-bound iodine (PBI) in offspring.

10. Myasthenia gravis.

11. Advanced maternal age is associated with an increased perinatal mortality rate; increased fetal distress in postterm pregnancies; and increased incidences of hydrocephalus, congenital heart disease, C, D, and E trisomies, and Klinefelter's syndrome.

Heredity

Heredity is the most important factor in certain congenital defects (see Appendix).

MULTIPLE BIRTHS

Twins may be monozygotic (identical) or dizygotic (fraternal). The intrauterine growth of each twin parallels that of a singleton until about 34 weeks of gestation. Thereafter, the fetal growth rate is less than that for a singleton. As a consequence, many twins (and triplets) are small for gestational age as well as preterm.

If the birth weights of twins are discrepant by 10% or more, the twins are regarded as discordant twins. If monozygotic twins are discordant, placental vascular anastomosis may have allowed one twin to chronically transfuse the other, resulting in a small, anemic donor and a large, plethoric recipient twin who may develop congestive failure.

PROGNOSIS

For Neonatal Survival

The prognosis for survival for a given newborn depends upon several factors:

A. Gestational Age: Mortality risk is approximately halved for every 2 weeks added to gestational age after 28 weeks.

B. Birth Weight: Small-for-gestational-age and large-for-gestational-age infants have increased mortality risks.

C. Multiple Births: The mortality rate is greater than for singletons; the second-born twin has a greater mortality risk than does the first-born.

D. Maternal Age: Neonatal mortality risk increases with very young and very elderly mothers.

E. Presence of Life-Threatening Condition: The presence at birth of severe congenital anomalies, erythroblastosis fetalis, hemorrhage, congenitally acquired infections, etc, affects the prognosis for survival.

For Neonatal Morbidity

Neonatal morbidity risk is increased by all factors that raise the mortality risk as well as by low Apgar scores at 5 minutes and by high-risk obstetric factors (antepartum hemorrhage, diabetes, preeclampsia-eclampsia, etc).

For Long-Term Development

In general, the more preterm the neonate, the greater chance the neonate has of showing some developmental handicap in later childhood (cerebral palsy; hearing, seeing, and learning disabilities). Twins have a higher risk of long-term disabilities than do singletons; small-for-gestational-age and large-for-gestational-age infants have a greater risk than do appropriate-for-gestational-age infants.

In long-term follow-up studies of infants born prior to 1953 and weighing less than 1500 g at birth, two-thirds had some developmental handicap. In infants who weighed less than 1000 g at birth and were 28–31 weeks' gestational age, the incidence of handicaps was about 75%. However, the advent of intensive care nurseries has resulted in an improved outlook for survivors of preterm births. Over 80% of infants weighing 1000–1500 g and about 60% of infants weighing less than 1000 g will be normal.

The Newborn Infant: Diseases & Disorders* | 9

Newborn infants are susceptible to a large number of diseases and abnormal conditions affecting older children, but they also may develop a number of problems peculiar to the neonatal period.†

DISEASES OF THE RESPIRATORY SYSTEM

RESPIRATORY DISTRESS OF THE NEWBORN

Respiratory distress is more common with maternal illnesses (maternal hypoxia, hemorrhage, shock, cardiorespiratory disease, preeclampsia-eclampsia, severe anemia, low blood pressure); abnormal uterine contractions; obstruction of the newborn's respiratory passages (aspirated material, especially meconium); congenital abnormalities, including choanal atresia, diaphragmatic hernia, lobar emphysema, lung cysts, tracheoesophageal fistula, macroglossia, glossoptosis, agenesis or hypoplasia of the lungs, laryngeal or tracheal web, tracheomalacia, vascular ring, and pressure on the trachea from without; injury to phrenic nerve, epiglottis, or larynx; depression of the respiratory center (anesthetics or analgesics to the mother, cerebral hemorrhage); drugs; fetal shock; and various diseases and congenital defects involving the infant, including intracranial hemorrhage, muscular weakness, cardiac disease, and pulmonary disorders such as idiopathic respiratory distress syndrome of the newborn (hyaline membrane disease), pneumomediastinum, pneumothorax, pneumonia, pneumonitis, pulmonary hemorrhage, persistence of fetal circulation, and transient tachypnea‡ of

*Revised with the assistance of Michael A. Simmons, MD.

†See also Chapter 8.

‡Transient tachypnea with respiratory distress in the newborn has been described. It lasts 2–4 days and is more common in males than females. It is characterized by tachypnea, costal or sternal retractions, grunting, and sometimes cyanosis. X-ray shows a pattern of symmetric parahilar pulmonary congestion. The possible cause is impaired lymphatic clearing of alveolar fluid.

the newborn. Immaturity of the respiratory system may be an important factor in premature infants.

Treatment is directed toward adequate oxygenation and elimination of underlying causes, if possible. Complete supportive care should include control of temperature and administration of fluids, glucose, etc. The use of an artificial respirator to administer intermittent positive pressure breathing or continuous distending pressure (continuous positive airway pressure [CPAP]) is helpful in certain situations.

Apnea lasting longer than 30 seconds occurs in about 25% of low-birth-weight infants. In most instances, cutaneous stimulation results in resumption of breathing; in the remainder, resuscitation with bag and mask is usually effective. Xanthines (eg, theophylline, caffeine citrate) and mechanical ventilation have been reported to be of value in the treatment of significant apnea of prematurity. Use of an oscillating waterbed has been reported to decrease the incidence of apneic episodes.

Endotracheal suction has been recommended to decrease the possibility of subsequent respiratory difficulty in meconium-stained infants.

Onset of significant respiratory distress in the first few hours of life, especially in infants of greater than 36 weeks' gestational age, should suggest the possibility of group B streptococcal pneumonia.

IDIOPATHIC RESPIRATORY DISTRESS SYNDROME (IRDS); HYALINE MEMBRANE DISEASE (HMD) OF THE LUNGS*

Hyaline membranes are found principally in lungs of newborn infants who have died between 1 hour and a few days after birth (especially premature infants, those delivered by cesarean section or from mothers with bleeding or diabetes, or infants who experience intrauterine distress).

The hyaline membrane is composed principally of fibrin derived from the pulmonary capillaries of the newborn infant and not from aspirated amniotic fluid. A deficiency of surfactant until about the 34th or 35th week of gestation has been described in these infants. A test has been devised to estimate the adequacy of effective surfactant production; when the ratio of lecithin to sphingomyelin in amniotic fluid is 2:1 or greater, the likelihood of IRDS is small. Infants who die have low concentrations of pulmonary phospholipid. Hypotension, diminished pulmonary blood flow, pulmonary artery vasoconstriction, vascular shunts, ventilation-perfusion imbalance, acidosis, and hypoxia may all result from primary alveolar collapse. Pulmonary lymphatics are larger in affected lungs than in normal lungs.

*See footnote on p 159.

Clinical Findings

The manifestations of IRDS are dyspnea, tachypnea, nasal flaring, retractions of costal margins and lower sternum, grunting respirations, and cyanosis. Symptoms are usually present immediately after birth but may be delayed for 2–4 hours. During this time, hypotension may be present. In the early stages, x-ray reveals a reticulogranular pattern throughout the lungs, with prominence of bronchial air shadows; generalized atelectases may occur later. The blood pH level may be low. Blood gas studies reveal hypoxemia (right-to-left shunting) and, later, hypercapnia. Systemic hypotension and hypothermia may be present. Cerebral, pulmonary, and visceral hemorrhages may develop in fatal cases. Marked coagulation defects and laboratory or pathologic evidence (or both) of disseminated intravascular coagulation are frequently found in ill infants. There is no evidence of postnatal adrenal hypofunction in infants with IRDS or evidence that steroid treatment of the newborn infant is beneficial. The incidence of subsequent umbilical hernia is increased.

Prophylaxis & Treatment

Administration of a corticosteroid (dexamethasone or betamethasone) to a pregnant woman without hypertension or edema between the 26th and 32nd week of gestation and at least 48 hours before the birth of the infant induces earlier activation of the pulmonary surfactant system and decreases the risk that HMD will develop. IRDS may be less common after prolonged rupture of the membranes, maternal heroin addiction, and antenatal bacterial infection.

Adequate and prompt resuscitation of all high-risk and premature infants is the most important preventive step. Regulate ambient oxygen concentration so that arterial P_{O_2} is 70–90 mm Hg (at sea level), and maintain humidity (at 60–80%) in the environment. (See Bronchopulmonary Dysplasia, below.) Maintain thermal balance. Give antibiotics if infection is suspected. Frequent blood pressure measurements and monitoring of urine output (> 2 mL/kg/h) can enable one to predict inadequate perfusion, which should be treated with whole blood transfusion (up to 10 mL/kg) or infusion of plasma or 5% albumin (up to 10 mL/kg). Infants with respiratory distress should have intravenous fluid support (10% dextrose in water, 65–100 mL/kg/24 h). Continuous positive airway pressure (CPAP) and intermittent mandatory ventilation are often required. Avoid rapid infusion of alkaline solutions. Documented metabolic acidosis may be corrected slowly with diluted $NaHCO_3$. Long-term umbilical vein catheterization may be associated with portal vein occlusion, embolization, sepsis, and local necrosis and thrombosis. Indwelling umbilical artery catheterization also has potential hazards. Wrapping the newborn infant and placing the infant in the intrauterine position have been suggested, but the effectiveness of this procedure has not been proved. Frequent arterial blood gas determinations are necessary to maintain and adjust the inspired oxygen concentration. In some cases, bronchopulmonary dysplasia and other serious complications have been reported after respirator therapy. Avoid unnecessary laryngoscopy and handling. Do not give oral feedings while the infant has unstable respiratory distress.

Course & Prognosis

Death may occur, or the condition may persist for 2–4 days and then improve rather rapidly. Infants with severe disease may have a prolonged recovery period (> 1 week). Occasionally, pulmonary sequelae may occur, apparently related to prolonged intermittent positive pressure ventilation, but the severity of disease and the use of continuous high concentrations of oxygen are also important factors.

PNEUMOTHORAX, PNEUMOMEDIASTINUM, SUBCUTANEOUS EMPHYSEMA, PNEUMOPERICARDIUM, & PULMONARY INTERSTITIAL EMPHYSEMA (Air Block)

Air block occurs in 1% of newborn infants but is asymptomatic in many. It is caused by the migration of air from a ruptured alveolus along perivascular sheaths into the mediastinum and thence to the pleural space, thoracic cavity, or pericardium.

Onset is abrupt. Sudden collapse is common. Signs include increased activity, dyspnea, tachypnea, grunting, flaring, shift in apical impulse, hyperpnea, and cyanosis. There may be minimal movement of the chest in spite of marked suprasternal and infrasternal retractions. Increase in chest size may be more prominent on one side. Other signs include tympany and hyperresonance to percussion, shift of mediastinum, and diminution in heart sounds, depending on the type and degree of involvement.

A chest x-ray is helpful for diagnosis, but if sudden collapse occurs, an attempt to remove pleural air by needle aspiration may be justified. Pleural air may also be demonstrated by transillumination and should be searched for in this way.

The majority of cases of pneumothorax (and almost all cases of pneumomediastinum) involve only small amounts of air and require no specific treatment. These conditions may be complications of assisted ventilation.

Treatment

Give oxygen. Aspiration of air from the pleural or pericardial space or thoracostomy is usually necessary only in infants with significant symptoms. Small pneumothoraces (10% of cases) in full-term infants may be managed by having the infant breathe 100% oxygen for 1–2 hours. Aspiration of the mediastinal air is ineffective.

Course & Prognosis

Absorption of air from abnormal locations occurs spontaneously in most cases, but removal of air may be necessary.

WILSON-MIKITY SYNDROME

Respiratory distress, primarily in low-birth-weight infants, may develop insidiously days or weeks after birth and is characterized by cyanosis, tachypnea, wheezing, coughing, apnea, a progressively greater need for oxygen, and radiologic changes. The condition may continue for months; clinical improvement may occur months before resolution of the radiologic changes. The cause is obscure; exposure to excessive oxygen may be a factor. Treatment is supportive.

BRONCHOPULMONARY DYSPLASIA

Bronchopulmonary dysplasia resembling the Wilson-Mikity syndrome is a chronic lung disease occurring during infancy. It appears to be associated with oxygen toxicity in small, severely ill infants who have received continuous high concentrations of oxygen over long periods of time, usually by prolonged positive pressure ventilation. Excessive fluid intake may also be a factor. Bronchopulmonary dysplasia may also occur with meconium aspiration syndrome, congenital heart disease, and tracheoesophageal fistula. Pulmonary problems may persist for many months.

Patent ductus arteriosus may also develop, and death may result, since infants with this condition often have cardiac enlargement, cor pulmonale, and pulmonary dysplasia with fibrosis, overexpanded lung, and infiltrates. Early ligation of the patent ductus arteriosus has been suggested to decrease the incidence and severity of bronchopulmonary dysplasia.

A syndrome of delayed respiratory distress with onset after 4–7 days in a previously healthy premature infant has been described. There is chronic pulmonary insufficiency with a mortality rate of 10–20% or complete recovery by 60 days of age.

DISEASES DUE TO PERINATAL FACTORS

FRACTURES

Fractures of the Clavicle

Fracture of the clavicle is the most commonly occurring fracture at birth and generally involves the middle third of the bone. Examination reveals limitation of motion on the affected side and absence of the Moro reflex on the side with fracture; crepitus may be elicited.

With immobilization of the arm and shoulder, healing is spontaneous and complete. Even when fracture is not recognized and without specific treatment, good callus formation and healing usually occur.

Fractures of Extremities

Fractures of extremeties usually are caused by a difficult delivery. Signs of fracture are generally present, and the Moro reflex is absent on the affected side.

Treatment consists of immobilization for fractures of the upper extremity or immobilization and traction for fractures of the lower extremity.

Fractures of the Skull

Skull fractures may be entirely asymptomatic. Only depressed fractures require surgical treatment; 10% of cephalhematomas are associated with linear fractures.

HEMORRHAGES

Cephalhematoma

Cephalhematoma is an accumulation of blood between the periosteum and a skull bone. The blood does not cross a suture line. The mass is soft, fluctuating, and irreducible and does not pulsate or increase in size with crying. During the first days of life, it may be obscured by superimposed caput succedaneum. (See Fractures of the Skull, above.) Absorption of a large quantity of blood may cause hyperbilirubinemia. No treatment is required (blood should not be aspirated). The condition generally clears within a few weeks or months.

During the healing process, a firm ring often can be palpated at the periphery of the hematoma and may simulate a skull defect.

Sternocleidomastoid Hemorrhage

Sternocleidomastoid hemorrhage may not appear until the third week of life and generally produces a mass in the midportion of the muscle, resulting in torticollis to the affected side. It is more common after breech presentations and is often associated with a fibromalike mass; its cause in many cases remains obscure.

Passive hyperextension of the neck should be started early and in most cases is all that is necessary. Surgical intervention may be indicated for those cases that do not resolve over a few months with conservative therapy.

Intracranial Hemorrhage

Intracranial hemorrhage can result from obstetric trauma, hypoxia, coagulation disorders, infections, circulatory disturbances, erythroblastosis fetalis, or hypernatremia; it occurs more commonly in premature than in full-term infants. The hemorrhage may be subdural or subarachnoid but occurs commonly in the subependymal region and may rupture into the ventricles or extend into the brain substance. It may arise from a tear of the tentorium. Symptoms and signs may be present at birth or may appear later and include apnea; somnolence; restlessness; irritability; opisthotonos; disturbed respiratory and cardiac function with cyanosis; high-pitched, shrill cry; failure to nurse well; muscular twitchings; and convulsions. The fontanelle may be bulging. Hemorrhage of the retina and abnormalities of the pupils may occur. Temperature regulation often is disturbed. The Moro reflex may be exaggerated at birth, disappearing later, or may be absent throughout. Paralyses generally do not appear for several days. Anemia may occur. Symptoms may be present at birth, clear for a day or so, and then reappear. Many subependymal and interventricular hemorrhages in asymptomatic low-birth-weight infants may be detected by ultrasonography and CT scan.

An increase in cerebrospinal fluid pressure may be of diagnostic significance, but the presence of bloody fluid in the cerebrospinal spaces is not of particular help in diagnosis in the newborn, since a small amount of bleeding may occur in the normal infant who has not had a particularly difficult delivery and is asymptomatic.

Rest, warmth, sedation, elevation of the head, minimal handling, and vitamin K may be helpful. There is disagreement as to the value of performing repeated spinal punctures. When a subdural hematoma is present, it should be evacuated if it is associated with persistent symptoms.

Most infants survive and recover completely, but cerebral palsy, mental deficiency, convulsive susceptibility, or hydrocephalus may result. With extensive or severe involvement, death usually occurs within the first 3 days.

Liver & Spleen Hemorrhage

Hemorrhage of the liver and spleen may result in formation of a palpable subcapsular hematoma that may not rupture for some time

(> 48 hours) after birth but then produce signs of rapidly progressive collapse. Liver and spleen hemorrhage occasionally results from vigorous attempts at resuscitation with flexion of the legs upon the abdomen. Treatment is with whole blood transfusions and surgical exploration, if necessary.

Adrenal Hemorrhage

See Chapter 22.

PERIPHERAL NERVE INJURIES

Brachial Plexus Palsy

In Erb-Duchenne (upper arm; C5 and C6 or their trunks) paralysis, simultaneous involvement of the phrenic nerve may occur. The arm is adducted, extended, and internally rotated with pronation of the forearm. The Moro reflex is absent on the affected side, and there is sensory loss on the lateral portion of the arm. The forearm and hand are not affected. In Klumpke's paralysis, the trauma involves nerves from C7, C8, and T1 or their trunks. There is loss of normal function of the small muscles of the hand. Sympathetic fibers of T1 may also be damaged, with resultant ptosis and miosis. Erb-Duchenne and Klumpke's paralyses may occur together.

Physical therapy and splinting to prevent deformity of the involved portions of the extremity are indicated in all cases.

Neuroplasty should be considered in persistent cases.

A period of several months may elapse before a definite prognosis can be given. In most cases, the paralysis is due to edema and hemorrhage about the nerve fibers or to nerve injury without laceration; in these instances, the outcome may be excellent. If laceration has occurred, return of function is not to be expected.

Phrenic Nerve Palsy

Phrenic nerve palsy is often associated with brachial plexus paralysis. There may be cyanosis and rapid, labored, irregular respirations with thoracic breathing. Fluoroscopy shows elevation of the diaphragm and paradoxic respirations on the affected side.

Recovery is possible if neither laceration nor avulsion of the nerve has occurred. If there is no spontaneous recovery from paralysis, good results can be obtained with diaphragm plication.

Facial Palsy

Facial palsy is generally due to injury to the peripheral portion of the facial nerve by pressure of forceps or of the shoulder or a foot during labor or delivery. When the infant cries, there is movement only on one side of the face and pulling to the unaffected side. The paralyzed side is smooth and may appear to be swollen. The forehead does not wrinkle. The eye on the affected side may not close.

Treatment is symptomatic.

The condition usually clears within a few weeks if nerve fibers have not been torn; in some infants with persistent paralysis, neuroplasty may be indicated. Permanent paralysis is more likely to occur when damage is due to pressure from the shoulder than when it is due to trauma from forceps.

INFECTIONS OF THE NEWBORN*

Common sources, manifestations, and treatment of infections in the newborn are shown in Table 9–1.

SEPSIS OF THE NEWBORN

Sepsis should be suspected in neonates born to mothers who have fever, prolonged ruptured membranes, frank amnionitis, or any suspected or treated infectious disease and in all cases of obscure illness in the infant. Appropriate specimens (blood, nasopharyngeal, urine, stool, cerebrospinal fluid) should be taken and cultured for bacteria and viruses.†

Infection may enter the bloodstream from a variety of sites. It may begin prenatally, perinatally, or in the newborn period and may be caused by any pathogenic organism. Localization may occur in any part of the body.

Elevated levels of IgM at birth are associated with an increased incidence of congenital infections, particularly subclinical infections with "silent" central nervous system involvement. However, the absence of IgM does not rule out congenital infection.

Clinical Findings

A. Symptoms: Onset is frequently insidious. Symptoms may be present at birth. Apnea, anorexia, poor weight gain, lethargy, or

*Conjunctivitis of the newborn is discussed in Chapter 19. For a description of group B streptococcal infections in newborn infants, see Chapter 25.

†Deliberate colonization of newborn infants with a coagulase-positive *Staphylococcus* of relatively low pathogenicity (502A) is now seldom employed as a means of controlling nursery outbreaks of pathogenic staphylococci.

Table 9–1. Common sources, manifestations, and treatment of infection in the newborn.*

Infection	Common Sources	Manifestations	Treatment
Diarrhea	*Enterobacter, Escherichia coli* (enteropathogenic types), *Klebsiella, Salmonella, Shigella, Staphylococcus,* many viruses.	Frequent explosive, water-loss stools with or without blood; poor feeding; vomiting; fever; weight loss; dehydration; acidosis. May progress to cardiovascular collapse. "Epidemic diarrhea of newborn," usually caused by *E coli,* spreads rapidly in nurseries and can be fatal. Illness varies in severity. Mortality rate may be high. Obstetric services and newborn nurseries may have to be closed.	Isolate the infant. Correct fluid and electrolyte imbalance. Give specific therapy when known.
Intrauterine infection†			
Herpes simplex	Herpesvirus hominis.	If acquired in utero, illness may be manifested at birth by skin vesicles. If acquired intrapartum, onset of illness is usually at 4–7 d, with lethargy and poor feeding. A few vesicles may appear. The infant then suddenly becomes quite ill, with jaundice, purpura, bleeding, pneumonia, seizures, and death. Cultures of vesicular fluid may grow virus in 48 h. Complement fixation titers peak at about 14 d.	Isolate the infant. Adenine arabinoside and acyclovir may be of value.
Meningitis	*E coli, Enterobacter,* enterovirus, *Haemophilus influenzae, Klebsiella, Listeria monocytogenes,* pneumococci, *Pseudomonas, Salmonella, Staphylococcus aureus, Streptococcus* (especially group B).	May be present at birth, may occur at any time as an isolated infection, or may be a manifestation of sepsis of the newborn. Symptoms of sepsis plus irritability, bulging anterior fontanelle, opisthotonos, seizures, and abnormal Moro reflex. Watch for rapidly increasing head circumference as a sign of hydrocephalus.	Give ampicillin and gentamicin until organism is identified.
Pneumonia	Coxsackievirus B, cytomegalovirus, *E coli, Enterobacter,* herpesvirus hominis, *Klebsiella, Pseudomonas,* rubella virus, *Staphylococcus, Streptococcus* (especially group B).	May be present at birth. Symptoms of sepsis plus tachypnea, nasal flaring, irregular respirations, and rales. Chest x-ray is essential.	Give specific therapy when known. Institute ventilatory support for respiratory failure.

Skin infection			
Cutaneous candidiasis	*Candida albicans.*	Erythematous maceration of skin in groin and perianal areas. May have oral lesions (thrush).	See Chapter 12.
Impetigo	*Pseudomonas, Staphylococcus, Streptococcus,* viruses.	Papules, pustules, or vesicles in moist areas or in skin creases. Vesicles often thin-walled, initially with clear fluid. *Pseudomonas* may produce punched-out necrotic ulcers. Infection may spread to other areas.	Give topical or systemic antibiotics (or both) as indicated.
Ritter's disease‡	*Staphylococcus* (phage type II).	Rapidly progressing cellulitis with loosening and sloughing of epidermal layers. May have positive Nikolsky sign.	Give specific antibiotic therapy.
Umbilical cord infection (omphalitis)	*E coli, Enterobacter, Klebsiella, Staphylococcus, Streptococcus.*	Erythema and edema of skin around umbilicus. Serous or purulent discharge from cord.	Give ampicillin and gentamicin pending cultures.
Urinary tract infection	*E coli, Enterobacter, Klebsiella, Proteus, Pseudomonas.*	Occasionally presents as sepsis but more often as abnormal weight loss in first few days, failure to gain weight, feeding difficulty, lethargy, fever, unexplained jaundice, vomiting, cyanosis, or pallor. More common in males and preterm infants. Urinalysis and culture of urine obtained by suprapubic aspiration are necessary. Pyuria is not a frequent finding.	Give specific therapy when indicated.

*Adapted from Morriss.

†The following intrauterine infections are discussed elsewhere in this book: cytomegalic inclusion disease (cytomegalovirus) and rubella, Chapter 24; syphilis, Chapter 25; toxoplasmosis, Chapter 26.

‡Scalded skin syndrome; toxic epidermal necrolysis.

restlessness may be the only findings. Temperature instability is a common manifestation, with hypothermia more common than fever. Gastrointestinal (vomiting, diarrhea, abdominal distention), central nervous system (restlessness, convulsions), or respiratory tract manifestations may be prominent. Respiratory distress in group B streptococcal pneumonia may occur early and be indistinguishable from idiopathic respiratory distress syndrome (see p 160).

B. Signs: Signs for bacterial and viral infections are similar. Hepatomegaly, splenomegaly, pallor, cyanosis, tachypnea, and jaundice (especially in the first 24 hours) often occur. Hemorrhage, with a petechial rash, is frequent. An associated meningitis or other focal infection is not uncommon.

Treatment

A. General Measures: Isolate the patient and give supportive therapy as indicated.

B. Specific Measures: Specimens should be obtained for culture, and antibacterial therapy in full dosage with appropriate antibiotics (see Chapter 6) should be instituted immediately. When herpes viral infection is suspected, antiviral therapy should be considered early.

C. Prophylactic Measures: An attempt to prevent infection with convalescent plasma should be considered for infants whose mothers have herpes.

Course & Prognosis

With early treatment, most infants recover. The mortality rate increases with delay in therapy. Careful observation should be made for localization of the infection.

DISTURBANCES OF THE BLOOD & BLOOD GROUP INCOMPATIBILITIES

Thrombocytopenia may be a manifestation of intrauterine infection, disseminated or focal intravascular coagulation, and platelet isoimmunization with or without maternal thrombocytopenia.

Polycythemia shortly after birth, with a central venous hematocrit level over 65% (or peripheral hematocrit level over 70%), may be due to placental-fetal transfusion, twin-twin transfusion in utero, or intrauterine growth retardation.

Anemia in newborn infants may be due to blood loss from fetoplacental transfusion at delivery; fetofetal transfusion in twins; chronic fetomaternal transfusion; ruptured liver or spleen; fracture; central nervous system, gastrointestinal, or pulmonary hemorrhage; hematoma; cord bleeding; hemolysis (erythroblastosis fetalis, red cell defects, hemoglobinopathies); or congenital aplastic or hypoplastic anemia.

HEMORRHAGIC DISEASE OF THE NEWBORN

Hemorrhagic disease of the newborn is a somewhat obscure disorder that may have a combination of causes. The essential feature is the accentuation of the coagulation defects that are found in all newborn infants. The major defect seems to be a deficiency of available prothrombin. The condition is more common in breast-fed infants who did not receive vitamin K.

Diarrhea, treatment with antimicrobial agents, and a diet low in vitamin K may produce hypoprothrombinemic bleeding in infants beyond the newborn period.

Clinical Findings

A. Signs: Bleeding of the skin, umbilical cord, mucous membranes, or viscera may occur spontaneously or following mild trauma, usually between the second and fifth days of life, when the available prothrombin is at its lowest level.

B. Laboratory Findings: The activity of prothrombin, plasma thromboplastin component, proconvertin, and Stuart-Prower factor may be decreased. Prothrombin time (one-stage) is usually prolonged. Coagulation time may be normal or prolonged.

Treatment

A. Vitamin K: Give vitamin K_1, 1–5 mg intravenously, to raise the prothrombin level. Repeat once if necessary. Avoid overdosage. (Vitamin K_1 may be given intramuscularly, but the effect will be slower.)

B. Blood or Plasma: Give transfusion of fresh, matched whole blood, 15–20 mL/kg, or fresh frozen plasma, 10 mL/kg.

C. Topical Measures: Use pressure dressings and topical application of coagulants (thrombin, fibrin foam) on accessible bleeding sites.

Prophylaxis

The intestine is sterile at birth, and it may take several days before the normal intestinal flora produces sufficient vitamin K for the infant. The administration of vitamin K to the mother will elevate the prothrombin level of the newborn infant, but it must be used with caution. Avoid overdosage. Vitamin K_1 (AquaMephyton, Konakion), 1 mg intramuscularly, should be given prophylactically to the newborn infant.

Prognosis

With adequate and early therapy, death is rare and complete recovery occurs.

ERYTHROBLASTOSIS FETALIS
(Hemolytic Disease of the Newborn)

1. DUE TO Rh INCOMPATIBILITY

Eleven percent of pregnancies among the white population occur as a result of the mating of an Rh-negative woman with an Rh-positive man. However, the incidence of erythroblastosis fetalis due to Rh incompatibility is much lower than 11% because not all women are capable of producing anti-Rh agglutinins and because immunization occurs slowly; one or more pregnancies with an Rh-positive fetus or previous transfusion with Rh-positive blood generally is necessary before a harmful degree of sensitization can develop. Severe Rh sensitization is less likely to occur when mother and infant have ABO compatibility.

Clinical Findings

A. Symptoms and Signs:

1. The placenta may be enlarged; the vernix is often yellow.
2. Marked edema (hydrops fetalis) and other signs of cardiac failure (pleural and pericardial effusions, ascites, etc) may occur in severe cases. The infant may be stillborn.
3. Jaundice appears during the first 24 hours.
4. Progressive anemia occurs.
5. Hepatosplenomegaly is common.
6. Central nervous system signs may be present (see kernicterus under Complications, below).
7. Bleeding tendency is occasionally seen.

B. Laboratory Findings:

1. The mother is Rh-negative; the infant is Rh-positive.
2. The anti-Rh titer of the mother is increased.
3. Sensitized Rh-positive infants may occasionally type as Rh-negative owing to "blocking antibodies."
4. Results of the direct Coombs (antihuman globulin) test on infant red cells are positive.
5. Reticulocyte and nucleated red blood cell counts in peripheral blood are increased.
6. Anemia may be present at birth or may appear within the first few hours or days of life. Other manifestations of erythroblastosis fetalis may occur in the absence of anemia.

7. The serum indirect (and, occasionally, direct) bilirubin level is increased (see Appendix).

8. Anti-Rh agglutinins may be present in the infant's serum.

9. Hypoglycemia (often asymptomatic) may occur.

10. After the 24th week of gestation, there may be an elevated peak at 450 nm in the spectrophotometric reading of the optical density of amniotic fluid.

Complications

Kernicterus may occur after any condition causing cerebral anoxia (even without severe hyperbilirubinemia) but generally follows erythroblastosis fetalis with marked elevation of unconjugated bilirubin level (> 20 mg/dL). It is characterized by destructive and degenerative changes of the brain associated with yellow staining with bile pigment in the nuclear areas of the midbrain and medulla. It is initially manifested by hypotonia, lethargy, and poor sucking in some cases. Spasticity, abnormal Moro reflex, deafness, mental retardation, opisthotonos, and fever may develop later. These findings may subside, but in many children there will be reappearance of permanent signs of extrapyramidal involvement. Death may occur in the early stages of the disease.

Premature infants appear to be more susceptible than mature neonates to the development of kernicterus at any given bilirubin concentration; they frequently are free of clinical signs and may not respond favorably to exchange transfusion. A decrease in the quantity of albumin or in its capability to bind bilirubin—or lowering of the blood-brain barrier to bilirubin—may be an important pathogenetic mechanism. Acidosis, drugs, hypoxia, hypothermia, hypoglycemia, or cold stress may facilitate the development of kernicterus at lower bilirubin levels.

Any Rh-negative mother with an Rh antibody titer of 1:32 or greater in the fourth or fifth month of pregnancy should have 2 amniocenteses at 1-week intervals, and the optical density of amniotic fluid (ΔOD) at 450 nm should be measured. (Some investigators recommend that serum Rh antibody titers greater than 1:32 should be present before performing amniocentesis.) If the ΔOD 450 is falling, the fetus may be left in utero safely. If the ΔOD 450 is found to be rising or staying the same and the levels are in arbitrarily defined upper zone II or lower zone III, the fetus should receive one or more intraperitoneal transfusions before the 32nd or 33rd week of gestational age.

Prenatal Care

The mother's Rh type should be determined in all pregnancies. The antibody titer (Rh or ABO) should be monitored throughout the pregnancy in all Rh-negative women or those with a possible history of disease in previous pregnancies. Minimum sedation should be used in sensitized women.

Prophylaxis

Rh sensitization may be prevented in almost 100% of cases by the administration of 1 mL of high-potency Rh_0 (D) immune globulin (RhoGAM) intramuscularly within 24–48 hours after delivery to an Rh_0-negative woman previously unimmunized to the Rh_0 antigen as determined by the absence of anti-Rh_0 in her serum prior to and at the time of delivery. The infant must be Rh_0-positive, and the Coombs reaction on cord blood specimen must be negative.

Treatment

A. Induction of Labor: Early induction of labor may be indicated if previous pregnancies have resulted in stillbirths, neonatal deaths, or hydrops due to erythroblastosis. It may also be indicated if serial evaluations of amniotic fluid demonstrate significant sensitization. If hydrops is suspected on the basis of ultrasonographic or x-ray findings, induction of labor should be considered. Excessive prematurity should, however, be avoided.

B. Specific Measures: Exchange transfusion with fresh type O, Rh-negative blood cross-matched with maternal serum may be indicated. In the presence of frank hydrops and anemia (hematocrit level < 30%), an initial partial packed red cell exchange transfusion should be done to raise the hematocrit level to greater than 40% prior to the 2-volume whole blood exchange.

Indications for exchange transfusion are as follows: (1) clinical illness at birth or significant jaundice within the first 12 hours of life, (2) cord bilirubin level over 4.5 mg/dL, (3) cord hemoglobin level under 14 g/dL, (4) rise in unconjugated serum bilirubin level greater than 0.5 mg/dL/h within the first 48 hours, (5) unconjugated bilirubin level greater than 20 mg/dL, and (6) early signs of kernicterus.

Extensive edema, effusions, and ascites may require paracentesis and thoracentesis. Positive pressure ventilation, digitalization, and the use of diuretics may be necessary.

C. Supportive Measures: Determine hemoglobin level daily until stabilized and then every 2 weeks until hematopoiesis develops. Breast feeding may be allowed, depending on the infant's state.

D. Prevention and Treatment of Complications: Exchange blood transfusions shortly after birth are said to lessen the incidence of kernicterus; these may be repeated as a therapeutic measure even after kernicterus has become established.

E. Phototherapy: Phototherapy may be a valuable adjunct to exchange transfusion and, when instituted early, will decrease the number of exchange transfusions required. Check for increased insensible and fecal water and electrolyte loss. Observe for anemia developing after several (2–6) weeks.

Course & Prognosis

The affected infant may be born dead or may die within the first few days of life. In other instances, complete recovery may occur without clinical evidence of the disease or after mild or severe manifestations. Sensorineural hearing impairment may develop. Residual damage of the central nervous system (kernicterus) may occur, particularly if the jaundice was prolonged and the serum was saturated with bilirubin.

The prognosis is good after the sixth day, although some increase in anemia usually occurs.

The disease is quite variable, and in any single instance no definite prognosis can be given. The overall mortality rate of exchange transfusion is approximately 1–3% but is considerably less in vigorous infants.

Multiple exchange transfusions are effective in preventing long-term sequelae due to hyperbilirubinemia.

Some patients become anemic from slow, persistent hemolysis even if their neonatal course was benign. Anemia following phototherapy is not uncommon. Simple transfusion is indicated if the hemoglobin level falls below 7 g/dL.

Intrauterine transfusions are associated with approximately 50% successful results. The risk to the fetus from a single intrauterine transfusion is between 5 and 12%. Even with fetal transfusion, the mortality rate in hydrops fetalis is still high.

No significant correlations have been found between the presence or absence of brain damage and the maximum bilirubin concentration, birth weight, sex, presence or absence of hemolytic disease, or use of exchange transfusion.

2. DUE TO ABO INCOMPATIBILITY

ABO incompatibility is the most common type of fetal-maternal blood group incompatibility.

The mechanism is the same as in hemolytic disease of the newborn due to Rh incompatibility except that the immunization is caused by the group A or B substance instead of the Rh substance. The disease commonly affects first-born infants. Most cases are subclinical and are due to incompatibility of A substance, but incompatibility of B substance may produce a more severe illness.

Clinical Findings

A. Symptoms and Signs: Jaundice may appear during the first 24 hours of life but is often delayed until 48–72 hours after birth. Hepatosplenomegaly may be present. Central nervous system signs are uncommon.

B. Laboratory Findings:

1. The mother is generally type O.
2. High anti-A or anti-B titer is present in the mother. The titer may not rise until several days after delivery. Correlation of severity of fetal sensitization with maternal titers is generally poor.
3. The serum bilirubin level is elevated (see Appendix).
4. The direct Coombs test is positive in most cases.
5. Anti-A or anti-B agglutinins may be present in the infant's serum.
6. The reticulocyte count is increased.
7. Spherocytosis and microcytosis are often present. Increased osmotic and mechanical fragility of red cells is often present.
8. The hemoglobin level is usually normal.
9. The erythrocyte acetylcholinesterase level is reduced.
10. There is increased in vitro hemolysis.

Treatment & Prognosis

In most cases, treatment is not necessary. Phototherapy is effective in lowering the bilirubin concentration. Check for increased insensible water loss and increased metabolic demands. Exchange transfusion is indicated for those infants whose indirect serum bilirubin level rises *significantly* above 20 mg/dL. Although similar in pathogenesis to the disorder caused by Rh incompatibility, this form of erythroblastosis fetalis is much milder.

JAUNDICE OF THE NEWBORN

"PHYSIOLOGIC" JAUNDICE OF THE NEWBORN (Jaundice of Undetermined Etiology)

"Physiologic" jaundice is a normal phenomenon, since almost all infants show some elevation of serum bilirubin level during the first week of life. Jaundice may be caused by many factors unique to the neonatal period, including relative deficiency of hepatic glucuronyl transferase activity, absence of bacterial flora to convert conjugated bilirubin to urobilinogen, increased enterohepatic circulation of bilirubin, inhibitory effect of maternal serum on bilirubin conjugation, and persistent patency of the ductus venosus.

The jaundice appears after the first day of life (generally between the second and fifth days) and clears within 1–2 weeks. Jaundice is the only sign, although some infants are lethargic and eat poorly at the height of jaundice. Dehydration and starvation may aggravate the condition;

lower serum bilirubin levels during the first week of life have been noted in low-birth-weight infants who are fed in the first 2 hours of life rather than after 24–36 hours. Infants who are small for gestational age have lower average mean serum bilirubin concentrations than do those with appropriate weight for age. Stools are normal in color. Jaundice is more severe in premature infants. The course is usually uneventful, and there are no sequelae.

No treatment is usually necessary. Recent reports indicate that continuous exposure of an infant with a bilirubin level greater than 10 mg/dL to artificial visible light will decrease the degree of hyperbilirubinemia, particularly in premature infants. There have been conflicting reports about the value of administration of small doses of phenobarbital to women during the last weeks of pregnancy—or administration of ethanol prior to delivery—in lowering bilirubin levels in their offspring during the first few days of life. The administration of phenobarbital may reduce the level of hyperbilirubinemia in the neonate, but the safety of this procedure is unproved.

Neonatal hyperbilirubinemia may be more severe in certain races (eg, Oriental) than others (eg, Caucasian) living in the same area, possibly owing to an increased incidence of red cell enzyme deficiencies.

There is no convincing evidence that nonhemolytic jaundice significantly affects ultimate intelligence and neurologic status.

PATHOLOGIC JAUNDICE OF THE NEWBORN

Abnormal jaundice may occur in a number of conditions, including (1) abnormalities of the blood (erythroblastosis fetalis due to Rh or ABO incompatibility, hemoglobinopathies [Bart's, Zurich], congenital leukemia, other hemolytic anemias); (2) defects involving enzyme activity (persistent deficiency of glycuronyl transferase [Crigler-Najjar disease], inhibition of enzyme activity [novobiocin], glucose-6-phosphate dehydrogenase deficiency [especially in premature black infants], deficiency of uridine diphosphopyridine glucose dehydrogenase, erythrocyte glutathione peroxidase deficiency); (3) infections (urinary tract infection, viral or bacterial sepsis, syphilis, congenital hepatitis, toxoplasmosis); (4) anatomic abnormalities (atresia of the bile ducts, choledochal cysts and bile plugs, high small bowel obstruction, congenital malformation of the intestine); and (5) other disorders, including those with unknown mechanisms (cystic fibrosis, cretinism, internal hemorrhage, hypoxia, galactosemia, tyrosinosis, α_1-antitrypsin deficiency).

Certain drugs may increase the risk of jaundice by competing for albumin binding (sulfonamides, salicylates, heme pigments, intravenous fat, sodium benzoate), by competing for the conjugating mechanism (salicylates, chloramphenicol, water-soluble analogs of vitamin K, sulfisoxazole, sulfamethoxypyridazine, sulfadimethoxine, steroids, caffeine with sodium benzoate), by increasing hemolysis (synthetic vitamin K), or by unknown mechanisms. Hyperbilirubinemia may occur following the use of oxytocin during labor.

In a few infants, breast feeding may be associated with hyperbilirubinemia that persists for 2–6 weeks.

Phototherapy may be of value in infants with nonhemolytic hyperbilirubinemia from a variety of causes.

GASTROINTESTINAL DISEASES OF THE NEWBORN

MECONIUM PLUG SYNDROME

Abdominal distention and lack of meconium passage with or without bilious vomiting may occur in infants who otherwise do not appear very ill but have a meconium plug obstructing the colon.

Expulsion of the plug may occur after digital examination or the use of enemas. Occasionally, Hirschsprung's disease may develop subsequently.

CONGENITAL BILIARY ATRESIA

Congenital biliary atresia may be associated with absence or obstruction of either intrahepatic or extrahepatic biliary passages. Biliary atresia and neonatal hepatitis may be different forms of the same basic disease process.

Clinical Findings

A. Symptoms and Signs: Jaundice (appearing shortly after birth or delayed for days or weeks) may be mild at first and then progresses and becomes severe. The skin eventually takes on a bronze, olive-green color. Stools are clay-colored or white and of puttylike consistency, although stools during the first days of life may have the appearance of normal meconium. Other symptoms include splenomegaly and progressive enlargement of the liver, hemorrhages due to deficiency of vitamin K, deficiencies of other fat-soluble vitamins, and dwarfing in long-standing cases.

Any or all of the clinical findings of congenital biliary atresia may be present also in **neonatal (congenital) hepatitis;** even liver biopsy may also give identical results. Juvenile cirrhosis may follow. Some infants with neonatal hepatitis may have α_1-antitrypsin deficiency.

B. Laboratory Findings: Stools occasionally contain small amounts of bile pigments or derivatives of bile pigments. The urine contains large amounts of bile pigments. Urine urobilinogen is generally absent. The bilirubin level and icterus index increase progressively (may be variable in first weeks). Prothrombin concentration is reduced. The radioactive rose bengal test is of value in determining complete obstruction to the outflow of bile.

In neonatal hepatitis, there may be fluctuating bilirubin levels. Alkaline phosphatase activity is a good indicator of disturbed parenchymal function in the follow-up period.

Treatment

A. General Measures: Give a diet low in fat, high in fat-soluble vitamins, and containing medium-chain triglycerides as the source of fat. Treatment with choleretics is sometimes of value in differentiating cases with blockage of the biliary system from those with atresia. Phenobarbital may reduce blood lipid, bile acid, and bilirubin levels.

B. Surgical Measures: Exploration is indicated if congenital biliary atresia is suspected. Hepatic portoenterostomy (Kasai procedure) appears to improve markedly the prognosis of many infants with biliary atresia (especially of the nonfamilial type) if it is performed in infants before age 2 months. Differentiation from neonatal hepatitis (using operative cholangiograms) should be carried out before that time.

Course & Prognosis

The patient's general condition may remain good for many months without surgery. Some cases apparently clear spontaneously. Improvement appears to be enhanced by surgical correction.

NECROTIZING ENTEROCOLITIS

Necrotizing enterocolitis is an idiopathic disease that occurs predominantly in low-birth-weight preterm neonates, who often have a history of maternal fever or amnionitis, postnatal respiratory difficulty (apnea, mild idiopathic respiratory distress syndrome), infection, high osmolar oral feedings, or exchange transfusion. It may be more common in orally fed infants who had an umbilical arterial catheter in place. Despite the history, they do well for 2–5 days before developing lethargy, vomiting, abdominal distention, hypothermia, recurrence of apnea, bloody stools, and finally cardiovascular collapse. Early abdominal x-rays show air-fluid levels, dilated loops of bowel, and separation of loops of bowel secondary to edema in the bowel walls. Linear streaks of intraluminal air (pneumatosis intestinalis) develop and are pathognomonic. If the disease continues to progress, pneumoperitoneum and gas in the portal vein may be seen. Cultures may reveal gram-negative bacteremia, but no specific organism is known to cause this disease.

Therapy consists of administration of antibiotics (ampicillin and gentamicin or kanamycin) and fluid (including colloid or whole blood), electrolyte, temperature, and circulatory support. Indications for laparotomy include perforation, persistent localized tenderness for over 12 hours, and abdominal wall cellulitis. Laparotomy for resection of necrotic intestine or for pneumoperitonitis may be necessary.

The disease has a high mortality rate. A spotty epidemiologic distribution has been noted.

Infants managed conservatively may develop late intestinal (usually colonic) stenosis, which requires resection.

PHYSIOLOGIC VOMITING

During the first day or 2 of life, vomiting of mucus or blood-streaked material occurs in many infants. It clears spontaneously, but improvement may be speeded if the stomach is lavaged.

For other causes of vomiting, see Table 16–1.

CONVULSIONS OF THE NEWBORN

Convulsions in the first few weeks of life are most commonly due to hypocalcemia, intracranial birth injury, central nervous system infection, congenital cerebral malformation, perinatal anoxia, polycythemia, pyridoxine deficiency, bilirubin toxicity, hypernatremia, mepivacaine toxicity, cerebral edema, hypomagnesemia, hypoglycemia, or unknown causes. The peak incidence of convulsions occurs on the first day of life, when perinatal anoxia is the most common cause, and on the second day of life, when intracranial hemorrhage and cerebral contusions are the most common causes. The seizures may vary in pattern and be clonic, myoclonic, focal, or generalized, or they may merely produce transient stiffening of the body. Momentary changes in respiratory rate, brief periods of apnea, slight posturing, chewing and sucking motions, abnormal cry, paroxysmal blinking, or localized twitching may also occur.

Treatment is directed toward correcting any deficiency or eliminating possible causes of the convulsive state. Until the cause is determined, intravenous therapy with pyridoxine, calcium, magnesium, and glucose should be tried, followed by anticonvulsant drugs (diazepam, phenobarbital, phenytoin, paraldehyde) as necessary.

Approximately half of neonates with convulsions will eventually be normal. The best prognosis is for those with normal electroencephalograms, hypocalcemia, intracranial birth injury, and convulsions due to unknown causes. Approximately one-fifth will die, and one-quarter will show neurologic deficits.

METABOLIC & ENDOCRINE DISEASES OF THE NEWBORN

NEONATAL HYPOCALCEMIA

Newborns, particularly those born prematurely or after complicated pregnancies or intrapartum periods, may demonstrate functional hypoparathyroidism. Hypocalcemia during the first 36 hours of life is associated with prematurity, asphyxia, infants of diabetic mothers, infants born to mothers with hyperparathyroidism (symptomatic or asymptomatic), difficult intrapartum periods, DiGeorge's syndrome, stress (infection, respiratory distress syndrome, exchange transfusion), and infants treated with sodium bicarbonate for acidosis.

Adaptation toward calcium homeostasis begins soon after birth in healthy infants and progresses without incident in breast-fed infants. In infants fed with cow's milk formulas, relatively high concentrations of phosphate may exceed the capacity of the kidney to secrete phosphate, and accumulation of phosphate may produce disturbances in calcium homeostasis, resulting in tetany. Late-onset hypocalcemia of this type (neonatal tetany) usually occurs near the end of the first week of life but may occur any time during the first 2 months.

Hypocalcemia in the neonate may be associated with hypomagnesemia and may fail to respond to calcium administration until the hypomagnesemia is corrected.

Clinical Findings

A. Symptoms and Signs: Increased irritability, localized twitching, periods of apnea, convulsions, vomiting, hypertonicity, high-pitched cry, and respiratory distress are the principal findings. Periods of immobility may occur. Laryngeal signs are uncommon. Chvostek's sign is of no value, since it is present in many normal infants. Carpopedal spasm is uncommon. The Moro reflex is not depressed. In premature infants with early-onset hypocalcemia, there are usually no symptoms or abnormal signs.

B. Laboratory Findings: The level of total serum calcium is low (< 7.5 mg/dL), as is that of ionized calcium (< 3.5 mg/dL). The serum phosphorus level is generally elevated.

Treatment

A. Severe Cases: Immediate treatment in severe cases consists of giving calcium gluconate, 0.1–0.2 g/kg, as a 10% solution slowly intravenously. Subsequently, add calcium lactate or gluconate, 0.5–1 g/kg/d, to the infant's formula. This regimen can usually be discontinued after 1 week. Do *not* give concentrated calcium solutions by mouth.

The severe local manifestations that may occur at the site of intravenous administration of calcium should be managed conservatively.

B. General Measures: A modified cow's milk formula with a more favorable Ca/P ratio—such as Similac PM 60/40—may be beneficial.

Prognosis

The prognosis is excellent in late-onset tetany unless anoxia, with resultant permanent brain damage, has occurred during episodes of convulsions; it is variable with early-onset tetany depending on the severity of predisposing factors. There is no evidence that hypocalcemia alone has an adverse effect in early-onset tetany.

NEONATAL HYPOGLYCEMIA

(See also Chapter 22.)

Asymptomatic physiologic hypoglycemia with blood glucose levels under 50 mg/dL occurs commonly in the neonatal period; blood glucose levels are higher if the infant is fed in the first hours after birth. Significant hypoglycemia (blood glucose < 30 mg/dL in low-birth-weight infants or < 40 mg/dL in full-term infants) may occur and be associated with irritability, lethargy, limpness, high-pitched cry, difficulty in feeding, sweating, apnea, cyanosis, tremors, and convulsions. Hypoglycemia is especially likely to occur in infants with low or increased birth weight or period of gestation, erythroblastosis fetalis, infection (especially with gram-negative bacilli), polycythemia, central nervous system injury or anomaly, galactosemia, leucine sensitivity, Beckwith's syndrome, neonatal cold injury, or trisomy 13–15 and in infants born to mothers with preeclampsia-eclampsia or diabetes. It may also occur in an idiopathic form. The smaller of twins is more likely to be hypoglycemic. The condition appears to be more common in males. Low blood glucose levels may occur within a few hours after birth and again on the third day. There may be associated hypocalcemia and polycythemia.

Prompt improvement usually occurs after intravenous administration of glucose. Rarely is more than 15% glucose at a rate of 125 mL/kg/24 h required, and rapid administration of hypertonic glucose should be avoided. In refractory cases, the administration of hydrocortisone (5 mg/kg/24 h) may be necessary. Do not discontinue glucose infusions abruptly.

INFANTS OF DIABETIC MOTHERS

Infants of diabetic mothers often present serious problems and have increased morbidity and mortality rates, an increased incidence of congenital anomalies, and an increased incidence of sudden intrauterine death. The exact mechanism is not known.

Clinical Findings

A. Symptoms and Signs: The infant is usually larger than average for the expected stage of maturity, with lethargy, round red face, cardiomegaly, hepatomegaly, splenomegaly, and a tendency to cyanosis, edema, and tetany. Large amounts of fluid are present in the trachea and bronchi and in the stomach. There is an increased incidence of congenital anomalies. Symptoms of hypoglycemia are sometimes but not always present. Infants of diabetic mothers have an increased incidence of hyaline membrane disease, hypocalcemia, impaired metabolism of bilirubin, and clotting abnormalities (renal vein thrombosis).

B. Laboratory Findings: Hypoglycemia often develops. In most infants, it may be no more marked than the physiologic hypoglycemia of the normal newborn. Hypoglycemia prolonged for several days has been reported in association with maternal chlorpropamide (Diabinese) therapy.

Additional findings may include erythroblastosis of peripheral blood or extramedullary hematopoiesis. There may be an increased incidence of hyperbilirubinemia. Also, there may be an abnormal placenta, increased insulin levels, reduced free fatty acid levels, disturbed adrenocortical and thyroid function, functional hypoparathyroidism with hypocalcemia, and reduced serum growth hormone levels.

Prophylaxis

Good control of the mother's diabetes and close observation of the infant are most important.

Treatment

Restrict maternal sedation. Aspirate the infant's upper respiratory tract and gastric contents as often as necessary. Oral or parenteral administration of dilute carbohydrate solutions may be indicated. Glucagon, 200 μg/kg intravenously, may be of value for hypoglycemia. Administer calcium if tetany develops. Correct serum electrolyte imbalance if present. Cortisone or hydrocortisone should be tried only in severe cases. See p 161 for treatment of hyaline membrane disease of the lungs. If gestational age is short, treat as a premature infant regardless of actual birth weight.

DISTURBANCES OF THE SKIN IN THE NEWBORN

TRAUMATIC SUBCUTANEOUS FAT NECROSIS

The cheeks and neck are most often involved as a result of trauma from forceps blades, but other parts of the body may also be involved. Lesions are isolated areas of firm induration that have sharply defined margins and are not attached to deeper tissues.

Traumatic subcutaneous fat necrosis generally clears spontaneously.

ERYTHEMA TOXICUM NEONATORUM

Erythema toxicum neonatorum is an extremely common eruption of unknown cause that is found during the newborn period only and usually occurs around 2–4 days of age but may develop later and persist for many days. The lesions are scattered and not numerous and consist of irregular, poorly circumscribed, erythematous spots with pale central zones (''flea-bite'' dermatitis). They contain many eosinophils. No treatment is indicated.

SCLEREMA
(Sclerema Adiposum)

Sclerema is characterized by diffuse hardening of the subcutaneous tissues that does not pit on pressure and begins in the lower extremities and rapidly spreads upward to involve almost the entire body. The skin is tense and cool. Sclerema may appear at any time during the first weeks of life and occurs most often in premature infants or those who are undernourished, dehydrated, and debilitated. The condition usually terminates fatally within a few days, although in some cases the administration of cortisone has been accompanied by recovery. Exchange transfusion has been effective in reversing the condition in some infants.

DISEASES OF THE UMBILICUS

The contents of the umbilicus include the umbilical vein, 2 umbilical arteries, the rudimentary allantois, the residual omphalomesenteric duct, and Wharton's jelly (gelatin).

CONGENITAL ABNORMALITIES

Persistence of the allantois causes patent urachus. Persistence of a portion of the omphalomesenteric duct may produce Meckel's diverticulum. Omphalocele with variable defects of the abdominal wall may occur. Increased quantity of Wharton's jelly is manifested by the persistence of a granuloma when the umbilical cord sloughs. Healing may be speeded by cauterization of the granuloma with a silver nitrate stick.

In approximately 1% of infants, only one umbilical artery is present; there is an increased incidence of congenital abnormalities in this group, especially of the gastrointestinal and urinary tracts in live-born infants.

UMBILICAL HERNIA

Umbilical hernia is a common finding, especially in black infants, and is due to weakness or faulty closure of the umbilical ring. It rarely causes incarceration or strangulation. Most infants clear spontaneously during the first 18 months of life.

• • •

INTRAUTERINE GROWTH RETARDATION
(Dysmaturity, Small for Dates, Small for Gestational Age)

Infants with intrauterine growth retardation are characterized by birth weights disproportionately low for gestational ages. A number of conditions may be associated with impaired intrauterine growth: (1) intrauterine undernutrition (placental insufficiency, multiple pregnancies, cardiovascular disease in the mother, preeclampsia-eclampsia, high altitude, arteriovenous anastomoses in identical twins); (2) congenital abnormalities (chromosomal trisomies, Turner's syndrome, Silver's syndrome, de Lange's syndrome, etc); and (3) intrauterine infection (rubella, cytomegalovirus, toxoplasmosis, syphilis).

Low birth weight may be suspected prior to delivery if the uterus is disproportionately small on palpation or if a small fetus is shown by ultrasonography or x-ray. Intrauterine undernutrition may occur in postterm infants. The infant's neurologic examination will reflect age, not size. These infants have a much higher incidence of asphyxia during labor, meconium aspiration, and transient symptomatic hypoglycemia as well as major congenital anomalies, massive pulmonary hemorrhage, polycythemia, and congenital infection.

"Postmaturity syndrome" may occur in full-term or postterm infants who show signs of intrauterine growth retardation. Growth in length and head circumference are usually not significantly affected unless involvement was prolonged. Mild involvement results in relatively thin, long infants with loose, flabby, dry, parchmentlike skin and deficient subcutaneous tissue. The infant often has an excellent appetite and gains weight at an excessive rate. More severe disturbance is frequently associated with intrauterine hypoxia, including passage of meconium into the amniotic fluid, green staining of membranes and skin, hypoglycemia, and hypocalcemia.

Overall, infants exhibiting intrauterine growth retardation have a poorer long-term prognosis for general development than do infants appropriate in size for gestational age.

Congenital Hypothyroidism

1. lg ant. fontanelle (also in Rickets, Ca^{++} diseases)
2. umbilical hernia (also in Down's)
3. thick, large tongue
4. thick skin, hair
5. slow reflexes
6. Slow bone growth
7. Constipation

Emotional Problems | 10

Ruth S. Kempe, MD

Through personal observation, the pediatrician or family practitioner* may become concerned about emotional difficulties in a young patient. Much more often, however, the pediatrician is consulted by adults, usually the parents or school personnel, who are worried about the child's behavior. Children tend to reveal in their developmental progress or their daily behavior that they are under stress, but these symptoms are often nonspecific and depend to a large extent on the child's stage of development. They may reflect aspects of the personality that are weak or not yet well integrated.

In assessing emotional problems in children, the pediatrician must be familiar with the child's developmental history, present mental and physical capabilities and handicaps, total emotional environment, and special crisis events in the child's life.

Very early in life, the infant's behavior—limited as it is by genetic endowment, temperament, and medical history—reflects the success with which bodily needs are recognized, interpreted, and satisfied, chiefly by the mother. Knowledge about and mastery of the infant's own body and physical environment develop simultaneously, and the interplay between development in the physical and emotional environments may be harmonious or conflictual. Serious conflict in either area is apt to affect performance in the other—eg, the motor development of emotionally deprived infants is slow. With time, experience becomes integrated and internalized, and the infant becomes a complex person capable of reacting in a highly individualized way to new experiences.

The child's emotional environment includes all of his or her relationships with others. For the very young child, emotional life is focused on the relationship with the parents, especially the mother. As the child grows, the environment expands to include siblings, extended family, baby-sitters, and peers. By 2 or 3 years of age, as contacts with outsiders increase, the child will already have developed many attitudes and learned ways of reacting to others. The environment will continue to

*In this chapter, the term "pediatrician" will be understood to include the family practitioner or other physician who undertakes responsibility for general medical care of a child.

expand to other relationships in school and outside the home. As these relationships develop, conflict is unavoidable and must be dealt with; how the conflict is resolved can contribute to the child's maturity and self-esteem or can create further difficulty.

For the parent, too, the child's development can present opportunities for emotional gratification or sometimes create problems. Parents often have difficulty in dealing with problems in their children that they themselves have resolved poorly or that caused difficulty when they were children. It is an attribute of maturity in parents if they are able to help a child develop freely without seizing on a "second chance" to gratify their own unfulfilled wishes.

ROLE OF THE PHYSICIAN

Pediatricians have a unique opportunity as physicians to promote emotional health as well as physical health and to practice preventive psychiatry. No other health professionals are in a position to be so knowledgeable about the interplay of genetic, physical, social, cultural, and interpersonal influences on the developing child.

Whether the pediatrician already knows the parents of a newborn or first becomes acquainted with them after the infant is born, the best chance to assess the relationship between parents and child is while mother and child are still in the hospital. If there are doubts about whether normal bonding between parents and infant will occur, the physician has an obligation to stop and think about whether the child might be abused or neglected. If that possibility exists, the physician should stand ready to help the parents adjust to their new roles and then stay alert for signs of abuse or neglect. The physician must be prepared to intervene promptly if necessary. In many cases, the pediatrician is the only contact the infant may have with the outside world. Child neglect and abuse, including sexual abuse, occur in families at all educational and economic levels. Many episodes can be prevented if the pediatrician schedules early and frequent office visits, encourages inquiries by telephone, and makes provision for extra visits by public health nurses or social workers in cases in which child abuse is considered to be a special risk. In the USA, physicians and nurses (and other specified classes of child care professionals) are legally required to report known or reasonably suspected cases of child abuse or neglect.

At each regular checkup, the pediatrician should inquire about the child's social and emotional adjustment. A useful question about a very young child might be, "What kind of baby is Johnny?" or "What kind of personality does Susie have?" Routinely checking the child's emotional adjustment during regular medical care makes it easier to give the parents appropriate information about variations in normal development, reassure them about common problems, and recognize serious parenting difficulties or emotional problems in the child.

Promotion of mental health is one of the most valuable services the pediatrician can provide. Families often ask for advice, and the pediatrician has the opportunity to further the child's healthy development by encouraging appropriate advances toward independence, providing reassurance when parental anxiety becomes restrictive, and reinforcing parental limit-setting when the child's impulses are self-destructive. The pediatrician can help parents anticipate and deal with questions about sex, drugs, death, etc, and make sure the parents are secure about their own knowledge. The pediatrician may discuss the use of contraceptives with a teenage girl and, in appropriate cases, encourage her to discuss the matter with her parents. Every physician should, of course, keep informed about the laws of the jurisdiction pertaining to such matters.

In times of family crisis, the pediatrician must be available to and supportive of the child, eg, by recognizing the child's need to mourn when the loss of one parent has made the other parent unavailable for a time. The physician can help prepare the child who needs hospitalization or surgery and can ensure liberal visiting hours and provide for appropriate activity in the hospital. The physician may be the only person involved who is not emotionally devastated by a fatal disease in a child and who thus is in a position to offer support. Not all patients or parents seek the kind of advice or support a pediatrician can provide, but when they do, they deserve the greatest consideration no matter how much time is required.

The pediatrician is often the first person the parents turn to for help with the emotional problems of their children. An interested physician can be very helpful; one who is uncomfortable in the role of psychologic counselor should be wary of giving casual advice and should find another professional for consultation or referral. No patient is a mere aggregate of physical symptoms; emotional ill health is often responsible for physical symptoms or can limit and retard recovery from physical illness. Many common problems that arise in families do not need the attention of a specialist in child psychiatry. Pediatricians practice much more psychologic medicine than is commonly realized.

No attempt is made here to present a formal psychiatric diagnostic outline, partly because diagnoses such as adjustment reaction or neurosis are difficult to establish and are not always useful in patient management. The concept of unconscious conflict (in which the individual responds with anxiety and defensive symptoms) remains valid; recognition of a complex history of stresses (internal and external) giving rise to these symptoms in children may result in a broader and more effective treatment approach than is offered by classic psychotherapy alone.

One of the pediatrician's first concerns will be to assess the severity of the problem and decide whether to refer the patient to a specialist for further care. The physician should be thoroughly familiar with normal development in children and the wide variations compatible with it. Since many children have transitory behavior difficulties during times of personal stress, the physician may wish to follow the patient for a time to see if the problem resolves spontaneously. Reassuring parents about normal behavioral variations can prevent intrusive and negative parental reactions. Such reassurances should never be given in a peremptory or derogatory manner but rather in the form of a discussion to which the parents are invited to contribute.

Severe emotional illness is usually easy to recognize, and the physician's goal in such cases will be to make a successful referral to a psychiatrist. Less obvious problems can be considerably more difficult to evaluate, and detailed examination is worthwhile.

If a detailed evaluation in the physician's office does not clarify possible treatment objectives, consultation with a psychiatrist may help. Some pediatricians meet regularly with a child psychiatrist or have developed an informal consultation relationship that can be educational for both and allows some patients to be treated in the setting of a pediatric practice. If little progress is observed after several interviews, referral can be discussed with the parents.

The role of the physician should also be considered from a more personal viewpoint. Physicians' attitudes undoubtedly influence their reactions to their patients' problems. Parents sometimes have difficulties helping their children with problems they themselves have not been able to overcome, and this is also true of physicians. Thus, physicians must be conscious of the part their personal attitudes play in their professional thinking. This does not mean, of course, that people with personal difficulties cannot help others; it does mean that we must understand how our personal concerns might influence our professional attitudes so we can minimize that influence to the extent possible.

Initial Interviews

It is often helpful to schedule 2 closely spaced interviews when evaluating a difficult emotional problem. The interval allows time to arrange for additional testing if needed and gives the parents an opportunity to ponder questions raised during the first interview, recall additional pertinent information, and perhaps view the child with greater insight, which may be revealing.

The history of an emotional problem is best taken in an unhurried, informal manner. For this reason, it is often wise to allow for a lengthy interview. The physician's ability to listen calmly, attentively, and with understanding is an important factor in determining the source of the problem. Parents should be encouraged to speak freely and to stress areas of greatest concern. Although there are questions that the physician must ask, the parents should only be interrupted for clarification or to emphasize statements. Noting the parents' modes of "body language" and other nonverbal communication can open unexpected channels of information. Nonverbal communications include facial expressions, hesitancy, restlessness, defensiveness, sudden angry tones of voice, tearfulness, and evidences of anxiety. It is appropriate, at some point, to make the parents aware of some of these forms of nonverbal communication.

The pediatrician needs to formulate an impression of the parents as individuals and an impression of the problems they face apart from those they have as parents. Care must be taken not to assume that only the parents are at fault; this is rarely true and can foredoom to failure any attempt at therapeutic intervention. Understanding the parents' own needs, even when they are in conflict with the child's needs, and recognizing their abilities as parents can do much to support and improve the quality of the parent-child relationship. Most people genuinely wish to be good parents. (Even people who cannot function adequately as parents and whose children must be permanently removed from their care may have a strong need to be parents and will be unhappy at the loss.) The anxiety and frustration aroused in parents by a child's difficult behavior need to be alleviated through supportive discussion and management. Because much of the physician's work will be with the parents, it is important to establish a good relationship with them. The physician also needs to recognize any emotional problems in the parents; their need for psychiatric therapy may be as urgent as the child's need for help.

The relationship between the child's presenting problem and coincident family events may be a clue to diagnosis. Thus, a brief family history should be taken to place the child's problem in a historic setting.

The child should be present for part of the evaluation to let the physician see how the child and parents interact in talking about the difficulty. This is also a time when the physician may wish to assure the child that his or her feelings of unhappiness or helplessness are recognized and to offer the parents an opportunity to recognize the child's point of view.

Pediatricians may tend to maintain the traditional authoritative role they feel is expected of them and to feel uncomfortable if they do not offer the parents something definite and concrete, even if it is only a diagnosis or prescription. Mutual exploration of the problem and a mutual decision about what to do about it are usually more constructive than an authoritative unilateral dispensation of advice.

When the pediatrician feels that help is needed from a psychiatrist or child psychologist, much can be done to ease the parents' anxiety about the referral. The apprehension many people have about psychiatry can be partially relieved before referral by explaining the problem and by outlining a general picture of psychotherapy. The parents' unrealistic feelings of failure as parents and their worries about their child being analyzed or about having a child who is "crazy" or "psycho" should be recognized. It is usually helpful to assure the parents that most people share these feelings before accepting a referral and to help the parents express their feelings. The realization that the physician understands these feelings can increase the parents' confidence in the program of management. Of course, the physician's own attitudes about psychiatry will influence the parents' feelings about the referral.

Evaluation of Emotional Problems in Children (Sample Outline)

A. Presenting Symptoms: Description of symptoms; duration and severity; time of onset and accompanying circumstances (possible precipitating cause); history of previous attempts to deal with the problem and attitudes toward it.

B. Other Symptoms: Description of past and present symptoms.

C. Adjustment of the Child: Description of overall and present adjustment; interactions in family, school, peer situations; description of personality traits, abilities, activities.

D. Developmental History: History of the pregnancy; mother's attitude toward pregnancy; initial reaction to infant; evidences of bonding. Child's psychomotor development; feeding, toilet training, sleep, or disciplinary problems; curiosity about sex and other topics.

E. Family History: Major events such as births of siblings, moves, illnesses, accidents, deaths, separations, parental discord.

F. Parent-Child Relationships: Past difficulties; parents' areas of special concern about the child; differences of opinion between parents about the child. Is child's symptom a reaction to serious problems in a parent?

G. Observation of the Patient: Child's reactions to the physician, to the medical examination, and to the parents with and without the parents present; feelings about the problem (if the child is old enough to confide and express them and has a sufficiently good relationship with the physician). An attempt by direct conversation to become acquainted with the child's general interests, some statement by the physician about desire to help, and an opportunity for the child to ask questions (with an explicit understanding about confidentiality) are certainly indicated in these circumstances.

H. Special Examinations: Indications, if any, for a screening examination for developmental problems, tests of vision or hearing, or referral for psychologic testing.

I. Outside Opinions: Advisability of soliciting opinions from teachers, psychologists, or others after obtaining a written release from the parents.

The following information is pertinent to the evaluation of emotional problems in children (outlined above): (1) Transitory or recent symptoms are usually more easily treated than those that have remained unchanged for months or years; they may even disappear spontaneously. If symptoms arise in response to a particular crisis event and can be understood as an appropriate response to the crisis, supportive counseling may lead to resolution and increasing maturity. When no precipitating causes are apparent, intrapsychic stress is more likely and a review of the history may show previous episodes of maladjustment. (2) Generalized adjustment difficulties—with several symptoms that affect performance in school, at home, and with peers—indicate a more pervasive pathologic process. (3) Two of the most common responses to stress in young children are the cessation of developmental progress and the partial reversal of developmental progress (regression). They occur with physical as well as with emotional illness and may be the only signs of problems in infants. (4) The parents' special concern about the child may not be shared by the child. If the symptom (eg, obesity or a phobia) produces little discomfort in the child and provides an effective mechanism for avoiding the child's underlying anxiety, the child may not want help until changes in life-style make the symptom less acceptable. If the symptom is disturbing only to the parents, a decision must be made about whether the parents' expectations are too high or the parents are reacting to personal intrapsychic distress, or whether therapy is indicated because of the nature of the symptom. A 4½-year-old child with encopresis may be responding to the mother's compulsive focus on bowel functions. A 9-year-old boy with a history of enuresis and firesetting needs psychiatric evaluation.

Diagnosis & Its Relation to Treatment

The following diagnostic categories are listed to give a rough indication of how mental illness develops and how opportunities for intervention exist throughout life.

A. Changes in Behavior Due to Normal Developmental Progress: For example, stranger anxiety in the infant 6–12 months of age is a symptom of normal developmental progress, and the parents can be reassured.

B. Delay in Developmental Progress: For example, if a parent dies during the child's latency period (6–10 years of age) and the child does not have an adequate opportunity to mourn, certain processes of ego development may come to a halt, leaving the child with residual areas of immaturity. When the child's needs are not met adequately or the child is under stress and cannot cope, delay in development may be pervasive or partial. With therapy, the child may rapidly resume normal ego development.

C. Temporary Adjustment Disorder: For example, a 5-year-old who moves to a new environment may have anxiety in the presence of strangers and enuresis for about 2 weeks. The symptoms disappear as the child adjusts and begins to make friends.

D. Emotional Disorder (as Personality Disorder): For example, a 10-year-old shows gradual onset of reluctance to meet strangers, anxiety, and excessive shyness, spending increasing amounts of time friendless and alone. This "avoidance disorder" may be a prelude to a lifelong personality disorder. Referral for psychotherapy is appropriate.

E. Emotional Disorder (as Neurotic Disorder): For example, an 8-year-old has separation anxiety with school phobia. The major problem is a dependent, ambivalent relationship with the parents, leading to anxiety at separation from them and from home; the parents participate in the child's fears and feel unable to enforce compliance. Aggressive treatment is necessary. The pediatrician should examine the child to be sure that complaints of illness have no significant physical basis and should then work with the school, the parents, and the child to ensure expeditious return to the classroom. The child may need to be accompanied to school by an adult (perhaps not the mother) or an older child, and a flexible schedule may be necessary until the child's and parents' anxieties are relieved. Referral for psychotherapy may be indicated, since these difficulties can return in more severe form near the onset of adolescence.

F. School Failure in Reading and Arithmetic: For example, evaluation reveals that the child has a normal IQ and that hearing and vision are normal. The child is well adjusted at home but does not like school except for lunch, recess, and music. On specialized testing, the child is found to have a developmental reading disorder (dyslexia) as well as a developmental arithmetic disorder (dyscalculia). Treatment must include remedial tutoring. It is important to make certain that teachers and parents do not become impatient or critical; that the child understands the problem and does not become discouraged; and that secondary behavioral symptoms do not develop.

G. Adolescent Adjustment Disorder: For example, a teenager who is failing in school experiences increasing isolation and anxiety about meeting people. These can be transient symptoms of preoccupation with identity problems and of "adolescent turmoil" or the first signs of suspicion and paranoid tendencies that on closer examination reveal the onset of delusions, hallucinations, and thought disorder characteristic of schizophrenia. These problems require evaluation and probably prompt referral for psychiatric consultation.

Principles of Treatment

As an understanding of the child's emotional difficulties develops during an evaluation, a further course of action may become self-evident. The evaluation itself can help parents and child to express their feelings openly, often for the first time, and to communicate them to one another, with the reassuring support of the physician. Exploration of the family's history and current situation can lead to better understanding, particularly when the physician helps interpret the relationship between events and the child's behavior. In such cases, interpretation would not center on unconscious dynamics but on educating the family about the usual limitations or capacities of children to respond to stress. With continued support from the physician, the parents and child may try new ways of coping with the problem, and the physician may be able, through subtle suggestion, to urge them in the direction of healthier behavior. Continued interest, follow-up, and support may lead to resolution of the problem. If not, psychiatric consultation can be recommended.

SPECIAL PROBLEMS OF PARENTING

Although everyone finds parenting tiring, stressful, and unrewarding at times, some parents seldom find it rewarding and some are unable to care adequately for a child. It is important to identify such people as soon as possible, keep track of their performance as parents, offer extra support, and intervene promptly if abuse or neglect occurs.

Some parents have great difficulty in bonding with one of their children but can love and respond well to the others. Even if physical abuse or gross neglect does not occur, the "unwanted" child may have developmental or behavioral difficulties brought on by unconscious or outright (overt) parental rejection. By encouraging day care or preschool placement and by early referral for psychiatric help, the pediatrician can be of help to a child whose parents offer no direct opportunity for intervention involving them.

Hints that a parent (or guardian or stepparent) may be at risk for poor parenting can be listed as follows:

(1) A history of abuse, neglect, or deprivation as a child.

(2) A suspected or explicit history of abuse or neglect of another child.

(3) Low self-esteem, depression, or social isolation.

(4) Signs of social stress, eg, marital discord, recent loss of an important personal relationship, frequent moves, layoffs or other financial difficulties.

(5) Unrealistic expectations of the child's performance and a lack of understanding of normal development in children.

(6) A belief that the child is willfully difficult or provocative and that physical punishment is "good for children."

(7) Difficulty in forming a bond with the child; a rejecting attitude.

(8) A history of mental illness, alcohol or drug abuse, or criminal activity.

(9) Violent outbursts of temper.

Child Abuse & Neglect

Physical abuse, neglect, emotional deprivation, and sexual abuse occur in families at all educational and economic levels. In the USA, physicians and nurses (and other specified classes of child care professionals) are legally required to report known or reasonably suspected cases of child abuse or neglect.

Cardinal signs of abuse are physical injuries inadequately explained by the history, injuries (including poisoning) that are implausible or discrepant with the child's developmental age, and delay in seeking medical care. In the USA, over 100,000 children are physically abused each year, and 3000–5000 children die; 100,000–150,000 children are grossly neglected each year, and there are indications that the number of deaths from neglect may be higher than that from physical abuse. Any combination of abuses may occur in a given family.

Signs of physical abuse include pathognomonic marks left by lashing, grabbing, slapping, tying, choking, and pinching. Forcible feeding of a crying infant may produce bruises of the frontal dental ridge. The pediatrician should recognize burns inflicted by cigarettes, heating grates, and dunking of the lower body in very hot water. Over half of subdural hematomas in infants occur without fractures or signs of scalp trauma and are the result of violent shaking. Retinal hemorrhages can usually be seen on ophthalmoscopic examination and their duration accurately estimated. Unexplained abdominal injuries such as ruptured spleen, ruptured bowel, intramural hematoma of the duodenum, or pseudocyst of the pancreas are usually inflicted injuries. A skeletal survey will often confirm the diagnosis by disclosing multiple bone changes due to fractures at different stages of healing that were caused by violent wrenching or pulling of the extremities. These findings may include metaphyseal chip fracture, subperiosteal calcification, epiphyseal displacement (''nursemaid's elbow''), and cortical thickening.

Signs of neglect include poor physical care, with inadequate nutrition, health care, and personal hygiene. Occipital baldness in an infant may be a sign that the infant is being left unattended in a crib for long periods. There may be failure to recognize and satisfy developmental and emotional needs and lack of supervision, exposing the child to a risk of accidental injury. These acts of omission may lead to growth retardation; frequent illnesses or accidents; and retarded motor, cognitive, or social development. Emotional deprivation may lead to severe distortions of personality development.

Nonorganic failure to thrive is common in infants during the first 2 years of life, with retardation or cessation of growth (especially of weight gain) in the absence of a discernible physical cause such as neurologic or heart disease. Unless the parent is cooperative and there is immediate response to initial outpatient treatment, the infant should be hospitalized for a basic physical evaluation and primarily for observation of the parent-infant interaction, especially in feeding. Some mothers have difficulties with breast feeding and need advice and support,

Others—through negligence or ignorance—have not obtained, understood, or followed instructions for good feeding techniques. A few infants are difficult to feed because of delay in development of motor (sucking) skills, chalasia, etc, and need special feeding techniques.

A high percentage of admissions for nonorganic failure to thrive reflect the mother's lack of adequate attachment to the infant, in some cases masked but occasionally expressed as overt rejection. This may lead to **reactive attachment disorder of infancy** (deprivation, hospitalism, or nonorganic failure to thrive), in which the deprivation of social interaction and love—which in these cases accompanies the inadequate feeding—causes severe delays in development. In addition to malnutrition, the infants show poor emotional development, with lack of early eye contact, smiling, affection, and the ability to be comforted. They are socially unresponsive, often even to the mother, and may ignore or look away from social contacts. They are apathetic and may show little or no interest in playing with toys. Physical development suffers and is characterized by weakness, poor muscle tone, and delayed gross and fine motor development.

This syndrome is a result of lack of attachment or of inadequate parenting, as can be demonstrated by placing the infant with an adequate substitute mother. Rapid recovery occurs when the infant's physical, emotional, and social needs are met. If the infant remains with the mother and parenting is only partially improved (eg, the infant is adequately fed but there is no improvement in the emotional relationship between parent and infant), delays in development and emotional difficulties may persist, making the infant even more vulnerable to stress at later periods.

Sexual abuse is the involvement of a dependent, developmentally immature person in sexual activities. A child or adolescent may be sexually abused by an adult or by another child or adolescent. When the data are extended to include minor episodes such as exhibitionism, it is estimated that over 250,000 children are sexually abused each year; 20% admit to an episode of abuse before adulthood. Sexual abuse includes exhibitionism (indecent exposure); molestation (pedophilia); seduction with oral, anal, or genital intercourse; forcible rape; incest; child prostitution; and child pornography. About 1–2% of all children are victims of incest at some time; 9 years is the average age at the time of the first experience. Most sexual abuse (75% of cases) involves an offender known to the child, and over half of cases of repeated abuse involve a member of the family.

Clinical signs of sexual abuse (eg, vaginal or anal lesions) may be present. However, symptoms may be primarily emotional and include anxiety, fear, depression, poor self-esteem, preoccupation, poor school performance, and seductive behavior. Depression, running away, promiscuity, prostitution, and substance abuse (eg, drugs, alcohol) in adolescents are often linked to sexual abuse. Masked sexual abuse presents as vague physical symptoms such as eating and sleeping problems, abdominal or joint pains, and depression. Boys who are victims of sexual abuse usually complain to no one. The pediatrician is often the only person with an opportunity to make the diagnosis of sexual abuse (including incest), which should be considered in children with poorly defined complaints.

Emotional abuse is recognized not only as an integral part of physical and sexual abuse but often as a devastating problem in itself. It is difficult to demonstrate, and the physician often must use the treatment of other symptoms as a means of aiding or arranging help for the child.

Intentional drugging or poisoning of children is rare but less so than may be supposed. Drugging or poisoning a child often involves a psychotic parent. It may continue during visiting hours while the child is in the hospital for diagnosis. Barbiturates, tranquilizers, alcohol, and heroin are among the substances implicated; salt feeding may also take place. Guarding the child and setting up a drug screen can assist in the diagnosis.

EMOTIONAL PROBLEMS ASSOCIATED WITH PHYSICAL HANDICAPS & CHRONIC ILLNESS

Nature of Handicaps & Illness

Emotional maladjustment frequently accompanies physical disability, particularly the obvious physical defects such as crippling (eg, cerebral palsy, paralysis following poliomyelitis), blemishes, cleft palate, and harelip. Chronic illness (eg, epilepsy, diabetes, cardiac disease, tuberculosis, orthopedic conditions such as osteochondritis) imposes an additional burden of adjustment, especially during adolescence. A young child with an acute illness may be quite disturbed if hospitalization is necessary. In the very young hospitalized child, separation from parents is the crucial problem; in the older child, fantasies about illness and procedures, especially of mutilation in surgery, become important.

Less obvious physical defects, such as impaired hearing and vision, place the child at a disadvantage both socially and educationally. If the defects are unrecognized, the child's difficulties may be attributed to other causes.

Attitudes Toward Handicaps & Illness

A physical condition that limits the child's activities can cause emotional problems if the child is unable to adjust to the limitations. Children seldom understand the reason for their condition and so may come to feel inferior or even guilty (assuming it to be a punishment). Competition with playmates actually becomes more difficult. If the condition requires restriction of activity, children may rebel against what seems to be unfair discrimination and blame the parents rather than the condition.

The attitude of the parents is often the single most crucial factor, since it usually influences the child's response to the handicap or illness. Irrational guilt on the part of the parents, who may feel somehow responsible for the physical problem, underlies much of the distortion in their attitudes. They may be ashamed of the condition and may resent having the child. They may make unrealistic demands for efforts to overcome the disability or illness, or they may be overprotective, reinforcing the child's impulse to self-pity and withdrawal. They may favor the child over their other children, causing resentment among them and further problems for the child.

Treatment

Treatment should begin with correction of the handicap or illness if possible, including carefully planned programs of physical or occupational therapy that include as much normal activity as possible. Adequate explanation of this regimen to parents and child will produce better cooperation.

Psychologic management consists primarily of allowing the child and parents to discuss their problems freely, followed by evaluation and redirection of parental and patient attitudes. In making the initial diagnosis of illness or handicap, the same kind of management will often prevent the development of unhealthy attitudes.

MENTAL RETARDATION

(See Chapter 21.)

The pediatrician is usually the professional in the best position to help the retarded child and the family over the course of years. Every pediatrician should be familiar with the procedures for confirmation of the diagnosis and should acquire skill in helping the parents understand the cause and nature of the child's disability. It is often helpful to refer the child for special services offered by the school system or community, governmental, or private facilities.

The support and understanding of the pediatrician may be important in helping the parents accept the idea of having a retarded child. The parents' feelings of grief, guilt, hopelessness, and resentment all need to be recognized and assuaged, not once but repeatedly. Genetic counseling and careful explanation of the causes of mental deficiency and the prognosis for best possible outcome provide a realistic foundation for family readjustment. Siblings may need help understanding these matters and with dealing with their own reactions. Most retarded children benefit from home and school environments that provide realistic expectations of performance, support the child's strengths, and reward appropriate achievement. The child's normal needs for affection and attention must be recognized and satisfied.

Emotional difficulties will arise from time to time and need to be explored; the child's diminished capacity for adaptation, however, should be kept in mind. Development of social judgment and interpersonal coping skills is an important goal for children who may find this difficult to do spontaneously.

Managing the child's special needs over the years requires knowledge of community resources and extra time for consultation and planning. Fortunately, most communities have special state or federally mandated and financed educational facilities and remedial training personnel and often provide special sports and social programs to meet the needs of retarded children and their families.

BORDERLINE MENTAL RETARDATION

There is a large group of children whose IQs range from 70 to 90 in whom a diagnosis of mental retardation should not be made but who do have a real intellectual handicap. Often this "slowness" is not recognized until the child is in the primary grades. The prognosis is excellent for successful social participation and unskilled job placement if emotional adjustment is good. However, these children are apt to be aware of their intellectual inadequacy, and this feeling of inferiority may make for resentful asocial behavior, particularly if the cause goes unrecognized and the child is considered lazy. A less demanding academic program for these children allows them the satisfaction of performing adequately in school. Aid in developing nonacademic skills and interests will help such a child become a more effective adult.

EDUCATIONAL UNDERACHIEVEMENT WITH NORMAL OR SUPERIOR INTELLIGENCE

Educational underachievement is extremely common during the early school years and may be due to various causes. The parents may assume that the child is lazy and impose a higher standard of performance. Such children may feel utterly inadequate in school and resent the pressure to achieve academically. The diagnosis usually depends on careful neurologic examination, individual testing by an experienced psychologist, and evaluation of the child's emotional status.

Educational underachievement may be generalized or specific, as in reading difficulty (dyslexia) with secondary generalized retardation. Neurologic examination may show mild neurologic dysfunction. Motor coordination and behavior may be poorly modulated. The following sections discuss specific and generalized forms of educational underachievement.

Specific Developmental Disorders of Reading, Arithmetic, or Speech

Specific causes of these special delays have not been identified. For example, in developmental reading disorder in young children, progress seems to be related to sensorimotor perceptual tasks; in older children, verbal intelligence and language skills reflect the potential for improvement. These disorders can be diagnosed by psychologic testing. Treatment is usually limited to remedial tutoring and helping the child and family understand the nature of the problem, especially the fact that the child is not "lazy" or "dumb." An important goal of the physician is to prevent the child's frustrations in school from leading to behavioral disorders. Some improvement may occur with maturation.

Attention Deficit Disorder, With or Without Hyperactivity

The attention deficit disorders (often called minimal brain dysfunction or hyperactive child syndrome) are developmental disturbances of unknown cause, usually noticed in a child by 3 years of age. They involve primarily problems of attention and impulse control; in addition, the child may be hyperactive. A child with attention deficit is easily distracted, has difficulty sustaining attention or completing tasks, and seems not to be listening. A child with impulsive behavior acts without thinking, works without planning, shifts activity frequently, has difficulty waiting for a turn, and requires supervision for satisfactory task completion. A hyperactive child is always "on the go," running about or moving constantly (sometimes even in sleep), and has difficulty sitting still. These problems make for poor school and social adjustment and often cause disciplinary problems or school failure. If attention deficit disorder is associated with mental retardation or with specific developmental disabilities (of reading, arithmetic, or speech), the educational handicap may be severe.

Children with attention deficit disorder may do well in a one-to-one situation, which can make the diagnosis difficult but which also can offer potential as a treatment method. These children seem to improve with a highly structured, somewhat restricted routine and an environment that provides few distractions and maximum opportunities for one-to-one supervision. Special remedial tutoring may be very helpful when educational failure is likely.

Treatment with methylphenidate (Ritalin) or dextroamphetamine, given in morning and noontime doses, may reduce hyperactivity and make the child more "reachable." Because these drugs have side effects, medication should be stopped periodically (usually during school vacations) to be sure it is still needed and to allow for possible reduction in dosage.

Other Causes of Educational Underachievement

Learning difficulties can be the result of prolonged social and cultural deprivation, especially in children who suffered early neglect with little verbal communication and no stimulus to learning.

Educational disability can also result from emotional disturbance. It may be the result of generalized inhibition in behavior or of a general oppositional pattern of behavior. A child who resists learning may be reacting unhappily to inappropriately high expectations from the parents. Depression or high levels of anxiety may cause a child to be too preoccupied to perceive and integrate new knowledge or to retrieve what has been learned.

Treatment depends on accurate assessment of the cause of underachievement. Relief from parental pressure can be of great benefit. If the parents have a realistic understanding of the nature of the child's difficulties, they can be helpful rather than critical.

SPEECH DISORDERS

As in many areas of developmental lag, all of the developmental speech disorders are more common in boys. Absence of other symptoms differentiates them from the speech delays of mental retardation, infantile autism, and neurologic disease.

Disorder of expression speech is characterized by immature articulation, restricted vocabulary, and poor sentence construction in a child who has normal comprehension and normal nonverbal communication.

Speech disorder of the receptive type denotes failure to develop comprehension as well as verbal expression. Sensory perception of auditory and visual symbols is poor.

Articulation disorder is failure to learn certain late-developing speech sounds, giving the speech an infantile quality.

Although it may not change the basic problem, the behavior of the parent in dealing with children with any of the above disorders is important. Overindulgent parents may respond too quickly, making distinct and accurate speech unnecessary; disinterested parents may fail to provide learning experiences or to reward communication. Realistic expectations and a supportive attitude are most helpful. The pediatrician must help by providing referral for diagnosis and remedial speech therapy.

Stuttering (compulsive repetition of certain syllables or words) is a transitory "normal" phenomenon that appears in some children during times of stress and is accompanied by incoordination of speech and breathing. When emotional tension is relieved, the stuttering disappears spontaneously. Speech therapy helps.

Elective mutism, as opposed to failure of development of speech (which is usually associated with severe mental retardation or the developmental childhood psychoses), is an emotional rather than a developmental disorder. A child with elective mutism understands what is said but refuses to speak at school and usually at home. The disorder is often accompanied by other symptoms, especially anxiety and negativism. The causes of the emotional disorder must be identified before therapy can be given.

FEEDING & EATING DISORDERS

Feeding difficulties of a minor nature are common in infants during the early months, especially infants with inexperienced mothers. The feeding process is often a good indicator of how the mother and infant are handling the early tasks of development, ie, regulation of the infant's feeding and sleep periods and ways to deal with crying; adaptation of mother and child to some kind of schedule; and development of social interactive behavior. An early effort by the pediatrician to make the feeding experience a success often enhances the whole mother-infant interaction. In the case of an infant with colic, for example, the pediatrician can support the mother and reduce her self-criticism and anxiety by discussing the problem of overactivity of the intestinal tract, suggesting ways of soothing the infant's discomfort, and explaining that symptoms will improve with maturation by 3 months of age.

A major feeding difficulty in infants between 6 and 15 months of age may involve the issue of autonomy. A mother who insists on putting food in the infant's mouth without allowing any awkward and messy self-feeding can deprive her infant of the opportunity to learn a satisfying skill. Cooperative feeding, in which both the mother and the infant participate, can provide mutual pleasure.

A normal decrease in the infant's appetite results from the slower growth that occurs during the second year of life. This decrease may arouse anxiety in the parent. Urging the child to eat produces resistance, which further decreases appetite. The physician can help by explaining this cycle to the parent, reassuring the parent about nutritional needs, and watching the infant's weight and growth curves (and perhaps prescribing vitamins). In severe feeding problems, the mother's anxiety about feeding is based on unconscious conflicts concerning nurturing or mothering, and psychiatric help may be required.

In children, eating difficulties may occur at any time.

Pica is the continued eating of nonnutritive substances, often unpleasant or dangerous, usually during the second or third year of life. Retardation, neglect, and iron or zinc deficiency may be implicated. Prevention of poisoning or bezoar formation and provision of additional companionship for the child may be important.

Deprivation dwarfism and **anorexia nervosa** are severe forms of eating disorders and usually require extended psychiatric evaluation of the child and family.

Obesity may be the result of urging of food in a food-oriented family, in which size is equated with strength and health or personal prosperity; or it may be due to the child's use of oral gratification as a means of assuaging feelings of inadequacy, depression, or being unloved. It may be useful to determine the difference (keeping in mind that the first could lead to the second) and then counsel the child and parents in developing not only a diet but also an exercise and social activity program. If the child is really unloved by peers or at home or is unable to use these more superficial methods, individual or group therapy may help.

SLEEP DISORDERS

Sleep disturbances are most marked in children between 2 and 6 years of age, but they may also occur during the first year of life if the parents are very uncertain or permissive about developing regularity in the family schedule. The young child who refuses to sleep alone may reflect normal fears concerning object constancy and separation. The physician may help by offering reassurances to the parents and child and by recommending sensible restrictions on the sleeping arrangements.

Nightmares are common in children after 3 years of age. They accompany rapid eye movement (REM) sleep, usually in the latter part of the sleep period, and can often be traced to some exciting or frightening event of the preceding day. Night terrors sometimes are called dreams but occur earlier in the sleep period and are associated with non-REM (NREM) sleep. They are accompanied by difficult arousal and signs of intense anxiety, agitation, and confusion, and the child is usually amnesic for the episode. Sleepwalking occurs also in NREM sleep and is accompanied by difficult arousal, poor coordination, and amnesia. Night terrors and sleepwalking have no reported associations with emotional disturbances in children.

Treatment involves soothing the child at bedtime and when sleep is interrupted. Encouraging the child to discuss nightmares may help. For sleepwalking, safety precautions to prevent accidents are important. However much the anxious child may want to sleep in the parents' bed, this is not the answer to sleeping problems, for it can encourage unconscious sexual fantasies and eventually increase the child's anxiety.

Children who sleep excessively during infancy may be reacting to deprivation (reactive attachment disorder of infancy; see Child Abuse and Neglect, above).

THUMB-SUCKING

In the young infant, thumb-sucking is related to the need for satisfaction of the oral drive, which is primary at this age. It occurs in both breast- and bottle-fed infants. Continued thumb-sucking after 2 years of age may be the result of boredom or of mild anxiety when a feeling of security is desired, as at bedtime.

Treatment in infants should require only reassuring the parents, explaining to them the infant's oral needs, and encouraging them to provide safe toys that will satisfy those oral needs. Physical restraints and scolding are not recommended. If the child is over 2 years of age, the pediatrician should explain to the parents that the activity is a sign of boredom or a wish for security. A happy bedtime should be provided. By the age of 4–5 years, malocclusion of the teeth may result from continued sucking; therefore, a dentist should be consulted if the child is over 3 years of age.

TEMPER TANTRUMS

Temper tantrums occur in most children during the latter half of the second year of life. (See Personality Development in Chapter 3.) From this point on, there is a gradual decrease in the frequency and severity of tantrums, with perhaps a second peak at about age 6 years. Early temper tantrums are uninhibited expressions of frustration and rage. Frustration is frequently due to unsuccessful attempts to perform complicated physical feats or due to inadequate linguistic resources that limit communication.

Treatment consists of relief of the child's frustrations whenever possible. Gradual education by the parents to teach more acceptable expressions of rage (usually verbal) is the second step. Isolation during the tantrum, as an aid to the child in achieving control of feelings, is usually helpful. Attempts to retaliate or to appease are both ineffective and counterproductive.

BLADDER CONTROL

Toilet training methods are in large part culturally determined; only recently have bladder function and children's physiologic and cognitive capacities for control been studied in any depth. Although some children can become continent before 2 years of age, many are not ready for toilet training before 3 years of age. They must first acquire bladder control (ie, the ability to retain a fairly large amount of urine and to be aware of the need to urinate). If they are able to understand the purpose of toilet training and are not in an oppositional phase, they are then presumably ready for training. If the child is spontaneously interested in body functions and self-control, this would be an optimal time for training. Toilet training, whatever method is used, must be noncoercive; modeling and praise are very helpful. Displeasure must be exhibited with caution, and angry shaming is contraindicated.

Enuresis is involuntary urination, usually at night, in children over 4–5 years of age; it is about twice as common in boys as in girls. If daytime "dribbling" is not due to organic factors, its use as a deliberate negativistic symptom must be suspected.

Causes of Enuresis

A. Maturational Delay: Longitudinal experience and sleep studies involving many children emphasize the importance of maturational delay in the development of bladder musculature and its ability to withstand increased intravesical pressure without involuntary voiding, particularly in children who have never achieved bladder control for prolonged periods.

B. Toilet Training: Toilet training may have been absent or, more often, too early or too coercive. If the only form of training was vague verbal instruction, the child may not know what is required. A child who was expected to perform before being physiologically ready may be confused or disheartened. If training was coercive, with shaming and punishment for accidents (which are often the nearly successful attempts to void that occur just before or after the child is placed on the toilet seat), the child may be confused, resentful, and resistant to further efforts. Retraining with positive, gentle encouragement is needed.

C. Emotional Disturbances:

1. Enuresis may be a temporary symptom of regression, and attention to the source of upset will usually result in improvement.

2. Enuresis sometimes seems to be a passive-aggressive response to parents who are thought to be too controlling, intrusive, or critical.

3. Enuresis may be associated with symptoms that indicate more difficult problems of adjustment, such as educational disability or an anxiety disorder. The evaluation of total adjustment is then indicated, with a referral for psychotherapy if the symptoms cannot be resolved readily by other means. Psychiatric evaluation is required when enuresis is associated with predelinquent behavior, firesetting, and problems of impulse control; the child's history is often one of emotional deprivation and long-standing family difficulty.

D. Physical Disease: Although physical disease is a rare cause, this should be ruled out.

1. Spina bifida or other lower spinal cord lesions, if significant, are usually accompanied by neurologic sensory changes that may be noted on physical examination.

2. Congenital anomalies of the genitourinary tract, especially the urethral valve, may be present. The test for residual urine is diagnostic. Urethral dilatations are psychologically very traumatic as a treatment procedure and should be avoided if possible.

3. Cystitis, tuberculosis, or other infections of the urinary tract usually produce dribbling during the day as well as at night.

4. Diabetes could be present, since enuresis may be an early symptom of diabetes.

5. Nocturnal epilepsy may rarely be accompanied by enuresis.

Treatment of Enuresis

The physician should discourage criticism, anger, and guilt in members of the child's family. Clarifying the motivational capacity of the child, evaluating the appropriateness of past toilet training, and reassuring the child and parents may be helpful in cases involving younger children.

Older children who are unhappy about enuresis may be helped by behavioral modification techniques or by the use for 5–12 weeks of a bell-alarm pad that awakens the child when the pad gets wet. When relapses occur, another period of treatment may be successful. In older children, treatment with imipramine has been useful in achieving rapid results. It is associated with a high relapse rate, however, and the patient's reaction to the drug must be monitored. In older teenage patients, the use of covert sensitization (a kind of negative conditioning) has sometimes been helpful. Psychotherapy is the treatment of choice when a clearly emotional cause of enuresis is recognized; behavioral modification may be used in conjunction with psychotherapy but not as a substitute.

BOWEL CONTROL

Permanent bowel control is usually more easily achieved than bladder control, probably in part because of individual differences in neurologic maturation. If movements are regular, training for bowel control may be begun after age 18 months, somewhat earlier than for bladder control. Many children, however, are not ready to start bowel training until almost age 2 years.

Constipation occurs frequently in children between ages 2 and 3 years and seems to be part of the "negative phase" of this period.

Withholding bowel movements seems to represent an attempt to exercise some autonomy against demanding, controlling parents. Treatment is aimed at diverting parental interest from the gastrointestinal tract; usually the child's interest will gradually decline as well. Physical causes for chronic constipation should be ruled out.

Encopresis is voluntary or involuntary passage of feces in an inappropriate place (eg, in the clothing) by a child over 4 years of age. The condition is called primary encopresis if bowel control has never been established and secondary encopresis if bowel control was established and incontinence recurred.

In primary encopresis, the difficulty may be traced to lack of toilet training or training that is inadequate, too early, or too coercive. These problems in training may cause a child who is physiologically or cognitively incapable of complying to be blamed by the parents for being uncooperative. Family, peers, and school contacts may react to encopresis with disgust and disapproval; the child may make great efforts to prevent discovery of the problem but nevertheless may have lost awareness of the need to defecate or of the smell after defecation has occurred.

Encopresis usually involves retention of hard fecal material in the colon, accompanied by pain, and passage of softer stool, usually involuntarily, around the impacted feces. The initial diagnosis should be confirmed by x-ray, and the retention problem should be explained thoroughly to the patient and family. Many children improve with bowel evacuation by enemas, institution of proper diet, reinstitution of toilet training involving toilet sitting twice a day and use of a stool softener, and much support. The pediatrician should urge patience and explain to the child the need to redevelop the "weakened" bowel muscles and "nerves"; this approach places the emphasis on a routine training task the child may find acceptable. It is of great importance that the parents support the child and refrain from criticism or discouragement. Frequent follow-up is necessary. If other indications of emotional disturbance are present or if encopresis is felt to be a deliberate behavior pattern, psychotherapy (with the parents involved) is recommended along with appropriate remedial training.

MASTURBATION & INTEREST IN SEX

Masturbation is damaging only because of the guilt and shame aroused by adult criticism. Aside from occasional slight irritation, there are no physical sequelae. Mental deficiency or psychosis is never caused by masturbation.

In the prepubertal child, masturbation is usually a transient habit, and parents should treat it with understanding. Reasonable restrictions (eg, emphasizing privacy) can be placed on the activity for social reasons. Continued or excessive masturbation may have limited sexual significance; in such cases, it can be viewed as a symptom of anxiety indicative of other emotional conflict. Excessive masturbation or sexually provocative behavior in young children, however, may also be a clue to sexual abuse, especially repeated abuse (see Child Abuse and Neglect, above).

In the postpubertal child, masturbation would undoubtedly be universal if adult prohibitions were not so strong. Here the conflict is more severe because of genital maturing and accounts for much of the "nonspecific" guilt found in adolescents. Treatment should be focused on the child's emotional needs, not on the act itself.

Interest in the genitals and in physical sex differences and pleasure in genital manipulation are normal in prepubertal children. Young children are aware of sex differences just as they are aware of social differences between the sexes in dress, games, and mannerisms. Parental anxiety about manifestations of sexuality in children is based on the unwarranted assumption that these are equivalent to adult sexuality and are abnormal.

Sexual concerns during childhood or early adolescence may be brought to the physician's attention by the parent or child if a good relationship exists, and the concerns should be taken seriously. Gender confusion and fears of being homosexual, for example, should not be dismissed but should be discussed confidentially with the pediatrician or with a mutually agreed upon consultant. If the adolescent requests a private consultation with the physician (ie, without the parents present), the physician should comply with the request. Homosexual fears may indicate that sexual abuse or adolescent homosexual activity has occurred.

TICS & OTHER STEREOTYPED MOVEMENTS

Atypical stereotyped movements include head banging, rocking, or other movements and are usually seen in children during infancy and preschool years. They are voluntary and repetitive; they seem to provide pleasure for long periods of time; and they are probably related to insufficient fondling, cuddling, and other expressions of affection. Head banging can have a self-punitive quality and in toddlers is sometimes a sign of frustration or anger.

Tics appear during childhood and are recurrent, involuntary, rapid movements, usually of facial or other small muscle groups. They can be voluntarily controlled for short periods and may disappear during periods of intense concentration or distraction; they are never present during sleep. Tics are made worse by stress, and although they may originate from some kind of physical irritation, they usually represent a response to emotional stress and tension. For example, an only child reared in a family in which aggression is rigidly controlled and conformity is expected in all areas of behavior may find no outlet for feelings of anger and worry. The facial tic allows some limited and distorted expression of tension but does not provide permanent relief. Treatment should be directed toward recognition and relief of tension.

Gilles de la Tourette's syndrome is a tic disorder, originating in childhood, that tends to persist throughout life. This condition is of unknown cause and usually presents with extensive hyperactivity and vocalizations. It will often be diagnosed as a severe behavior disorder, temper tantrum, or hysteria. Familial cases are common, and the disease is particularly frequent in Eastern European Jewish families. It may be severely disabling in social situations, at school, or at work. This disorder involves more extensive involuntary movements than do other forms of tic. Most of the movements are accompanied by involuntary vocal sounds, including grunts, barks, crying, and shouted or choked-off obscenities. They are worsened by stress and can sometimes be voluntarily controlled for a time; they do not occur during sleep. The impact upon the family can be profound. Haloperidol (Haldol), 0.5–1.5 mg given 1 to 3 times daily, may produce some relief. The effect of clonidine on patients who do not respond to treatment with haloperidol is currently under investigation. Psychologic support for the child and the family is also important.

PSYCHOSOMATIC PROBLEMS & CONVERSION DISORDERS

The close relationship between the emotions and physiologic functions is established during early infancy and persists throughout life. It is necessary to recognize the physical components of emotional states ranging from mild physiologic deviations such as urinary frequency accompanying apprehension over an approaching examination to such life-threatening conditions as anorexia nervosa. A comfortable working relationship between psychiatrist and pediatrician can contribute to the successful treatment of patients with underlying emotional conflicts and physical symptoms.

There have been many efforts to categorize personality types according to susceptibility to certain illnesses. Dependency conflicts are often seen in patients with ulcers, and conflicts involving expression of anger are seen in patients with ulcerative colitis. Problems associated with sexual maturation, control of instinctive behavior, and acceptance of femininity are common in girls with anorexia nervosa. However, these correlations are too simplistic even when correct, and treatment does not consist simply of making conscious the patient's underlying conflicts. Participation of the parents in the patient's problem may be a major issue. It is often difficult to find a solution to the conflict that will be healthier than the somatic malfunction. Prolonged psychiatric and pediatric treatment, sometimes with hospitalization, may be needed.

Conversion disorder is characterized by physical complaints with no apparent bodily change noted on physical examination. Complaints involve functions controlled by the voluntary nervous system (as opposed to psychosomatic illness, which involves functions controlled by the autonomic nervous system). Symptoms of conversion disorder represent a neurotic use of physical complaints (pain, anesthesia, paralysis, blindness, etc) as a substitute for expression of unconscious impulses. It is important to rule out physical illness in order to emphasize the role of psychiatric treatment. For example, hysterical partial blindness or tunnel vision in a prepubertal girl may be related to conflicts about "seeing" sexual phenomena; when this diagnosis is made, physical methods of treatment can be bypassed in favor of psychiatric management.

DELINQUENCY (CONDUCT DISORDERS)

Delinquency includes behavior that violates societal rules in a major way, such as stealing, repeated truancy, running away, and persistent lying. In addition to these nonviolent types of behavior, there are aggressive ones, which include vandalism, robbery, battery, rape, and firesetting. Drug and alcohol abuse, precocious sexual behavior, and prostitution can occur in all delinquent children, male or female.

Children who show repeated delinquent behavior frequently come from a chaotic or disturbed family and very often from a neglectful or abusive one. Runaways often have good reasons for leaving their homes. Some parents of delinquent children may appear upright and give the child strict scoldings or severe punishment but demonstrate by their own behavior that they have unrecognized conflicts in the same area as the child.

Delinquent children are often classified not only by the presence or absence of aggressive, violent behavior but also on the basis of whether they have close relationships with others. The children in the nonrelating group tend not to feel guilty about their behavior and to have no empathy for their victims, while those who relate, even if only through friendships among their own circle (or gang), have some potential for guilt. Attempts to treat the nonrelating aggressive group are discouraging; these young people are apt to have antisocial personalities and get into serious trouble as adults. The outcome for delinquents who are able to relate to others depends on how well the environment meets their needs for emotional warmth and increased self-esteem and helps them control their behavior. Because delinquent children are often depressed and have health and educational handicaps as well, individual comprehensive evaluations are needed to determine whether they can benefit most from remaining at home, perhaps with counseling or psychiatric treatment, or whether a group home, hospital, or institutional placement is necessary, as in severe cases.

Isolated episodes of delinquent behavior often occur during adolescence, and if the family quickly mobilizes to understand and help, recurrences will be rare.

DRUG & SUBSTANCE ABUSE

In recent years, children have abused alcohol, cigarettes, marihuana, sedatives, cocaine, heroin, hallucinogens, nitrous oxide, and paint and glue solvent vapors. Suspecting that the problem may exist is often the best clue to diagnosis. Sometimes their use begins during the latency or prepubertal years, usually as experimentation or at the instigation of an older child, but most drug and substance abuse begins during adolescence and may rapidly progress to severe abuse. Many of these children fail in school and become truant, and they may become alienated from family and friends. Drug abuse may be part of the regular behavior of a child's peer group, or it may be an individual activity that severely isolates a child. Marked personality change comes with continued intoxication, and activities are often focused on how to obtain the drug even at the expense of important relationships or work progress. Thefts, prostitution, and other forms of delinquency may be the means of paying for drugs.

Although the drug problem may be limited to episodic use, the decision on how to help the child involves a complete evaluation. Treatment ranges from supportive counseling of the child and family to psychotherapy or hospitalization for more severe difficulty.

DEPRESSION

Depression may occur in children at any age from infancy through adolescence. It is often unrecognized, because the depressed child does not usually complain of feeling sad and may attempt to avoid behavior that reflects unhappy feelings.

Depression in Infants & Young Children

In infants, depression is usually the result of object loss (eg, loss of the mother, caretaker, or sibling), lack of attention, or depreciation and rejection by the parents. A good mother substitute may reverse the mood, which is expressed in apathy and lack of interest in surroundings.

Depression takes 3 forms in children:

Reactive depression is an acute reaction, often caused by sudden object loss (especially of a parent or sibling), in a child who previously appeared to be fairly well adjusted. Sadness may be evident but is often not sustained, leading to the false assumption of quick recovery. Young children may need help to mourn.

Chronic depression is sometimes expressed in sadness, in signs of unhappiness, in poor self-image, and in apathy. The life history of children with chronic depression often reveals why they are depressed.

Masked depression often takes the form of aggressive or difficult behavior, which may be a mechanism to avoid feelings of hopelessness and helplessness or may be an expression of some of the child's angry feelings leading to depression; the behavior does not relieve the feeling of sadness or promote love and acceptance. During early childhood, depressive feelings may be channeled into fantasy and play as a way of masking sadness. During acute and chronic depression, children often do not express unhappiness in tearfulness or sad rumination; they may show apathy, psychomotor retardation, poor appetite, or sleep disturbances.

Depression in Adolescents

Depression is common in adolescents, partly because of the stress of biologic maturation, dependence-independence conflicts with parents (who may be critical or rejecting), and anxiety-provoking school and social demands. The discrepancy between an adolescent's self-image and ideal (changeable as the latter may be) results in feelings of anxiety, inadequacy, and helplessness. The reality of the inability to change oneself quickly or to alter circumstances may lead an adolescent to feel hopeless and depressed, especially when the environment presents difficult stresses. Symptoms may include vague psychosomatic complaints, withdrawal, boredom, anorexia or overeating, and insomnia or excessive sleeping. Preoccupation with the self and excessive guilt or depressive rumination may lead to school failure by a child with a record of being a good student. Acting-out behavior may take the form of alcohol or drug abuse, running away from home, or delinquency; in these cases, the adolescent often denies the depression.

Supportive psychotherapy is probably the most helpful treatment, especially if environmental stresses can be reduced. Antidepressant drugs should be used with caution but can be effective. Hospitalization is sometimes indicated.

Manic-depressive illness of the bipolar type occurs occasionally during adolescence, sometimes first as a full-blown manic episode. An adolescent going through a manic episode displays an elevated or expansive mood, a marked increase in activity with less need for sleep, marked talkativeness with flight of ideas, inflated self-esteem, distractibility, and poor judgment. Hospitalization, psychotherapy, and the use of lithium are probably the most effective methods of management. Patients must be followed continuously, because of the episodic and sometimes progressive nature of the disorder.

SUICIDE

Suicide can occur in children during the latency period, although the incidence increases dramatically during adolescence, when it becomes the second or third most frequent cause of death.

Suicidal ideation occurs in young children, mostly in terms of retaliation against people who have made them unhappy. ("How sorry they'll be when I'm dead!") Some children who feel unloved and unwanted assume it is their fault and thus have a poor self-image. Some attention-getting suicide attempts may be accidentally successful. The angry, impulsive suicidal gesture of the adolescent usually indicates a need for help from others or a need for environmental change. Gestures are more common in girls; successful suicides are more common in boys, perhaps because of the methods used. All suicidal threats or ideation should be taken seriously, especially when they occur after a major bereavement or in an adolescent with a major depressive illness. Protection, psychotherapy, and the use of an antidepressant medication may all be needed. It is also important to evaluate the family's response and to prevent family members from giving the child the unconscious message, "We don't really want you."

PSYCHOSIS

Psychosis is rare in prepubertal children. The very early psychoses of infantile autism and symbiotic psychosis (discussed below) are categorized as pervasive developmental disorders, an appropriate description of their natural history.

When a young child presents with apparent psychosis, it is important to rule out organic disease; this includes certain metabolic diseases, neurologic disease, brain tumor, and chronic poisoning. A psychiatric evaluation alone is not necessarily sufficient to make the diagnosis, for symptoms of emotional disorder and a pathogenic environment can coexist with organic disease.

Example: A 6-year-old boy, referred for probable migraine and school phobia, exhibited severely regressive behavior during episodes of pain. Findings were normal on neurologic examination. During an interview, he seemed comfortable until asked about school adjustment, whereupon he began to whine and complain of a headache. The next day, papilledema was noted for the first time, and a brain tumor was diagnosed soon thereafter.

Some autistic symptoms occur in children with severe mental retardation. Recent studies of psychoses have produced evidence of biochemical and physiologic brain malfunction, but the significance of these studies cannot yet be fully assessed. In patients with infantile autism, the level of the developmental defect that usually accompanies the disease makes brain malfunction a strong possibility.

Psychoses in Infants & Young Children

Infantile autism is diagnosed within the first 30 months. The infant may form little or no emotional attachment to the mother or other persons, although these persons may be recognized as providers of food and useful for other purposes. On the other hand, the infant may form strong attachments to inanimate objects and be more interested in object manipulation and repetitive motor activity than in social interaction. There is usually rigid adherence to routine and manifestations of anxiety when change is enforced. Speech may be absent; when present, it has poor communicative value, with echolalia, reversal of pronouns, and use of rote repetitions.

The prognosis for children with infantile autism depends mainly on the child's IQ and ability to speak, which reflect the severity of symptoms. Only 30% of these children attain an IQ of 70, and studies show that a much smaller percentage can live independently. Some children with higher IQs may develop highly specialized and rote skills, but these are rarely adaptable enough to be useful. Treatment consists of psychotherapy or counseling for the family. For the child, a highly structured and individualized educational program that uses behavioral modification techniques, social training, and special techniques to "make contact" may be useful. A few children must be institutionalized, and treatment should be continued in these cases. Psychotropic drugs may help to control symptoms, without sedative effects. In later years, drugs may be needed to control late-developing seizures.

Symbiotic psychosis or **interactional psychosis** is diagnosed after age 30 months and apparently involves a "normal" mother-child relationship during the first year. Separation from the mother occurs with great difficulty and is marked by anxiety and regression; the child gradually withdraws, presents an autistic and bizarre clinical picture, and develops unevenly and poorly, as in infantile autism. Unprovoked extremes of behavior, stereotyped movements, abnormal speech patterns, and self-mutilation may all occur. Prognosis and treatment are similar to those of infantile autism.

Schizophreniform psychosis occurs during later prepubertal childhood and tends to be shorter in duration than the later schizophrenias. Symptoms include delusions, auditory hallucinations, thought disorder, inappropriate affect, and isolation and withdrawal. Severe "neurotic" symptoms such as phobias or compulsions may occur. Bizarre behavior may also take place and includes unusual motor activity, such as twirling, and destructive behavior directed outward or at the self. There is clear deterioration from the child's previous level of behavior. Psychiatric care with hospitalization is needed.

Psychoses in Older Children & Adolescents

Acute confusional state is usually a fairly brief psychotic episode characterized by anxiety, depression, confusion, and feelings of depersonalization and diffusion of identity. Hospitalization, with a delay in the use of antipsychotic drugs (which may exacerbate confusion and feelings of helplessness), usually helps; the psychotic episode is generally followed by a need for intensive psychotherapy to aid in the support and reestablishment of identity.

Schizophrenia of the type found in adults may have its early onset in postpubertal children. Occasionally, only one psychotic episode occurs. The illness may have all the characteristics of adult schizophrenia and is often gradual in onset. Characteristics include thought disorder, delusions, and hallucinations, followed by disorganized behavior, combativeness, withdrawal, or depression. Hospitalization, use of neuroleptic drugs, and supportive psychotherapy help bring about some integration. A long period of regression then follows, accompanied by ongoing reintegration and requiring long-term therapy. Even after the acute symptoms have improved, the adolescent is still vulnerable, and long-term support and psychotherapy are recommended.

USE OF PSYCHOTROPIC DRUGS IN CHILDREN

(For anticonvulsant therapy, see Chapter 21.)

The response to drugs given to modify behavior may be different and less satisfactory in children than in adults. The best long-term results are obtained by using drugs very conservatively and helping the parents to use behavioral modification techniques in specific repetitive situations and to improve interpersonal relationships. The following drugs have been helpful.

For sedation or treatment of anxiety in acute situations, the benzodiazepines (chlordiazepoxide and diazepam) in small doses are probably the safest and best-known drugs. These agents should not be used for long periods; symptoms are better controlled by diagnosis and treatment of the underlying causes. The use of tranquilizers such as thioridazine for treatment of sleep disorders in young children is not justifiable.

In children who have attention deficit disorder with hyperactivity, methylphenidate or dextroamphetamine, in morning and noontime doses, can be effective in reducing hyperactivity and allowing the child to attend better to classroom activity.

Haloperidol is effective in suppressing the more severe symptoms of Gilles de la Tourette's syndrome. In patients with enuresis, imipramine is useful for short periods when rapid achievement of continence is an important first step in treatment. Imipramine has also been used in children with school phobia, but its potential toxicity probably outweighs its usefulness.

The major antipsychotic tranquilizers can be of great benefit for the treatment of patients with psychosis during late childhood and adolescence. They are also used extensively in the management of aggressive behavior in institutionalized children who are retarded or who have antisocial conduct disorder. There is evidence that better management techniques can help by allowing lower doses and therefore less sedation. Children with antisocial conduct disorder who have symptoms of major depression—and perhaps attention deficit disorder as well—may benefit from antidepressant drugs such as imipramine.

All of these drugs should be monitored for toxicity, and pediatric doses should always be calculated carefully.

11 | Adolescence*

PSYCHOLOGIC ASPECTS OF ADOLESCENCE

During adolescence, an acceleration in ego development occurs concurrently with growth acceleration. Although generally socially competent and able to assume increasing responsibility, the early adolescent may make unrealistic demands for privileges that represent being "grown up." Areas of conflict through which the child has passed at an earlier stage of emotional development can be reawakened and intensified in late adolescence. Concerns about parental love, sibling rivalry, and the adolescent's own real or imagined physical or intellectual shortcomings make adolescence a time of great doubt and insecurity.

Characteristically, adolescents swing quickly from the desire to be more mature to the desire to resort to a childlike state, protected by those who love them. While they seek greater responsibilities at one moment, at the next they may want to be freed of the responsibilities and the demands made upon them because they are "growing up." These lightning changes from childish to more mature behavior are frequently puzzling and frightening both to the adolescent and to the parents. The adolescent's constant posing in a great variety of different roles must be regarded as experimentation rather than taken seriously by physicians, parents, and teachers. In general, problems of this nature will be minimized if the adolescent's adult associates can maintain a consistent, realistic, and supportive attitude.

The rapid acceleration of somatic growth during this period may give rise to a variety of fantasies and fears about the body and its functions and disorders. This, as well as the fears that may accompany the awakening of sexual drives, concerns about masturbation, and increasing social and academic pressures, may make adolescence a time of intense emotional turmoil.

Concern with bodily changes may be expressed as a fear of being physically imperfect. An understanding of this fear of imperfection is of great importance to the physician in the management of adolescent patients. Fears of real or imagined physical imperfections may not be

*Revised with the assistance of Ida Nakashima, MD.

verbalized by the adolescent patient, but they can be brought out into the open by the understanding physician. For example, an adolescent's overt concerns about being too tall, too short, too fat, or too thin or worries about acne or dysmenorrhea may symbolize more than anxiety about the specific complaint; they may instead represent a general intense concern about being less than physically perfect. Known imperfections or chronic disease such as diabetes, epilepsy, asthma, or rheumatic fever may present a tremendous emotional problem to the adolescent desiring to be physically perfect. Rebellion against previously well accepted medical advice is not uncommon, even when the advice is offered by a physician whose relationship with the patient has always been good.

Concern with physical perfection may result in various degrees of hypochondriasis. However, suspicion of hypochondriasis should not prevent the physician from carrying out a complete and careful examination to determine the presence of any specific disease. Undue anxiety about minor symptoms for which no organic causes can be found should alert the physician to the possibility of underlying psychologic problems. The physician can then discuss the findings with the patient and gently and sympathetically ask about other aspects of the patient's life that may be causing anxiety and depression (ie, sexual abuse).

During middle and late adolescence, some degree of conflict with authority will probably occur no matter how satisfactory the parent-child relationship has been. An adolescent needs firm, clear-cut, and above all consistent limits. Adolescents striving for independence and greater maturity will invariably test limits and push imposed restrictions. They are skilled in marshaling both arguments and emotional appeals to tax the endurance of even the most loving parents. Parents, teachers, and physicians need to be aware of the adolescent's need for definite limits so they can be sympathetic with unreasonable demands but not yield to them, particularly when these demands impinge on the rights of others or conflict with parents' values. Parents should realize that an overly compliant adolescent may simply be postponing a process that is essential to maturation.

The Physician's Attitude Toward the Adolescent Patient

It is impossible to deal adequately with adolescent patients in a hurried manner. The problem of providing sufficient time makes the medical care of adolescents extremely difficult. In general, it is desirable for the physician to assume a friendly and supportive attitude, to avoid prying, and to take the adolescent patient's complaints seriously. In performing the physical examination, the physician should take into consideration the shyness and acute self-consciousness often present both in boys and in girls. Adolescent girls should be draped by nurses and should be chaperoned throughout the examination. Explanations and reassurances of normal findings can be given as the examination progresses. Pelvic examination is done only when specifically indicated.

In opening the conversation with the adolescent, the physician may simply ask the patient why he or she is being seen. Often it is easier with an apprehensive patient to inquire about the medical history first, particularly if the real reason for the visit is emotional problems. Then, when the patient is more at ease and reassured by the physician's warmth and accepting manner, questions regarding difficulties with parents or school problems may be asked and answered more readily.

The actual purpose of the visit should always be clearly and openly stated by the physician if the adolescent is reluctant to state it, ie, "Your parents are worried about your rebelling at home and fighting a lot with your brothers." This establishes the fact that the physician understands why the patient is there and establishes a setting of frankness and honesty in all the physician's subsequent contacts with the adolescent.

The Physician & the Parents of the Adolescent Patient

Counseling of parents is an indispensable part of the management of the adolescent's problem. Parents can often be helped to make a more realistic evaluation of their child's behavior if they understand the normal physical and psychologic changes that occur during adolescence. One should not "take sides" in conflicts relating to discipline and behavior; however, by showing parents that their child's behavior is common during adolescence, the physician may help them to assert authority. Adolescents, in spite of demands for freedom from control and in spite of a natural desire for independence, are actually afraid that they may not be able to maintain adequate control over themselves. Parents can help by providing realistic standards and good examples of behavior and by insisting upon cooperation in matters of discipline and conduct in the home and community. Firm but fair parental authority is of tremendous therapeutic value; even though adolescents may complain about it at length, they find it a reassuring demonstration of their parents' interest in their future welfare and development.

Medical Problems of Adolescence

A. Hypochondriasis: Once a careful medical examination has ruled out physical causes as the basis of headache, dizziness, palpitations, insomnia, vague abdominal pains, or other complaints that the adolescent may have, the physician should attempt to determine whether the complaints might have a psychosomatic basis.

These vague, ill-defined complaints may represent anxiety about a variety of concerns: guilt and anger about the impending divorce of parents, depression over the loss of a close friend or relative, unspoken fear about a possible pregnancy, or sexual abuse.

Physical complaints are easier to face and discuss than the true psychologic sources of anxiety. Some adolescents, when reassured that the symptoms are not serious, can then openly discuss their emotional difficulties under a physician's tactful guidance. Other adolescents use a minor symptom to seek the attention they feel they deserve but do not receive from adults. The trivial nature of the complaint should never cause the physician to reject the patient. Interviews with an understanding and kindly practitioner can be of great therapeutic value in improving hypochondriacal symptoms.

B. Obesity: The diagnosis of obesity during adolescence should not be based simply upon a variation in weight from that indicated on standard charts. Attention should be paid to the total body configuration, pattern of growth, and weight in the preceding years. Rapid increase in weight during the adolescent period may be related to emotional stress if the adolescent resorts to food as a source of immediate satisfaction and comfort. Obesity on this basis may be helped by repeated interviews with a sympathetic physician; the objective of these conferences should be to allay underlying anxieties and to seek more constructive sources of satisfaction. In families where obesity is common, "good food" may be considered to be important as a source of health and satisfaction or as part of a cultural pattern. Therapy in these cases may be extremely difficult unless the adolescent has a strong desire to lose weight. The caloric intake of very active adolescents may be extremely high without excessive gain in weight (3500–4000 kcal and 100–125 g of protein per day for boys; 2500–3000 kcal and 75–95 g of protein per day for girls). On the other hand, if activity is markedly reduced, obesity may occur even though the caloric intake is not high. In these cases, increased physical activity must be encouraged.

Care must be taken to provide an adequate intake of protein, calcium, and vitamins with all dietary regimens.

In general, the results of attempting to correct obesity in adolescents have been disappointing.

PHYSICAL ASPECTS OF ADOLESCENCE

Physical, psychologic, and endocrine changes during adolescence follow an orderly sequence, but wide individual variations in time of appearance of the changes may occur. The first signs of adolescent sexual maturation appear between ages 8 and 14 years (Table 11–1). They seem to be initiated by neural or neurohumoral stimuli from the hypothalamus; these stimuli cause secretion of gonadotropic hormones by the anterior pituitary, with resultant growth of genital organs and appearance of secondary sex characteristics.

Table 11–1. Normal pattern of sexual maturation.

Approximate Age (yr)	Sexual Characteristics		Status of Hormone Production
	Boys	Girls	
3–7	Infantile.	Infantile. Vaginal pH alkaline.	Very small amounts of 17-ketosteroid (both sexes) and estrogen (females) in urine.
7–9		Uterus begins to grow.	Amounts of 17-ketosteroid and estrogen begin to increase.
9–10		Growth of bony pelvis. Budding of nipples.	
10–11	Increased vascularity of penis and scrotum.	Budding of breasts; may be unilateral at first. Pubic hair appears.	Estrogen excretion greatly increased in the female.
11–12	Prostatic activity. Pubic hair appears.	Cornification of vaginal epithelium. Vaginal pH acid. Growth of genitalia.	Gonadotropins demonstrable in urine (both sexes). Estrogen excretion cyclic (females).
12–13	Rapid growth of testes and penis.	Axillary hair. Menarche (average age, 12½ yr). Anovulatory menstruation.	
13–15	Axillary hair. Down on upper lip. Voice change.	Earliest normal pregnancies can occur.	Pregnanediol in urine during luteal phase (females).
15–16	Mature spermatozoa (average age, 15 yr; range, 11–17 yr).	Acne.	
16–17	Acne.	End of skeletal growth.	
17–21	End of skeletal growth.		

General Biologic Considerations

Growth during adolescence is a function of biologic rather than chronologic age. Growth of different parts of the body may be uneven, and the adolescent may be living on various levels of maturity in different organ systems and functional processes.

A. Variations Between Boys and Girls:

1. Height and weight–Before puberty, boys tend to be taller than girls; then from ages 11 to 14 years, girls are taller than boys, because of the earlier female growth spurt. The adult male is about 15 cm taller than the adult female.

The adolescent growth spurt begins about 2 years earlier in girls (at about age 11–12) than in boys, is slower and less extensive than that of boys, and accounts for a gain of 5–20 cm in height and 7–25 kg in weight. Boys start their growth spurt between ages 12 and 16 years and gain 10–30 cm in height and 7–30 kg in weight.

2. Shape–One of the most obvious sex-related differences between boys and girls is the distribution of subcutaneous fat. At birth, girls have a little more total fat than boys do, and the difference increases gradually during childhood. During adolescence, trunk fat increases and continues to do so steadily into adulthood. Boys experience a "fat spurt" between ages 8 and 10 years and then lose subcutaneous fat as they progress into adolescence.

The most marked sexual dimorphism of the skeleton occurs at puberty, involving hips and shoulders. In females, estrogen produces a large increase in hip width, whereas in males, testosterone causes a large increase in shoulder width.

B. Variations in Girls: The menarche occurs between ages 10 and 17 years (average, age 12½ years). It generally takes place within 2 years of the time when the sesamoid at the distal end of the first metacarpal appears. Irregularities of menstruation are common during adolescence, and cycles are anovulatory for the first 1–2 years; consequently, pregnancy during this period is very unlikely. Periods of amenorrhea are more likely to occur during summer than winter.

Girls who menstruate late eventually become taller than those with early onset of menses. The menarchial ages of mothers and daughters are positively correlated.

Physiologic Considerations

It is important to keep in mind that the exact timing and duration of pubertal growth vary from individual to individual and that young people grow at a faster rate during adolescence than at any other time except during infancy. Pubertal growth varies in time of onset, duration, and extent.

Pubertal growth occurs at an earlier age today than it did 100 years ago, and sexual maturity is achieved at a younger age than in previous generations. This is most dramatically illustrated by the fact that the age at which menarche occurs has decreased by 3–4 months per decade over the last 100 years. For unknown reasons, this decrease in pubertal age appears to have reached a plateau during the last 10 years.

Sexual changes in males and females usually proceed according to a predictable pattern, called **sequencing.** This is the orderly appearance of secondary sexual characteristics, which appears to follow the same pattern from generation to generation and from culture to culture and can therefore be used to stage development despite the wide range in appearance of some of the characteristics. Thus, the growth of the penis and testes in boys, pubic hair in both boys and girls, and breast size in girls can be staged from 1 (childlike) to 5 (full development).

In boys, the sequence is (1) growth of testes and changes in the texture and color of the scrotum; (2) initial penile growth; (3) development of pubic hair; (4) accelerated penile growth, continued growth of the testes and scrotum, and growth of seminal vesicles and prostate; (5) peak growth in height; (6) development of full facial hair; and (7) voice change. In girls, the sequence is (1) broadening of the bony pelvis; (2) breast development; (3) development of the uterus, vagina, labia, and clitoris; (4) growth of pubic hair; (5) maximum height spurt; and (6) menarche, which occurs late, following the maximum height spurt. The average age of menarche is 12.8–13.2 years.

In both sexes, there is an increased need for vitamins (especially vitamin D), calcium, and protein during adolescence. There is an increased incidence of thyroid disturbances (enlargement of the thyroid as well as hypothyroidism and hyperthyroidism), tuberculosis, disturbances of epiphyses, anemia, dental caries, and circulatory instability.

Preceding the onset of menstruation, basal metabolism rises and nitrogen and calcium retention increase; this is followed by a postmenarchial decrease in retention of these substances and a fall in metabolism.

Striae, particularly about the breasts and hips, are common during adolescence even in the nonobese child. They appear to be associated with normally increased adrenocortical function.

The unilateral development of breast tissue in young girls is often disturbing and worrisome to them. This tissue appears as a firm, often painful mass just under the nipple, about 2 × 2 cm, and usually disappears as the girl goes on to develop fully formed breasts bilaterally. Boys also often undergo unilateral or bilateral breast enlargement during puberty, with firm, tender masses 1–2 cm in diameter similarly located just beneath the areola. This is often seen in boys who have well-developed testes and are virilizing rapidly and is called adolescent gynecomastia; it is usually transitory, subsiding spontaneously in about 6 months.

In girls, estrogens are responsible for changes in the labia minora, vagina, uterus, and uterine tubes as well as for changes of the nipple and duct structures. Androgens are responsible for pubic and axillary hair and enlargement of the clitoris and labia majora.

DISTURBANCES OF MENSTRUATION

ANOVULATORY BLEEDING

Irregular, acyclic anovulatory bleeding (metropathia hemorrhagica) is most frequently functional in nature and may merely represent a variation from normal. It is common during the first 1–2 years following menarche.

This entity occurs frequently and, in exceptional cases, may be associated with serious acute and chronic blood loss. Endometrial hyperplasia is the only pathologic finding.

Metropathia hemorrhagica is a diagnosis of exclusion and is reached after a careful history, physical examination, and pelvic examination have been performed and after laboratory tests (including complete blood count, Papanicolaou's test for maturation index, and thyroid function tests) are done.

Other diagnoses that must be considered when menses are irregular and erratic include complications of pregnancy (early or threatened abortion, ectopic pregnancy); malignancies of the uterus or ovaries; benign lesions of the pelvic organs (cervicitis, polyps, vaginal adenosis); systemic disorders (blood dyscrasias, anticoagulant therapy); bleeding caused by sporadic and incorrect use of oral contraceptives and occasionally from use of intrauterine devices; and, more rarely, a miscellaneous group that includes endocrine abnormalities (polycystic ovary syndrome, thyroid disorders), psychotropic drugs, obesity, and emotional stress.

Treatment

A. Minor Bleeding: Bleeding may be corrected by use of a progestin (eg, medroxyprogesterone acetate [Provera], 10 mg orally for days 15–20 of each menstrual cycle). Bleeding occurs 3–6 days after discontinuance and is usually limited to 5 days. Monthly treatment is continued until the patient establishes her own cycles. Normal sexual maturation will not be altered by these doses of hormone.

B. Moderately Severe Bleeding: Patients who suffer persistent, moderately severe blood loss may be given combined estrogen-progestin oral contraceptives. Any of the relatively high dose preparations (eg, mestranol, 80 μg, plus ethinyl estradiol, 50 μg) may be used, starting with 4 tablets a day for the first 5–7 days. Flow will cease within 12–24 hours; this is followed by a heavy flow 2–4 days after cessation of therapy. The patient can then begin a low-dose 28-day oral combination contraceptive (eg, one containing mestranol, 50 μg, such as Ortho-Novum 1/50) on the fifth day of flow and continue taking the oral contraceptive for a total of 3 cycles. Menstrual periods will often be normal thereafter.

C. Severe Hemorrhage and Anemia: If the patient presents with severe hemorrhage and anemia, bleeding may be stopped rapidly by the use of sodium estrone sulfate (Premarin), 20 mg intravenously, repeated at 6-hour intervals for 3 doses. Ethinyl estradiol, 0.5 mg, and medroxy-progesterone, 10 mg, are given orally daily at bedtime, and this larger dose of oral estrogen is continued for the first 24 days of the first cycle. After the first month, the usual dose of combined estrogen-progestin (eg, Ortho-Novum 1/50 or Norinyl 1+50) can be given for a total of 3 cycles.

D. Curettage: Curettage should be used only for severe bleeding that cannot be cured by nonsurgical measures. It is not useful for diagnosis unless an incomplete abortion is suspected. Curettage can be particularly hazardous to adolescent patients, because their uteri are small and the myometrium is not well developed. Dilatation of the cervix can injure the thin musculature about the internal os.

DYSMENORRHEA

Dysmenorrhea (painful menstrual periods) is one of the most common menstrual complaints in adolescent girls. Most frequently it is primary, ie, there is no demonstrable pelvic disease. Secondary dysmenorrhea is associated with organic pelvic disorders, including endometriosis, adenomyosis, uterine myomas, polyps of the cervix or uterus, and chronic pelvic infections, and with use of an intrauterine device (IUD).

Dysmenorrhea reportedly affects up to 80% of women, depending on the population studied and the criteria used. About 10% of adolescent girls fail to attend classes because of menstrual pain.

Painful menses almost always follow an ovulatory cycle, and since early postmenarchial menstrual cycles are generally anovulatory, dysmenorrhea is uncommon during the first 1–2 years after the menarche.

The pain of menstrual cramps is sharp and colicky and usually begins on the first day of menses, seldom lasting longer than the second day. It generally occurs in the midline in the lower abdomen and can radiate to the lower back and thighs. Severe menstrual pain can be accompanied by nausea and vomiting, diarrhea, and syncope.

The causes of menstrual pain are still unclear, although recent evidence strongly suggests that prostaglandin $F_{2\alpha}$ produced in the endometrium during the secretory phase of the menstrual cycle causes painful uterine contractions, nausea and vomiting, and diarrhea.

A careful history and physical examination, including a pelvic examination, are essential to rule out other organic causes of pelvic pain before a diagnosis of primary dysmenorrhea can be confirmed. It is helpful to assess the girl's understanding of the menstrual cycle and related body functions, the possible importance of secondary gains (secondary gains from being unwell include staying home from school and receiving special attention from the parents), and psychologic factors (the girl may have been reared to expect menses to be a painful and disabling experience). Reassurance and education can help allay anxiety arising from a distorted understanding of menstruation.

Treatment

Mild dysmenorrhea responds well to analgesia with aspirin or phenobarbital and belladonna compounds given every 6 hours. Nonsteroidal anti-inflammatory drugs have been found to actively inhibit prostaglandin synthesis and are used in the treatment of moderate to severe pelvic pain. One of the following may be used: indomethacin (Indocin), 25 mg 3–4 times daily; naproxen sodium (Anaprox), 250 mg twice daily; ibuprofen (Motrin), 400 mg 3 times daily; or mefenamic acid (Ponstel), 250 mg 4 times daily. Side effects, including nausea and vomiting, are few. These drugs should not be given to patients with gastrointestinal ulcers.

If these drugs are ineffective, aspirin or acetaminophen with codeine, 30 mg, may be given every 6 hours. Promethazine (Phenergan), 25 mg every 8 hours, may help control vomiting. If oral medication is not tolerated, promethazine, 25 mg rectally every 6 hours, may be prescribed.

DELAYED MENARCHE & AMENORRHEA

Delayed menarche may be difficult to differentiate from primary amenorrhea. However, well-developed (or developing) secondary sexual characteristics and a family history of late menarche are helpful in making this diagnosis; and a policy of watchful waiting, with reevaluation every 6 months until onset of menses, is recommended.

Etiology

A. Primary Amenorrhea: Primary amenorrhea is failure of onset of menarche. Rarely, it may be due to pregnancy. Other causes include central nervous system or hypothalamic-pituitary disorders, including panhypopituitarism and Laurence-Moon-Biedl syndrome; hypogonadotropic hypogonadism; polycystic ovary syndrome; and neoplastic disorders such as suprasellar and intrasellar tumors (craniopharyngiomas, gliomas). The only psychogenic basis for primary amenorrhea is anorexia nervosa. Genetic causes are Turner's syndrome and variants, adrenogenital syndrome, testicular feminizing syndrome, and true hermaphroditism. Endocrine abnormalities associated with primary amenorrhea include hypothyroidism, diabetes mellitus, Cushing's syndrome, and functioning ovarian tumors. Anatomic reasons for primary amenorrhea include imperforate hymen, vaginal agenesis, congenital absence of the uterus and vagina, and atresia of the uterine cervix. Chronic debilitating conditions and autoimmune disorders may also be a cause of primary amenorrhea.

B. Secondary Amenorrhea: Secondary amenorrhea is cessation of menses following menarche and absence of spontaneous bleeding for at least 120 days. The most common cause in adolescents is pregnancy. Temporary cessation of menses, often for as long as 2–3 months, may also occur when birth control pills are stopped. Other causes include anovulatory cycles; ovarian tumors, both estrogen- and androgen-producing; polycystic ovary syndrome; and premature ovarian failure.

Nonovarian causes may be of psychogenic origin, such as environmental or emotional trauma. Nutritional deficiencies, such as those due to anorexia nervosa or crash diets, may produce secondary amenorrhea. Other causes include organic brain disease (suprasellar and intrasellar tumors), end-organ disease following too vigorous curettage or severe uterine infection postoperatively, and systemic illness such as thyroid disorders, adrenal disease, and Cushing's and Addison's disease.

Treatment

Rational therapy obviously depends on precise diagnosis. History, physical examination (including pelvic examination), and assessment of secondary sexual characteristics are essential. In addition, buccal smear for Barr bodies, vaginal smear for estrogen effect, a bone age determination, and thyroid function tests are helpful in diagnosis.

A progesterone withdrawal test with progesterone in oil, 100 mg intramuscularly, may be given. Withdrawal bleeding should occur within 5–7 days. This shows that a source of estrogen exists and that the uterine cavity, cervix, and vagina are patent and functional. If bleeding does not occur, then more definitive and refined diagnostic tests are in order; these include tests to determine plasma follicle-stimulating hormone (FSH), luteinizing hormone (LH), and prolactin levels. If FSH, LH, and prolactin levels are low, pituitary tumor should be suspected, and visual field tests, skull films of the sella, and CT scan should be done.

VAGINITIS

Vaginal discharge is a common complaint among adolescent girls. A patient with physiologic leukorrhea, which occurs during early adolescence as the cervical and vaginal epithelium responds to increasing levels of estrogen, needs only simple reassurance and no treatment,

The diagnosis can be made by looking at the vaginal aspirate under the microscope; no white or red cells are seen, but there are many desquamated epithelial cells.

Trichomonas vaginalis Vaginitis

Vaginitis due to *Trichomonas* infection is seen in sexually mature and frequently sexually active girls. It can be transmitted by sexual intercourse. Characteristically, it produces a malodorous, frothy, thin, yellow-green discharge. When a wet mount is made (1 drop of discharge with 1 drop of saline) and examined under the microscope, the motile pear-shaped organisms with flagella are seen, larger than pus cells. Treatment is with metronidazole (Flagyl), 250 mg given as a single 2-g dose (see Chapter 6). The sexual partner should also be treated.

Candidal Vaginitis

The discharge in candidal vaginitis is thick, white, and curdlike, often accompanied by intense itching and reddening of the vulva. A wet mount will show yeastlike budding cells and hyphae. Treatment can be with one of the following: nystatin vaginal suppositories inserted twice a day for 14 days; miconazole nitrate (Monistat), 2% vaginal cream, 1 applicatorful at bedtime for 10 days; or clotrimazole (Lotrimin, Mycelex-G), 1% vaginal cream, inserted at bedtime for 7 days.

Gardnerella vaginalis (Formerly *Haemophilus vaginalis*) Vulvovaginitis

Gardnerella vaginalis thrives in an estrogenic vagina, producing a gray malodorous discharge, often with little discomfort other than pruritus. A wet mount shows "clue cells," superficial vaginal cells with a stippled or granulated look due to *G vaginalis*. Treatment can be with metronidazole (Flagyl), 500 mg twice a day for 7 days; cephradine (Anspor), 250 mg 4 times a day for 7 days; ampicillin, 500 mg 4 times a day for 7 days; or tetracycline, 500 mg 4 times a day for 7 days. The sexual partner should also be treated.

Herpes Simplex Type 2

Pain, swelling, itching, and burning in the perineal area, often with dysuria and bilateral tender inguinal nodes, can be caused by herpesvirus type 2. Examination reveals clusters of vesicles on the vulva that rupture in 1–3 days, leaving painful ulcerations that heal in 3–15 days, with spontaneous clearing. Treatment is symptomatic, as there is no cure. Sitz baths twice a day, Burow's soaks to the area, and fresh moist tea bags applied to the perineum may help relieve pain and swelling. Local anesthetics such as lidocaine, 2.5%, may reduce discomfort, particularly with voiding. An antiviral agent, acyclovir (Zovirax), 5% ointment, is now available. Applied to lesions every 3 hours, 6 times a day for 7 days, it decreases viral shedding, shortens healing time, and decreases duration of pain, but it is most effective in primary infections only and does not seem to affect the number of recurrences or their clinical course. Better methods of administration of acyclovir may soon be available. A male partner who is infected must use condoms to prevent transmission of the virus during intercourse; vaginal spermicidal contraceptives should be used at the same time.

Foreign Body

Foreign bodies in the vagina can produce a malodorous and copious discharge. In the adolescent, a forgotten or irretrievable menstrual tampon is the most common object. Vaginal discharge will clear spontaneously within a few days following removal of the object.

Allergic Vaginitis

Allergic vaginitis (contact vaginitis) may occur from reaction to bubble bath, douches, contraceptive foam, or deodorant sprays. It can be treated with topical hydrocortisone cream and oral antihistaminics.

CONTRACEPTION

Of the 29 million teenagers in the USA, 7 million young men and 5 million young women have had sexual intercourse. One-third of girls age 15–17 years are sexually experienced. By age 19, 70% of young women report having had sexual intercourse. Most teenagers seek contraception after they have been sexually active, usually following a bad scare. Moreover, half of premarital pregnancies in this age group occur within 6 months of first intercourse. Eighty percent of premarital teenage pregnancies and two-thirds of premarital teenage births are unintended. With such alarming statistics, contraception becomes of primary importance in preventing unwanted pregnancies in unready and immature young women.

Counseling about birth control can be initiated during history-taking, when questions about menses can lead to inquiries about sexual activity. If the girl is sexually active, the physician can offer advice about different methods of birth control. Any fears or anxieties the girl may have about various methods should be elicited, and any questions she may have should be fully answered. The physician should remember that adolescence is an age of rebellion and testing-out behavior and that teenagers have a feeling of being immune to risk, so that the final decision to use contraception should be left to the girl. It is sometimes difficult for even the most understanding practitioner to remain nonjudgmental when a teenager admits sexual activity but does not wish to use birth control because she "will not get pregnant." A friendly, interested demeanor and a return visit scheduled within a month will help maintain an open-door policy so the girl can return if she changes her mind.

Oral contraceptives are probably the safest and certainly the most effective method of birth control among teenagers. As a group, teenage girls are least vulnerable to the risks of pill use. No significant difference has been found in the mortality rate due to the pill as compared with that for other methods of birth control. Teenagers are 5 times more likely to die of pregnancy-related causes than they are from use of the pill.

The use of the IUD also poses a minimal mortality risk to teenagers. However, nulliparous women are known to have more difficulty in using IUDs successfully. Moreover, the risk of pelvic inflammatory disease and possible subsequent infertility must be considered, particularly since teenagers, unless they are married or with a stable partner, are likely to have multiple partners. Ectopic pregnancy also occurs more frequently in IUD users. These factors raise doubts about the suitability of the IUD for teenagers.

Oral Contraceptives

Before prescribing oral contraceptives, the physician should obtain a medical history to rule out recent hepatitis, thrombophlebitis, cerebral vascular accident, undiagnosed genital bleeding, any history of breast or genital neoplasms, and possible pregnancy. These are all absolute contraindications to use of oral contraceptives. Diabetes and epilepsy are usually not contraindications to the use of birth control pills. It is felt that the hazards of pregnancy far outweigh the risks of taking oral contraceptives. Girls who have migraine headaches, however, probably should not take birth control pills, as the risk of cerebral vascular accidents is increased 6-fold for migraine sufferers who use steroid contraceptives.

A physical examination, including blood pressure measurement, examination of the breasts and pelvis, Papanicolaou's test, culture for gonoccoci, and a wet mount for yeast or trichomonads, should be done. A return appointment should be made for 6 weeks after the first pill is taken. On this visit, the girl's blood pressure should be checked, and she should be asked about her first menses while taking the pill (normally shorter and scantier than usual menses) and any side effects she may have noted. Return visits should be scheduled in 3 months and again in 6 months. One year after starting oral contraceptives, the girl should have a repeat of the initial examination. Adolescents seem to do better with closer supervision and more frequent visits.

A. Dosage and Administration: Commonly prescribed preparations are compounds that contain enough estrogen and progestin to ensure good protection but pose minimal complications. Since teenagers often take medicines erratically, the use of a 28-day package (which contains 7 inert or iron-containing pills) is recommended; this will eliminate the need to count the days between cycles and is more likely to ensure continued daily usage. These preparations include Norinyl 1+35 28-Day, Norinyl 1+50 28-Day, Ortho-Novum 1/50 28-Day, and Norlestrin Fe 1/50, all of which contain 35–50 μg of ethinyl estradiol or mestranol and 1 mg of progestin per tablet. They are begun on day 5 to day 7 of the menstrual cycle. A menstrual period should occur between days 21 and 28 of the package. When one 28-day package is finished, the girl begins the next 28-day package.

B. Complications:

1. Breakthrough bleeding–Bleeding that occurs at any time in the cycle except during days 21–28 is probably the most common complication. If bleeding occurs in the early part of the cycle, estrogenic stimulation may be inadequate, and a compound containing more estrogen, eg, Norinyl 1+80 or Ortho-Novum 1/80, can be prescribed. If bleeding occurs late in the cycle, the progestin effect may be deficient, and a compound containing more of this steroid, eg, Norlestrin 2.5/50, may be prescribed. However, breakthrough bleeding is common in the first 1–2 cycles and often will cease thereafter.

2. Pregnancy–Accidental pregnancy can occur when a woman takes her pills irregularly; thus, if there is a history of sporadic intake of pills and an active sexual life, the patient should always have a pregnancy test and a pelvic examination. The ingestion of oral contraceptives during early pregnancy has been reported to produce birth defects, but recent evidence suggests that this hazard is minimal and probably only occurs in predisposed persons.

3. Rise in blood pressure–If rising blood pressure is noted after the patient begins taking oral contraceptives, they should be discontinued. Other reasons for elevated blood pressure should be considered and ruled out with appropriate laboratory tests. Alternative methods of birth control should be advised.

Barrier Contraceptives

Vaginal foam and a condom used together provide a safe and very effective method of contraception. The condom has the added advantage of protecting against venereal disease. Recently, vaginal foam has been packaged in convenient purse-size containers and in suppository form, to be inserted 10 minutes before intercourse. While easier to use, the suppositories contain somewhat less spermicide than does the foam. Because the combined use of foam and condom requires some forethought and preparation, this method of contraception is not popular among teenagers, and some males complain that condom use decreases sensation. The diaphragm has become more popular with older teenage girls who are concerned about the long-term effects of birth control pills and wish to use an alternative method of contraception.

Skin | 12

PRINCIPLES OF TREATMENT

Sensitivity of Skin

The child's skin is more sensitive than the adult's, and areas treated with topical medications must be carefully observed for evidence of irritation from too great a concentration of drug.

Choice of Topical Medication

Choice of medication is determined as much by the presenting morphology of a lesion as by the diagnosis. Treat the stage as well as the type of dermatitis.

Becoming familiar with a limited number of types of medication will prove more useful than attempting to try the immense variety of skin remedies endorsed by others.

Medications useful in the treatment of skin diseases in childhood are shown in Table 12–1.

Application of Medications

(1) Undertreatment is sometimes more effective than overtreatment. Improvement in a skin disease sometimes occurs with dicontinuance of all therapy.

(2) The medication itself may produce a skin lesion (treatment dermatitis), and frequent observation is necessary when a new therapy is tried. Especially when treating allergic conditions such as eczema, the physician should know the antigenic potentialities of the medication in use. Corticosteroid ointments will produce local side effects with prolonged use, especially in areas where the skin is thin. The local effects are those of telangiectasia, which may become permanent.

(3) Adequate and complete instructions should be given. The anxious parent must be cautioned against overenthusiastic application of medication.

(4) Topical corticosteroids vary widely in potency, eg, hydrocortisone, 1% (low potency); fluocinolone, 0.01% (medium potency); and halcinonide, 0.025% (high potency). Always use the lowest

potency that is effective. Ointments are more effective than creams because they stay on the skin longer and retain moisture in the skin.

Special Diagnostic Procedures

A. Microscopic Examination:

1. Types of specimens–Specimens include scrapings from the edge of an active lesion in suspected fungous infection of the skin and hair shafts in suspected tinea of the scalp.

2. Preparation of specimens–Put the scrapings from the possible fungous lesions on a glass slide, and add a few drops of 20% potassium or sodium hydroxide solution. Allow the slide to stand for 20 minutes, and then examine it under the "high-dry" lens of the microscope by diffuse light. In a properly cleared specimen, fungous elements, if present, will be seen as fragments of mycelium and spores of various types.

B. Examination With Hand Lens: In suspected scabies, examine a nonexcoriated burrow with a hand lens, and look for the female mite at the end of the burrow or for small black dots of feces along the burrow. The mite may be demonstrated under the microscope by teasing it out of the burrow with a delicate needle or by slicing off the top of the burrow and placing the whole specimen on a slide.

C. Wood's Light: Ultraviolet irradiation passed through a Wood's filter is used for the diagnosis of *Microsporum* infections only. In a darkened room, examine the specimen for fluorescence. This technique is useful for scalp or axillary infection but is not satisfactory in the study of infection on glabrous skin.

D. Patch Tests and Scratch Tests: These are sometimes useful in determining the possible source of an allergic skin reaction.

1. Patch test–A piece of gauze containing a solution or suspension of the suspected allergen is applied to the skin of the forearm, thigh, or lower back and covered with a piece of plastic material. The test is read after 48 hours, and erythema with or without vesicular reaction is significant. The test may become positive as late as 7 days after removal of the test material.

2. Scratch test–Solutions of potentially allergenic substances are applied to the skin of the same areas of the body as in the patch test. The test solutions are best obtained from commercial sources. A drop of solution is placed on the skin, and the tip of a pin or scalpel is drawn through it without causing bleeding. The test is read after 15 minutes. Significant reactions are erythema and edema.

CONGENITAL DISEASES OF THE SKIN

PIGMENTED NEVI

Types

A. Simple Forms: These include ephelides, or freckles; Mongolian spots, found in most black, Oriental, and Amerindian infants; and café au lait spots, which are oval and light brown on white skins or dark brown on black skins.

B. True Pigmented Nevi: True pigmented nevi (moles) are of 3 basic types: (1) nevus spilus—smooth, flat, no hair; (2) nevus pilosus—with a growth of downy or stiff hair; and (3) nevus verrucosus—hyperkeratotic, raised, sometimes wartlike areas.

Treatment

Excision may be for cosmetic reasons or if the lesion is subject to trauma or repeated irritation. Tissue removed should be submitted in every case for pathologic examination to rule out malignant melanoma. Lesions with changes in color to blue, white, or red with irregular borders or ulceration and bleeding should be removed because of the greater possibility of malignant melanoma.

Prognosis

The prognosis is good for all types except when there is microscopic evidence of nevus cell invasion of the epidermis.

VASCULAR NEVI

Vascular nevi consist of an abnormal mass of blood vessels of the skin, which may be discolored or tumorlike.

Nevus Flammeus ("Port Wine Mark")

Nevus flammeus is a smooth, flat, superficial angioma that varies in color from red to dark purple. It is located most often on the face or neck and varies in size from a few millimeters to an area that covers most of the face and neck.

Use of a cosmetic cream (eg, Covermark) to mask lesions of small size is the only treatment indicated.

The less intensely colored nevi often disappear spontaneously during infancy or early childhood.

Capillary Hemangioma ("Strawberry Mark")

Capillary hemangioma is a slightly raised, sharply demarcated, bright red spot varying from several millimeters to 2–3 cm in diameter; it does not blanch completely on pressure. Although it usually appears during the first 6 weeks of life, it is occasionally present at birth. Commonly, there is an increase in size for a few months, but few such nevi will continue to increase after age 12 months.

Treatment is rarely indicated and is only for those lesions of the face, scalp, and areas where trauma or infection may produce bleeding, ulceration, and scarring. Carbon dioxide freezing is the treatment of choice.

Most hemangiomas will spontaneously regress and disappear by adolescence.

Cavernous Hemangioma

Cavernous hemangioma is formed from large, sinuslike blood vessels in the skin and often has a capillary component. The lesions are raised, poorly circumscribed, blue to purple, and readily blanched by pressure. Distribution and behavior are similar to the capillary type. The cavernous type will heal spontaneously, usually before age 5 years. When a cavernous hemangioma is situated where trauma can be common or is located around the mouth or on the oral mucous surfaces, there may be ulceration, infection, or serious hemorrhage. In addition, disseminated intravascular coagulation may be a complication (see Chapter 17). With any of these complications, treatment may be indicated.

Surgical excision or radiation therapy requires experienced specialists. Prednisone given orally and accompanied by compression may be tried before these measures and will occasionally be successful.

Most lesions will involute spontaneously. However, some persist, and some may become arteriovenous fistulas. They occasionally accompany retrolental fibroplasia or internal hemangiomas in vital organs.

ICHTHYOSIS

The ichthyoses are inherited skin diseases characterized by generalized thickening, scaling, and marked dryness. Inheritance is autosomal or X-linked.

Types

A. Excessive Production of Scales:

1. Epidermolytic hyperkeratosis–Yellow scales are present in the flexural areas and on the palms and soles.

2. Lamellar ichthyosis–Red skin and thickened palms and soles are characteristic.

B. Increased Retention of Scales:

1. Ichthyosis vulgaris–This develops during childhood, with fine scales and prominent palmar and plantar markings.

2. X-linked ichthyosis–Apparent at birth, the ichthyosis spares the palms and soles. Corneal opacities are seen in the patient and the carrier mother.

Treatment

Patients should bathe infrequently with synthetic, nonfat soap and lubricate the skin with mineral oil daily. Topical administration of tretinoin, 0.05% cream (Retin-A), has been most promising. Control of keratinization through the use of 5% pyruvic, citric, lactic, or salicylic acid in petrolatum, applied once or twice daily, has been reported to be successful.

Prognosis

Improvement may occur with simple treatment measures, but the prognosis for recovery is hopeless for some cases and very poor for moderate cases.

UNCOMMON CONGENITAL SKIN DISORDERS

Acrodermatitis Enteropathica

Acrodermatitis enteropathica is an autosomal recessive disorder characterized by erosive lesions around the mouth, nails, eyelids, anus, genital areas, elbows, knees, and ankles; alopecia; diarrhea; and malabsorption. Zinc sulfate is effective therapy.

Anhidrotic Ectodermal Dysplasia

Anhidrotic ectodermal dysplasia is a rare familial syndrome characterized by marked inhibition of sweating; sparse hair; alteration of the nails; dry, white, smooth, glossy skin; saddle nose; prominent supraorbital ridges; and faulty dentition. Convulsions with fever occur owing to decreased ability to dissipate heat through evaporation. A hearing defect may also be present. The sodium chloride level in the sweat is elevated (see Appendix).

Epidermolysis Bullosa

Epidermolysis bullosa, a sometimes familial disorder, appears at any age but most commonly in early infancy. Hemorrhagic bullae develop following trauma to the skin. The prognosis is variable depending on the form of the disease.

Cutis Hyperelastica

Cutis hyperelastica is characterized by extreme elasticity of the skin. The skin may appear normal but can be extended by pinching and pulling. When released, it snaps back as though it were a sheet of rubber. No treatment is necessary.

Ehlers-Danlos Syndrome

Ehlers-Danlos syndrome consists of skin hyperelasticity and friability, fragility of blood vessels, and hyperextensibility of the joints. Multiple, freely movable subcutaneous fatty nodules are sometimes present. Protection against injury is most important. No specific therapy is available.

Adenoma Sebaceum

Adenoma sebaceum consists of pinhead-sized to pea-sized, rounded, elevated papules or nodules situated particularly upon the nose, cheeks, and chin. The color may be that of normal skin, waxy, or reddish, and there may be an associated telangiectasia. Adenoma sebaceum may occur in association with tuberous sclerosis. Mental deficiency and convulsions may be associated with either condition in a familial pattern.

Treatment consists of applying carbon dioxide snow to the lesions. Surgical planing is the treatment of choice. Larger adenomas may require electrodesiccation. Recurrence of lesions is common.

Ritter's Disease (Dermatitis Exfoliativa Neonatorum)

See Table 9–1.

INCONTINENTIA PIGMENTI

Incontinentia pigmenti is a rare hereditary disorder, most common in females, characterized by developmental defects of the skin, anomalies of dentition (pointed, wide teeth), concomitant neurologic symptoms, osseous deformities, and alopecia. In the neonatal period, linear skin lesions are erythematous and vesicular; these become verrucous and then pigmented, and they eventually fade.

DEPIGMENTATION
(Albinism, Vitiligo)

Generalized depigmentation (albinism) is rare. Localized depigmentation (vitiligo) may occur on any part of the body, and the hair of the affected area is white. The cause is not known, but these disorders may be associated with endocrine abnormalities. Treatment is unsatisfactory.

COMMON SKIN DISORDERS IN INFANCY

Miliaria Crystallina & Miliaria Rubra

Miliaria is due to obstruction of sweat ducts and occurs in most infants. It appears as very small vesicles (miliaria crystallina) or as erythematous papules over the chest and neck (miliaria rubra). Heat and high humidity predispose to miliaria. No treatment is indicated.

Erythema Toxicum

In erythema toxicum, erythematous macules appear over the face, chest, and back at age 1–4 days and disappear by age 8 days.

Sucking Blisters

Sucking blisters result from sucking in utero. They appear at birth as bullae or eroded areas on the infant's arms and hands.

DISEASES DUE TO BACTERIA

IMPETIGO

Types

A. Impetigo of the Newborn: See Table 9–1.

B. Impetigo Contagiosa: In older children, impetigo is due to group A streptococci or staphylococci. There are multiple lesions of varying sizes and shapes, with vesicles, blebs, and yellow crusts on an erythematous base. With healing at the center of the lesion, circinate lesions may be mistaken for ringworm.

C. Ecthyma: Ecthyma differs from impetigo only in that the lesions are more deep-seated and are therefore likely to leave pigmentation and slight scarring.

Treatment

A. Impetigo of the Newborn: See Table 9–1.

B. Impetigo Contagiosa and Ecthyma: Rupture all intact vesicles or mature pustules, and remove crusts and other debris by washing with antiseptic detergent (pHisoHex) and water. Wet dressings to soak the crusts may be necessary before crusts can be removed.

Systemic antibiotics are indicated. Give procaine penicillin, 100,000–300,000 units intramuscularly every 24 hours for 7 days. With penicillin sensitivity, give erythromycin (see Chapter 6) for 10 days.

Antibiotic ointments in a water-soluble base, eg, bacitracin, neomycin, or bacitracin-polymyxin combination, may be used in addition to systemic antibiotics but are not usually effective when used alone.

Prognosis

Impetigo generally responds well to therapy, but skin lesions may act as primary sites for metastatic infections.

Observe for nephritis and other complications of staphylococcal or streptococcal infections.

EPIDERMAL NECROLYSIS

Epidermal necrolysis is usually associated with *Staphylococcus aureus* infection, but some cases may be drug-induced. The age range is from the neonatal period to 5 years. Onset is with conjunctivitis or rhinorrhea, with purulent discharge. After 2–4 days, generalized erythema and bullae appear, principally on the face and upper trunk. Exfoliation begins 4 days after onset of the rash and lasts 7–14 days.

Dicloxacillin should be given systemically because of possible sepsis, but treatment will not alter the course of the skin manifestation.

The prognosis is good for complete healing.

FOLLICULITIS

Follicle infections may be superficial or deep. The lesion consists of pinhead-sized or slightly larger pustules surrounded by a narrow area of erythema. Many pustules are usually present in the same area. The most common cause is staphylococci.

Folliculitis is most often secondary to intertrigo and chronic irritation of the skin (eg, from diapers), but it may be secondary to drainage of chronic otitis media or a similar source of purulent material.

Treatment is essentially the same as for impetigo, with rupture of all localized pustules and application of antibiotic ointment. The systemic use of antibiotics is reserved for cases with fever and complicating cellulitis. For prophylaxis, see under Furunculosis, below.

FURUNCULOSIS

Furuncles usually start as painful, deep-seated infections of a sebaceous gland or hair follicle. They gradually approach the surface and appear red and elevated. After several days, the skin in the center becomes thin, and a pustule may form. With rupture or after careful incision, a "core" of necrotic material, together with liquid pus, is discharged.

The fusion of several furuncles produces a carbuncle.

Multiple, recurrent furuncles may occur in certain children (usually over age 5 years). The cause is unknown. Bouts may continue to recur over several years and usually cease after adolescence.

Treatment

A. Local Measures: Measures include immobilization of the affected part if an extremity is involved, application of heat (in the form of warm moist saline dressings frequently renewed; see Table 12–1), and drainage after the lesions become localized and fluctuant. Deep incisions are not necessary; a small incision with a needle or scalpel is sufficient. A furuncle must never be squeezed. During drainage, an antibiotic ointment dressing may be applied.

Daily bathing and cleansing of the entire body with pHisoHex is most important. This should be vigorously carried out for at least 1 month.

B. Prophylactic Measures: For prophylaxis of folliculitis and furunculosis, treat possible contributory skin disease such as seborrhea or excessive oil on the skin, excessively dry skin, and acne. Rule out diabetes in recurrent cases.

Control of the nasal carrier state is most effective in preventing recurrent furunculosis. Instill as ointment 5 mg of neomycin per gram of water-soluble base, twice daily for 1 month.

C. Specific Measures: Systemic antibiotics are sometimes necessary in cases of recurrent furunculosis. Erythromycin (see Chapter 6) is the drug of first choice. Vaccines and toxoids have not proved to be effective.

DISEASES DUE TO FUNGI

Principles of Treatment & Prophylaxis

(1) Treat acute active fungous infections initially as for any acute dermatitis; it may be necessary to treat the dermatitis before using fungicidal medication.

(2) Many fungicidal agents may be strong skin irritants. Undertreat rather than overtreat.

(3) Keep skin dry. Moist skin favors the growth of fungi.

TINEA CIRCINATA, TINEA CORPORIS, TINEA CRURIS, & TINEA CAPITIS

Lesions begin as one or more irregular erythematous, slightly raised, scaly patches that are soon covered with small vesicles. The lesions tend to spread, but central clearing occurs and results in the typical ring-shaped lesion with the active process around the healed center. Itching, if present, is usually mild. During adolescence, lesions in the inguinal region may become acutely inflamed and macerated as a result of perspiration and bacterial contamination. Common causative fungi include *Trichophyton mentagrophytes* and *Microsporum canis*. Tinea capitis infections are common in children and rare in adults. Lesions consist of rounded, hairless, slightly reddened areas covered with grayish scales and broken stumps of hair. Common causative fungi are *Trichophyton tonsurans, M canis,* and *Microsporum audouini*. The active lesions can be seen to fluoresce under Wood's light in *Microsporum* infections. *Trichophyton* species do not fluoresce.

Treatment

A. Local Measures:

1. Secondarily infected or inflamed lesions may be treated with potassium permanganate, 1:10,000, or aluminum acetate solution, 1:20, as wet compresses.

2. Dusting powders may be used 2–3 times a day on involved areas where perspiration is excessive. Avoid powders containing starch, which encourages the growth of fungi.

3. Tolnaftate (Tinactin) ointment or 1% powder is the treatment of choice. Apply twice daily for 2–4 weeks.

4. Haloprogin (Halotex), 1% cream; miconazole (Micatin), 2% cream; and clotrimazole (Lotrimin), 1% cream, are all effective when applied to affected areas twice daily for 2–4 weeks.

B. Specific Measures: When hair is involved (tinea capitis), fingernails or toenails are involved, or disease is severe and widespread, the treatment of choice is griseofulvin (Fulvicin, Grifulvin), 20 mg/kg/d in 3 divided doses. Continue for 4–8 weeks, depending on the response. Leukopenia may be an indication to stop the drug.

C. Follow-up Measures: Check results for several months by observation and by examining with Wood's light.

Prophylaxis

It is essential to treat infected individuals or household pets, with reexamination to determine cure. Advise patients to avoid exchange of clothes and headgear that have not been adequately laundered. In epidemics, examine all potential tinea cases with Wood's light and treat infected individuals.

Prognosis

The chief complication of tinea is formation of kerions (abscesslike swellings). *T tonsurans* infections, which are now extending over the USA from west to east, are resistant to simple forms of treatment and usually require griseofulvin.

EPIDERMOPHYTOSIS, DERMATOPHYTOSIS
("Athlete's Foot," Tinea of Palms & Soles)

Fungous infection in the interdigital areas is probably very widespread in older children and adults and does not always produce clinical manifestations. The causative organisms are *Trichophyton* and *Epidermophyton*. Three basic types of lesions are found: (1) red, dry, scaly, and fissured eruptions between the toes; (2) acute, tense, papulovesicular, and bullous eruptions on the soles or on the sides of the feet; and (3) dry, scaly, thickened areas between the toes or on palms.

Treatment

A. Local Measures: Do not overtreat.

1. Acute stage–If the infection is in the acute stage (1–10 days), treat as for any acute dermatosis, using soaks (see Table 12–1) for 20 minutes 2–3 times daily. If mild secondary infection is present, use 1:10,000 potassium permanganate soaks.

2. Subacute stage–Use fungicidal medicaments as for tinea corporis (see above) and Whitfield's ointment, ¼- to ½-strength.

B. General Measures: Put special emphasis on personal hygiene. Advise the patient to wear well-ventilated shoes, if possible; dry carefully between the toes after bathing; change socks frequently; and use dusting and drying powders on affected areas as required.

TINEA VERSICOLOR

Tinea versicolor is an uncommon childhood disease caused by *Malassezia furfur* and characterized by small yellowish-brown macules that slowly spread and coalesce to form large brownish patches covered with a fine, furfuraceous, mealy scaling, usually over the chest and back. Treatment with sodium thiosulfate, 25%, applied to affected areas 2 or 3 times a day for 2 weeks is usually effective. Full-strength suspension of selenium sulfide (Selsun), applied to the entire body overnight, may be tried in resistant cases. Another alternative is to treat as for other forms of tinea (see p 242).

CANDIDIASIS
(Moniliasis)

Candidiasis is common in early infancy and is usually the result of candidal infection *(Candida albicans)* in the mother's vagina. The eruption may resemble eczema and may be scaly, papulovesicular, and erythematous, with a sharp border. It usually occurs in moist areas of the body that are subject to rubbing, most often in the diaper area, axillae, and the inguinal regions. Erythematous satellite lesions outside the area of main involvement are characteristic. However, candidiasis may cause a generalized skin eruption or become invasive and produce a variety of visceral lesions. It is often associated with candidal infection of the mouth ("thrush") and may be a complication of hypoparathyroidism, diabetes mellitus, or prolonged antibiotic therapy.

Treatment

A. Local Measures: Use moist soaks (aluminum acetate solution) if the lesions are acute, inflamed, and wet. Nystatin (Mycostatin) cream, 100,000 units/g, or haloprogin (Halotex), 1% cream, is applied to the lesions 3 times daily. Keep area dry.

B. Specific Measures: For treatment of thrush, any of the following may be used: a suspension of nystatin (Mycostatin), 100,000 units/mL, 10 drops applied to the mouth 4 times daily after ingestion of food or milk; gentian violet, 1:10,000 in 10% alcohol (or 1% aqueous solution), applied locally to lesions in the mouth twice daily for 3 or 4 days (avoid prolonged use); or a solution of vinegar, 10 mL/1000 mL, applied locally twice daily.

DISEASES DUE TO VIRUSES

VERRUCAE

While not all types of warts have definitely been shown to be infectious or to be caused by viruses, the evidence of apparent autoinoculation and person-to-person spread in the various types of warts is most suggestive.

Types

A. Verruca Vulgaris (Common Wart): This wart is a sharply circumscribed, firm, round elevation of the skin that may have a roughened, thick surface or papillary protuberances. It is common in childhood and usually appears in multiple distribution on the hands or feet.

B. Verruca Plana Juvenilis (Flat or Plane Wart): This wart is a small, round, slightly elevated, flat lesion, usually the color of the surrounding skin. It is common in children and usually occurs in linear distribution on the face or neck or on the backs of the hands.

C. Verruca Plantaris (Plantar Wart): This represents a common wart (verruca vulgaris) modified by pressure, which forces the hypertrophied epithelium into the skin and by irritation stimulates further cornification. It is located on the soles of the feet and appears either singly or in groups.

Treatment

Treatment of all warts is not entirely satisfactory. Cases have been reported of spontaneous disappearance after psychotherapy ("suggestion" therapy), but this corresponds to the rate of spontaneous disappearance without psychotherapy.

A. Verruca Vulgaris and Verruca Plana Juvenilis: These warts should rarely be surgically excised. Cryotherapy with liquid nitrogen is usually most successful after the first application. A second application, however, may be necessary.

B. Verruca Plantaris: Application of liquid nitrogen or chemical cauterization may be attempted and has a better than 50% chance of at least partial success. Carefully apply trichloroacetic acid to the center of the wart, with the surrounding skin protected by petrolatum. Several applications may be required, with removal of the desiccated area before each procedure. When salicylic acid is used, a 40% plaster is applied for 24 hours, followed by removal of macerated material and reapplication of the plaster.

Surgical removal by scalpel or electrodessication may be necessary in persistent lesions. The patient will be incapacitated for about a week after each such operation.

HERPES SIMPLEX CUTANEOUS INFECTION

(See Chapter 24.)

ECZEMA HERPETICUM
(Kaposi's Varicelliform Eruption)

Eczema herpeticum in children results from a primary infection with herpes simplex virus or from secondary infection with vaccinia and is characterized by a vesicular eruption and a febrile reaction complicating a preexisting atopic dermatitis or eczema. The lesions go through the same stages as those of herpes simplex (vesiculation, umbilication, and crusting). Death may result.

Dye-light procedures may be useful, but there is much recent controversy about their safety and effectiveness.

MOLLUSCUM CONTAGIOSUM

Molluscum contagiosum is an uncommon contagious virus infection characterized by scattered pinhead-sized to pea-sized, waxy, white or pale pink, centrally umbilicated papules that contain a white, cheesy material. They occur mainly on the face and trunk but may occur on the extremities as well. They have a characteristic histologic picture (molluscum bodies).

Treatment

The individual lesions may be excised with a sharp curet and cauterized with tincture of iodine or phenol solution, or they may be treated by electrodesiccation. The patient should be examined subsequently to make certain that autoinoculation has not recurred. All lesions will usually disappear within 2–3 years.

DISEASES DUE TO PARASITES

PAPULAR URTICARIA

Papular urticaria is a very common skin eruption of infancy and early childhood. It is associated with the bite of common dog or cat fleas, bedbugs, or human fleas and is the result of sensitivity to these types of insects. It is commonly seen during the warmer months and usually disappears if the child is removed from exposure to the insect source. Lesions are distributed mostly on arms, legs, and exposed areas of the face and neck. The initial lesion is a small papule that itches and is soon excoriated. Secondary infection is very common.

Papular urticaria must be differentiated from varicella, scabies, and pediculosis.

Treatment

Remove or at least partially control insect sources in and around the house by use of spray or dusting powder (Raid, Off, etc) on dogs, cats, cushions, and rugs and around baseboards. Powder may be dusted on bedclothes and mattresses.

Topical corticosteroids and oral antihistamines may be used to control symptoms.

SCABIES

Scabies is an infestation of the skin with *Sarcoptes scabiei,* an insect mite rarely visible with the naked eye. It occurs cyclicly in pandemics and is at a peak at present.

Clinical Findings

The initial lesion consists of a small vesicle at the point of entrance of the parasite into the skin and a linear elevation of the skin caused by the burrowing of the insect through the superficial layers. The subsequent reaction consists of vesicles, papules, scaling, and excoriations in linear distribution. These ''runs'' are found most frequently on the interdigital surfaces; the axillary, cubital, and popliteal folds; and the inguinal region. Facial lesions are rarely observed except in nursing infants whose mothers have scabetic lesions on the breasts. *Itching is intense,* especially at night and with warmth, and excoriation from scratching is commonly seen. Secondary infection is common.

The intense itching is almost diagnostic. Confirmation is by dissection of a burrow and microscopic examination of the scrapings for the mite (see p 234).

Treatment

A. Local Measures: Any of the following may be used.

1. Gamma benzene hexachloride (Kwell), 1% in cream base, applied to the entire body for 4 hours and thoroughly rinsed off with water, is satisfactory treatment. In small infants, absorption of gamma benzene hexachloride, which is concentrated in the central nervous system, has been suspected; alternative treatment may be advisable.

2. Crotamiton, 10% cream (Eurax), is applied once daily for 2 days to the entire body. With small infants, there may be many more organisms, and this treatment should be repeated in 5 days.

3. Benzyl benzoate emulsion (see Table 12–1) is applied morning and evening for 2 days, using a paint brush or an ordinary hand insecticide spray. Give instructions for preliminary and follow-up shower and changes of linens.

4. Sulfur may be used if the above measures are not available. After preliminary bath or shower, sulfur ointment, 5–10%, is rubbed in from neck to toes each night for 3–5 nights. The patient should not change clothing or bed linen or bathe during this period. On the day after the final application of sulfur, bath and shower are repeated, and clothing and linen are changed. Soothing baths or shake lotion (see Table 12–1) may be necessary during treatment in patients with sensitive skin.

B. General Measures: Itching may persist for 5–7 days after initial treatment as an allergic response to killed insect antigen. If intense, treat with corticotropin (ACTH) gel, 0.5 unit/kg, in 2 doses 12 hours apart.

Check all contacts and treat as indicated. Dogs may be a source of infestation. Infestation may be present for several days before itching begins, and person-to-person spread can occur during this period.

PEDICULOSIS
(Louse Infestation)

Types

A. Pediculus Capitis: Infestation produces severe itching of the scalp, with excoriation, secondary infection, and enlargement of occipital and cervical nodes. Ova are attached to hairs as small, round, gray lumps (''nits'').

B. Pediculus Corporis: Infestation produces intense itching, with multiple scratch marks and excoriations. Close examination will reveal hemorrhage points or spots where the lice have extracted blood. Lesions are most common on the upper back, sides of the trunk, and the upper outer arms. The insect lives in the folds of clothing and is present on the skin only when foraging.

C. Pediculus Pubis: Pediculus pubis is extremely rare in children. It may affect eyebrows or axillary areas.

Treatment

Gamma benzene hexachloride (Kwell), 1% cream, lotion, or shampoo, is the treatment of choice in the USA. However, a warning has been issued by the FDA regarding the potential neurotoxicity of this substance; its use in infants and overuse should be avoided.

Pyrethrin preparations are highly effective as an alternative treatment. A-200 Pyrinate, liquid or gel, is applied to the scalp or body for no longer than 10 minutes, followed by thorough rinsing. It is repeated once only, in 24 hours.

Chlorophenothane (DDT) is not available as a pharmaceutical preparation in the USA for use as a pediculocide but may be so used in other parts of the world in the form of an emulsion (2–5%) or a 10% powder in talc or other diluent dusted onto the body and into the folds of clothing.

A. Head Lice: For head lice, Kwell shampoo is left on the scalp for 5 minutes and rinsed thoroughly, followed by combing with a fine-tooth comb to remove nits. This may be repeated in 24 hours. Alternatively, treat with pyrethrin preparation, as above.

B. Body Lice: Kwell cream or lotion, applied to the body for 24 hours, may be necessary for body lice. Alternatively, treat with pyrethrin preparation, as above. Washing the clothing in boiling water followed by ironing the seams with a hot iron usually eliminates the parasites.

C. Pubic Lice: Kwell cream or lotion, applied to the affected area for 4–6 hours, is sufficient. It may be repeated in 4–5 days if necessary. Alternatively, treat with pyrethrin preparation, as above.

Prophylaxis

Lice and their eggs live for days in carpets, bedding, and upholstery and can reinfest the patient or others. A spray of pyrethrins, eg, R & C Spray, can be applied liberally to such locations to kill the lice and eggs.

DISEASES DUE TO PHYSICAL & CHEMICAL AGENTS

DIAPER DERMATITIS (Intertrigo, Diaper Rash)

Diaper dermatitis is a condition to be expected in at least a mild form at some time during the diaper-wearing stage of infancy.

Clinical Findings

A. Mild Form: The mild form is essentially a chafing reaction that occurs where 2 moist skin surfaces are in apposition or where normal skin is subjected to the prolonged irritation of a wet diaper. The lesion consists of a patch or a diffuse erythematous reaction covering the perineal area, the buttocks, and the genitals. If the region about the external urethra is involved, there may be pain on urination.

B. Severe Form: The severe form is characterized by shallow ulcerations throughout the diaper area, with a general erythema of the entire area covered by the diaper. There may be papular vesicular lesions with excoriation in the folds of skin, especially in the inguinal area.

C. Infection: Infection may occur as any of the following.

1. Candidal infection–This probably plays a role in almost every severe diaper dermatitis.

2. Folliculitis–This is due to skin and intestinal bacteria and may be confirmed by microscopic examination of a smear or culture. There is marked erythema with a sharp border.

3. Vaccinia–Vaccinia of the diaper area was formerly associated with primary vaccination against smallpox and resembled very severe dermatitis. It is now rare.

Treatment

A. Mild Form: The diaper area should be exposed during the day to warm, dry air. This is best accomplished when the infant is asleep and lying on folded diapers. An incandescent lamp may be placed *at a safe distance* over the exposed buttocks. Zinc oxide ointment may be applied (see Table 12–1).

B. Infection: For antifungal treatment, use of nystatin, haloprogin, miconazole, or clotrimazole is effective. These preparations should be applied at least 4 times daily. For antibacterial treatment, use the same topical agents as for impetigo (see p 239).

Prophylaxis

Preventive measures are more important than treatment and should be a part of any treatment regimen.

A. Local Measures:

1. Change diapers as frequently as feasible.
2. Wipe diaper area 2–3 times daily with 1:1000 quaternary ammonium chloride solution.
3. After fecal soiling, cleanse diaper area with cottonseed oil or mineral oil instead of water.
4. Avoid tight-fitting waterproof pants.
5. Apply protective ointment such as zinc oxide paste (see Table 12–1) or petrolatum at the earliest sign of erythema.
6. Avoid use of starch powders or ointments that will encourage the growth of *Candida*.

B. Washing of Diapers: Use mild detergent soap, and rinse diapers thoroughly. After washing, rinse in ammonium chloride solution (1:10,000–1:25,000 concentration) and allow to dry. Cloth diapers should be boiled at least once a week.

DERMATITIS VENENATA
("Poison Ivy" or "Poison Oak")

Dermatitis venenata is a contact type of dermatitis due to a vegetable antigen found in *Rhus toxicodendron* (ivy) and *Rhus diversiloba* (oak). Dermatitis venenata may also result from contact with contaminated clothes or the fur of a dog or cat.

Clinical Findings

The eruption appears from several hours to a few days after contact with the plant. The lesion consists of multiple vesicles, papules, and blebs on an erythematous base and is accompanied by intense itching and burning. There may be swelling of the involved area. Vesicles often appear in linear streaks from brushing against twigs or leaves. In the severe forms, the nephrotic syndrome may occur.

Treatment

A. Local Measures: For treatment of small areas, symptomatic relief is obtained with a soothing antihistaminic lotion or calamine lotion with phenol. For treatment of larger areas of dermatitis, where exudation and swelling may be present, give cold, moist compresses of Burow's solution or instruct the patient to bathe in a tub with potassium permanganate solution (see Table 12–1).

B. General Measures: In severe forms, apply hydrocortisone cream, 1–2.5%, 2–4 times a day locally. Corticotropin (ACTH) gel, 0.5 unit/kg intramuscularly daily in 2 equal doses 12 hours apart for 3 days, may be necessary.

Prophylaxis

(1) Destruction of plants may be carried out by manual removal or by chemical means (2,4-D or 2,4,5-T) near dwellings and in areas frequented by people.

(2) Avoid *Rhus*-infested areas or wear adequate protective clothing.

(3) Thorough washing of the skin with detergent soap and water within a few minutes of exposure may be of value in preventing the development of lesions.

(4) Desensitization procedures are of no value and may produce serious complications.

DISEASES OF UNKNOWN ETIOLOGY

ACNE

Acne is the most common skin disease of humans. Minor involvement is probably normal for both sexes, especially during the adolescent years. The normal flow of sebum from the pilosebaceous glands in the skin of the face, shoulders, chest, and upper back is blocked by clumps of epithelial cells under the influence of hormonal and hereditary factors. The resultant accumulation of sebum under the skin will appear as a "whitehead." When the pigmented cells from the lining of the gland accumulate in sufficient concentration, the lesion is called a "blackhead."

Bacteria, principally *Corynebacterium acnes,* break down the sebum to irritating free fatty acids, causing an intense inflammatory response. Further bacterial infection with pustulation and eventual scarring represents the most serious complication of this condition.

Clinical Findings

The primary lesion is the comedo, a plug of sebum filling the pilosebaceous orifice, which produces a "blackhead" or "whitehead."

The other common clinical characteristics of acne are due to modifications of the comedo by inflammation, pustulation, cyst formation, and scarring. There may also be an associated seborrheic scaling and greasy skin. The openings of the pores are prominent.

Treatment

Acne patients require emotional support and an active, enthusiastic approach to therapy. Small papules and blemishes not arising from the pilosebaceous mechanism involved in true acne should be carefully explained to the young patient and should not be treated as acne.

A. Tretinoin: Topical tretinoin (Retin-A) will help to prevent the epithelial cells from clumping and blocking the flow of sebum. It is applied once daily in the morning for early uncomplicated acne eruption consisting only of comedones, "whiteheads," or "blackheads."

B. Benzoyl Peroxide: Benzoyl peroxide, 5%, is available in a wide variety of commercial preparations and will produce drying, scaling, and desquamative action. Apply at bedtime.

C. Isotretinoin: For severe cystic acne, give isotretinoin (Accutane), 1–2 mg/k/d orally in 2 doses for 15–20 weeks. The course may be repeated in 2 months if severe lesions persist or recur.

D. Tetracycline or Erythromycin: For inflammatory acne with pustular formation, give tetracycline or erythromycin. These antibiotics concentrate around the hair follicle and specifically interrupt the formation of irritating free fatty acids. Tetracycline may be given in a dosage of 250 mg 3 times daily for 10 days and then reduced to 250 mg daily for maintenance therapy. This may be continued for at least 3 months and sometimes for over a year. The dosage of erythromycin for adolescent patients is 2 g/d in 3 doses.

Prophylaxis

Good skin hygiene should be encouraged in adolescence. Patients should be instructed to scrub the face vigorously with a washcloth and soap twice a day and to avoid greasy cleansing creams and occlusive cosmetics. The scalp should be shampooed once or twice a week.

Foods associated with flare-ups of skin eruption should be avoided. Although this recommendation is controversial, many physicians feel that avoidance of chocolate, nuts, fried foods, and some carbonated drinks will minimize the acne experience.

Exposure of the skin to ultraviolet rays, either from sunshine or by the careful use of sunlamps sufficient to produce the mildest erythema level, will minimize the eruption.

Squeezing comedones with the fingers should be avoided. If comedones are large, they should be extracted with a "comedone extractor," an instrument with a small round loop at the end that produces equal pressure around the circumference of the plug.

SEBORRHEA, SEBORRHEIC DERMATITIS

Seborrhea is a relatively common skin eruption during infancy and childhood; it may also occur during adolescence.

Clinical Findings

A scaling, erythematous, poorly circumscribed rash, covered with oily, yellowish scales, is especially prominent over the scalp. In young infants, this is called "cradle cap;" in children and adults, "dandruff." The lesion may spread downward over the forehead, ears, eyebrows, nose, and back of the neck.

Erythematous, moist, scaly areas may be seen in the flexural zones such as the elbows, axillae, and, particularly in infants, behind the ears. Papular, erythematous, scaly, and moist lesions may also occur on the forehead and face.

Treatment

Treatment usually produces relief in less than 1 week.

A. Scalp: Treatment depends on the age group. For "cradle cap" in infants, scrub the scalp vigorously each day with the fingers or with a soft brush and soap and water. For "dandruff" in children, shampoo carefully once or twice a week with green soap or soapless detergent shampoo. Selenium sulfide suspension (Selsun) or zinc pyrithione shampoo (Head and Shoulders) may be most effective when used twice a week for 2 weeks.

B. All Areas: Hydrocortisone, 1% cream or ointment, applied twice daily is most effective. If hydrocortisone preparations are not available, use coal tar lotion (see Table 12–1) applied twice daily for more severe cases.

LEINER'S DISEASE

Leiner's erythroderma is considered a severe generalized seborrheic dermatitis. It occurs principally in breast-fed infants between the fourth and twelfth weeks of life, and the symptoms include, in addition to seborrhea of the scalp, generalized erythema and diarrhea. Desquamation is also a prominent symptom.

Leiner's disease must be differentiated from atopic dermatitis, which does not usually include diarrhea.

Treatment is with topical corticosteroids such as 1% hydrocortisone cream 3 times a day.

Table 12–1. Medications useful in the treatment of skin diseases in childhood.

Name	Action	Prescription	Instructions and Remarks
Baths			
Starch and soda	Cleansing and soothing.	¼ cup each of cornstarch and soda in bathinette or ½ cup starch and 1 cup soda to tub. Use tepid water.	Do not use soap. Bathe child for 15 min and then dab (do not rub) dry. Do not use for candidiasis.
Lotions			
Basic lotion (Sulzberger)	Soothing; used as vehicle for other agents.	Zinc oxide 20 Talcum 20 Glycerin 15 Water, qs ad 120	May add active medication: phenol, ¼%; benzocaine, 3–10%; coal tar solution, 3–20%; ichthammol, 2–10%. May add color. Apply 2–3 times daily.
Benzyl benzoate lotion	Scabicide.	Benzyl benzoate 40 Soft soap liniment 40 Alcohol, 95%, qs ad 120	After thorough bathing, apply over whole body from neck to toes twice daily for 2 days.
Calamine lotion	Soothing, antipruritic, and drying.	Prescribed with or without ¼% phenol.	Apply as a lotion 3–6 times daily. *Caution:* If phenol is added, frequent application may cause serious burn.
Coal tar solution	Keratoplastic and healing.	Add to starch lotion, 0.5–4%.	Apply with cotton twice daily.
Olive oil lotion	Soothing and protective.	Zinc oxide 10 Olive oil Lime water $\overline{aa}$, qs ad 120	Apply 4–6 times daily.
Starch lotion	Soothing, antipruritic, and drying.	Zinc oxide 24 Corn starch 24 Glycerin 12 Lime water, qs ad 120	Apply as a lotion 3–6 times daily. Do not use for candidiasis.

Ointments			
Ammoniated mercury ointment	Keratoplastic and bactericidal.	Prescribed as 2 or 5%.	Apply 3–5 times daily. Mercury sensitivity may be induced by too frequent use.
Hydrophilic ointment as base for:	Vehicle for water-soluble medications.		Apply sparingly with fingertips twice daily.
Ammoniated mercury	For psoriasis and seborrhea.	5%.	
Sulfur, salicylic acid	Fungicidal.	1% salicylic acid, 3% sulfur.	
Ichthammol ointment	Keratoplastic and keratolytic.	Prescribe as such.	Apply 3 times daily as a paste. Apply to not more than ¼ body surface. Remove at least once a day with mineral oil. Avoid exposure to direct sun.
Salicylic acid–sulfur ointment	Keratolytic and fungicidal.	Sulfur, 1%, and salicylic acid, 5%, in anhydrous wool fat.	Apply 2 or 3 times daily.
Sunscreen ointment	Protects from actinic burn; good for small infants and blond children exposed to sunlight.	5% *p*-aminobenzoic acid in cream or ointment base. Many proprietary preparations are available.	Apply every 3–4 hours. Remove with water.
Whitfield's ointment	Fungicidal.	Use ¼ strength for children.	Apply 3 times daily. Watch for signs of increased irritation.
Zinc oxide paste	Protective and soothing.	Prescribe as such.	Apply locally twice daily.
Paints			
Gentian violet	Antiseptic (*Candida*, gram-positive cocci) and astringent.	1% aqueous solution.	Apply to affected areas with swab of cotton once daily. May be used in the mouth. Will stain clothing.
Powders			
Zincundecate	Fungicidal.	Prescribe as such.	Apply twice daily to affected area.

Table 12–1 (cont'd). Medications useful in the treatment of skin diseases in childhood.

Name	Action	Prescription	Instructions and Remarks
Wet dressings			
Aluminum subacetate solution (Burow's solution)	Mildly astringent and cleansing.	Use 4 Domeboro tablets, or 1 tsp Domeboro powder, or 50 mL Burow's solution to 1 qt water.	Wring out a washcloth or Turkish towel and lay it on affected areas for 15 min twice daily or continuously. Use no waterproof covering, as the usefulness of these agents is due to the cooling effect of evaporation. Permanganate is poisonous and should not be used internally or on large denuded areas. Keep solution away from children.
Normal saline solution (0.9%)	Cleansing and soothing.	2 tsp (9 g) salt to 1 qt water.	
Potassium permanganate solution (1:10,000)	Antipruritic, antiseptic, astringent, and deodorizing.	Dissolve one 0.3-g (5-gr) tablet in 3 qt warm water. For bath, 15 tablets in 1 qt water and add to full tub.	
Sodium bicarbonate solution (3%)	Cooling, soothing, and antipruritic.	2 tbsp (30 g) to 1 qt water.	
Magnesium sulfate solution	Promotes blood flow; localizes infections and aids phagocytosis.	2 tbsp (30 g) to 1 qt hot water.	Wring out a washcloth or Turkish towel and lay on affected areas for 15 min twice daily or continuously. Cover with plastic material and keep warm with hot water bottle. Do not use electric heating pad.

ERYTHEMA MULTIFORME

Erythema multiforme is commonly a manifestation of sensitivity to some drug acting as the antigenic stimulus, but in many cases the cause is undetermined. It is rare in infancy and uncommon before the fourth year of life.

Clinical Findings

A. Skin Eruption: The onset is sudden; in its earliest form, it is usually macular and erythematous, with irregular distribution over any area of the body. This progresses rapidly to papular and vesicular phases, with polymorphous lesions. Some lesions may appear as concentric rings of variegated tints or as concentric rings of vesicles. Sites of predilection are the backs of the hands, the forearms, and the sides of the neck. Lesions may erupt in "crops" and persist over 2–4 weeks, and they may recur. Itching is slight.

B. Systemic Symptoms: Fever, joint pains, malaise, or nausea may accompany or precede the skin manifestation.

C. Severe Form: Erythema multiforme bullosum (Stevens-Johnson syndrome) may include the following additional findings: marked inflammation of one or more mucous membrane-lined cavities (mouth, nose, urethra, vagina) or eyes; pneumonitis, apparent by x-ray and manifested by cough; and necrotic changes in bullous lesions of the skin, which may slough out.

Treatment

Eliminate causative stimuli, if identified. Soothing lotions (see Table 12–1) or antihistaminic drugs may be of some value.

In the bullous type, prescribe peroxide rinses after eating, broad-spectrum antibiotics for prophylaxis of infection in necrotic areas of the skin or mucous membranes (see Chapter 6), and corticosteroids (see Chapter 22).

PITYRIASIS ROSEA

Pityriasis rosea, an acute self-limited disease of unknown cause, must be differentiated from other erythematous eruptions; it is not common in childhood.

A primary lesion or "herald patch" may precede the generalized rash by 3–10 days; it is usually larger and has a more intensely red border than subsequent lesions, which consist of pink to red erythematous oval patches that may be flat or slightly raised and have a pale, wrinkled central area. Patches show wide variation in size and shape and are often covered with thin scales that are adherent at the center but tend to separate at the edges. There may be some itching. The rash is usually confined to clothed areas of the body. The lesions tend to be parallel to the ribs.

Treatment

Treatment is rarely necessary; complete healing generally occurs in 1–8 weeks. Itching may be relieved with starch lotion (see Table 12–1).

PSORIASIS

Psoriasis is characterized by bright red, tiny, circumscribed spots that become covered with dry, silvery scales shortly after onset. With increase in size, the central area becomes less red and more thickly covered with scales. Fingernails may be wrinkled. Itching is not a prominent symptom. The pathologic process seems to be a rapid proliferation of epidermal cells, with resultant accumulation of scales. Eruption is common on extensor surfaces of the extremities, trunk, and scalp. Recurrence and remission are the rule.

Psoriasis is extremely rare before age 3 and uncommon before age 10 years.

Treatment

Treatment is guided by the local condition of the eruption. Soothing wet dressings (see Table 12–1) and bland ointments are useful during the acute stage. In the chronic stage, therapy consists of a combination of coal tar ointments and ultraviolet light. Crude coal tar ointment (2%) is applied to the skin for 12–18 hours. Coal tar substitutes such as anthralin, 1% ointment, may be more convenient and do not stain the clothing. The ointment is then removed and the skin exposed to gradually increasing doses of ultraviolet light, avoiding erythema. The combination of methoxsalen and high-intensity ultraviolet light may be successful in severe cases but requires highly experienced personnel.

Prognosis

Prognosis is for persistence and recurrence of skin lesions, sometimes over several decades. Most treatment measures available at the present time have limited value.

KERATOSIS PILARIS

Keratosis pilaris is a fairly common condition characterized by a fine papular eruption limited to the pilosebaceous orifices, giving the skin a rough, granular texture. It occurs especially in cold temperatures

Table 12–2. Cutaneous signs of systemic disease in infants and children.*

Sign	Disease
Acnelike erythematous papules in mid face; white ash-leaf macules on trunk; shiny thickened patch on back; subungual fibromas.	Tuberous sclerosis.
Café au lait macules.	Neurofibromatosis, Albright's disease.
"Chicken skin"—yellow rows of soft papules with wrinkled valleys in between in neck, axillae, groin.	Pseudoxanthoma elasticum.
"Dirty" neck and axillae (hyperpigmented, velvety flexural papules).	Acanthosis nigricans and obesity (endocrinopathies).
Eczematous erosions around the mouth, eyes, perineum, fingers, toes; alopecia; diarrhea.	Acrodermatitis enteropathica (zinc deficiency).
Erythematous flat-topped papules over knuckles.	Dermatomyositis.
Erythematous isolated papules on elbows, knees, buttocks, face.	Papular acrodermatitis (antigen-positive hepatitis).
Erythematous truncal macules with central pallor.	Juvenile rheumatoid arthritis.
Hemorrhagic (1–2 mm) macules on lips, tongue, palms (epistaxis, gastrointestinal bleeding).	Hereditary hemorrhagic telangiectasia (Rendu-Osler-Weber syndrome).
Hyperpigmentation in palmar creases, knuckles, scars, buccal mucosa, linea alba, scrotum.	Addison's disease.
Linear or oval vesicles on hands or feet; erosions on soft palate; tonsillar pillars.	Hand, foot, and mouth syndrome (coxsackie A16 and others).
Palpable purpura.	Vasculitis.
Pigmented macules on oral mucosa.	Peutz-Jeghers disease (benign small intestinal polyps).
Pruritic blisters on buttocks, elbows, knees, scapula.	Dermatitis herpetiformis (celiac disease).
Purpuric lakes.	Purpura fulminans—disseminated intravascular coagulation.
Purpuric (petechiae) seborrheic dermatitis.	Histiocytosis X.
Purpuric pustules on hands and feet.	Gonococcemia.
Sebaceous (multiple) cysts on face and trunk.	Gardner's syndrome (premalignant polyps of colon and rectum).
Stretchy skin; healing with large purple scars.	Ehlers-Danlos syndrome.
Tight, hard skin; telangiectases; hypo- and hyperpigmentation.	Scleroderma.
Ulcers with undermined, liquifying borders.	Pyoderma gangrenosum (ulcerative colitis, regional enteritis, rheumatoid arthritis).
Vitiligo (completely depigmented macules with hyperpigmented borders).	Pernicious anemia, Hashimoto's thyroiditis, Addison's disease, diabetes mellitus.
Yellow papules (lower eyelids, joints, palms).	Xanthomas, hyperlipidemias.

*Reproduced, with permission, from Weston WL: Skin. Chapter 8 in: *Current Pediatric Diagnosis & Treatment,* 7th ed. Kempe CH, Silver HK, O'Brien D (editors). Lange, 1982.

and in individuals with naturally dry skin. It is most common on the extensor surfaces of the arms and legs. Some cases are associated with a deficiency of vitamin A, but in others no cause can be determined. Mild, emollient keratolytic agents may be helpful. Bathing should be restricted, and only synthetic nonfat soap should be used.

• • •

CUTANEOUS SIGNS OF SYSTEMIC DISEASE

Cutaneous signs of systemic disease in infants and children are outlined in Table 12–2.

Heart | 13

PHYSICAL EXAMINATION OF THE HEART

Point of Maximum Cardiac Impulse

The point of maximum cardiac impulse varies considerably. In infants, it is the third or fourth interspace, just outside the nipple line; in children 2–5 years of age, it is the fourth interspace at the nipple line; and in children over 5 years of age, it is the fifth interspace, at or within the nipple line.

Percussion

Percussion may be difficult in young children.

Auscultation

A. Heart Sounds: The first and second sounds are of equal intensity during the first year of life. The second sound is usually split; it is best heard in the left second interspace.

B. Murmurs: Innocent ("functional") murmurs are heard in more than 50% of children, may persist for many years, and have no pathologic significance. These innocent murmurs usually change in character with changes in position, exercise, phases of respiration (inspiration and expiration), and the location of the stethoscope. They are well localized and transmit a low-intensity vibratory grade, usually grade I–II.

There are 5 main types of murmurs, which may be coexistent or occur separately:

1. Systolic, musical, vibrant murmur–A murmur that is heard best in the fourth left interspace but that may also be heard toward the apex.

2. Venous hum–A continuous, variable humming sound or roar heard best in the second left or right interspace. It is usually present when the child is in the sitting position and disappears if there is a change in position of the head, if pressure is applied to the jugular vein, or if the child lies down.

3. Pulmonary ejection murmur–A soft, early systolic ejection murmur localized to the pulmonary area and more audible when the child is in the supine position. The second heart sound (S_2) is usually split and varies with respiration. This murmur must be differentiated from that of the atrial septal defect, which is similar but has a widely split and fixed S_2 sound together with a middiastolic murmur along the left lower sternal border.

4. Carotid bruit–An early to midsystolic murmur heard over the supraclavicular fossa or carotid artery, accentuated by exercise and unaffected by posture.

5. Cardiorespiratory murmur–A rare murmur heard over the entire precordium and varying with respiration and with changes in position. It disappears when respiration is voluntarily stopped for a brief moment.

Cardiac Rate & Rhythm

In infants and children, the cardiac rhythm and rate vary widely, and multiple determinations must be made.

In infants, the rate may vary from 70 in sleep to 180 when crying. In older children, emotional factors (including the medical examination) may affect the pulse. Any rate over 150 requires investigation.

Blood Pressure

Children 3 years of age and older should have their blood pressure measured annually as part of continuing health assessment. Hypertension detection should be part of a total child health care program.

A. Method: Cuff size must be carefully chosen (Table 13–1). For infants, the following "flush method" should be used: Wrap rubber sheeting or a rubber glove snugly around the foot or hand, starting distally, so that the blood is pressed from the extremity. Inflate cuff to a pressure slightly above suspected systolic pressure (Table 13–2). Remove rubber bandage and reduce pressure in cuff slowly, noting the level at which blood reenters the foot or hand, causing a sudden flush. This is the mean pressure.

B. Diagnosis: Comparison of blood pressure in upper and lower

Table 13–1. Recommended cuff widths.

Patient	Cuff Width (cm)
Premature infant or newborn	2–3.5
Child 1–5 yr	5–8
Child 6–10 yr	8–10
Child 11 yr	12
Obese child	14

Table 13–2. Percentile values for blood pressure by age.*

Age	Systolic Pressure		Diastolic Pressure	
	50%	95%	50%	95%
0–6 mo	80	110	45	60
3 yr	95	112	64	80
5 yr	97	115	65	84
10 yr	110	130	70	92
15 yr	116	138	70	95

*Reproduced, with permission, from Mitchell SC et al: The pediatrician and hypertension. *Pediatrics* 1975;**56**:3.

extremities simultaneously is of great importance in the diagnosis of coarctation of the aorta. Systolic pressure in the lower extremities is higher than that in the upper by 20 mm Hg. In coarctation of the aorta, blood pressure is lower in the legs than in the arms. Excitement and struggling will increase systolic pressure as much as 50 mm Hg. Heavy pressure from the stethoscope will cause errors. The term "high normal blood pressure" should be used during evaluation and follow-up to avoid adverse psychosocial and economic implications.

ELECTROCARDIOGRAPHY

The upper limits of the normal P–R interval in children are shown in Table 13–3.

Normal Configurations

A. P Wave: P wave is upright in lead I; it is inverted in aVR when sinus rhythm is present.

B. QRS Complex: In children, the height may vary greatly. Prominent Q waves in lead III are not unusual.

Table 13–3. Upper limits of the normal P–R interval in children.*

Age	Pulse Rate				
	<70	71–90	91–110	111–130	>130
Birth–18 mo	0.16	0.15	0.145	0.135	0.125
18 mo–6 yr	0.17	0.165	0.155	0.145	0.135
6–13 yr	0.18	0.17	0.16	0.15	0.14
13–17 yr	0.19	0.18	0.17	0.16	0.15

*Reproduced, with permission, from Ashman R, Hull E: *Essentials of Electrocardiography for the Student and Practitioner of Medicine,* 2nd ed. Macmillan, 1941.

C. T Wave: T wave is inverted in V_{4R}–V_2 in all children from 48 hours to approximately 8 years of age; it is upright in all other leads.

Axis Deviation Patterns

A. Right Axis Deviation: S wave is deep in lead I; R wave is high in lead III. Right axis deviation is a common finding in young infants.

B. Left Axis Deviation: R wave is high in lead I; S wave is deep in lead III. Left axis deviation is associated with various congenital lesions (eg, ostium primum defect, tricuspid atresia) and with left ventricular hypertrophy.

SPECIAL STUDIES

Circulation Time

In infants and children, circulation time is difficult to measure by any method that requires cooperative effort on the part of the patient and is rarely useful except in following the progress of congestive failure, especially in rheumatic heart disease.

For older children, inject 3–5 mL of 20% sodium dehydrocholate (Decholin Sodium) rapidly by intravenous route. Circulation time is considered to be normal if 8–15 seconds lapse before the appearance of a sour taste in the mouth.

X-Ray Examination

X-ray examination of the chest for cardiac evaluation should include posteroanterior, oblique, and lateral views. Films taken after barium swallow or fluoroscopy will show greater detail. The overall heart size of a normal newborn infant is greater than that of an older child, and cardiothoracic ratios up to 0.6 are normal. An enlarged heart on x-ray examination is a significant finding that calls for further study.

Echocardiography

Echocardiography is of great value in evaluating heart disease, especially in the newborn. Cross-sectional techniques provide special information on the relationships of intra- and extracardiac structures. Echocardiographic diagnoses include tricuspid atresia; hypoplasia of the ascending aorta with or without mitral atresia or aortic valve atresia; transposition of the great vessels; and endocardial cushion defect. The echocardiogram will provide strong evidence for tetralogy of Fallot, cor triatriatum, aortic stenosis, mitral valve deformities, and aortic valve deformities.

Catheterization of the Heart

Catheterization, which consists of the passage of an opaque catheter of small caliber through the vein into the right side of the heart or through an artery to the left side of the heart, is useful in the diagnosis of congenital heart lesions (Table 13–4). X-ray localization of the catheter may demonstrate defects in the heart and relative size of the right atrium and right ventricle. Catheterization can be used to determine pressures in the atria, ventricles, and pulmonary vessels and the oxygen content of blood withdrawn from the various chambers. Special techniques using dyes or catheters sensitive to special substances (eg, hydrogen) may be used to detect small communications between heart chambers and great vessels.

Risks associated with catheterization include thrombosis of great vessels and irreversible renal damage.

Phonocardiography

Phonocardiography is a device for making recordings of heart sounds and murmurs and is frequently an aid to diagnosis.

Respiratory Function & Exercise Tolerance Tests

These studies are useful in determining the degree of functional impairment that has been caused by the heart lesion.

Venous Pressure

Venous pressure is of little diagnostic aid in infants because of technical difficulties and because normal values have not been established. In children over 4 years of age, normal is 40–120 mm of water.

Cineangiography

The dynamic behavior of radiopaque material in the great vessels and chambers of the heart recorded on motion picture film allows more detailed study.

CONGENITAL HEART DISEASE

The incidence of congenital heart disease is estimated to be 6–8 cases per 1000 live births. In the USA, about 25–30 thousand children are born each year with congenital heart disease. Of the children surviving infancy, almost half have either ventricular septal defects or pulmonary stenosis. Atrial septal defects and aortic stenosis affect another one-third of these children, and the remainder have a wide variety of other types of congenital heart disease.

A history of the following may indicate the possibility of congenital heart disease: (1) poor weight gain, with a history of a feeding problem;

Table 13–4. Relative pressures and oxygen content as obtained during cardiac catheterization.*

Heart Condition	Pressure			Oxygen Content			
	Right Atrium	Right Ventricle	Pulmonary Artery	Right Atrium	Right Ventricle	Pulmonary Artery	Systemic Artery
Normal heart	5/0	25/2	25/8	Equals vena cava	Equals right atrium	Equals right ventricle	95–100% saturated
Atrial septal defect	Normal or slightly increased	Normal or increased	Normal or increased	Greater than vena cava	Equals right atrium	Equals right ventricle	Normal†
Ventricular septal defect	Normal	Normal or increased	Normal or increased	Equals vena cava	Greater than right atrium	Equals right ventricle	Normal†
Patent ductus arteriosus	Normal	Normal or increased	Normal or increased	Equals vena cava	Equals right atrium	Greater than right ventricle	Normal†
Tetralogy of Fallot	Normal	Increased	Decreased; lower than right ventricle	Equals vena cava	Equals or is greater than right atrium	Equals right ventricle	Decreased
Eisenmenger's complex	Normal	Increased	Increased	Equals vena cava	Greater than right atrium	Equals right ventricle	Decreased
Valvular pulmonary stenosis	Normal	Increased	Decreased	Equals vena cava	Equals right atrium	Equals right ventricle	Normal
Valvular pulmonary stenosis with patent foramen ovale	Increased	Increased	Decreased	Equals vena cava	Equals right atrium	Equals right ventricle	Decreased

*Modified from Marple CD: Congenital heart lesions: Study, diagnosis, and surgical treatment. *Postgrad Med* 1951;9:239.

†May be decreased if there is associated pulmonary hypertension.

(2) attacks of fainting or "blackouts," which in a small infant may appear as "sighing attack"; (3) difficulty in swallowing, with frequent regurgitation of uncurdled milk; (4) respiratory difficulties, including stridor, and preference for a position of hyperextension when having difficulty breathing; (5) exercise intolerance, with the child frequently assuming a squatting position when tired at play; (6) cyanosis, intermittent or continuous; or (7) a history of maternal illness during the first trimester of pregnancy, including bleeding, rubella, excessive vomiting, severe anemia, and excessive sweating.

General treatment measures, in addition to specific recommendations in the discussion of specific diseases, are as follows: (1) Institute a high-protein, high-vitamin diet and avoid excessive weight gain. (2) Maintain hydration. (3) Prevent common childhood infections by avoiding exposure to known infectious disease, by active immunization, and by appropriate passive immunization when exposure has occurred. (4) Administer prophylactic penicillin or other appropriate antibiotics before dental procedures. (5) Meticulously evaluate the child's personality development. (6) Advise the parents of the prognosis and of particular symptoms of importance, and encourage them to allow the child to live as normal a life as possible.

CONGENITAL HEART DISEASE WITHOUT SHUNT

Dextrocardia

Dextrocardia consists of right-sided heart, with or without reversal of position of other organs. If there is no reversal of other organs, the heart usually has other severe defects. With complete situs inversus, the heart is usually normal.

A. Clinical Features: Apical pulse and sounds are heard on the right side of the chest. Reversal of position of other organs (ie, situs inversus) may be present. X-ray shows the cardiac silhouette on the right side. On ECG, the P waves are usually inverted in lead I; QRS is predominantly down in lead I; lead II resembles normal lead III and vice versa.

B. Treatment and Prognosis: With situs inversus and no heart defects, the prognosis is excellent. If severe heart defects are present, definitive diagnosis is imperative, since corrective surgery is frequently beneficial.

Coarctation of Aorta

Blood pressure is high in the head and upper extremities, low in the lower part of the body and in the legs. In the "infantile" ("preductal") type, there is a constriction between the subclavian artery and the ductus arteriosus (incompatible with life if the ductus closes). In the "adult" ("postductal") type, there is a constriction at or distal to the ductus arteriosus.

A. Clinical Features: There may be minimal findings in early childhood. The older child may have numbness of the legs, headaches, and epistaxis. Femoral or dorsalis pedis pulsation is absent, weak, or delayed. Systolic murmurs may be present over the sternum and left back. Cardiac enlargement may or may not be present on routine x-ray examination. The site of coarctation and dilatation may be seen on a PA film. Coarctation is the commonest cause of heart failure from the first week through the first month of life. Older children may show notching of the ribs by collateral vessels. ECG may be normal or show left ventricular hypertrophy. Symptomatic infants show combined ventricular hypertrophy.

B. Treatment and Prognosis: Surgical correction is ideally postponed until the patient is 8–15 years of age. Onset of cardiac failure requires vigorous treatment, including digitalis, diuretics, and oxygen. Response to such medical treatment allows further postponing surgery to a more ideal age. The prognosis is excellent with successful surgery.

Aortic Stenosis

In this outflow tract lesion of the left heart, constriction of the aortic valve causes the left ventricle to hypertrophy. Systolic blood pressure is lower than normal, and pulse pressure is low unless there is associated aortic insufficiency.

A. Clinical Features: A loud, harsh murmur is heard in the second or third right interspace, with transmission to neck and prominent thrill. The second heart sound is normal or weak. Pulse pressure is narrow. X-ray may show slight left ventricular enlargement. ECG is frequently normal but may show left ventricular preponderance.

B. Treatment and Prognosis: Surgical valvulotomy is indicated in the severe case with a high-pressure gradient across the valve (as determined by catheterization of the left ventricle). Operative mortality is less than 10%. Restriction of activity will postpone failure. The prognosis is guarded. Sudden death may occur, and life expectancy is only about 30 years.

Vascular Rings

Vascular anomalies that may compress the trachea are double aortic arch, right aortic with right brachial arch, anomalous right subclavian artery, anomalous innominate artery, and anomalous left carotid artery.

A. Clinical Features: There are usually no symptoms. Constriction of the esophagus and trachea may cause vomiting, dysphagia, and stridor and predispose to recurrent respiratory infections. The child's head may be held in hyperextension. X-ray of the heart with barium in the esophagus will establish the diagnosis. Outlined trachea with contrast material will add to diagnostic detail. Electrocardiographic examination is noncontributory.

B. Treatment and Prognosis: Surgical correction is indicated if the trachea or esophagus is constricted. The prognosis is excellent.

Abnormal Origin of the Left Coronary Artery

The left coronary artery arises from the pulmonary artery.

A. Clinical Features: With decrease in pulmonary arterial pressure during the first 2 months of life, there is a marked decrease in blood flow to the left coronary artery. The child appears normal at birth, and growth and development are normal in the early months. With the onset of myocardial ischemia, the child will have intermittent episodes of what appears to be severe colic with pallor and sweating, especially during feeding. Examination may reveal a mitral murmur. X-ray shows cardiac enlargement. The ECG is diagnostic, with findings of myocardial infarction. Cardiac catheterization and angiocardiography will demonstrate the absence of the left coronary artery originating from the aorta. The right coronary artery is usually enlarged, and the contrast medium will flow from the right coronary system into the left coronary system.

B. Treatment and Prognosis: Transplantation of the coronary artery has been carried out successfully. Prognosis is good with successful surgical correction. Massive infarction of the heart occurring during early infancy is often fatal.

Endocardial Fibroelastosis

Endocardial fibroelastosis is a myocardial disease of unknown cause involving marked thickening of the endocardial tissues of the left ventricle and occasionally the left atrium. This disease has been postulated to follow intrauterine infection with mumps or coxsackievirus.

A. Clinical Features: In about half of the cases, the infant appears normal at birth and develops symptoms within the first 5 months of life. Almost all patients are symptomatic by age 1 year. The symptoms and signs are those of left ventricular heart failure (see p 279). X-ray shows generalized cardiac enlargement, and the ECG indicates left ventricular hypertrophy.

B. Treatment and Prognosis: Early and vigorous treatment of cardiac failure is most important. Treat as for myocardial failure (see pp 279–280), using digitalis and diuretics. Treatment for several years may be necessary. The prognosis is poor in children who do not improve initially and who have recurrent myocardial failure.

Valvular Pulmonary Stenosis

This outflow tract lesion of the right heart may occur with other anomalies but commonly occurs with an otherwise normal heart. If this is the sole lesion, right ventricular pressure is increased. Pulmonary blood flow is normal. With failure, cyanosis may result from stagnant blood flow.

A. Clinical Features: Symptoms are rare during infancy. Many children are asymptomatic. Dyspnea, fatigue, and, rarely, cyanosis develop after age 2 years. A loud, harsh, systolic murmur, often with thrill, is heard in the second to fourth left interspaces, usually with a prominent ejection click. X-ray shows right ventricular enlargement with a dilated main pulmonary artery. Pulmonary vascular markings are normal in the absence of cyanosis. ECG shows right ventricular hypertrophy.

B. Treatment and Prognosis: Pulmonary valvulotomy should be undertaken between the ages of 5 and 10 years in all severe cases. The operative mortality is about 10%. Treat cardiac failure with digitalis (see p 284) and other measures (see p 140). The prognosis is poor without surgical repair. Death occurs within 2–4 years after the first attack of failure. The long-term prognosis with repair is not known at present.

CONGENITAL HEART DISEASE WITH SHUNT: ACYANOTIC

Persistent Patent Ductus Arteriosus

High aortic pressure shunts blood through the ductus into the pulmonary artery systole and diastole. Left ventricular output, blood volume, and pulse pressure are increased.

A. Clinical Features: A murmur in the second or third interspace to the left of the sternum appears during infancy. At first it may be systolic alone, but by 2 years of age, most patients will show a diastolic component with a "machinery" sound and thrill. Pulse pressure is wide. X-ray shows enlargement of the left atrium and ventricle, increased pulmonary vascular markings, and expansible pulsation of the pulmonary arteries. ECG may be normal or may show left ventricular or combined hypertrophy.

B. Treatment and Prognosis: Surgical division and ligation of the ductus may be indicated. Operative mortality is so low that the procedure should be undertaken as soon as possible after diagnosis. With surgical repair, the prognosis is excellent. Without repair, subacute infective endocarditis or cardiac failure may develop.

Interatrial Septal Defect

Interatrial septal defect is very common, particularly in girls. There are 3 types: (1) foramen secundum defect (high in the atrial septum); (2) foramen primum defect (low in the septum, often with deformity of the mitral or tricuspid valve and with persistent atrioventricular canal); and (3) Lutembacher's syndrome, which consists of atrial septal defect in association with congenital or acquired mitral stenosis. In foramen secundum and foramen primum defects, oxygenated blood shunts from the left to the right atrium.

A. Clinical Features: Linear growth may be retarded, and the chest may bulge in time owing to the enlarged right ventricle. Murmur is systolic. Primum defect is common in Down's syndrome. Secundum defect causes a grade III, blowing, systolic murmur. Primum defect causes a grade IV, harsh murmur. Murmurs are loudest near the second left interspace in secundum defect and transmitted to the apex or back in primum defect. The second heart sound is widely split and fixed. X-ray shows slight cardiac enlargement in secundum type and globular enlargement in primum type. Pulmonary vessels are enlarged and may show pulsation on fluoroscopy. The aortic shadow is small. ECG shows right ventricular hypertrophy with an incomplete right bundle branch block in secundum defects and right ventricular hypertrophy with left axis deviation in primum defects.

B. Treatment and Prognosis: Surgical closure is recommended for secundum defect. Primum defect is more difficult to repair. With pulmonary vascular obstruction, surgery is not recommended.

With repair, life expectancy is prolonged beyond the 35 years expected without repair.

Interventricular Septal Defect

Interventricular septal defect is the most common congenital heart disorder. In half of the cases, the defect is small and asymptomatic and will probably close spontaneously before the patient is 18 years of age. Oxygenated blood passes from the left to the right ventricle. (A large defect may lead to Eisenmenger's complex, which is discussed below under cyanotic types.)

A. Clinical Features: A systolic, harsh, loud murmur, often with thrill, is heard in the third left interspace. There may be a diastolic inflow murmur at the apex. The x-ray may be normal or show cardiac enlargement with increased pulmonary vascular markings. The ECG may show left or combined ventricular hypertrophy.

B. Treatment and Prognosis: With moderate to large defects producing intractable congestive heart failure during infancy or early childhood, surgical closure should be done at age 2–5 years. The prognosis following surgery is good. Surgery is not indicated if obstructive pulmonary vascular disease is present.

CONGENITAL HEART DISEASE WITH SHUNT: CYANOTIC

Valvular Pulmonary Stenosis With Interatrial Septal Defect (Patent Foramen Ovale)

Venous blood from the right atrium is shunted into the left atrium before oxygenation, causing cyanosis. The right atrium and ventricle are enlarged.

A. Clinical Features: Clinical features may simulate those of tetralogy of Fallot (see below). Differentiation is often possible only by cardiac catheterization (Table 13–4). The ECG shows right ventricular hypertrophy.

B. Treatment and Prognosis: Surgical repair of the stenotic valve is possible, and the prognosis is good after repair.

Cor Triloculare Biatriatum

Characteristics of cor triloculare biatriatum include failure of development of the right ventricle; cyanosis at birth; a soft, systolic murmur over the precordial area; and dyspnea. X-ray and electrocardiography demonstrate a large left ventricle. Life expectancy is limited. Treat as cardiac failure.

Cor Biloculare

Cor biloculare is an interatrial septal defect, with small right ventricle or a large interventricular septal defect. Marked cyanosis, dyspnea, and cardiac failure are seen early in life. Death usually occurs within a few months.

Tetralogy of Fallot (Pulmonary Stenosis With Interventricular Septal Defect)

Tetralogy of Fallot is the most common cyanotic type of congenital heart disease. It may include overriding dextraposition of the aorta. Right-to-left shunt is fundamental to the lesion. A small amount of blood flows through the pulmonary artery, and the blood is poorly oxygenated.

A. Clinical Features: Cyanosis occurs early as the ductus closes ("blue baby"). Lips and nail beds may be blue. Dyspnea is apparent early. The older child may squat or lie down during play. "Spells" may occur owing to cerebral anoxia. Clubbing of the digits usually appears after 2 years. Congestive heart failure rarely occurs. A loud, harsh systolic murmur is heard at left base, frequently with thrill. Blood findings consist of polycythemia and increased hematocrit and red blood cell counts. The circulation time is short as a result of overriding aorta. X-ray usually shows a typical "wooden shoe" contour of the heart. The heart is not enlarged. The apex is blunt and elevated above the diaphragm. The pulmonary artery segment is concave. The right ventricle is enlarged. Pulmonary vessels appear to be scarce, and the lung fields are unusually clear. The ECG shows marked predominance of the right ventricle and peaked P waves.

B. Treatment and Prognosis: Surgery is usually indicated. Procedures available are anastomosis of the subclavian artery (Blalock-Taussig) and side-to-side anastomosis of the pulmonary artery to the aorta (Potts). Open heart surgery with repair of the ventricular septum and pulmonary stenosis is being attempted at present. If the pulmonary artery is absent or too small, no surgery is possible. Without surgery, death occurs within 20 years. With surgery, the prognosis is probably markedly improved toward a normal life.

Eisenmenger's Complex

Eisenmenger's complex consists of a ventricular septal defect without pulmonary stenosis but with increased pulmonary vascular resistance and resultant right-to-left shunt.

A. Clinical Features: Severe symptoms develop early with congestive failure, sometimes first in infancy. Dyspnea, repeated infection, and cyanosis are all common. Hemoptysis may occur in older children. The systolic murmur is not so loud as with smaller ventricular septal defects. No thrill is noted. The second pulmonic sound is accentuated. X-ray shows cardiac enlargement, apparently involving both ventricles and the left atrium. Pulmonary vessels are engorged, with pulsation on fluoroscopy. ECG shows right ventricular hypertrophy and, occasionally, right bundle branch block.

B. Treatment and Prognosis: No specific treatment is indicated, and surgery is not possible. Restrict activity and treat cardiac failure. The prognosis is good with restricted life. Long-term prognosis is poor.

Transposition of Great Vessels

The aorta arises from the right ventricle; the pulmonary artery arises from the left ventricle. Blood from the right heart goes through the systemic vessels and returns to the right side. Blood from the left heart goes through the lungs to return to the left side. This anomaly is incompatible with life unless patent foramen ovale, ductus arteriosus, or interventricular septal defect is also present. The coronary arteries arise from the aorta and carry anoxic blood.

A. Clinical Features: Marked cyanosis is apparent at birth or shortly thereafter. Dyspnea, engorged neck vessels, and an enlarged liver become apparent during the neonatal period. Murmurs are not typical or always present. The heart enlarges rapidly during the first few weeks of life. X-ray shows enlargement of ventricles with a narrow base on PA view and a wide base on lateral and oblique views. Pulmonary vascular markings are increased. ECG may show myocardial damage, due to ischemia, and right ventricular hypertrophy.

B. Treatment and Prognosis: Palliative surgery for the enlargement of an atrial septal defect by balloon catheter or by the Blalock-Hanlon procedure is sometimes carried out. Corrective surgery by the Mustard procedure is recommended before the patient reaches 1 year of age. If a ventricular septal defect and pulmonary stenosis are present, the prognosis is poor, although the patient may survive to early adulthood.

Tricuspid Atresia

Tricuspid atresia consists of marked stenosis of the tricuspid valve and a small right ventricle, with or without pulmonary stenosis. Blood from the right atrium goes through the septal defect to the left atrium and into the systemic arteries. The pulmonary circulation goes through a patent ductus arteriosus or interventricular septal defect. Collateral circulation through bronchial arteries must develop to sustain life.

A. Clinical Features: Cyanosis is apparent shortly after birth. The neck vessels and the liver are engorged and pulsating. Murmurs are not typical or always present. If the blood supply to the lungs is by way of an open ductus or large bronchial arteries, a continuous murmur is present. X-ray shows enlargement of the left ventricle, a concave left border, and small pulmonary vessels. The aorta is continuous with the cardiac shadow in left anterior oblique views. ECG shows left ventricular hypertrophy and left axis deviation (the only cyanotic type of congenital heart disease with this finding).

B. Treatment and Prognosis: Pulmonary anastomosis, as in tetralogy of Fallot, is palliative. In older infants, anastomosis of the superior vena cava to the right pulmonary artery may be carried out. The prognosis is poor.

DISEASES OF ENDOCARDIUM & MYOCARDIUM

ACUTE RHEUMATIC HEART DISEASE

Acute rheumatic heart disease may involve all parts of the heart and accompanies an attack of active rheumatic fever. For discussion of diagnosis and treatment of acute rheumatic fever and heart disease, see Chapter 29.

CHRONIC RHEUMATIC HEART DISEASE

The chronic rheumatic heart is the residuum of rheumatic fever with persistent damage to the valves.

Clinical Findings

The mitral and aortic valves are the most commonly involved.

A. Mitral Valve Involvement: Involvement occurs early in the course of almost every case of rheumatic carditis. The appearance of an apical murmur in the course of an obscure febrile illness may be the first sign of the rheumatic cause of the disease.

Mitral regurgitation usually occurs first. A moderate, blowing, pan-systolic murmur is present at the apex or slightly to the right and may merge with the first heart sound. A soft, low-pitched murmur in mid diastole, loudest at the apex, may be present; it does not indicate organic stenosis.

Stenosis of the mitral valve is a late change appearing with the passage of years. A rumbling, moderate, mid- or late-diastolic murmur is present, sometimes with a palpable thrill. The first heart sound usually is sharp, preceded by the crescendo presystolic murmur. A visible bulge of the chest wall may be apparent in long-standing cases.

B. Aortic Valve Involvement: Aortic involvement may occur with mitral involvement.

Regurgitation is the only change observed in childhood. A soft or moderate, blowing, diastolic murmur is present, occurring immediately after the second sound and heard best just to the left of the sternum in the second to fourth intercostal interspaces. It may be transmitted to the neck and to the apex. "Corrigan" pulse, with wide pulse pressure, capillary pulsation, and loud systolic impact, is present in the femoral area. Systolic blood pressure may be elevated and diastolic pressure lowered, giving a wide pulse pressure.

Complications

Complications include cardiac failure (see Myocardial Failure, below) and subacute infective endocarditis. Atrial fibrillation in mitral stenosis due to dilatation of the left atrium may occur in the older child.

Treatment

The treatment of chronic rheumatic heart disease consists of preventing progress of the disease and treating the complications.

A. Specific Measures: None available.

B. General Measures:

1. Antibiotics–Prevent recurrences of acute rheumatic fever by treating upper respiratory tract infections promptly with appropriate antibiotic agents (see Chapter 6) and maintaining a prophylactic antibiotic program (see Chapter 29). Attempt to prevent further valvular damage during a recurrent bout of rheumatic fever by adequate and careful treatment of the rheumatic fever (see Chapter 29).

2. Established routine–Avoid fatigue and overexertion by restricting play activities to sedentary games and exercise within the individual's tolerance. Rest 9–10 hours every night, and rest after lunch.

C. Surgical Measures: Valvulotomy of the stenosed mitral valve is rarely indicated in children.

D. Treatment of Complications: Treat congestive heart failure, atrial fibrillation, and infective endocarditis.

Prognosis

Prognosis depends upon the presence and extent of valvular damage. If the heart is greatly enlarged or cardiac failure occurs early in the disease, the 10-year survival rate is about 70%. If enlargement of the heart occurs after adolescence has passed, survival to 30 years of age is rare. If there is little or no enlargement of the heart early in the disease and maximum care in follow-up is taken, the prognosis is excellent. In the absence of recurrences, the murmur may decrease and the heart size return to normal limits.

SUBACUTE INFECTIVE ENDOCARDITIS

Subacute infective endocarditis is rare in children under the age of 3 years. It generally develops in the heart or great vessel that already is diseased. The 2 common predisposing diseases are rheumatic heart disease and congenital heart disease.

Endocarditis may develop in children with rheumatic valvular damage or congenital heart disease and in children with surgical repair of congenital defects.

Clinical Findings

A. Symptoms: The patient may have a history of predisposing heart disease. There is usually insidious onset of chronic, low-grade fever, anorexia, or malaise, but fever may be spiking. There may be a history of preceding infection (respiratory, skin, dental abscess, etc), dental extraction, or tonsillectomy.

B. Signs: There may be signs of associated heart disease. New murmurs may appear or existing ones be altered. Petechiae may be present on skin, under nail beds, or in conjunctiva. The spleen may be palpably enlarged.

C. Laboratory Findings: Blood culture should be repeated several times. If the clinical picture is suggestive, it is extremely important that the causative organism be identified if possible. Leukocytosis may not be marked, but sedimentation rate is elevated. Progressive anemia and hematuria may occur.

Treatment

A. Specific Measures: Specific measures depend upon the causative organism and, where possible, the results of the determination of this organism's sensitivity to various antibiotics or combinations of antibiotics.

1. *Streptococcus viridans*–Give penicillin daily for at least 4 weeks. If sensitivity is known to be less than 0.1 unit/mL, use procaine penicillin G, 600,000 units 2–3 times daily. If sensitivity is not known or is known to be greater than 0.1 unit/mL, give penicillin G, 2–10 million units intramuscularly daily in 4–6 doses, depending upon body weight and organism resistance. If fever persists, the initial dosage should be doubled and, if necessary, redoubled.

2. Hemolytic streptococci, group D (*Streptococcus faecalis*, or enterococci)–Combined therapy is indicated. Give penicillin G as above for at least 4 weeks and streptomycin, 60 mg/kg/d in 3–4 doses for the duration of penicillin therapy.

3. Hemolytic *Staphylococcus aureus*–If the organism is sensitive to penicillin, give this drug in large doses for at least 10 days and continue therapy for 2 months with methicillin, oxacillin, nafcillin, or cloxacillin orally. If the organism is resistant to penicillin, use cephalothin or oxacillin. In patients allergic to penicillin, use vancomycin, 20–30 mg/kg/d intravenously in 2 doses; continue treatment for 4–6 weeks (see Chapter 6).

4. Unidentified organism–If the organism is unknown, all cultures are negative, and clinical evidence is strong, treat as for group D streptococci or with a combination of vancomycin or ristocetin plus kanamycin or neomycin, or with bacitracin plus kanamycin or neomycin (see Chapter 6). If the patient is very ill and clinical evidence is strong, treatment should not be unduly delayed pending positive blood culture.

B. General Measures: General measures include transfusion of fresh whole blood, especially if anemia is severe; oral or parenteral iron therapy (see Chapter 17); adequate treatment of infections of skin, teeth, tonsils, etc; and institution of a high-protein, high-vitamin diet.

C. Surgical Measures: Congenital heart lesion, if present, may be corrected surgically.

D. Follow-Up Measures: Sedimentation rate should be determined at periodic intervals. If elevated initially, it should decrease toward normal. Blood culture should be repeated at intervals over the course of the following 3 months. Leukocytosis should be absent before stopping antibiotic therapy.

Prognosis

Prognosis depends upon the organism producing the disease, the presence of congenital heart disease that cannot be corrected surgically, damage to other organs by emboli, the presence and results of treatment of cardiac failure, and the rapidity with which diagnosis is made and treatment started. In the absence of specific factors preventing a favorable outcome, the prognosis for the single occurrence is excellent. Prognosis for recurrence should be guarded.

CARDIAC ENLARGEMENT IN NEWBORN INFANTS

Cardiac enlargement unassociated with any other malformation of the heart has been observed in newborn infants. It is most commonly associated with erythroblastosis fetalis and diabetes mellitus in the mother and may also occur in newborns with high hematocrit levels.

Cardiac failure should be treated if present. The prognosis depends on the associated diseases. With survival, the heart will return to normal size.

MYOCARDITIS

Myocarditis is an inflammation or degeneration of the heart muscle, usually secondary to systemic infections. It may occur in conjunction with a severe infection, but certain infections are more prone to cause myocardial injury. The most common causes of myocarditis are rheumatic fever, coxsackievirus infection, and diphtheria. It also occurs in some viral diseases (eg, rubeola, poliomyelitis, influenza) and rickettsial diseases (typhus) and in other severe bacterial infections. Collagen diseases and endocardial fibroelastosis may have an associated myocarditis.

Clinical Findings

Diagnosis is difficult because the myocarditis may be masked by the primary disease. There may be no cardiac symptoms or there may be precordial oppression, pain or tenderness, tachycardia out of proportion to fever, and abnormalities of rhythm. In severe cases, evidence of congestive failure is present (see below). The pulse is usually weak and rapid, the blood pressure low, and the heart frequently enlarged. Findings on ECG are occasionally normal but usually show partial to complete atrioventricular block and intraventricular conduction defects. If the patient survives, there is usually no permanent myocardial damage.

Complications

Complications include congestive failure and arrhythmias.

Treatment

A. Specific Measures: No specific measures are known, and treatment is aimed at the primary disease. In nonspecific acute myocarditis where other measures have failed, corticotropin (ACTH) or cortisone should be considered.

B. General Measures: The patient should be kept at bed rest until all evidence of active myocarditis has disappeared and the ECG has returned to normal or is no longer changing. Oxygen, digitalis, and other supportive treatment should be given as indicated.

C. Treatment of Complications: For congestive failure, see below. Treat specific arrhythmia, if indicated.

MYOCARDIAL FAILURE

Myocardial function may be impaired by a variety of disorders; if this impairment is great enough, myocardial failure results.

The most common of these disorders are myocarditis, rheumatic heart disease, congenital heart disease, hypertension (eg, of renal origin), and pulmonary heart disease (following chronic respiratory disease). Contributing factors in myocardial failure include severe anemia and certain acute and chronic diseases.

Clinical Findings

The symptoms and signs of myocardial failure in children will vary with the age of the child and with the nature of the associated conditions.

A. Symptoms: Symptoms include dyspnea and weakness, which may be manifested during infancy as episodes of gasping or sighing; loss of appetite; nausea and vomiting, especially during infancy; and chronic nonproductive cough.

B. Signs: Signs include pallor or cyanosis (first perioral) and distention of the veins of the neck. The heart is usually enlarged; arrhythmias may occur. Heart sounds are of poor quality, with the normal sharp difference between the 2 sounds becoming less distinct. There may be an increase in the pulse rate above that expected for the age group and the associated disease. Rales of pulmonary edema may be heard. Enlargement of the liver is one of the earliest and most accurate signs; the degree of enlargement reflects the severity of cardiac failure. Failure may be relatively rapid in onset in infants and may be heralded by fever, tachycardia, and minimal increase in respiratory rate. Slight generalized edema may occur. Previously heard heart murmurs may become weaker or disappear owing to low output.

C. X-Ray Findings: An x-ray usually demonstrates enlargement of the cardiac silhouette and congestion of pulmonary vessels.

D. Electrocardiographic Findings: Although it is neither specific nor diagnostic, the ECG may show tachycardia, low amplitude of QRS and T waves, and an abnormal shape of the RS–T segment.

Treatment

A. Specific Measures: If possible, treatment of myocardial failure should start with the underlying cause. However, treatment of myocardial failure very often represents the only contribution the physician may make to the comfort of the patient in severe cases.

B. General Measures:

1. Bed rest–Bed rest is essential in patients with all types of heart failure. In many children, this may only be accomplished with the aid of sedatives, especially the longer-acting types such as phenobarbital (see Appendix). Narcotics may be necessary.

2. Oxygen–Oxygen is extremely important and should be used even when dyspnea and cyanosis are absent.

3. Digitalis–Digitalis is of great assistance but should be used with caution in the presence of diphtheritic myocarditis or acute rheumatic fever with severe myocarditis. For dosage and preparations, see Table 13–5.

4. Diuretics–Diuretics may be used to accelerate the removal of edema, especially following digitalization. Spironolactone should be given to prevent hypokalemia. Check potassium levels every 3 days. The dosage for chlorothiazide is 20 mg/kg/d; for hydrochlorothiazide, 2 mg/kg/d; and for furosemide, 2 mg/kg/d.

5. Morphine–Morphine may be of value for use in a patient with paroxysmal dyspnea or in any restless infant with myocardial failure.

6. Diet–A low-sodium diet may be of some value in older children with edema but is rarely indicated in infants.

DISORDERS OF RATE & RHYTHM

Certain changes in the rate and rhythm of the heart occur as part of a specific heart disease or congenital defect. Many of these changes will be corrected with successful treatment of the underlying disease state.

Sinus arrhythmia, with accelerated pulse on inspiration, is common during childhood. Marked arrhythmia may require electrocardiographic study to rule out other causes.

Gallop rhythm, with 3 heart sounds heard in each cycle, usually occurs as an ominous sign in the course of heart disease and failure. This should not be confused with the normal, physiologic third heart sound, which is heard best at the apex.

PAROXYSMAL TACHYCARDIA

Paroxysmal tachycardia may occur at any age. The cause is unknown in most cases. There are 2 types: paroxysmal atrial tachycardia (PAT) and paroxysmal ventricular tachycardia (PVT). PAT is the most common, occurring in young patients with normal hearts and recurring throughout a long life. It may be secondary to an infectious disease, associated with various congenital heart lesions, or stimulated by nervous or physical exhaustion. PVT is usually the result of myocardial infarction or digitalis intoxication. Some individuals with PVT have a short P–R interval and prolonged QRS complex (Wolff-Parkinson-White syndrome).

Clinical Findings

A. Symptoms: Onset is sudden. It is a frightening experience in older children. Symptoms include pallor, sweating, vomiting, restlessness, labored respirations, fever, and sometimes, in infants, cyanosis.

B. Signs: High pulse rate (may be 180–400) may be too rapid to count, requiring ECG for accurate determination. The rate in PAT is steady; in PVT, the rate may show variations. The heart is often enlarged, with murmurs in one-third of patients. Cardiac failure, with dyspnea and orthopnea, may develop if serious heart disease is present or if the arrhythmia is particularly rapid and long in duration. The liver may become enlarged with the onset of cardiac failure.

C. Electrocardiographic Findings: The PAT shows abnormal P waves, which at times may be difficult to identify because of the rapid rate. The QRS complex is usually normal. In PVT, P waves show no relation to QRS complexes, which are wide and bizarre. The P–R interval is shortened and QRS duration prolonged in Wolff-Parkinson-White syndrome.

Treatment

Spontaneous return to normal rhythm is common. If symptoms persist, the need for treatment is urgent. Give oxygen.

A. Mechanical Measures: Vagal stimulation by pressure on the eyeballs or on the carotid sinus (of particular value in supraventricular tachycardia) may be attempted. ***Caution:*** Bilateral simultaneous carotid sinus pressure is dangerous and should not be used. The child may be induced to gag or vomit as a means of vagal stimulation.

B. Drugs:

1. PAT–Digitalis is used in full digitalizing doses (Table 13–5).

2. PVT–Quinidine sulfate has rapid action. First give 15–30 mg orally. If this is tolerated, give 6 mg/kg orally every 2 hours. Procainamide may be used. Continuous ECG monitoring is essential.

Prognosis

Prognosis depends upon success of treatment and duration of attack. Death is due to cardiac failure. Attacks usually disappear as the child grows older. Prophylactic digitalis may be given over several months' time and then withdrawn under observation for recurrence. Wolff-Parkinson-White syndrome is generally not harmful.

ATRIAL FIBRILLATION

Atrial fibrillation usually occurs as a complication of rheumatic heart disease. Thyrotoxicosis, infection, shock, or poisoning may cause attacks of atrial fibrillation in normal hearts.

Clinical Findings

There are no symptoms. The rhythm is irregular, and sounds vary in intensity. A variable pulse deficit is present.

Treatment

Give digitalis in a full digitalizing dose, preferably parenterally (Table 13–5), to slow the rate and assist the ventricle. Give quinidine to convert to regular atrial sinus rhythm; the drug may be discontinued in 24 hours (see Appendix).

HEART BLOCK

First-Degree Heart Block

The P–R interval is prolonged in first-degree heart block. The block may be the result of a myocarditis, as in rheumatic fever. It should be suspected if, in the course of observing such a case, the first heart sound at the apex suddenly is noted to diminish in intensity. Diagnosis is established by repeated ECGs.

Complete Heart Block

In complete heart block, the atria and ventricles beat independently. Complete block occurs as a congenital lesion associated with other types of congenital heart disease, usually a septal defect, and, at times, after surgical repair of septal defects.

Symptoms are minimal, consisting only of occasional mild syncope. Signs include a slow but regular ventricular rate, 40–60/min. The diagnosis is established by ECG, which shows dissociation of the P wave and the QRS complex.

Treatment

Treat underlying heart disease. An electric pacemaker may be necessary. The prognosis depends on the underlying disease.

DISEASES OF THE PERICARDIUM

PERICARDITIS & PERICARDIAL EFFUSION

Etiology

A nonsuppurative effusion may occur during acute rheumatic fever and other collagen diseases. Purulent pericardial effusion may result from sepsis. Coxsackievirus causes an acute pericarditis as an isolated phenomenon. In advanced uremia, pericarditis may be a complication.

Clinical Findings

A. Symptoms: There may be pain, which the older child will describe as being less severe in the upright position. Symptoms of cardiac failure, as a result either of the primary disease process or of the constrictive effect on the heart of the pericardial fluid, may be present.

B. Signs: Signs are most often encountered with effusion. Pulse may be paradoxic owing to a fall in systolic blood pressure during inspiration. High diastolic blood pressure, with low pulse pressure, may be present. Neck veins may be distended and nonpulsating. The area of cardiac dullness may be enlarged to percussion. Apical pulsation may be absent. On auscultation, the heart sounds are distant.

C. X-Ray Findings: X-ray shows an enlarged mediastinal shadow. Pulmonary vessels may appear normal despite apparent presence of marked cardiac failure. Fluoroscopy reveals absent or diminished marginal pulsations.

D. Electrocardiographic Findings: The amplitude of all waves, especially of the QRS complex, may be decreased. T waves may be exaggerated at first but later are rounded, lower in voltage, and occasionally inverted.

Complications

Chronic adhesive pericarditis may result from pericardial inflammation. The bands of scar tissue that are produced may result in stress on the myocardium during systole.

Treatment

A. Specific Measures: Paracentesis should be performed if the volume of fluid accumulated in the pericardium is producing tamponade or if the nature of the infecting organism is unknown. The location of the left cardiac border is determined by percussion or x-ray. The site for introduction of the needle is 1–2 cm within the area of cardiac dullness in the fourth or fifth interspace (depending upon the size of the child). Other sites, more difficult to utilize, are to the right of the sternum in the fourth or fifth intercostal interspace and through the diaphragm cephalad under the xiphoid process. Insert a 20-gauge needle on a sterile 10-mL syringe, with suction as the needle passes through the chest wall. Fluid, if present in the pericardium in abnormal quantities, will readily flow into the syringe. Withdraw as much as can be obtained with ease. This amount may total 250 mL in a child who is 6 or more years of age and has acute pericarditis with effusion such as that caused in rheumatic fever.

B. General Measures: Measures are the same as those used for cardiac failure. The underlying condition should be treated. Corticotropin (ACTH) and cortisone have been used in the treatment of severe cases of acute benign pericarditis of unknown cause, with apparently good results.

C. Surgical Measures: Surgery may be indicated to cut fibrous bands of chronic adhesive pericarditis.

• • •

USE OF DIGITALIS

Action

In cardiac failure, digitalis increases the force of the contraction of the myocardium, thereby increasing the cardiac output and decreasing venous pressure. In arrhythmias, it slows the conduction time between atrium and ventricle and depresses the AV and SA nodes. Digitalis prolongs the refractory period of the AV node and thereby slows ventricular rate in atrial fibrillation.

Digitalization

Digitalis must be administered in large initial doses in order to achieve tissue saturation. When this has been accomplished, smaller doses will maintain saturation by replacing that part of the drug which is utilized and excreted.

Criteria of Adequate Digitalization

The dose of digitalis preparations given to children must be determined individually. In general, children require more digitalis in proportion to weight than do adults. Premature infants require relatively less than full-term infants. Changes in the dose may be necessary in the course of digitalization on the basis of signs of toxicity, inadequate digitalization, or gain in weight.

Decreasing signs of cardiac failure, especially slowing of the heart rate, are criteria for adequate digitalization. However, even in the absence of such signs, if electrocardiographic changes due to digitalis (eg, ST depression) are present, it can be assumed that digitalization has been accomplished and an increase in dosage is not indicated.

Table 13–5. Digitalis preparations and dosages for pediatric use.

Drug	Age	Total Digitalizing Dose (TDD)	Division of TDD	Maintenance
Digoxin*†	Premature infant	0.04 mg/kg orally	1st dose, 1/2 of TDD; 2nd dose, 1/4 of TDD after 6–8 h; 3rd dose, 1/4 of TDD after 6–8 h.	1/4–1/3 of TDD in 2 divided doses in 24 h.
	Newborn	0.05 mg/kg orally		
	1–12 mo	0.08 mg/kg orally		
	1–5 yr	0.06–0.07 mg/kg orally		
	5–15 yr	0.05–0.06 mg/kg orally		
Digitoxin	<2 yr	0.035 mg/kg orally	Same as digoxin.	1/5–1/10 of TDD given every 12 h.
	>2 yr	0.025 mg/kg orally or 0.02 mg/kg IV or IM		
Deslanoside‡	<2 yr	0.03 mg/kg orally	Give 3/4 of TDD IV or IM: 1/4 in 3–4 h and repeat every 3 h until effect is obtained.	Initial digitalization only. Maintain with digoxin or digitoxin.
	>2 yr	0.01–0.02 mg/kg orally		

*Use 2/3 of calculated dose when administering IM or IV.

†Purified digitalis preparations have very narrow margins of safety. Give too little rather than too much. The entire dose may be given immediately, parenterally or orally, or may be divided in half and given 4 h apart. For slower digitalization, distribute over a 24-h period.

‡The margin of safety for lanatoside products is *very narrow* in children.

Toxic Effects

Toxic effects are difficult to evaluate in small children. Slight effects include anorexia, nausea and vomiting, and headache. Moderate effects include diarrhea, excitement, and disorientation. Marked effects include abdominal pain, conduction defects as noted on ECG (coupling of rhythm and slowing of heart rate), and atrial or ventricular fibrillation.

Relationship of Digitalis to Potassium Ion

Potassium and digitalis have antagonistic pharmacologic properties. Digitalis toxicity is more likely to occur in any clinical disorder in which decreased potassium is present. In these circumstances, reduce the dose of digitalis or give potassium.

HYPERTENSION*

Blood pressure patterns in children and adolescents show wide variations without evidence of sustained hypertension. Therefore, a single determination of hypertension is unreliable. Periodic measurement should be part of routine preventive health assessments in a child over 3 years of age.

Clinical Findings

Children with blood pressure levels above the 95th percentile (Table 13–2) on 3 or more occasions require diagnostic study.

A. History: A history of renal disease, corticosteroid usage, use of oral contraceptives, smoking, obesity, possible aldosteronism (see Chapter 22), or pheochromocytoma (see Chapter 22) may be an important factor. A family history of hypertension or target organ damage such as stroke may be significant.

B. Physical Examination: The patient should be examined for secondary causes or target organ damage.

C. Laboratory Studies: Studies may include urinalysis with culture; complete blood count; determination of serum electrolyte, lipid, creatinine, and blood urea nitrogen levels; and electrocardiography.

Treatment

Vigorous effort at weight reduction is recommended in children 7–18 years old. The vascular fluid volume can be decreased by reduction in salt intake or diuretics (or both). Initially, either chlorothiazide or hydrochlorothiazide may be used in the following dosage: chlorothiazide, 10 mg/kg/d, increasing in 14-day intervals to a maximum of 20 mg/kg/d if necessary; or hydrochlorothiazide, 1 mg/kg/d, increasing in 14-day intervals to a maximum of 2 mg/kg/d if necessary. Methyldopa may be added as the next step; the dosage is 10 mg/kg/d, increasing in 5-day intervals to a maximum of 40 mg/kg/d if necessary. A vasodilator agent may be added, if necessary, as the final step, eg, hydralazine, 1 mg/kg/d, increasing at 4-day intervals to a maximum of 5 mg/kg/d.

Prognosis

The best predictor of hypertension in adult life is blood pressure at an early date. Primary hypertension probably has its onset in childhood. Control of weight and salt intake may offer great potential for prevention of hypertension in later life. Prognosis for secondary hypertension depends upon the primary incitant.

*Based on National Heart, Lung, and Blood Institute: Report of the Task Force on Blood Pressure Control in Children. *Pediatrics* 1977;**59(Suppl)**.

CARDIAC EVALUATION FOR PARTICIPATION IN SPORTS*

Children and adolescents with previously recognized cardiac defects should be evaluated by a cardiologist before they participate in sports. Evaluation includes taking a history of heart disease in the family and of experience with exercise tolerance and previous heart problems in the child or adolescent. Many children and adolescents with congenital and rheumatic heart defects that do not cause hemodynamic impairment are capable of full, active competition in sports.

There are 3 major areas for concern in the evaluation of the child or adolescent for participation in sports:

A. Heart Murmur: Heart murmurs are commonly found and are usually of the ejection type (see p 262). Normal findings on palpation of femoral and brachial pulse will rule out coarctation of the aorta. Auscultation is performed to evaluate S_1 and S_2 sounds. If S_1 is heard clearly, any murmur that may be present is not related to a ventricular septal defect. If S_2 is normal and there is no ejection click, the majority of possible pathologic heart conditions are ruled out. Any suspected abnormality should be further evaluated by x-ray and electrocardiography.

B. Elevated Blood Pressure: Children and adolescents with mild elevations of blood pressure (see p 262 and Table 13–2) should be reevaluated every week to establish the range of values. Limitation of sports participation is not warranted in these individuals. Studies in adults show that there is a lowering of blood pressure associated with the increased cardiovascular fitness induced by moderate to intense exercise. Children and adolescents with mild to moderate hypertension should have a maximum exercise stress test, simulating a pulse rate of 150–200, to determine the blood pressure and electrocardiographic response. A systolic pressure above 200 mm Hg in response to such exercise is probably a contraindication for sports participation. Isometric sports activities, weight lifting, wrestling, or gymnastics should not be allowed if mild to moderate hypertension is present.

C. Arrhythmia: Arrhythmias in the school age population are generally caused by ectopic beats of atrial, junctional, or ventricular origin. Paroxysmal atrial tachycardia is also observed. Supraventricular arrhythmias are usually considered benign or of little or no consequence especially if they disappear with exercise. Children and adolescents who have ectopic beats that do not disappear or who show an increase in premature ventricular contractions during low-intensity exercise (eg, when doing 10 sit-ups or deep knee bends) should be further evaluated by exercise electrocardiography. If the premature ventricular contractions

*Modified from the report of the Committee on Pediatric Aspects of Physical Fitness, Recreation, and Sports of the American Academy of Pediatrics.

disappear when the cardiac rate reaches 140–150/min, the contractions are probably benign and do not preclude full competitive participation. Frequent, sporadic ectopic ventricular beats or bigeminy may be associated with myocarditis. Confirmation of this association requires electrocardiography. Complete heart block is a contraindication to participation in competitive sports.

A cardiologist familiar with the problems of children and adolescents should be consulted before the young person is completely excluded from sports.

Ear, Nose, & Throat* | 14

Examination of the ear (including visualization of both eardrums) and a test of hearing are essential parts of the pediatric examination. In children under the age at which hearing can be tested reliably, pneumatic otoscopy (or tympanometry) is an essential test.

HEARING LOSS & DEAFNESS

Hearing is as important to speech as sight is to reading. Hearing is the means by which individuals control the articulation and sound quality of their own voice. Deafness ranks with mental retardation as one of the main causes of delay in normal speech development.

Hearing loss of any degree over 20 dB in the speech frequency range (500–2000 Hz) can interfere with both education and speech development. Children with symptoms indicative of brain injury, mental retardation, speech problems, or autism should have their hearing checked, because hearing loss may simulate any of these disorders.

It is of the utmost importance that severe hearing loss or deafness be detected as early as possible so that habilitative procedures may be instituted immediately. It is now possible in audiology clinics to test infants as young as 3 months old. Referral to an audiology facility is essential whether the suspected loss is mild or severe.

Etiology

As in adults, there are 3 types of hearing loss in children. They are directly related to cause (Table 14–1) and can be classified as (1) sensorineural hearing losses, which involve the organ of Corti, the eighth nerve system, the midbrain area, or a combination of these; (2) conductive hearing losses, which involve only the middle ear structures (tympanum, ossicles, eustachian tube) or the external auditory canal; and (3) mixed losses, which involve both the sensorineural and the conductive apparatuses.

"Psychogenic" hearing loss (hearing loss apparent on audiometry but with no organic basis) is occasionally seen.

*Revised with the assistance of Barton D. Schmitt, MD.

Table 14–1. Causes and types of hearing loss.

Source	Cause	Type	Degree of Loss
Congenital			
Endogenous	Hereditary (recessive, X-linked, or dominant)	Sensorineural (organ of Corti)	Usually severe to profound
Exogenous	Asphyxia	Sensorineural (organ of Corti)	Moderate (high-frequency deficits)
	Erythroblastosis	Sensorineural (brain stem)	Mild to severe (high-frequency deficits)
	Maternal rubella and other viruses	Sensorineural (organ of Corti)	Moderate to severe
	Ototoxic drugs (quinine, kanamycin, dihydrostreptomycin)	Sensorineural (usually organ of Corti)	Moderate to profound
Either endogenous or exogenous	Congenital atresia, stenosis, or ossicular deformity	Conductive (may be unilateral)	Moderate
Acquired			
	Labyrinthitis	Sensorineural (cochlear)	Mild to profound
	Measles	Sensorineural (usually cochlear)	Moderate to profound
	Meningitis	Sensorineural (cochlear and 8th nerve)	Moderate to profound
	Mumps	Sensorineural (usually cochlear and unilateral)	Profound
	Trauma	Conductive, sensorineural, or mixed	Moderate to profound
	Tumors	Sensorineural (8th nerve)	Moderate to profound
	Cerumen	Conductive	Mild to moderate
	Cholesteatoma		
	Foreign bodies		
	Otosclerosis		
	Perforated tympanum		
	Serous otitis media		
	Suppurative otitis media		

Clinical Findings

A. Symptoms: Hearing defects are often noticed, sometimes very early, by the child's family; if there is any question, the child should be referred to an audiology center.

B. Signs: Findings on otologic examination may include abnormalities of the external ear canal and eardrum; presence of middle ear fluid (retraction, decreased mobility of the eardrum); or evidence of obstructive adenoids.

Tuning fork tests may reveal abnormalities.

1. Weber test–Lateralization to one ear indicates either a conductive loss in that ear or a sensorineural loss in the other ear.

2. Rinne test–If the tuning fork is heard louder by bone conduction than by air conduction, a conductive loss is certain.

The child's behavior patterns should be observed for signs of sensorineural and conductive losses.

1. Sensorineural losses (mild to profound)–

a. Up to 4 months of age–Signs include failure to sit or to be aroused by a voice or noises when sleeping, failure to become quiet when spoken to, and failure to startle to loud noise.

b. Four months to 1 year of age–Signs include failure to orient (localize) to soft, interesting sounds on both sides and failure to respond when the child's name is called softly from out of the child's vision.

c. One to 2 years of age–Signs include failure to have varied vocalizations of consonants and vowels and failure to recognize that some sounds stand for certain things. A strident, loud voice quality (which begins only after 9 months of age) may be noted, with only simple vowel sounds being voiced (a harsh "ah" is typical). Often, the use of "a-mah," "a-mah," sounding like "mama," is noted in children at about 1 year of age. (This use develops from vibrations felt when being held closely, but after walking starts, it is lost.)

d. Two years of age and over–Signs include speech development retarded or faulty for age group (speech may sound like "jargon"; the only problem may be continued substitutions for consonant sounds); language development retarded for age group; educational problems (slow learning, behavior problems in school, restlessness, nervousness); and frustration and tantrums with communication failures.

2. Conductive losses (mild to moderate)–

a. Up to 1 year of age–Signs include a soft voice quality and the failure to respond to softer sounds, although there is good awareness of louder sounds.

b. One to 2 years of age–Signs include a soft voice quality; failure to respond to a very soft voice when the child's name is called; and a subtle retardation in speech and language development, although speech articulation is normal.

c. Two years of age and over–Signs include measurable retardation in language and speech skills and the failure to respond to the child's name when whispered very softly or from far away.

Treatment

A. Specific Measures: Medical correction (eg, cerumen removal) or surgical correction (eg, insertion of tympanostomy tubes) may be indicated.

B. Hearing Aids: A significant hearing loss as mild as 20 dB may be considered for amplification via wearable hearing aids. Proper audiologic habilitation should always be secured when a hearing aid is applied. Children as young as 1 month of age may be fitted with a hearing aid. Referral to a competent audiology center should be made.

C. Educational Measures: The hard-of-hearing child (20–65 dB average loss) may, if trained early enough, succeed in regular school settings with supplementary help. (Tutoring, curriculum help, and speech and hearing therapy are indicated for the more severe cases.) Children with very severe losses (65–100 dB average loss) may do best in oral schools for the deaf and hard-of-hearing, where the residual hearing is used in combination with other approaches. Profoundly deaf children, such as those with postmeningitis deafness or total congenital deafness, may not benefit from acoustic treatment of any sort and may benefit most from manual language techniques in schools for the deaf. Occasionally, a hard-of-hearing child also has central perception disorders that make the child a candidate only for such schools.

CONGENITAL MALFORMATIONS OF THE EXTERNAL EAR

Congenital malformation of the auricle is a cosmetic problem; associated abnormalities of the urogenital system or inner ear may be present. Hearing should be tested in children with congenital malformation.

A small skin tag, fistula, or cystic mass in front of the tragus is a characteristic remnant of the first branchial cleft. These are best treated surgically.

Protruding auricles are a dominant hereditary characteristic. If the defect is severe, otoplasty should be performed for cosmetic purposes when the child is 5–6 years of age.

Agenesis of the external auditory canal or ear can be corrected surgically. If agenesis is bilateral, a hearing aid is fitted when the child is 2–4 weeks of age so that the child is not deprived of auditory stimulation during early development. Surgery is performed before school age in patients with bilateral agenesis and after childhood in patients with unilateral agenesis.

OTITIS EXTERNA
(Inflammation of the External Ear Canal)

The most common cause of otitis externa is maceration of the ear canal lining due to frequent swimming or shower bathing. Trauma, reactions to foreign bodies, and accumulation of cerumen are other contributing factors. Pyogenic (especially *Pseudomonas* or staphylococcal) and mycotic superinfections are common.

Recurrent otitis externa is usually caused by the frequent use of cotton-tipped applicators or frequent swimming in chlorinated pools (or both).

Treatment

A. Pyogenic Infections: Treatment is aimed at keeping the external ear canal clean and dry and protecting it from trauma. Debris should be removed from the ear canal by gentle irrigation. Topical antibiotics combined with a corticosteroid applied on a wick or as eardrops are essential. Give systemic antibiotics (usually penicillin) in full doses for 10 days if there is evidence of extension of the infection beyond the skin of the ear canal (fever or adenopathy). During the acute phase, swimming should be avoided if possible.

B. Removal of Foreign Bodies: Removal should always be done under direct vision and never done blindly. A stream of lukewarm saline directed past the foreign body into the external canal may float it out. Vegetable matter, such as peas and beans, swells in the presence of water and should instead be removed with a wire loop; care should be taken not to push the object farther into the canal. If the object is large or is wedged in place, the patient should be referred to an otolaryngologist.

C. Removal of Impacted Cerumen: Cerumen in the external ear must be removed before the examination can continue. It may be removed with a wire loop or with cotton on the end of a thin wire applicator. Cerumen may be softened, if necessary, by instilling mineral oil or Cerumenex. (***Caution:*** Cerumenex can cause contact dermatitis if left in the ear canal for over 30 minutes.) It may also be washed out with warm water or saline, using a syringe. Irrigation is contraindicated if any possibility of a perforated eardrum exists.

Prognosis

After removal of a foreign body, rapid improvement occurs.

ACUTE SUPPURATIVE OTITIS MEDIA

Acute otitis media is common during infancy and childhood. Intelligent use of antibiotic therapy has diminished the frequency of progression to severe illness and perforation. Inadequate therapy is responsible for most of the present-day complications.

The most common bacterial pathogens are pneumococci, *Haemophilus influenzae* (especially in children under 12 years of age), and the β-hemolytic streptococci. *Escherichia coli, Staphylococcus aureus, Klebsiella pneumoniae,* and various anaerobic organisms may be predominant in newborns. *Staphylococcus epidermidis* may be the primary pathogen. In one-third of cases, no pathogen can be found and a viral cause is likely. Nasopharyngeal cultures frequently fail to recover the organism found in the middle ear. Acute otitis media in infants may be related to feeding the bottle to the infant in the horizontal position. Sudden altitude changes may force organisms into the middle ear.

Clinical Findings

A. Symptoms: Irritability and restless sleep may be the only signs in an infant, or the infant may also rub or pull the ears. Older children will complain of pain, dizziness, and headache. Fever in infants may be very high, sometimes with convulsions, or it may be absent. Symptoms of an upper respiratory tract infection are usually present. Occasionally, vomiting may be prominent.

B. Signs: Examination of the ear may reveal distortion or absence of light reflex and impaired mobility of the drum. The drum is diffusely red rather than the normal pearl-gray; it is usually bulging. If the tympanic membrane has ruptured, an opening discharging pus or serous fluid may be seen. A conductive type hearing loss is always present.

Note: Mild redness of the drum in the presence of high fever often is entirely nonspecific and related only to the fever. Hyperemia of the drum may also occur with crying.

Treatment

A. Specific Measures: Full doses of systemic antibiotics for 10 days are indicated. (See Table 6–2 for drugs of choice.) Penicillin is the drug of choice for streptococcal or pneumococcal otitis. Penicillin with triple sulfonamide or ampicillin alone is preferred in children under 12 years of age or for those proved by ear culture to be infected with *H influenzae*.

B. General Measures: Aspirin or other analgesics should be given to reduce the discomfort and fever. Recent studies have shown that antihistamines and decongestants are of no value in reducing the duration or severity of acute or chronic otitis media. Analgesic eardrops are generally contraindicated because they obscure physical findings; however, a single application is often diagnostic. Vasoconstrictor nose drops are also of questionable efficacy, since they cannot be delivered to the eustachian tube.

C. Surgical Measures: Myringotomy during the early, acute stage is usually not necessary when full doses of antibiotics are used, but it may provide immediate relief if pain is severe and there is pronounced bulging of the eardrum. Later, myringotomy may be indicated if there is no response to antibiotics within 48 hours or when mastoiditis is present.

Tonsillectomy and adenoidectomy do not significantly affect the later occurrence of otitis media.

Complications

Complications include perforation of the drum, resulting in chronic otitis media; mastoiditis; occasionally, meningitis or brain abscess; and chronic serous otitis ("glue ear").

Course & Prognosis

Untreated, the disease is self-limited unless complications occur. Spontaneous perforation leads to prompt systemic improvement, but infection may become chronic. Prompt and prolonged (10 days) antibiotic therapy usually prevents perforation and complications.

Continuing drainage in spite of adequate antibiotic therapy usually indicates that the infection has become chronic or that mastoiditis has developed. Mastoid x-rays showing clouding of the air cells or demineralization of the bony trabeculae may indicate the need for mastoidectomy. External otitis may be treated as described above.

The incidence of deafness in children does not have a significant relationship to acute otitis media.

SECRETORY (SEROUS) OTITIS MEDIA

Secretory (serous) otitis media is a comon cause of mild hearing loss in children, most often between the ages of 2 and 7. The middle ear contains sterile fluid that varies from a thin transudate to a very thick consistency ("glue ear"). Eustachian tube obstruction is usually due to primary congenital tube dysfunction. Other possible contributing factors are allergic rhinitis, adenoidal hyperplasia, supine feeding position, or a submucous cleft.

Onset is usually sudden, with a slight conductive hearing loss. Symptoms may include slight earache, a feeling of watery bubbles in the ear, or a sensation that the head is full. If the ear is not completely filled with fluid, there may be air bubbles or a meniscus visible through the tympanic membrane. The eardrum shows a loss of translucency, diminished movement, and a change in color from the normal gray to a more pale or even bluish hue.

Antihistamines and decongestants are of no value and may be harmful. Management of allergies may be of value in the allergic child.

If the duration has been over 8 weeks, the child should be referred for myringotomy, suctioning, and the insertion of plastic ventilation tubes. Unilateral serous otitis media can be treated conservatively for a longer period of time.

CHRONIC PERFORATION OF THE EARDRUM

Pyogenic organisms are usually the causative agents.

Clinical Findings

A. Symptoms: Recurrent or persistent ear drainage may be present. Chronic otitis media may be painless, and the child may be afebrile in the intervals between acute exacerbations.

B. Signs: The eardrum is perforated. Peripheral perforations provide a greater risk of cholesteatoma formation. Marked scarring of the drum signifies previous perforations. Mastoid tenderness may be present. A conductive type hearing loss will be present.

C. Laboratory Findings: Bacteriologic study is imperative. Specific etiologic diagnosis must be made by culture of drainage fluid. Secondary invaders following perforations are frequent causes of chronic drainage and are much more resistant to therapy. These include *Pseudomonas, Escherichia coli, Klebsiella pneumoniae,* and staphylococci.

D. X-Ray Findings: X-ray studies for evidence of mastoid involvement are indicated in selected cases.

Treatment

Keep water out of the ear by plugging the ear with cotton impregnated with petrolatum when washing or bathing. Swimming should be forbidden. Instill appropriate antibiotic drops for any serous drainage; systemic antibiotics are also indicated for purulent drainage or systemic signs.

Myringoplasty or tympanoplasty is performed when the child is about age 10 or older. Cholesteatoma is a pocket of skin that invades the middle ear and mastoid spaces from the edge of a perforation. This type of chronic otitis should be treated surgically when diagnosed.

Complications

Complications include hearing loss, mastoiditis, brain abscess, meningitis, and labyrinthitis (with dizziness).

Course & Prognosis

With massive and prolonged antibiotic treatment and surgical drainage of the mastoid bone when indicated, the prognosis is good. If no treatment is given, hearing loss is certain.

ACUTE BULLOUS MYRINGITIS

In acute bullous myringitis, bullae form between the outer and middle layers of the tympanic membrane. Though this condition was previously thought to be viral, recent studies demonstrate that 50–75% of patients with acute bullous myringitis have underlying acute suppurative otitis media. The organisms are very similar to those found in isolated acute suppurative otitis media, with the exception that *Mycoplasma pneumoniae* is occasionally involved. The patient complains of ear pain on the involved side. Examination reveals 1–3 bullae containing straw-colored fluid. Antibiotics are prescribed as for acute suppurative otitis media. The bullae do not have to be opened unless they cause severe pain.

MASTOIDITIS

Mastoiditis is an inflammation of the mastoid antrum and air cells, with bone necrosis. Pyogenic bacteria, chiefly streptococci, staphylococci, and *Pseudomonas* species, are the causative agents.

Clinical Findings

A. Symptoms: Pain behind the ear, irritability, and fever may be present.

B. Signs: Signs include tenderness over the mastoid bone and reddening and swelling over the mastoid area. The eardrum usually shows the changes of acute suppurative otitis media.

C. Laboratory Findings: In the acute phase, the white blood cell count and sedimentation rate are elevated. Myringotomy is indicated to define the offending organism.

D. X-Ray Findings: In the acute phase, there is diffuse inflammatory clouding of the mastoid cells; there is no evidence of bone destruction. With accumulation of the exudate, there is resorption of the calcium of the mastoid cells so that they are no longer visible. Subsequently, there is destruction of the cells, with areas of radiolucency representing abscesses.

In chronic mastoiditis, there is an increase in thickness of the mastoid cells and sclerosis of the bone. This is associated with a reduction in size of the cells. Small abscess cavities may persist in the sclerotic bone.

Treatment

A. Specific Measures: Intravenous administration of an antibiotic likely to affect the β-hemolytic streptococci and pneumococci (the most common causative organisms) may be indicated.

B. Surgical Measures: In the presence of increasing toxicity and extension of the disease process, surgical intervention and drainage may be necessary. Mastoidectomy is seldom necessary when adequate amounts of antibiotics are employed early in the course of the disease.

Complications

Complications include bacterial meningitis and brain abscess.

Course & Prognosis

If appropriate antibiotics are given in sufficient dosages over an adequate period, complete cures can be expected. Chronic infections usually require surgical intervention to eradicate the infectious focus. Prognosis is generally good.

DISEASES OF THE NOSE & SINUSES

COMMON COLD

Nonbacterial upper respiratory tract infections are exceedingly common in the pediatric age group; about 2–4 such infections per year (6–8 in younger children) are considered usual in the USA.

A number of viruses are specific agents. Secondary bacterial invaders (β-hemolytic streptococci, pneumococci, *Haemophilus influenzae*) frequently contribute to prolongation of illness (beyond 4 days).

Clinical Findings

A. Symptoms: Malaise, sneezing, "stuffiness" of head, sore throat, and cough may be present.

B. Signs: Signs include serous nasal discharge and moist and boggy nasal mucous membranes. Fever is generally slight but may be high in an infant.

C. Laboratory Findings: The white blood cell count is normal or low.

Treatment

A. General Measures: Usually, no medications are needed. Give acetaminophen for pain or fever. Humidifying the air (vaporizer or bathroom shower water) is helpful in relieving nasal and pharyngeal discomfort and cough.

B. Local Measures: Topical vasoconstrictors, nose drops, or nasal sprays may provide symptomatic relief of nasal congestion but should not be used for more than 1 week. Overuse of any topical medication may result in irritation and "rebound" congestion. Oral decongestants cause jitters, and oral antihistamines cause lethargy; their use for treatment of the common cold is questionable.

Course & Prognosis

The usual course is of 4 days' duration. Continuation of rhinitis, regardless of whether it is serous or purulent, considerably beyond this period suggests bacterial complications or sinusitis that might respond to antibiotic therapy. A culture should confirm the superinfection. Prognosis is excellent, but reinfections occur throughout life.

RECURRENT RHINITIS

A child with a chief complaint of "constant colds" is not uncommonly seen in office practice.

Differential Diagnosis & Treatment

A. Common Cold: The most common cause of recurrent runny nose is repeated viral upper respiratory tract infection. The onset is usually after 6 months of age. The bouts of rhinorrhea are usually accompanied by fever. Cultures are negative for bacteria. There is usually some evidence of contagion within the family.

Serum immunoelectrophoresis is an excessively ordered test. Children with immune defects do not have an increased number of colds.

Treatment consists of specific reassurance. The parents can be told that their child's general health is good; that the child will not have a great number of colds for more than a few years; that exposure to colds is building up the body's supply of antibodies; and that the child's problem is not the parents' fault.

B. Allergic Rhinitis: The onset of "hay fever" usually occurs after 2 years of age, ie, after the child has had adequate exposure to allergens. There is no fever or contagion among close contacts. The attacks include frequent sneezing, rubbing of the nose, and a profuse clear discharge. The nasal mucosa is pale and boggy. Smear of nasal secretions demonstrates over 20% of the cells to be eosinophils. Oral decongestants and antihistamines should be prescribed.

C. Chemical Rhinitis: Prolonged use of vasoconstrictor nose drops beyond 7 days results in a rebound reaction and secondary nasal congestion. The nose drops should be discontinued.

D. Vasomotor Rhinitis: Some children react to sudden changes in environmental temperature by manifesting prolonged congestion and rhinorrhea. Oral decongestants can be used periodically to give symptomatic relief.

Unwarranted Therapy

Administration of immune globulin injections is the most common error made in treatment of recurrent rhinitis. The injections may be initiated without determining the serum IgG level or as a consequence of misinterpreting the results by comparing them with adult levels rather than with norms for age. Many studies show that immune globulin injections do not benefit patients with frequent upper respiratory tract infections. In addition to being painful and expensive, they may cause anaphylaxis or isoimmunization. Other worthless approaches to this problem include administration of bacterial vaccines or prophylactic antibiotics and tonsillectomy and adenoidectomy.

PURULENT RHINITIS

Purulent rhinitis caused by pathogenic bacteria is an occasional aftermath of nonbacterial upper respiratory tract infections. In infants with persistent rhinitis, consider congenital syphilis.

Etiology & Clinical Findings

Pyogenic infection is usually due to group A hemolytic streptococci, *Haemophilus influenzae,* or pneumococci. Infection with these organisms is characterized by purulent nasal discharge, dried pus about the nares, and inflamed nasal mucous membranes.

Nasal diphtheria is characterized by chronic serosanguineous nasal discharge.

Foreign bodies usually cause mucopurulent discharge from one nostril only, and that discharge often has a foul odor.

Treatment

If purulent rhinitis is due to infection, an appropriate antibiotic in the adequate dosage (see Chapter 6) should be given. For treatment of nasal diphtheria, see Chapter 25. Cases of rhinitis due to foreign bodies should usually be referred to a specialist.

Prognosis

The prognosis is excellent. Improvement is prompt with specific therapy.

ACUTE SINUSITIS

Acute sinusitis is an inflammation of the mucous membrane lining of the paranasal sinuses. In early infancy, the ethmoid and maxillary sinuses are most frequently inflamed. The frontal sinuses rarely become infected until the child is 6 years of age.

Sinuses are involved in most cases of upper respiratory tract infection, but sinus infection usually does not persist after the nasal infection has subsided. In superinfection, the most common bacterial pathogens are *Haemophilus influenzae*, β-hemolytic streptococci, and pneumococci. *Staphylococcus aureus* is occasionally responsible.

Clinical Findings

A. Symptoms: Symptoms include mucopurulent discharge from the nose, with persistent postnasal drip; fever; headache; and malaise.

B. Signs: Signs include tenderness over the involved sinus; pain upon percussion; cellulitis in the area overlying the affected sinus; periorbital cellulitis, edema, and proptosis (especially with acute ethmoiditis); failure to transilluminate; and hyponasal voice.

C. Laboratory Findings: Culture of nasal discharge should be performed to determine the causative agent. Eosinophils in the nasal secretion suggest allergy.

D. X-Ray Findings: Clouding of the affected sinus region is often present, or a fluid level may be observed.

Treatment

A. Specific Measures: Systemic use of ampicillin (with dicloxacillin in severe cases) for 10 days in full doses is indicated for signs of superinfection (fever, purulent discharge, or overlying cellulitis).

B. General Measures: A combination of oral decongestant and antihistamine may be used. Use of vasoconstrictor nose drops, followed by repeated high nasal suction, may be indicated. Aspirin may be used to decrease discomfort.

Course & Prognosis

A single attack of sinusitis does not predispose to recurrences unless contributing underlying abnormalities (nasal allergy, deflected septum, obstructing adenoid, etc) remain uncorrected. The immediate prognosis is good.

CHRONIC SINUSITIS

Repeated episodes of sinusitis may be due to allergic causes, cystic fibrosis, anatomic deformity resulting in poor sinus drainage, or recurrent irritating factors (eg, repeated diving).

Clinical Findings

A. Symptoms: Symptoms may be minimal and include stuffy nose, nasal discharge of variable amount and character, and headache or face pain.

B. Signs: Signs may be minimal and include moderate or mild tenderness over the infected area, with pain on percussion of the affected part, and intermittent low-grade fever.

C. Laboratory Findings: White blood cell count and sedimentation rate are elevated or normal. Culture for bacterial pathogens should be made. Numerous eosinophils in the nasal smear suggest an allergy.

D. X-Ray Findings: The most common finding is membrane thickening, which may be associated with fluid and cysts or polyps. The bone surrounding the sinus may be thickened.

Treatment

A. Specific Measures: Chronic infection may be primary or secondary; in either case, the patient should be treated with full doses of a suitable antibiotic (see Chapter 6).

B. General Measures: Good drainage should be established by use of nasal vasoconstrictors and frequent nasal suction or voluntary sniffing; correction of anatomic deformity; or use of a combination of oral decongestant and antihistamine.

Allergic irritants must be removed. Humidification may be beneficial.

Complications

In persistent sinusitis, bronchitis may occur from the bronchial aspiration of infected material from the draining sinuses. This clinical combination is known as the sinobronchitis syndrome; it is frequently associated with a chronic cough, and chronic bronchitis may develop.

Course & Prognosis

The course is usually protracted, especially in those children who suffer from a combination of an allergy and an infection. When the therapeutic approach encompasses all possible causative factors, the ultimate prognosis is good. Recurrences during adulthood are frequent, however. Sinus surgery for correction of chronic sinusitis is uncommon in children, but if complications of extension of the infection into the orbit (orbital cellulitis or abscess) or intracranial cavity (meningitis or brain abscess) occur, prompt surgical treatment is essential.

EPISTAXIS

Etiology

The most common cause of epistaxis during childhood is trauma to the nose due to nose picking or nose rubbing, which results in abrasion of the anterior inferior part of the nasal septum (Kiesselbach's area). Trauma to the nose may also be due to falls or blows. Bleeding diseases such as hemophilia, leukemia, von Willebrand's disease, and hereditary hemorrhagic telangiectasia (Rendu-Osler-Weber disease) may present as epistaxis. Other causes include presence of infection (a bloody, purulent nasal discharge is found in syphilis and diphtheria), foreign bodies, and allergic rhinitis. Severe epistaxis may occur with many tumors (eg, angiofibroma, lymphoma, sarcoma).

Clinical Findings

In addition to the bleeding from the nose, blood may be swallowed and produce nausea, vomiting of coffee-ground vomitus, and tarry stools. Blood may be found under the fingernails.

Treatment

A. Mild Bleeding: Either of the following methods is usually successful.

1. Compress the nose between the fingers for at least 10 minutes. Place the child in a sitting position. Do not release the nose intermittently to see if bleeding has stopped.
2. Insert a cotton plug with petrolatum into the nose, and allow it to remain for 4 hours.

B. Persistent Bleeding: A pledget of cotton with 0.25% phenylephrine, a 1:1000 solution of epinephrine, or 1% cocaine, placed in the nose for 5 minutes, will stop most bleeding from Kiesselbach's area. Cauterization with silver nitrate sticks, chromic acid bead, or trichloroacetic acid or by electrocautery should be limited to selected cases.

Prophylaxis

Application of petrolatum ointment to the irritated and crusted regions of the nasal septum and discouragement of nose picking will prevent recurrences in cases due to such local trauma.

Prognosis

Epistaxis may recur but rarely leads to serious difficulties.

DISEASES OF THE THROAT

ACUTE TONSILLITIS & PHARYNGITIS

(See Table 14–2.)

Acute tonsillitis and pharyngitis are usually recurrent and are almost invariably associated with systemic manifestations. They are most prevalent during winter and may occur at the onset of scarlet fever.

Table 14–2. Differential diagnosis of exudative tonsillitis and acute pharyngitis.*

Etiology	Fever	Exudate	Adenopathy	WBC (per μL)	Splenomegaly	Heterophil Titer
β-Hemolytic streptococci	High	Can be wiped off	Cervicals only	$\geqslant$ 15,000	Occasionally	No change
Adenoviruses	Moderate	Can be wiped off	Minimal or none	$\leqslant$ 10,000	Never	No change
Infectious mononucleosis virus	Moderate	Resists wiping	Generalized	Abnormal lymphocytes	Frequently	Elevated
Corynebacterium diphtheriae	Moderate	Resists wiping, extends beyond tonsil	Cervicals only	$\geqslant$ 15,000	Never	No change

*Mouth lesions are also seen in agranulocytosis, thrush, herpes simplex, coxsackievirus, and syphilis infections.

Etiology

The primary cause of bacterial infection is β-hemolytic streptococci. Diphtheritic membranes may simulate tonsillar exudate but differ from it in being more firmly adherent, grayish in appearance, and usually extending across the tonsillar pillars. Tonsillar membranes are also seen in infectious mononucleosis.

The adenovirus group of viruses may cause exudative tonsillitis.

Clinical Findings

A. Symptoms: Fever, malaise, and pain on swallowing may be present.

B. Signs: The febrile child appears flushed and usually moderately toxic. Tonsils are enlarged and infected and are frequently covered with a whitish exudate. Cervical lymph nodes may be enlarged and tender.

Note: Look for deformity of the tonsillar pillars, suggesting peritonsillar abscess (very uncommon during early childhood), and for swelling in the midline of the pharynx, suggesting retropharyngeal abscess (usually occuring in children before 2 years of age).

C. Laboratory Findings: In bacterial infection, leukocytosis with a shift to the left may be present. The white blood cell count may be as high as 20,000/μL. With viral tonsillitis and pharyngitis, the white blood cell count is normal or low. Throat culture should be performed to identify significant bacterial pathogens.

Complications

Complications include otitis media, cervical adenitis, sinusitis, peritonsillar abscess, pneumonia, and delayed hypersensitivity reaction (rheumatic fever, glomerulonephritis).

Treatment

A. Analgesics: Aspirin is usually adequate. Do not overdose.

B. Local Measures: Gargles or throat irrigations with hot, nonirritating solutions (saline or 30% glucose) often relieve pain. Hard candy usually reduces symptoms also.

C. Antibiotic Treatment: A single dose of benzathine penicillin given intramuscularly or penicillin V given orally 4 times daily for 10 days should be used only if β-hemolytic streptococci are cultured.

TONSILLECTOMY & ADENOIDECTOMY

Very few children require tonsillectomy and adenoidectomy. If possible, surgery should be deferred for 2–3 weeks after an acute attack has subsided.

A. Indications for Surgery: Persistent nasal obstruction, persistent oral obstruction, cor pulmonale, recurrent peritonsillar abscess, recurrent pyogenic cervical adenitis, suspected tonsillar tumor, and sleep apnea syndrome are indications for surgery.

B. Contraindications to Surgery: Contraindications include tonsillitis in the acute phase, uncontrolled systemic disease (diabetes mellitus, tuberculosis, heart disease), hemorrhagic disease, and polio epidemics. Great care must be taken in evaluating the child with cleft palate, submucous cleft palate, or bifid uvula for adenoid and tonsil surgery, because there is a risk of aggravating the defect of the short palate. Tonsillectomy and adenoidectomy do not significantly affect the later occurrence of otitis media.

C. Invalid Reasons for Surgery: "Large" tonsils, recurrent colds and sore throats, recurrent streptococcal pharyngitis, parental pressure, school absence, and "chronic" tonsillitis are invalid reasons for surgery. Over 95% of tonsillectomies and adenoidectomies are performed for these unjustified reasons.

ACUTE CERVICAL ADENITIS

The classic case of acute cervical adenitis involves a large, unilateral, isolated tender node. About 60% of such cases are due to β-hemolytic streptococci, 20% to staphylococci, and the remainder perhaps to viruses.

The most common site of invasion is from pharyngitis or tonsillitis. Other entry sites for pyogenic adenitis are periapical dental abscess (usually producing a submandibular adenitis), impetigo of the face, infected acne, and otitis externa (usually producing preauricular adenitis). The problem is most prevalent among preschool children.

Clinical Findings

A. Symptoms and Signs: The chief complaints are a swollen neck and high fever. The mass is often the size of a walnut or even an egg; it is taut, firm, and exquisitely tender. If left untreated, it may develop an overlying erythema. Each tooth should be examined for a periapical abscess and percussed for tenderness.

B. Laboratory Findings: The white blood cell count is usually about 20,000/μL with a shift to the left. A tuberculin skin test should be given and a throat culture obtained.

Differential Diagnosis

Four general categories can be distinguished on the basis of the clinical findings. (Acute unilateral adenitis has been described above and is usually pyogenic.)

A. Acute Bilateral Cervical Adenitis: Painful and tender nodes are present on both sides, and the patient usually has fever.

1. Infectious mononucleosis–This diagnosis can be aided by the finding of over 20% atypical cells on the white blood cell smear and a positive mononucleosis spot test.

2. Tularemia–There is a history of wild rabbit or deerfly exposure.

3. Diphtheria–This only occurs in children who have not been immunized.

B. Subacute or Chronic Adenitis: An isolated node usually exists, but it is smaller and less tender than that in acute pyogenic adenitis. Occasionally, bilateral adenopathy is present.

1. Nonspecific viral pharyngitis–This accounts for about 80% of subacute cases.

2. β-Hemolytic streptococci–Streptococci can occasionally cause a low-grade cervical adenitis; staphylococci never do.

3. Cat-scratch fever–The diagnosis is aided by the finding of a primary papule in approximately 60% of cases. Cat scratches are present in over 90% of cases.

4. Atypical mycobacteria– The node is generally nontender and submandibular. If the PPD test is positive, infection with atypical mycobacteria is the probable cause of adenitis.

C. Cervical Node Cancers: These tumors usually are not suspected until the adenopathy persists despite treatment. Classically, the nodes are painless, nontender, and firm to hard in consistency. Cancers that may appear in the neck are reticulum cell sarcoma, leukemia, Hodgkin's disease, lymphosarcoma, and cancers that have an occult formation in the nasopharynx (eg, rhabdomyosarcoma). The patient with a cervical node that has been enlarging for more than 2 weeks despite treatment or is still large and unchanged for more than 2 months should be referred to a surgeon for biopsy.

D. Imitators of Adenitis: Several structures in the neck can be infected and resemble a node.

1. Mumps–The most common pitfall in diagnosis is mistaking mumps for adenitis.

2. Thyroglossal duct cyst–When superinfected, this congenital malformation can become acutely swollen. An aid to diagnosis is the fact that it is in the midline and that it moves upward with tongue protrusion.

3. Branchial cleft cyst–Aids to diagnosis are its location along the anterior border of the sternocleidomastoid muscle and its smooth and fluctuant consistency. Occasionally, it is attached to the overlying skin by a small dimple.

Complications

The most common complication in the untreated case is suppuration of the node. In the preantibiotic era, extension sometimes occurred internally, resulting in jugular vein thrombosis, carotid artery rupture, septicemia, and compression of the esophagus or larynx. Poststreptococcal acute glomerulonephritis has also been reported.

Treatment

Penicillin for 10 days is the drug of choice unless *Staphylococcus aureus* is suspected. The patient should be referred to a dentist if a periapical abscess is suspected. Analgesics (even codeine) are necessary during the first few days of treatment.

Early treatment with antibiotics prevents most cases of pyogenic adenitis from progressing to suppuration. However, once fluctuation occurs, antibiotic therapy alone is insufficient. When fluctuation or pointing is present, the physician should incise and drain the abscess.

A good response includes resolution of the fever and a decrease in the tenderness after 48 hours of treatment. Reduction in size of the nodes may take several more days. If there is no improvement within 48 hours and the PPD test is negative, it can be safely assumed that the infecting organism is penicillin-resistant *S aureus;* dicloxacillin, 50 mg/kg/d orally, should then be added to the treatment regimen. Aspiration of the node with an 18-gauge needle and 0.5 mL of normal saline in the syringe to obtain material for Gram's stain and culture may be helpful at this stage.

Prognosis

After the infection clears, the node may remain palpable for several months but will gradually decrease in size unless it is scarred. Recurrent pyogenic adenitis is rare. When it occurs, it is usually due to diseases such as granulomatous disease of childhood or to an immunologic disorder. More often, it is a misdiagnosed branchial cleft cyst or thyroglossal duct cyst.

15 | Respiratory Tract

*John G. Brooks, MD**

Most lung disease in children is due to infection, allergy, congenital anatomic abnormalities, or a combination of causes. Airway obstruction is a manifestation of many different pediatric lung diseases, whereas degenerative changes are unusual. Only rarely is the clinical presentation pathognomonic of a single disease process, and a given organism or allergic process may present in a variety of different clinical syndromes.

DISEASES OF THE LARYNX, TRACHEA, BRONCHI, & BRONCHIOLES

Most diseases of the conducting airways present with signs and symptoms of airway obstruction such as stridor, rhonchi, wheezing, or prolongation of inspiratory or expiratory time. Clinical comparison of the relative severity of inspiratory and expiratory obstruction can help localize the major site of the airway narrowing to either the extrathoracic airway (inspiratory obstruction more severe than expiratory obstruction) or the intrathoracic airway (expiratory obstruction more severe than inspiratory obstruction).

EXTRATHORACIC AIRWAY OBSTRUCTION

1. CONGENITAL EXTRATHORACIC AIRWAY OBSTRUCTION

Congenital causes of inspiratory obstruction may present at birth or may not cause significant symptoms until the first upper respiratory tract infection. The most common causes are congenital laryngeal stridor, due to underdevelopment of the supporting tissues of the epiglottis, glottis, and larynx; and vocal cord paralysis, usually due to birth trauma. Other

*Associate Professor of Pediatrics, University of Rochester School of Medicine and Dentistry, Rochester, NY.

causes are fixed anatomic airway narrowing due to intrinsic webs, stenosis, tumors, or cysts; extrinsic compression from neck masses or aberrant or enlarged vessels; and macroglossia or micrognathia.

Clinical findings consist of inspiratory stridor and intercostal and supraclavicular retractions, which are more severe with crying. A hoarse cry is present if the vocal cords are involved. Direct laryngoscopy usually reveals the anatomic cause.

The primary abnormality should be corrected by operation if possible, and an adequate airway must be maintained. Extending the neck and placing the infant prone may decrease inspiratory obstruction. Bilateral vocal cord paralysis usually requires an artificial airway.

Congenital laryngeal stridor disappears when the child is 6–18 months of age. The prognosis in cases of severe stridor due to other causes depends on whether the underlying abnormality is spontaneously reversible or amenable to surgical treatment.

2. CROUP SYNDROME
(Acquired Acute Upper Airway Obstruction)

(See Table 15–1.)

Croup syndrome may be due to infection, allergy, trauma (especially postextubation), or laryngeal or high tracheal foreign body. The chief bacterial cause is *Haemophilus influenzae*; the most common viral

Table 15–1. Croup syndrome.

	Bacterial Epiglottitis	Nonbacterial Croup
Common cause	*Haemophilus influenzae.*	Parainfluenza virus, respiratory syncytial virus.
Most common age range	3–7 yr.	<3 yr.
Seasonal occurrence	Not seasonal.	Late fall, winter.
Clinical onset	Rapid; acutely ill.	Preceded by rhinitis and cough for several days.
Dysphagia	Marked; may be drooling.	None.
Fever	$>39.4\ ^{\circ}C$ (103 °F).	Variable, usually $<39.4\ ^{\circ}C$ (103 °F).
White blood cell count	High ($>18{,}000/\mu L$).	Usually normal.
Criteria for diagnosis	"Cherry-red" epiglottis on direct visualization or enlarged epiglottis on lateral neck roentgenogram.	Clinical presentation and exclusion of other diagnoses.
Treatment	IV chloramphenicol, artificial airway.	Cool mist, nebulized racemic epinephrine.

causes are parainfluenza virus and respiratory syncytial virus. Less common infectious causes are measles and diphtheria. Hypocalcemic laryngeal tetany and angioneurotic edema of the larynx are unusual causes.

Clinical Findings

A. Viral Croup: This is the most common form. There is a gradual onset of respiratory symptoms: barking cough, inspiratory stridor, and suprasternal and intercostal retractions. There may be hoarseness and low-grade fever. Systemic involvement is mild or absent. The white blood cell count is normal. Children under age 3 years are most frequently affected.

B. *H influenzae* Epiglottitis: This is characterized by a rapid onset of high fever, early dysphagia, salivation (drooling), and a toxic appearance. The voice may sound muffled. Leukocytosis is marked, and blood culture is usually positive. Lateral neck x-ray shows an enlarged epiglottis. On inspection, the epiglottis is "cherry-red" and swollen. Children 3–7 years old are most frequently affected.

C. Postextubation Croup: This may develop within minutes to hours after removal of an endotracheal tube and is characterized by inspiratory stridor and chest wall retractions and sometimes by decreased breath sounds and cyanosis.

D. Bacterial Tracheitis: This presents with inspiratory stridor and brassy cough. Fever and leukocyte count are higher in bacterial tracheitis than in viral croup. Tracheitis is commonly due to *Staphylococcus aureus,* and the diagnosis is usually made after the patient fails to respond to treatment for croup.

Treatment

A. Viral Croup: Many cases can be managed on an outpatient basis by providing mist from a hot shower or cool humidifier, along with close observation for signs of increasing airway obstruction. If there is persistent stridor at rest, hospitalization is required. In the hospital, provide cool mist and ensure adequate hydration. Symptoms can be relieved with racemic epinephrine (2.25% diluted 1:8 in preservative-free distilled water to a total of 4 mL) delivered by nebulization. Avoid sedation and minimize anxiety by means of reassurance.

Indications for artificial airway include marked agitation or unresponsiveness to treatment, severe or unremitting cyanosis, and markedly decreased breath sounds. Endotracheal intubation is preferable to tracheostomy. Leave the tube in place at least 2–3 days, and remove it when the patient is breathing around the tube without effort.

A brief course of parenteral corticosteroids (eg, dexamethasone, 0.5 mg/kg/d in 4 doses) may be beneficial in cases of *severe* croup.

B. *H influenzae* Epiglottitis: Give chloramphenicol, 100 mg/kg/d intravenously in 4 divided doses for 7–10 days. An endotracheal tube should be inserted by an experienced person and left in place until epiglottic swelling has receded and the patient can breathe around the tube (usually 1–3 days).

C. Postextubation Croup: Provide mist and racemic epinephrine by nebulization. Low levels (2–4 cm of water) of continuous positive airway pressure delivered by nasal prongs are helpful in some young infants.

D. Bacterial Tracheitis: Antistaphylococcal antibiotics and close observation are essential. Many patients will require tracheal intubation to remove profuse, thick, purulent tracheal secretions and to reestablish the airway.

Course & Prognosis

A. Viral Croup: An artificial airway is rarely required, and gradual recovery over 2–7 days is the rule. The prognosis is generally good.

B. *H influenzae* Epiglottitis: Overwhelming and fatal sepsis may occur when antibiotic therapy is not promptly instituted. The course is stormy initially, but, with specific antibiotic therapy and early, skillful intubation, the prognosis is good.

C. Postextubation Croup: Inspiratory obstruction usually clears in several hours, although it may last several days in young infants.

D. Bacterial Tracheitis: With appropriate therapy, recovery is prompt.

INTRATHORACIC AIRWAY OBSTRUCTION

1. FOREIGN BODY ASPIRATION

Children between 6 months and 4 years of age are at high risk for aspiration of small objects such as seeds, nuts, pins, or pebbles. This diagnosis should be suspected in any young patient presenting with an acute onset of wheezing or chronic unexplained cough, localized atelectasis, chest infiltrates on x-ray, or hyperinflation. A careful history should be taken of episodes of coughing, choking, or wheezing of acute onset.

Extrathoracic foreign body (in larynx or high trachea) is unusual but very serious and presents with marked inspiratory and often expiratory obstruction.

Clinical Findings

There may be a history of playing with or near a small foreign body and a subsequent acute onset of choking, gagging, coughing, and wheezing, often followed by a temporary or prolonged decrease in symptoms.

A. Symptoms and Signs: A child with intrathoracic foreign body (usually in a main stem or lobar bronchus) presents most commonly with a localized expiratory wheeze or decreased breath sounds over the obstructed lung. The percussion note over the affected lung may have increased resonance or increased dullness. There may be tracheal shift, asymmetric chest movement, and some inspiratory stridor.

B. X-Ray Findings: The foreign body itself is usually radiolucent and therefore not visible. Initially—and in some cases for several weeks—the foreign body will serve as a "ball valve" obstruction, with resultant localized hyperinflation. The findings on chest x-ray in such cases may be normal during full inspiration, but the film during forced expiration will show mediastinal shift away from the affected side, which will remain hyperinflated. Similar changes may be seen during fluoroscopy. A forced expiratory film can be obtained in a patient of any age by manual pressure on the abdomen. When the foreign body has completely obstructed an airway, there will be distal resorption of air and resultant atelectasis. This is the most likely finding if the foreign body has been in place for several weeks, and there will be no hyperinflation on forced expiration. If the signs, symptoms, and history are strongly suggestive, this diagnosis should be pursued with bronchoscopy even if results of repeated x-ray studies are normal.

Treatment

Every patient with an aspirated foreign body should be hospitalized.

Bronchoscopy, performed by an experienced endoscopist, is the best treatment for most cases of aspirated foreign body. When the foreign body is lodged between the larynx and the carina, bronchoscopy should be performed as an emergency procedure. For bronchial lesions, it can usually be done electively within 12–24 hours.

After the foreign body is removed, vigorous chest percussion over the affected lung should be continued until the chest examination shows normal findings.

Prophylaxis

Small objects such as beads, buttons, and certain foods (nuts, seeds, popcorn) must be kept out of the reach of small children. Children should not be allowed to run with food or other objects in their mouths. Siblings may have to be taught not to force-feed infants in play.

Prognosis

Prompt diagnosis and removal of the entire foreign body usually results in complete recovery. Prolonged presence of a foreign body may result in bronchiectasis or lung abscess and irreversible destruction of lung tissue.

2. ANATOMIC NARROWING OF THE INTRATHORACIC CONDUCTING AIRWAY

The airway can be narrowed by intrinsic tumors; by fixed stenosis (congenital or acquired), dynamic compression, or extrinsic compression by abnormal vessels (eg, anomalous innominate artery, double aortic arch, enlarged pulmonary artery); or by other mediastinal masses (Table 15–2).

Clinical Findings

Patients with fixed intrathoracic airway narrowing may present with a barking crouplike cough, more expiratory than inspiratory difficulty, and an inspiratory and expiratory wheeze. There may be a history of recurrent, possibly localized pneumonia and increased respiratory distress with apparently mild respiratory infections. Chest x-ray may show infiltrates and possibly a mediastinal mass. Tomograms, x-ray films appropriately exposed to demonstrate the airway, and thoracic CT scans, which better delineate the tracheobronchial air column, may demonstrate localized airway narrowing. If localized intrinsic narrowing is strongly suspected but cannot be proved, diagnostic bronchoscopy is indicated. Bronchography is a dangerous procedure in young children and is rarely necessary.

Most mediastinal masses do not cause airway narrowing.

Table 15–2. Differential diagnosis of mediastinal mass according to anatomic location.

Superior mediastinum	Anterior mediastinum
Aortic aneurysm	Intrathoracic thyroid
Cystic hygroma	Lymphadenopathy
Esophageal lesion	Lymphoma
Intrathoracic thyroid	Pleuropericardial cyst
Mediastinal abscess	Teratoma
Neurogenic tumor	Thymic cyst
Teratoma	Thymic hyperplasia
Thymic tumor	Thymoma
Vascular tumor	Vascular tumor
Mid mediastinum	**Posterior mediastinum**
Aortic aneurysm	Aortic aneurysm
Bronchogenic cyst	Gastrointestinal tract duplication
Gastrointestinal tract duplication	Neurogenic tumor
Granuloma	Thoracic meningocele
Great vessel anomaly	
Hypertrophic lymph nodes	
Lymphoma	
Metastases	
Pericardial cyst	

Treatment

Treatment is directed toward the specific obstructing lesion. Surgery is indicated for most mediastinal masses (except inflammatory lymph node enlargement secondary to lung infection or sarcoidosis), intrinsic tumors, and severe stenosis.

Additional diagnostic tests to specifically characterize a mediastinal mass depend on the location of the mass within the mediastinum and might include chest CT scan, electrocardiography, esophagogram, angiography, skin tests for fungal infections and tuberculosis, urinary catecholamine assay, peripheral lymph node biopsy, and mediastinoscopy.

Prognosis

The prognosis is that of the specific mass or intrinsic airway lesion. The prognosis is generally good for most nonmalignant lesions, although if tracheal resection and reanastomosis are required, the narrowing and obstruction may recur.

3. TRACHEOMALACIA

Because of incomplete development of cartilage and other supportive tissue, the infant's trachea is more compliant and therefore more compressible than that of the adult. However, pathologic "tracheomalacia" in the absence of other lung disease is probably very rare. Tracheal collapse can occur in any patient with obstruction in smaller airways, necessitating forced expiration to empty the lungs of air. The positive intrathoracic pressure thus developed causes "dynamic compression" of the larger intrathoracic airway. Other causes of tracheal compression (eg, vascular ring) must be ruled out.

Treatment is directed toward the small airway disease. An artificial airway is rarely required.

4. BRONCHITIS

Bronchitis can be acute or chronic, and it can be infectious (viral or bacterial) or due to chemical or mechanical irritation of the bronchial epithelium. The chief symptom is cough, which is generally productive except for the first 4–6 days of acute bronchitis. The temperature is normal or only slightly elevated. Diffuse expiratory rhonchi are present on auscultation. Chest x-ray shows increased bronchial markings in chronic bronchitis and in some cases of acute bronchitis.

General treatment for all types of bronchitis includes postural drainage and chest percussion, preceded by inhalation of a bronchodilator, and avoiding inhalation of irritants such as cigarette smoke. Antibiotics are, of course, required for treatment of bronchitis due to bacterial infection.

5. BRONCHIECTASIS

Bronchiectasis is chronic dilatation and infection of one or more bronchi. It usually begins in early childhood and may be either generalized or localized to one or 2 lobes. The lower lobes are more commonly affected than are the upper lobes.

Bronchiectasis is most often due to recurrent lower respiratory tract infections, usually secondary to some underlying abnormality such as cystic fibrosis, defects of the immune system or cilia, bronchial stenosis, congenital deficiency of bronchial cartilage, pulmonary sequestration, bronchogenic cyst, or Kartagener's syndrome. It is often progressive to irreversible bronchial damage. Acute pneumonia due to adenovirus types 7 and 21, measles, *Bordetella pertussis,* or, less frequently, *Haemophilus influenzae* type B, pneumococci, or *Staphylococcus aureus* may be followed by chronic recurrent symptoms of bronchiectasis rather than the usual complete resolution. Occasionally, localized bronchiectasis may develop in a chronically collapsed lobe—owing to, for example, an unrecognized foreign body, a mucus plug, or right middle lobe syndrome.

Bronchiectasis is classified as cylindric, varicose, or saccular, depending on the nature and severity of the bronchiectatic changes on bronchography or histologic examination. In cylindric bronchiectasis, the bronchi are dilated, with regular outlines. In the varicose form, irregular dilatation and constriction of bronchi occur. In saccular bronchiectasis, the bronchial diameter increases progressively in the more distal airways, and the airways end in large blind sacs.

Clinical Findings

A. Symptoms and Signs: Bronchiectasis is characterized by chronic productive cough, worse in the morning and with vigorous exercise. Sputum may be foul-smelling in older children. There may be associated sinusitis, producing copious nasal and postnasal drainage and headache. Dyspnea on exertion may develop, and a few children will have hemoptysis and bronchospasm.

Recurrent low-grade fever is the rule. Moist rales are usually heard over the involved area. Digital clubbing may develop with prolonged lung involvement.

B. X-Ray Findings: Findings on plain chest film are almost always abnormal. Findings range from mildly increased bronchovascular markings to cystic changes or complete lobar collapse. High-kilovoltage chest x-rays may demonstrate the dilated airways. Bronchograms may help determine whether the disease is localized or diffuse; however, a normal finding on bronchogram does not necessarily rule out bronchiectatic changes. Bronchograms can be dangerous in children and should be performed only if surgery is seriously considered, to support an impression of localized disease, and after at least 3–6 months of maximal medical therapy.

Treatment

A thorough search for underlying causes must be made, including cultures, immune system evaluation, a sweat test, a Mantoux test, sinus x-rays, and in some cases bronchoscopy and electron microscopy. (Electron microscopy may reveal abnormal ciliary morphologic features.) Systemic antibiotics selected on the basis of the bacterial culture results must be administered for at least 2–4 weeks. Optimal pulmonary therapy is essential and consists of giving a bronchodilator drug by inhalation followed by postural drainage and chest percussion to the affected lung. This should be performed at least 2–4 times daily. Sinusitis should be vigorously treated.

Surgical removal of one or 2 lobes with severe saccular bronchiectasis may be indicated if prolonged optimal medical therapy has been ineffective and if the rest of the lung appears to be normal. Only a very small number of children with bronchiectasis are appropriate candidates for surgery.

Prognosis

The prognosis is variable depending on the cause, severity, and distribution of the bronchiectasis. Cylindric bronchiectasis is potentially reversible; the saccular type causes irreversible tissue destruction. Some patients improve significantly after lobectomy or treatment of sinusitis, and most show some improvement with optimal medical management.

6. ACUTE BRONCHIOLITIS

Acute bronchiolitis is a potentially serious disease, characteristically occurring during the winter months and affecting children under 2 years of age. The widespread bronchiolar inflammatory exudate, mucosal edema, and resultant airway narrowing can be due to infection or an allergic process (or a combination of both). An allergic component is likely in infants with recurrent acute bronchiolitis or a strong personal or family history of allergy. Respiratory syncytial virus is by far the most frequent cause.

Clinical Findings

A. Symptoms and Signs: After 1–2 days of mild coryza, the infant develops gradually increasing respiratory distress with rapid shallow respirations. Cough is often present, as well as tachypnea and tachycardia, diffuse rales, expiratory wheezes, decreased breath sounds, and prolonged expiratory time. There may be inspiratory intercostal, subcostal, and suprasternal retractions, nasal flaring, and intermittent cyanosis. Pulmonary hyperinflation due to air trapping produces increased chest expansion, depression of the diaphragm, and easy palpation of the liver edge. **Note:** This should not be confused with cardiac failure, which may or may not be present.

B. Laboratory Findings: The white blood cell count is usually normal.

C. X-Ray Findings: Chest x-ray reveals hyperinflation (loss of diaphragmatic doming on lateral x-ray). There may be increased bronchovascular markings.

Treatment

Hospitalization is recommended for infants with bronchiolitis meeting any of the following criteria: patients under 2 months of age, a history or clinical signs of cyanosis or apnea, a history of a previous severe attack, a resting respiratory rate of 60/min or more, and arterial P_{CO_2} level greater than 45 mm Hg or P_{O_2} level less than 60 mm Hg of breathing room air.

Arterial blood gases should be monitored, and humidified gas of increased oxygen concentration should be administered. Avoid under- and overhydration by monitoring fluid intake (orally, intravenously, or both) and urine output and specific gravity.

Since bronchospasm is responsible for part of the airway obstruction in some infants with acute bronchiolitis, a trial of subcutaneous epinephrine (0.01 mL/kg of 1:1000 solution to a maximum dose of 0.3 mL) with or without oral theophylline (2–5 mg/kg every 6 hours) should be considered. Because young infants metabolize theophylline slowly, low doses should be used. The infant should be observed closely for side effects or toxicity (eg, vomiting, decrease in appetite or sleep, irritability). Chest percussion and postural drainage may be useful.

Antibiotic therapy is indicated in more severe cases because of the possibility of secondary bacterial infection. High fever, significant leukocytosis, significant infiltrates on chest x-ray, respiratory failure, and positive bacterial cultures are indications for parenteral antibiotics.

There is no evidence that exogenous corticosteroids influence the course of this disease. Pharmacologic sedation should not be used.

Endotracheal intubation and mechanical ventilation are required for the occasional infant who develops respiratory failure. Respiratory acidosis with pH less than 7.25 and inability to maintain the arterial P_{O_2}

level over 60 mm Hg are both indications for intubation and ventilation. The time course and progression of the disease may necessitate modification of these guidelines.

Course & Prognosis

The acute symptoms usually clear over 2–7 days. With prompt optimal therapy, the prognosis is usually excellent, although rare deaths occur despite good treatment. About half of infants with bronchiolitis will have subsequent episodes of wheezing and are likely to be atopic or have hyperreactive airways.

DISEASES OF THE ALVEOLI & PULMONARY INTERSTITIUM*

PNEUMONIA

In patients with pneumonia, it is not possible to reliably predict the causative organism from the clinical findings. Therefore, for successful treatment, an educated guess about the etiologic agent is of greatest therapeutic importance.

Etiology

A. Bacteria: Especially pneumococci, staphylococci, *Haemophilus influenzae, Klebsiella, Mycobacterium tuberculosis, Mycoplasma pneumoniae, Chlamydia.*

B. Fungi: *Candida, Histoplasma, Coccidioides,* and, in immunodeficient patients, *Aspergillus.*

C. Viruses: Respiratory syncytial virus, adenovirus, influenza, and parainfluenza viruses.

D. Protozoa: *Pneumocystis carinii.*

E. Chemicals: Especially inhalation of hydrocarbons, food, or gastric contents.

Clinical Findings

A. Bacterial: The onset is often fairly rapid, with fever, tachypnea, cough, and chills in older children. There may be pain in the chest, or it may be referred to the abdomen. There may be cyanosis, localized or generalized dullness and decreased breath sounds, rales, rhonchi, wheezing, and a prolonged expiratory phase. Abnormal physical findings in the chest may precede chest x-ray abnormalities. The white blood cell count is high (18,000–30,000/μL), sputum or tracheal aspirate

*Tuberculosis is discussed on p 332.

cultures are positive, and blood culture is often positive.

B. Fungal: Fungal pneumonia occurs in a wide variety of clinical and x-ray presentations and degrees of severity.

C. Viral and Chlamydial: Pneumonia due to these causes is generally more insidious in onset and slower in progression, often preceded by upper respiratory tract infection. Severe pulmonary symptoms may develop (tachypnea, retractions, rales, poor breath sounds, cyanosis) as well as respiratory failure. The white blood cell count may be slightly elevated early in the disease but later drops to normal. Cold hemagglutinins may be demonstrated during convalescence in cases of *M pneumoniae* pneumonia. Complement-fixing antibodies show specific rises in patients with pneumonia due to *H influenzae,* adenoviruses, and *Chlamydia*.

D. Protozoal: *P carinii* pneumonia (interstitial plasma cell pneumonia) occurs in immunodeficient patients and in premature infants and is often fatal, especially if the initiation of treatment is delayed. The onset is insidious but progresses to marked dyspnea, cyanosis, and extreme tachypnea. Severe hypoxemia is present. There may be minimal chest findings with good breath sounds, and there is little or no fever. The chest x-ray findings are variable, but typically there are diffuse miliary or reticular nodular shadows that may become confluent throughout both lung fields.

E. Chemical: The usual history is of choking on food, sometimes during vomiting, or ingestion of hydrocarbon with or without choking. The onset of increased respiratory distress (tachypnea, retractions, perhaps cyanosis), rhonchi, and rales is abrupt with food aspiration and more gradual (over 2–8 hours) following hydrocarbon ingestion. High fever, leukocytosis, and diffuse patchy infiltrates or atelectasis may develop.

Complications

A. Bacterial: Complications include empyema, pleural effusion, lung abscess, pneumatocele, hemoptysis, atelectasis, local hyperaeration, and bronchiectasis.

B. Viral and Chlamydial: Complications include atelectasis, bronchiectasis, hyperlucent lung, and interstitial fibrosis.

C. Chemical: Complications include lung abscess, bronchiectasis, and pneumatocele.

Treatment

A. General Measures: Give supplemental humidified oxygen as needed to maintain the arterial P_{O_2} level over 60 mm Hg. Tracheal intubation and mechanical ventilation may be required to prevent severe respiratory acidosis (arterial pH < 7.25) or to ensure adequate oxygenation. Vigorous pulmonary physiotherapy is indicated.

B. Specific Measures: Give appropriate antibiotics as outlined in Table 6–2. Antibiotics may be useful in the acute phase of chemical pneumonia also. There is no benefit from corticosteroids given after aspiration.

Prognosis

The prognosis for children without underlying disease who do not develop serious complications is excellent. Viral pneumonia during infancy may resolve very slowly over 3–12 months or, especially in the case of adenovirus pneumonia, may leave permanent obliterative and fibrotic changes.

HYPERSENSITIVITY PNEUMONITIS

Allergic pulmonary disease can be divided into 4 groups: (1) Type I, or IgE-mediated immediate hypersensitivity, produces clinical asthma (see Chapter 28). (2) Type II involves the reaction of cytotoxic antibody with lung cell or lung cell-bound antigen, producing cellular destruction. This may be the mechanism causing lung damage in Goodpasture's syndrome. (3) Type III disease results from deposition of complexes of antigen and precipitating antibody in the presence of complement. (4) Type IV responses are of the delayed hypersensitivity type and are involved in pulmonary tuberculosis, sarcoidosis, and some fungal lung infections.

Hypersensitivity pneumonitis is a type I or type III allergic response to inhaled organic antigen. This is the mechanism of diseases such as farmer's lung, bird breeder's lung, humidifier lung, and allergic bronchopulmonary aspergillosis.

Clinical Findings

Hypersensitivity pneumonitis usually results from intermittent exposure to organic dust and can present in acute, chronic, and subacute forms.

A. Acute: Acute hypersensitivity pneumonitis presents with fever, chills, malaise, chest tightness, nonproductive cough, and dyspnea 4–6 hours after antigen exposure. There may also be cyanosis, tachypnea, and basilar rales, usually without wheezing. Leukocytosis is common. The chest x-ray findings may be normal, or there may be diffuse small nodules or patchy interstitial infiltrates. Most of these findings begin to resolve within 12–24 hours after antigen exposure. Prolonged antigen exposure may be associated with weight loss.

B. Chronic: Chronic hypersensitivity pneumonitis occurs after prolonged, usually intense antigen exposure and is characterized by the insidious onset of progressive dyspnea with eventual cyanosis and digital clubbing. Chest x-rays show progressive increases in interstitial markings, and markings may develop a cystic appearance with decreased lung volume.

Treatment

Optimal treatment for both the acute and chronic forms is avoidance of the antigen. Treatment of both forms with cromolyn sodium and corticosteroids may also be helpful.

IDIOPATHIC FIBROSING ALVEOLITIS (Chronic Interstitial Pneumonia)

Liebow has described 3 main classes of interstitial pneumonia seen in children on the basis of the histologic appearance of lung biopsy material. The 3 classes differ in degrees of fibrosis and inflammation of the interalveolar septa and in degree of alveolar infiltration. They undoubtedly represent a final common pathway for a variety of lung diseases and may actually be different stages of a single pathologic process (fibrosing alveolitis). The diagnosis can only be made by lung biopsy.

Desquamative Interstitial Pneumonia (DIP)

DIP (rare in children) is characterized histologically by widespread proliferation and desquamation of type II alveolar pneumocytes. The distal air spaces are filled with these cells and alveolar macrophages. Mild interstitial infiltration with lymphocytes, plasma cells, and eosinophils may be noted. Later in the course, interstitial fibrosis may be present. There is an insidious onset of cough and dyspnea with subsequent tachypnea, weight loss, and cyanosis. Chest x-ray may show normal findings but is usually characterized by irregularly distributed, homogeneous "ground glass" infiltrates that may be migratory.

The disease generally responds well to corticosteroids, which must be given for several years.

"Classic" or "Usual" Interstitial Pneumonia (UIP)

UIP is characterized by some interstitial mononuclear cell infiltration, extensive necrosis of alveolar lining cells, and accumulation of hyaline membranes and necrotic cells within alveoli. This results in increased linear markings on chest x-ray, progressing in some cases to honeycomb changes. The initial symptoms, which in children usually develop gradually during infancy, consist of nonproductive cough and dyspnea with progression to marked tachypnea, anorexia, weight loss, cyanosis, and digital clubbing over a period of weeks or months.

It is not clear whether corticosteroids and immunosuppressive drugs are beneficial to children with this disease.

Lymphoid Interstitial Pneumonia (LIP)

LIP is the rarest of the 3 types and consists of infiltration of the pulmonary interstitium by lymphocytes and plasma cells. Chest x-ray reveals "feathery" infiltrates with progressively increasing densities. The disease begins with cough and dyspnea, with gradual progression (years) to basilar rales, cyanosis, and death. The course is unaffected by corticosteroids.

PULMONARY ALVEOLAR PROTEINOSIS

Pulmonary alveolar proteinosis is a rare disease in childhood characterized by accumulation of eosinophilic, granular, PAS-positive material within alveoli and bronchioles. Cough, dyspnea, low-grade fever, and poor weight gain are early findings, with subsequent yellow sputum production in older children. Cyanosis and death usually occur several months later. Physical findings are few, with scattered rales and occasional cases of digital clubbing. Characteristic laboratory findings are elevation of serum lactic acid dehydrogenase, PAS-positive material in sputum, and diagnostic lung biopsy. Fine perihilar densities are seen on chest x-ray. No therapy has been proved to be beneficial, although lung lavage with heparinized saline may be helpful in some cases.

ATELECTASIS

Atelectasis is collapse of alveoli, often associated with more proximal airway destruction. It may result from complete intrinsic airway obstruction (eg, from mucus plug, mucosal inflammation, foreign body, endobronchial tuberculosis, tumor), extrinsic airway obstruction (eg, hilar lymphadenopathy, enlarged or aberrant blood vessels, cyst or tumor), airway smooth muscle spasm, direct local parenchymal compression (eg, secondary to lobar emphysema or pleural effusion), chronic shallow respirations (eg, diaphragmatic paralysis or muscular dystrophy), or diminished alveolar surfactant (eg, hyaline membrane disease).

Atelectasis is apt to be present in cystic fibrosis and asthma. Allergic children have a tendency toward right middle lobe atelectasis, which may be chronic or recurrent.

The clinical findings depend on the distribution and extent of atelectasis and may include rales, wheezing, localized decreased breath sounds, mediastinal shift, and dyspnea. Chest x-ray may show diffuse patchy lobar or linear infiltrates, signs of unilateral volume loss, and areas of compensatory hyperinflation. A Mantoux test should be included in the work-up.

The therapy includes appropriate treatment of any underlying lung disease, vigorous chest percussion, and postural drainage combined with bronchodilators given orally or by inhalation (or by both routes). If foreign body is suspected, treatment should be given as described on p 311. If localized lobar or segmental atelectasis persists for 1–2 months despite optimal medical therapy, bronchoscopy may be indicated for diagnosis and treatment. Lobectomy is indicated only if the lung has failed to expand after at least 1–2 years of optimal therapy. Children with right middle lobe atelectasis should be evaluated for asthma, and chronic bronchodilator therapy should be considered.

DISEASES OF THE PLEURA & PLEURAL CAVITY

Most pediatric diseases in this category involve abnormal accumulation of air (pneumothorax), fluid (effusion), pus (empyema), inflammatory tissue, or some combination of these within the pleural space. There is likely to be associated chest, shoulder, or abdominal pain, especially with deep breathing or coughing in most affected patients.

PLEURISY

Pleural inflammation can be classified as dry pleurisy, pleurisy with effusion (serofibrinous pleurisy), and empyema (purulent pleurisy).

1. DRY PLEURISY

Dry pleurisy is usually associated with other respiratory tract infection due to viral (especially coxsackie), mycobacterial, or bacterial (especially pneumococcal) causes. It may also occur with rheumatic fever or systemic lupus erythematosus. The chief symptom is chest pain, especially with coughing, though abdominal pain is reported occasionally. The signs are variable and may be absent: guarded and grunting respirations and diminished respiratory excursions on the affected side. The child may lie with the affected side down. Chest x-ray findings may be normal, or there may be thickening of the pleural shadow along the thoracic wall.

Treatment is that of the associated disease, plus analgesia for chest pain.

2. PLEURISY WITH EFFUSION (Serofibrinous Pleurisy)

Pleural effusion in children is most commonly associated with infections of the lung (especially pneumococcal pneumonia). Other causes are systemic lupus erythematosus, rheumatic fever, polyarteritis nodosa, cancer, pulmonary infarction, ascites, pancreatitis, or any cause of increased venous pressure or decreased plasma osmotic pressure.

Clinical Findings

A. Symptoms and Signs: In larger effusions, there may be cough and dyspnea. A secondary rise in temperature in the course of an acute pulmonary infection is characteristic of the development of pleural effusion. There may be dullness to chest percussion and decreased breath sounds over the effusion, cyanosis, asymmetric chest movements with respiration, and mediastinal shift.

B. Laboratory Findings: Thoracentesis should be performed and the fluid cultured for aerobic, anaerobic, and acid-fast organisms; stained with Gram's and acid-fast stains; and analyzed for cell count and differential, specific gravity, glucose, pH, protein, and lactate dehydrogenase (LDH). If appropriate, determine hematocrit and amylase level and perform cytologic examination. Serum samples from blood drawn at the same time as thoracentesis should be analyzed for protein, glucose, LDH, and, if appropriate, amylase.

1. Exudate–Exudate is characterized by either a pleural fluid/serum protein ratio of greater than 0.5, a pleural fluid LDH level of greater than 200 IU/mL, or a pleural fluid/serum LDH ratio of greater than 0.6. An exudate results from disease (usually inflammation) of the pleural surface, as may occur with tuberculosis, pneumonia, cancer, pancreatitis, pulmonary infarction, or systemic lupus erythematosus. It may be infected or sterile.

2. Transudate–Transudate is usually a clear, sterile yellow fluid not meeting any of the above criteria for an exudate and may result from a decrease in plasma oncotic pressure or an increase in pulmonary or systemic hydrostatic pressures such as may occur in congestive heart failure, renal disease, or malnutrition.

3. Hemothorax–Hemothorax may result from chest trauma, clotting disturbances, or tumors, especially neuroblastoma.

4. Chylothorax–Chylothorax generally results from trauma to or obstruction of the thoracic duct.

C. X-Ray Findings: Chest x-rays taken with the patient both upright and lying on the affected side (lateral decubitus) will show an area of uniform density completely or partially obscuring underlying lung. Small effusions may only blunt the costophrenic or cardiophrenic angles or widen the interlobar septa. Loculated fluid will not move with changes in body position.

Treatment

Check the Mantoux reaction, and treat underlying disease. Thoracentesis is indicated in all patients for diagnosis and should be done as therapy when the presence of the effusion is causing significant respiratory distress.

Prognosis

The prognosis depends on the underlying cause of the effusion but is generally good.

3. EMPYEMA
(Purulent Pleurisy)

Empyema is pus in the pleural space, usually associated with bacterial pneumonia, most commonly due to staphylococci. Pneumococci and *Haemophilus influenzae* are slightly less common causative organisms. Trauma or rupture of a lung abscess may also cause empyema.

Clinical Findings

A. Symptoms and Signs: There may be a secondary rise in fever or persistent high fever in the course of pneumonia. Signs include dyspnea, dullness to percussion, and decreased breath sounds over the affected lung. Toxicity may be marked.

B. Laboratory Findings: The white blood cell count is usually high, and blood culture is often positive. Thoracentesis is necessary to distinguish between empyema and serofibrinous effusions.

C. X-Ray Findings: Chest x-ray shows diffuse density, especially in the dependent part of the pleural space. Purulent pleural exudates are usually loculated except in the early stages of infection.

Treatment

A. Antibiotics: Appropriate antibiotics for systemic administration should be selected on the basis of the Gram-stained smear and culture of fluid obtained by thoracentesis. (For choice of drugs, see Table 6–2.) Instillation of appropriate antibiotics into the pleural cavity is indicated (if ever) only in the most severe cases.

B. Evacuation of Empyema: Continuous closed drainage of the empyema by use of a large chest tube should be initiated promptly. Several chest tubes simultaneously or sequentially may be required to drain loculated areas. Chest tubes are rarely required for more than 1–2 weeks.

C. Surgical Measures: Use of thoracotomy, with open drainage and decortication, is almost never required in children.

Prognosis

Empyema is a serious disease, especially in young children. When appropriate therapy is initiated promptly, the prognosis is generally good, although chest x-ray findings may not return to normal for 6–12 months.

PNEUMOTHORAX

Pneumothorax is not common in pediatric patients except in newborns, where the incidence is 1–2% in term infants and higher in premature infants. Pneumothorax may be spontaneous but more commonly is associated with trauma, with obstructive lung disease such as asthma, cystic fibrosis, or pneumonia, or with mechanical ventilation.

Clinical Findings

A. Symptoms and Signs: Pneumothorax may be asymptomatic, or there may be dyspnea, chest pain, and cyanosis. Hyperresonance and decreased breath sounds may be noted on the affected side. There may be a shift of the point of maximal cardiac impulse, hypoxemia, and occasionally decreased blood pressure.

B. X-Ray Findings: The definitive diagnosis is based on x-ray demonstration of air in the pleural space. Small amounts of pleural air are best detected using a cross-table lateral chest x-ray or a lateral decubitus chest x-ray with the affected side up.

Treatment

In the newborn infant, tension pneumothorax is an emergency requiring immediate needle aspiration of the pleural air (see p 769) followed by chest tube insertion and underwater drainage for several days.

In older children, spontaneous resorption will usually occur if activity is minimized (bed rest). This may sometimes be hastened if the patient breathes 100% oxygen. Significant respiratory distress is an indication for chest tube drainage of pleural air.

DISEASES OF THE PULMONARY CIRCULATION

PULMONARY HEMORRHAGE

1. ACUTE PULMONARY HEMORRHAGE

Acute pulmonary hemorrhage and hemoptysis may be associated with bronchiectasis (especially in cystic fibrosis), lung abscess, foreign body aspiration, tuberculosis, heart disease, esophageal duplication, and clotting disorders. In addition to treatment of the underlying disorder, bed rest and blood transfusion may be indicated.

2. PULMONARY HEMOSIDEROSIS

Pulmonary hemosiderosis, or the accumulation of hemosiderin in the lung due to chronic or recurrent hemorrhage, usually from pulmonary capillaries, may be associated with glomerulonephritis (Goodpasture's syndrome), myocarditis, polyarteritis nodosa, systemic lupus erythematosus, rheumatoid arthritis, rheumatic fever, Wegener's granulomatosis, heart disease causing elevated pulmonary capillary or pulmonary venous pressure (especially mitral stenosis), purpuric disease, or possibly milk allergy. It may also be an isolated finding unassociated with other pathologic processes.

Clinical Findings

Intermittent episodes of dyspnea, cough, hemoptysis, wheezing, and fever are seen in a patient with iron deficiency anemia who may have melena and occasionally jaundice and splenomegaly. Hemosiderin-laden macrophages in gastric washings are evidence of pulmonary hemorrhage. Chest x-ray shows soft perihilar infiltrates, often with diffuse speckling in the periphery of the lung. Infiltrates may change rapidly during an episode of acute bleeding.

Treatment

Treatment is that of the associated disease. Oxygen and blood transfusion may be required during episodes of acute bleeding. Oral iron may be necessary. Steroids and azathioprine may be helpful. In rare cases of characteristic milk allergy (Heiner's syndrome) in infants, milk elimination should be tried.

Course & Prognosis

The course and prognosis depend on the associated disease. Idiopathic pulmonary hemosiderosis is characterized by episodes of acute intrapulmonary hemorrhage separated by asymptomatic intervals. The long-term course is variable, and about half of patients die within 5 years after onset.

PULMONARY EMBOLISM

Pulmonary embolism is rare in children and is usually a consequence of venous stasis or trauma. The clinical onset is abrupt if major pulmonary vessels are involved and may include dyspnea, chest pain, cyanosis, hemoptysis, tachycardia, chest splinting, rales, and a pleural friction rub. Chest x-ray may show a peripheral infiltrate, small pleural effusion, and elevated diaphragm. The lung perfusion scan will show nonperfused areas and is a key to diagnosis. Treatment includes oxygen and anticoagulation. Survival of the acute embolic period depends on the size of the embolus. The long-term prognosis is related to the underlying disease.

PULMONARY EDEMA

Pulmonary edema results from changes in hydrostatic or oncotic pressure gradients across the vessel walls or increased permeability of the pulmonary capillaries. Thus, it may be associated with heart disease, a wide variety of infectious and toxic primary lung insults, and hypoproteinemia due to many causes. Neurogenic pulmonary edema may follow severe insults to the central nervous system such as head trauma. Severe pulmonary edema produces dyspnea, tachypnea, rales, wheezing, chest wall retractions, and cyanosis. There is prominent pulmonary vascularity, with diffuse haziness on chest x-ray. Milder pulmonary edema, especially when associated with another underlying lung disease, may be difficult to identify but may contribute to the patient's respiratory difficulty. Depending on the severity of the edema and the age of the patient, appropriate therapy may include oxygen, diuretics, digitalis, morphine sulfate, phlebotomy, mechanical ventilation, rotating tourniquets on the extremities, placing the patient in a semierect position, and treating the underlying disease.

CONGENITAL ABNORMALITIES OF THE LUNG

Congenital abnormalities of the respiratory tract, some of which have been discussed above, may present clinically at any time from birth through adulthood depending on the lesion. Others may never cause symptoms.

PULMONARY APLASIA

Pulmonary aplasia, or the absence of any pulmonary tissue beyond a rudimentary bronchus, is a rare anomaly of unknown cause often associated with other congenital anomalies. There may be symptoms referable to the decreased amount of lung tissue, from recurrent lower respiratory tract infections, or from associated anomalies. Chest x-ray shows total or partial opacification of one hemithorax, with mediastinal shift toward the affected side. The absence of pulmonary arteries and airways is documented by angiography and bronchoscopy. The prognosis is generally poor, with death usually occurring as a result of associated anomalies.

PULMONARY HYPOPLASIA

Pulmonary hypoplasia—small lung with relatively normal bronchial anatomy—can be an isolated finding or may be associated with congenital diaphragmatic hernia, renal agenesis (Potter's syndrome), or abnormal pulmonary arterial and venous anatomy of the right lung (scimitar syndrome). Unilateral pulmonary hypoplasia is associated with normal body growth and an increased frequency of lower respiratory tract infections in some young patients and no symptoms in others.

PULMONARY SEQUESTRATION

Pulmonary sequestration is an area of lung tissue without normal connections to the pulmonary arteries or tracheobronchial tree. This multicystic tissue, composed of poorly developed alveoli and airways, is supplied by a systemic artery from the thoracic or abdominal aorta. It is usually associated with the lower lobes (left more frequently than right) and may be intralobar (usually surrounded by normal lung tissue) or, less commonly, extralobar (separate from normal lung, with its own pleural covering). Sequestration may present with recurrent or chronic localized pulmonary infection or as an incidental finding of cystic or consolidated density on chest x-ray. The anatomy can be defined by bronchography and aortography. When infection occurs, there is usually some connection between the sequestration and surrounding airways.

After the diagnosis is confirmed, the sequestered tissue should be surgically removed. Care should be taken to avoid severing one of the related systemic arteries.

The prognosis following surgery is good.

INFANTILE LOBAR EMPHYSEMA (Congenital Lobar Emphysema)

Infantile lobar emphysema refers to progressive overdistention of lung, usually a single lobe, producing respiratory distress within the first 6 months of life—especially during the first 2 weeks. Chest x-ray reveals a hyperinflated area with poorly defined borders, mediastinal shift, and compression of other lung tissue. The upper lobes and right middle lobe are most commonly involved. There is usually no identifiable causative large airway obstruction, but aberrant or large pulmonary arteries (especially associated with large left-to-right shunt), mucus plugs, foreign body, and other causes of intrinsic and extrinsic large airway narrowing (see above) should be considered. The respiratory distress typically progresses rapidly over several days or a few weeks, necessitating lobectomy.

Surgery is probably not indicated in patients who are asymptomatic or have only mild and intermittent symptoms. After surgery, there may be intermittent cough and wheezing with no evidence of hyperinflation, but 10% of the patients may develop hyperinflation of another lobe.

PULMONARY CYSTS

Pulmonary cysts can be congenital or acquired; associated with the trachea or main bronchi (ie, extrapulmonary) or with the smaller airways or alveoli (ie, intrapulmonary); and symptomatic or asymptomatic. Distinguishing between congenital and acquired (usually postinfectious) causes may be difficult but is crucial, since surgery is indicated in the former category and generally contraindicated in the latter. The differential diagnosis of pulmonary cysts includes congenital cysts, cystadenomatoid malformation, pneumatoceles, lung abscess, sequestration, loculated pyopneumothorax, and infantile lobar emphysema.

CONGENITAL CYSTS

Congenital extrapulmonary cysts (bronchogenic cysts) usually present with cough and wheezing due to external irritation and compression of the airway. Congenital intrapulmonary cysts present with increasing respiratory distress, with manifestations of secondary infection, or as incidental findings on chest x-ray.

ACQUIRED PULMONARY CYSTS

Pneumatocele

Pneumatoceles are round or oval radiolucencies with thin, well-demarcated borders that appear on chest x-ray during the course of pneumonia, most commonly staphylococcal or measles pneumonia, though pneumonia due to other causes listed on p 318 may also be associated with pneumatocele. Pneumatocele is characterized by sudden onset, rapid changes in extent and site of pulmonary involvement, and a tendency toward rapid resolution, although it may persist for several months.

Conservative therapy is indicated and consists of pulmonary percussion and drainage and appropriate antibiotic therapy for the primary pneumonia. Bronchoscopic or surgical treatment is indicated only in rare cases where the pneumatocele becomes infected and fills with purulent material or is life-threatening because of its size or location.

The prognosis for eventual complete resolution is excellent.

Lung Abscess

Abscess may occur in several sites in the lung (especially in chronic lung disease such as cystic fibrosis) or at a single site. It may be a complication of bacterial pneumonia (especially due to staphylococci, *Klebsiella,* or pneumococci), secondary to aspiration of a foreign body or infected material, secondary to penetrating chest trauma, or due to infection of pulmonary sequestration, pneumatocele, or congenital cyst. There is usually a rapid onset of fever, dyspnea, cough, chest pain, and leukocytosis. The abscess may contain some air if it communicates with the airway. If the abscess is in peripheral lung tissue, there may be a pleural reaction, and rupture may occur into the pleural space, producing empyema and a bronchopleural fistula.

Treatment includes appropriate parenteral antibiotics, vigorous pulmonary physical therapy, and bronchoscopy to recover material for culture, to rule out foreign body aspiration, and to drain the abscess. If there is no significant improvement after about 1 month of optimal therapy (repeated bronchoscopy may be necessary), lobectomy should be considered. With vigorous optimal therapy and in the absence of underlying disease, the prognosis is good for complete recovery.

PULMONARY TUBERCULOSIS*

Infection with *Mycobacterium tuberculosis* results in a lifelong relationship between the host (humans) and the tubercle bacillus; dormant organisms are alive in the host for years but are kept under control by the host's defense mechanisms. The organisms remain capable of "reactivating" and causing a progressive, potentially life-threatening disease known as tuberculosis. Therapy can alter the host-organism relationship in favor of the host, whether infected or diseased.

Tuberculosis is a contagious disease transmitted by coughing that produces droplets containing organisms that are inhaled by noninfected persons. The disease is most commonly transmitted by adults with cavitary pulmonary lesions. Children are infected by close contact with such a person, usually a relative. Children rarely transmit infection to others. When an infected child is detected, it is imperative to do a thorough contact investigation to find the index case (usually an adult) so that spread of infection to others can be stopped.

Atypical mycobacteria have been shown to cause drug-resistant cervical adenitis and skin lesions (swimming pool granuloma). Children with these infections may have a positive reaction in the tuberculin skin test, but more commonly the reaction is equivocal ($<$ 9 mm of induration). Pulmonary or disseminated disease rarely occurs and is usually related to underlying immune deficiencies.

Types

Disease following initial infection, the most common form in children, varies from that seen in reactivation, which occurs uncommonly in children under 10 years of age but may occur in adolescents.

A. Initial Infection (Primary Complex): The initial infection consists of a peripheral lung lesion usually in the lower lobes or the base of the upper lobes, with involvement of the lymphatics draining the area and enlargement of the regional (hilar) lymph nodes.

B. Progressive Disease: The initial lesion often heals spontaneously, but the disease may progress with the following results: (1) direct extension to adjacent lung tissue, causing tuberculous pneumonitis; (2) erosion into the bronchus with seeding of distal lung (endobronchial disease); (3) extrinsic pressure on the bronchus from a large node, which may cause collapse of lung tissue; and (4) lymphohematogenous spread to both lungs (miliary pulmonary tuberculosis), pleura, bone, kidney, or brain, with spread to the brain causing meningitis or tuberculoma.

C. Reactivation: Reactivation of dormant disease usually causes slowly progressive apical pulmonary lesions with no lymph node in-

*Revised with the assistance of C. Henry Kempe, MD, and James W. Bass, MD (COL, MC, USA).

volvement. Fibrosis and calcification occur as healing proceeds. Cavitation is common if the disease progresses.

Clinical Findings

Most initial infection is found during tuberculin skin testing where the reactivity has changed from negative to positive. Most children are tested routinely or in relationship to a history of exposure to an adult with active tuberculosis. The presence of a positive result in the tuberculin skin test and the demonstration of tubercle bacilli in gastric washings confirm the diagnostic impression obtained by x-ray examination.

A. Symptoms: Initial infection in children often is asymptomatic. Symptoms are nonspecific but include fatigue, malaise, low-grade fever, anorexia, and weight loss. Cough is not a common symptom of tuberculosis in children.

B. Signs:

1. Primary lesion–No pulmonary signs are found if the lesion is small even if mediastinal lymphadenopathy is marked.

2. Tuberculous pneumonitis–Tuberculous pneumonitis may be a segmental lesion of the collapse-consolidation type or progressive pneumonitis with cavitation. Minimal physical findings or symptoms may occur, with extensive pulmonary disease seen on x-ray.

3. Miliary infection or disseminated disease–Findings on pulmonary examination are usually normal. The patient may have irregular spiking fevers, extreme toxemia, malaise, and splenomegaly.

C. Laboratory Findings: The white blood cell count may be normal. Leukopenia or leukocytosis may occur. Erythrocyte sedimentation rate is commonly elevated during tuberculous activity. It is usually necessary to isolate acid-fast organisms from gastric washings, since infants and children swallow rather than expectorate sputum. Gastric washings should be collected in the morning before the patient arises and then concentrated and cultured. Three specimens on 3 separate days are recommended. The yield of positive results is low. Where drug resistance is suspected or the clinical circumstances allow, more vigorous efforts should be attempted to culture organisms from gastric aspirates. Other specimens (eg, spinal fluid, biopsy material) should be carefully cultured for tuberculosis where this diagnosis is suspect.

D. X-Ray Findings: Serial chest x-rays are the most important single method for following the course of the disease.

1. Tuberculous pneumonitis–Tuberculous pneumonitis, the early x-ray manifestation of pulmonary tuberculosis, may involve all or part of a lobe. It is always accompanied by lymphadenopathy and sometimes by pleural thickening and pleural effusion. There is a diffuse infiltrative lesion that is indistinguishable from pneumonitis due to other bacteria or other causes except for striking lymphadenopathy.

2. Healing–There may be complete resorption of the exudate and disappearance of the lymphadenopathy without residual scarring. Fibrosis and calcification of the primary lesion and lymph nodes (Ghon complex), as well as pleural thickening, may occur.

3. Miliary infection or disseminated disease–Miliary tuberculosis cannot be seen on x-ray in its earliest stages. As the disease progresses, small, nodular densities throughout the lungs appear as a faint stippling. Later, the small nodules coalesce, producing larger nodular densities scattered throughout the lung fields and giving the characteristic "rice grain" or "snowflake" appearance. (This may be indistinguishable from the picture produced by pertussis pneumonitis, Löffler's pneumonia, coccidioidomycosis, histoplasmosis, metastatic tumor, hemosiderosis, berylliosis, or pulmonary alveolar microlithiasis.)

4. Reactivation–Apical lesions usually occur with reactivation tuberculosis but are quite uncommon with primary tuberculosis. Hilar lymphadenopathy may not be demonstrable. Cavitation is infrequent in the pediatric age group.

Complications of Primary Tuberculosis

Complications include pleural effusion, disseminated (miliary) tuberculosis, tuberculous meningitis, tuberculosis of the bones and joints or of the kidneys, and tuberculous cervical lymphadenitis.

Treatment

A. General Measures: Except for acute symptomatic illness or diagnostic work-up, it is unnecessary to hospitalize the child with tuberculosis. Bed rest is not indicated. Nutrition consists of the normal diet for the child's age. Clinical aids in following the course of disease include monitoring the temperature, the child's general condition (including the presence or absence of malaise and changes in weight), sedimentation rate, and serial chest x-rays.

B. Antituberculosis Drugs:

1. Primary drugs–Primary drugs used for treating tuberculosis in children are as follows:

a. Isoniazid (INH), 10–20 mg/kg/d orally, usually up to 300 mg/d. (Up to 500 mg/d may be necessary in some cases.)

b. Rifampin, 10–20 mg/kg/d orally to a maximum of 600 mg/d.

c. Streptomycin, 20–40 mg/kg/d intramuscularly to a maximum of 1000 mg/d.

d. Ethambutol, 15 mg/kg/d orally to a maximum of 1500 mg/d.

2. Other drugs–Other antituberculosis drugs that may be substituted when drug resistance to primary antituberculosis drugs is present include:

a. Aminosalicylic acid (PAS), 200 mg/kg/d orally to a maximum of 12 g/d.

b. Ethionamide, 10–20 mg/kg/d orally to a maximum of 1000 mg/d

c. Pyrazinamide, 15–30 mg/kg/d orally to a maximum of 2000 mg/d.

C. Specific Measures: The pretreatment work-up may include the tuberculin skin test, gastric specimens for culture, an early morning urine specimen for culture, x-rays of the chest (posteroanterior and lateral), and examination of pleural and spinal fluid as appropriate.

1. Positive tuberculin reaction–Infants, children, adolescents, and young adults up to 35 years of age who have a positive reaction in the tuberculin test should be treated with INH for 12 months.

2. Primary tuberculosis–For treatment of children with primary tuberculosis (ie, those with abnormal x-ray findings or progressive lesions), 2 drugs, usually INH and rifampin, should be given for 12–24 months. If the immediate response is unsatisfactory or the disease is extensive, streptomycin should be added to the treatment regimen and continued for 1 month.

3. Extrapulmonary tuberculosis–For treatment of patients with extrapulmonary tuberculosis, a minimum of 2 drugs should be used, usually INH and rifampin.

a. Miliary infection including tuberculosis meningitis–Streptomycin, 20–40 mg/kg/d intramuscularly to a maximum of 1 g/d, should be added as a third drug to the treatment regimen and continued for 1 month. Duration of INH and rifampin treatment should be 18–24 months.

b. Superficial lymph node infection–Surgical excision may be necessary if response to the antituberculosis drug regimen is unsatisfactory. Excision is the treatment of choice for node disease caused by atypical mycobacteria.

c. Skeletal and renal infection–Patients with these infections may also be treated with a combination of INH plus ethambutol or INH plus PAS. Skeletal infections should be treated for 12–18 months and renal tuberculosis for 24 months.

d. Bone and joint infection–Patients with these infections should be treated for 18–24 months. The necessity for immobilization of involved joints is in question. Current studies suggest it is not necessary. Surgery is reserved for improving joint function or reversing cord compression and may include drainage of superficial and accessible abscesses.

e. Meningitis–Streptomycin, 20–40 mg/kg/d intramuscularly to a maximum of 1 g/d, should be added to the treatment regimen and continued until 1 month after a satisfactory clinical response. Other antituberculosis drugs should be continued for a full course.

4. Reactivation tuberculosis–For treatment of patients with reactivation tuberculosis, a 2- or 3-drug regimen for 2 years after sputum culture conversion is best. INH, PAS, rifampin, and ethambutol are the drugs of choice. If the tuberculosis is resistant to INH or other drugs, these drugs should not be used. Drug susceptibility studies are helpful to determine the best drugs. Cycloserine, ethionamide, pyrazinamide, capreomycin, viomycin, and kanamycin are useful drugs in drug-resistant tuberculosis.

5. Use of steroids–In treatment of patients with tuberculosis, prednisone, 1 mg/kg/d orally to a maximum of 60 mg/d, may be useful under the following circumstances:

a. Endobronchial disease–Use for 6–12 weeks.

b. Miliary tuberculosis–Use only during periods of extreme dyspnea.

c. Pleurisy with effusion–Use until effusion is controlled. Steroids may reduce immediate morbidity.

d. Acute pericardial effusion with tamponade–Use until effusion is controlled.

e. Meningitis–Use for 6–12 weeks is strongly recommended.

D. Epidemiologic Considerations:

1. Contagion–Children with primary tuberculosis generally are noncontagious and may return to regular activities when clinical symptoms have disappeared and effective chemotherapy has been started.

2. Examination of contacts–Identification of contacts is imperative. The local health department should be notified so that effective and complete case-finding can be carried out. This should proceed from the immediate household contacts to more peripheral contacts including relatives, baby-sitters, school personnel, etc. Skin testing should be done and chest x-rays obtained on all positive reactors. Exposed tuberculin-negative children should be skin tested every 2 months for 6 months after contact has been terminated.

3. Skin testing–Routine skin testing of all tuberculin-negative children should be done as recommended by the American Academy of Pediatrics: prior to administration of the measles immunization at approximately 15 months of age and thereafter as determined by community risk. We feel that testing at school entry and at adolescence is wise as a minimal control measure. If a child has no reaction to 0.001 mg of purified protein derivative (PPD) or its equivalent, there is little possibility of tuberculosis. However, there is considerable skin test cross-reactivity between *Mycobacterium tuberculosis* and members of the atypical mycobacterial group in some geographic areas.

4. Risk factors–Persons at risk for developing tuberculosis include infants born of mothers with tuberculosis; infants and children under 3 years of age, in whom the complications of disseminated disease and meningitis are more likely to occur; and adolescents (especially young girls at the time of menarche), in whom reactivation or more severe progressive disease is noted.

E. Prophylaxis:

1. BCG vaccination–Use of BCG (see Chapter 7) is an attempt to artificially stimulate immunity against tuberculosis. It may be administered by the intradermal route and usually results in the appearance of a positive result in the tuberculin test. The use of BCG in pediatric practice is limited to tuberculin-negative children living in areas where there is a high incidence of tuberculosis or in households where the risk of exposure to tuberculosis is high.

2. Chemoprophylaxis–Preventive treatment has been recommended by many for all children and adolescents who have positive results in the Mantoux test but no manifest disease. Treatment with INH for 1 year has been shown to significantly reduce the risk of developing future active disease.

3. Protection of newborn infants at risk–Infants born to mothers with active tuberculosis are highly likely to become infected unless protection is provided. They should be separated from the mother until she is considered noncontagious. The infant should receive prophylactic INH until the mother's tuberculosis is well controlled and it is certain that she is no longer contagious. If compliance in INH prophylaxis is considered doubtful, the infant should be vaccinated with BCG as soon after birth as possible. The BCG vaccine should not be given to any infant with acquired or congenital immunologic deficiency.

16 | Gastrointestinal Tract*

There are, in pediatrics, many diseases that do not specifically involve the gastrointestinal tract but that may have presenting manifestations referable to the digestive system. These symptoms frequently require the immediate attention of the physician. The underlying cause may not be immediately apparent.

ANOREXIA

Anorexia may occur as a passing phase of normal development (Spock's "anorexia of runabouts") or may be a presenting manifestation of almost any acute febrile illness and of some chronic illnesses. Most frequently, and especially when protracted, it is of psychogenic origin.

Treatment

A. Physiologic Anorexia: In physiologic anorexia accompanying an acute or chronic illness, avoid overenthusiastic forcing of fluids, especially in the acute phase of illness. Give the usual minimum daily requirements of vitamins for the age group.

B. Psychologic Anorexia:

1. The physician and the parents should have a clear understanding of psychologic mechanisms. The parents' definition of "lack of appetite" must be determined and clarified, and parents should be encouraged to discuss their interpretation of the symptom.
2. Careful history and physical examination should allow the physician to assure the parents that no organic disease exists. Reassure with regard to weight gain.
3. Parents should offer a normal diet at regular mealtimes and depend upon the child's nutritional needs to "dictate" his or her appetite. There should be no coaxing, bribing, or threatening and no insistence on a special diet or special foods.
4. Excess intake of milk should be avoided; 1 pint per day is adequate for most children over 1 year of age.

*Revised with the assistance of John R. Lilly, MD.

5. Small feedings of fruit or crackers may be given between meals, without comment or discussion.

6. Psychiatric consultation is indicated only for persistent or severe cases.

RECURRENT ABDOMINAL PAIN

Recurrent abdominal pain is frequent in children. It may result from a number of conditions but is most commonly a manifestation of functional gastrointestinal illness with a varied and erratic history. Extensive diagnostic investigations have shown that significant abdominal disease is present in fewer than 8% of cases of this syndrome. Recurrences usually diminish or disappear during puberty. Pain seems to be precipitated by emotional stress. The pain may be of varied intensity and duration and is frequently associated with headache, pallor, nausea, vomiting, constipation, dizziness, and anorexia. There may be tenderness on deep palpation over varying sections of the abdomen. Results of laboratory and x-ray examinations are usually normal. Proctoscopic examination may reveal mucosal pallor, prominent vascular markings, dilated rectal lumen, and lymphoid hyperplasia. Various behavioral disturbances may occur.

The child is often described as being "very good," sensitive, insecure, and very close to other members of the family. Treatment is primarily directed toward a clearer understanding of the psychologic factors involved in producing the symptoms. The multiple diagnostic studies often required must be carefully managed to minimize the development of preoccupation with illness by both parents and child. Restriction of lactose ingestion should be tried.

VOMITING

(See Table 16–1.)

Vomiting is a common symptom throughout childhood and may be associated with a wide variety of diseases of all degrees of severity. A serious disease must always be considered if vomiting is protracted or severe.

The presence of other cases of vomiting or diarrhea (or both) in the family and community may have diagnostic significance.

Physical examination should emphasize the ears, throat, and chest in a search for infectious processes. Examination of the abdomen should include auscultation, which may show the high-pitched, tinkling diastolic sounds associated with intestinal obstruction. Central nervous system infection (see Chapter 25) may first manifest itself by vomiting.

Treatment is discussed below.

Table 16–1. Causes, characteristics, and treatment of vomiting.

Cause	Usual Age Group	Appears Ill	Relation to Intake	Fever	Diarrhea	Treatment*
Acute infectious diseases ("parenteral vomiting"), almost any disease with fever at onset, pertussis	< 10 yr	Moderately to severely	Immediate	Yes	Occasional in younger children	Treat specific disease. Nothing by mouth, then liquid diet, and finally soft diet.
Central nervous system disorder						
Acute meningitis	All ages	Severely	None	Yes	Occasional in younger children	Treat specific disease. Parenteral fluids.
Expansile lesions, tumor, hematoma, edema	All ages	Moderately	None	No	None	Surgery and parenteral fluids.
Motion sickness	All ages	Mildly	Immediate	No	None	Meclizine sedation (see dosage in Appendix).†
Epidemic vomiting (viral)‡	All ages	Mildly	Varies	Yes	Occasional	Restrict intake. Liquid diet, then soft diet.†
Obstruction of gastrointestinal tract						
Appendicitis or Meckel's diverticulitis	All ages	Moderately	None	Yes	Occasional	Surgery.*
Congenital anomalies	Infants	No	Varies	No	None	Surgery.*
Ileus with peritonitis	All ages	Severely	None	Yes	Yes	Chemotherapy, surgery, or both.
Pyloric stenosis	2–8 wk	No	Varies	No	None	Surgery.*
Physiologic; faulty feeding technique	Infants	No	Immediate	No	None	Instruct mother (see Chapter 4).

Specific enteric infection‡ Bacterial: Salmonellae, shigellae, enteropathogenic or enterotoxigenic Viral: Epidemic vomiting and diarrhea virus, reoviruses	All ages	Moderately	Immediate	Usual	Usual	Nothing by mouth, then liquid diet, then soft diet. Chemotherapy in salmonellae and shigellae infections.
Toxic vomiting						
Diabetic acidosis	All ages	Severely	None	No	None	Treat diabetes (see Chapter 22).
Food poisoning‡ (See Table 16–4.)						
Poisoning	All ages	Moderately	None	No	Occasional	See Chapter 31.

*For details of treatment, see under specific disease or infection in this chapter.

†Chlorpromazine suppository.

‡Check for other cases in family or community.

REGURGITATION IN INFANCY
(Physiologic Vomiting or Chalasia)

(See Table 16–1.)

Partial regurgitation or return of ingested milk or food from the stomach during or shortly after feeding ("spitting up") is considered regurgitation rather than vomiting, in which a large portion of the stomach contents is expelled. Regurgitation probably occurs in over half of infants in the first 6 months of life, particularly active infants, and it may accompany the colic syndrome (see p 351).

Treatment involves minor modifications of feeding techniques with emphasis on adequate expulsion of swallowed air during and after eating and avoidance of loud noises and excitement during feeding. Placing the infant in the crib on the right side with the head slightly elevated may also be useful. Excessive crying before feeding may result in a large amount of swallowed air and will stimulate regurgitation. In persistent cases where large volumes are regurgitated, it may help to keep the infant in a semi-upright position for about an hour after feeding.

Complications of aspiration pneumonia and poor weight gain are extremely rare. The prognosis is good for relief by 6 months of age.

RECURRENT (CYCLIC) VOMITING

Recurrent cyclic vomiting is a syndrome characterized by recurrent attacks of violent vomiting without apparent cause, sometimes associated with headache and abdominal pain. A family history of migraine is frequently obtained. The onset is sudden, and all types of food, including water, will be vomited during a period of several hours to several days. Dehydration and electrolyte depletion, together with starvation ketosis, must be treated with intravenous fluids. Sedation may be of value.

Differential diagnosis must exclude other causes of vomiting (see Table 16–1).

DIARRHEA

(See Tables 16–2, 16–3, and 16–4.)

Diarrhea is a common symptom in children. In the infant under 2 years of age, it may be the first or only symptom of a very serious infection such as pneumonia, sepsis, or meningitis. The physician should always consider diarrhea a serious symptom and must begin general treatment measures as soon as results of diagnostic studies are obtained. Because a simple, mild diarrhea may gradually become se-

Table 16–2. Causes, characteristics, and treatment of noninfectious diarrhea.

Cause	Age	Stool Examination	Symptoms	Treatment
Acrodermatitis enteropathica	1 yr	Profuse and watery, with mucus.	See Chapter 12.	See Chapter 12.
Allergy				
Cow's milk allergy	6 mo	Stool watery, with mucus; eosinophils on smear.	Cramping stools with each feeding.	Eliminate cow's milk from diet (see text).*
Other food allergy	6 mo	Stool watery, with mucus; eosinophils on smear.	Cramping; symptoms associated with new food in diet.	Eliminate food causing allergy.
Celiac syndrome*	5 yr	See text.*	Abdominal distention, failure to thrive.	See text.*
Irritable colon	3 yr	Watery, with mucus and undigested food.	May follow fright, other illness, or painful injury.	Dietary management; liquid diet, then soft diet, then regular diet.
Malrotation or stenosis of large or small bowel	3 mo	Profuse and watery, often with blood.	Vomiting, cramping, abdominal distention.	Surgery (see text).*
Nonspecific enterocolitis	4 mo	Watery.	Profuse cramping; vomiting common.	Parenteral fluids.
Parenteral infection (otitis, sepsis, urinary tract infection)	2 yr	Soft to runny, with little mucus.	Symptoms relate to underlying disease.	Treat primary disease.
Regional enteritis (Crohn's disease)	2 yr	With blood and mucus.	Cramping; see text.*	See text.*
Starvation or malnutrition	1½ yr	Soft to runny, with little water.	Failure to thrive, weakness, apathy.	Dietary management; attention.
Ulcerative colitis	2 yr	Loose, with blood; often nocturnal.	See text.*	See text.*

*See under specific disease or infection in this chapter.

vere, the patient should be under careful observation. If the child is being kept at home, parents should be instructed to observe and report the child's progress.

In addition to the findings presented in Tables 16–2 and 16–3, the following information should be routinely obtained: (1) Duration, frequency, and description (consistency and color) of diarrheal stools. The parents may interpret a watery stool as urine. (2) Incidence and character of vomiting and its relation to the ingestion of food. (3) Incidence,

Table 16–3. Causes, characteristics, and treatment of infectious gastroenteritis.

Cause	Source	Incubation Period	Stool Examination	Symptoms	Treatment
Bacteria (invasive)					
Campylobacter fetus	Carrier, ?poultry.	2–7 d	Watery, with mucus.	Cramps, diarrhea, nausea.	Erythromycin.
Salmonellae	Carrier.	1–2 d	Stool bloody; white blood cells present.	Diarrhea, fever, nausea.	See Chapter 25.
Shigellae	Carrier.	1–3 d	White blood cells present.	Cramps, diarrhea, fever, nausea.	See Chapter 25.
Staphylococcus aureus	Carrier, skin.	Unknown	Watery, with pus.	Cramps, diarrhea.*	Oral neomycin.
Bacteria (toxic)					
Clostridium difficile	Bowel.	Unknown	With mucus.	Cramps, diarrhea, prolonged antibiotic therapy.	Oral vancomycin (see Chapter 6); cholestyramine.†
Vibrio cholerae	Carrier.	6 h–2 d	Profuse and watery.	Diarrhea, fever, epidemic.	See Chapter 25.
Protozoa					
Amebas	Carrier.	Unknown	Bloody. Cysts or trophozoites.‡	Cramps, diarrhea.	See Chapter 26.
Giardia	Carrier.	Unknown	Soft. Cysts or trophozoites.‡	Cramps, diarrhea.	See Chapter 26.
Viruses					
Adenovirus	Airborne.	2–5 d	With mucus.	See Chapter 24.	Fluid and electrolyte replacement.
Parvovirus, enterovirus, calicivirus	Carrier, fecal-oral route.	1–3 d	Watery, with mucus.	Diarrhea, vomiting.	Fluid and electrolyte replacement.
Rotavirus	Carrier, fecal-oral route.	2–3 d	Watery, with pus and blood.	Diarrhea, fever, vomiting, respiratory infection, age < 5 yr.	Fluid and electrolyte replacement.

*Commonly in association with prolonged antibiotic therapy or debility due to any cause.

†See p 349.

‡Detection may be difficult.

Table 16–4. Causes, characteristics, and treatment of acute foodborne gastroenteritis (food poisoning).

Cause	Source	Mechanism of Action	Incubation Period	Symptoms	Treatment
Bacillus cereus	Contaminated food.	Emetic and necrotizing toxins are produced.	1–12 h	Abrupt onset of vomiting and cramping; diarrhea follows; symptoms continue for 24 h.	Treatment nonspecific.
Clostridium botulinum	Anaerobic nonacid foods canned or processed at 115 °C (239 °F).	Absorbed toxin blocks neuromuscular junction.	24–96 h	See Chapter 25.	See Chapter 25.
Clostridium perfringens	Meat preparations.	Enterotoxin causes hypersecretion of fluid in small bowel.	8–18 h	Abrupt onset of profuse diarrhea; occasional vomiting.	Fluid and electrolyte replacement.
Escherichia coli	Contaminated food.	Organism grows in intestinal tract; toxin causes hypersecretion of fluid in small bowel.	24–72 h	Abrupt onset of diarrhea; rare vomiting.	Fluid and electrolyte replacement required in small infants. Neomycin, 100 mg/kg/d in 3 doses, may be useful. Dietary management.
Staphylococci	Meats, dairy products, gravy, cream preparations.	Enterotoxin produced in food acts on intestinal receptors that transmit to medulla.	1–18 h	Abrupt onset of violent vomiting; vomiting continues for 48 h. Occurs in groups eating same food.	Fluid and electrolyte replacement occasionally indicated.
Vibrio parahaemolyticus	Fish, shellfish, crabs.	Toxin causes hypersecretion of fluid in small bowel.	6–96 h	Abrupt onset of diarrhea; diarrhea continues for 1–3 d and is sometimes bloody. Occurs in groups eating same food.	Treatment nonspecific.

Table 16–5. Differential diagnosis of rectal bleeding in infants and children.

Cause	Usual Age Group	Additional Chief Complaints	Amount of Blood	Type of Blood	Blood With Movement	Treatment
Allergy	Infants	Colicky abdominal pain.	Moderate to large	Dark or bright	Yes	Eliminate allergen.
Anal fissure or proctitis	< 2 yr	Pain.	Small	Bright	No	Soften stool; anal dilatation; habit training.
Bacterial enteritis	All ages	Diarrhea, cramps.	Small	Usually bright	Yes	See Chapter 25.
Duplication of bowel	All ages	Variable.	Usually small	Usually dark	Yes	Surgery.
Esophageal varices	> 4 yr	Signs of portal hypertension.	Variable	Usually dark	Yes	Acute: medical. Portal hypertension: surgery.
Hemangioma or telangiectasia	All ages	Usually none.	Variable	Dark or bright	Yes or no	None.
Hemorrhagic disease of the newborn	Newborns	Other evidences of blood.	Variable	Dark or bright	Yes or no	Vitamin K, transfusion.
Idiopathic	All ages	Variable.	Variable	Dark or bright	Yes or no	Surgery for diagnosis; vitamin K, transfusion.
Inserted foreign body	Children	Pain.	Small	Bright	No	Removal.
Intussusception	< 18 mo	Abdominal pain; mass.	Small to large	Dark or bright	Yes	Barium enema or surgery.
Meckel's diverticulum	Young children	None or anemia.	Small to large	Dark or bright	Yes or no	Surgery.
Peptic ulcer	All ages	Abdominal pain.	Usually small	Dark	Yes	Bland diet.
Swallowed foreign body	All ages	Usually none.	Small	Dark	Yes	None.
Swallowed maternal blood	Newborns	None.	Variable	Dark	Yes	None.
Systemic blood disease	All ages	Other evidences of blood.	Variable	Dark or bright	Yes or no	As indicated.
Volvulus	Infants or young children	Abdominal pain, intestinal obstruction.	Small to large	Dark or bright	Yes or no	Surgery.

volume, and frequency of urination. Dehydration will decrease the volume and frequency of urination, and more severe dehydration will cause urination to cease. (4) Estimate of weight loss. In the infant or young child, weighing at the onset of diarrhea will provide an index with which subsequent weights can be compared. (5) Incidence of other cases of diarrhea or vomiting in the family, nursery, or school.

Examine the abdomen for tenderness, either localized or generalized, and abnormal masses. Examine rectally for further localization.

For treatment, see Tables 16–2 and 16–3.

GENERAL SYMPTOMATIC TREATMENT MEASURES FOR VOMITING & DIARRHEA

(See Tables 16–1, 16–2, and 16–3.)

General Considerations

The young child loses more weight through vomiting and diarrhea than from a marked reduction in caloric intake when on a controlled diet. For purposes of treatment, all cases of vomiting or diarrhea should be assumed to require strict control of diet. Fats and cereal starches aggravate early cases of diarrhea or vomiting and should not be given for at least 24 hours. Lactose intolerance is common. Symptomatic medications (see below) are secondary to diet control in therapy.

Avoid overuse of fluids or foods containing salt; hypernatremia may result. Exclusive intake of water may produce hyponatremia.

The electrolyte status of infants and small children with diarrhea or vomiting should always be followed carefully in the laboratory when these facilities are available (see Chapter 5).

Treatment Methods

A. Parenteral Fluid Therapy: Parenteral fluid therapy (see Chapter 5) is indicated in the following circumstances: (1) if vomiting or weakness prevents oral therapy; (2) in the presence of shock due to severe dehydration and acidosis; or (3) if surgical procedures are contemplated.

B. Oral Glucose/Electrolyte Therapy: Patients of all ages, if strong enough to drink and not vomiting, will ingest a volume of a glucose/electrolyte mixture sufficient to produce rehydration and maintenance. Stool output may increase temporarily.

1. Glucose/electrolyte mixture–Mix 3.5 g of sodium chloride, 2.5 g of sodium bicarbonate, 1.5 g of potassium chloride, 20 g of glucose, and enough water to make 1 L. Sucrose (cane sugar) may be used if glucose is not available.

2. Dosage–Give up to 20 mL/kg/h. (Adult dosage is 750–1000 mL/h.)

C. Liquid Diet: Introduce a liquid diet when diarrhea and vomiting subside. If the diet is tolerated without increase in symptoms, proceed to a soft, low-residue diet (see D, below).

1. Lytren solution–Give on the basis of daily maintenance requirements for fluid (see Table 5–3) plus replacement of losses due to diarrhea (see p 77).

2. Grape or apple juice–Mix 500 mL of juice, 500 mL of water, and ½ teaspoon of table salt.

3. Orange juice–Mix 250 mL of juice, ½ teaspoon of table salt, 1–2 oz of corn syrup, and enough water to make 1 L.

4. Dosage–***Caution:*** Give no more than 150 mL/kg/d (68 mL/lb/d) of the above juices.

D. Soft, Low-Residue Diet: This diet should be appropriate for age and dietary preference. The following are suggested: gelatin desserts; frozen, fruit-flavored ice sticks or sherbets; segments of fresh orange or grapefruit; carbonated beverages; clear soups, bouillon, or clear chicken broth without fat; and custards.

1. Infants–Apple purée, 2–4 tablespoons as desired (not oftener than every 2 hours), is an excellent way of providing pectin, which is often effective in relieving diarrhea. Other sources of pectin include bananas, pears, cranberries, lemons, grapefruits, and various jellies. The diet may also include crushed ripe banana or prepared banana flakes, 2–4 tablespoons every 4 hours. Boiled skimmed milk in a quantity equal to that of regular formula may be tried. **Note:** Temporary lactose intolerance is common following severe diarrhea.

2. Children age 1 and over–The diet may include any item mentioned above, plus boiled egg, toast or soda crackers, whole ripe bananas, puréed vegetables and fruits, lean meats, and custards and puddings.

E. Specific Symptomatic Therapy:

1. Suspension of kaolin–This is best used as diarrhea subsides. Give 30–60 g/d in 4–6 doses.

2. Paregoric (camphorated tincture of opium)–This is not tolerated in a young child with vomiting; it is sometimes useful in an older child with diarrhea and tenesmus. Because of the danger of "masking" a surgical condition, paregoric should never be used if this possibility exists. The dosage varies with age: 0.2 mL per month of age every 6 hours for infants up to 1 year of age; 2–4 mL every 6 hours for children 1–10 years of age; and 5–10 mL every 6 hours for children over 10 years of age.

3. Diphenoxylate with atropine (Lomotil)–Do not use in patients under 2 years of age. For patients 2–12 years of age, use liquid preparation as follows: 2–5 years, 2 mg (4 mL) 3 times daily; 5–8 years, 4 mL 4 times daily; and 8–12 years, 4 mL 5 times daily.

4. Cholestyramine–Cholestyramine (Questran), a resin that absorbs bile acids, has been reported to be highly effective in persistent or chronic diarrhea in infants and small children refractory to other treatment. It contains 4 mEq of sodium per gram of resin, and hypernatremia is a risk in prolonged therapy (see Chapter 5). Give 2–15 g/d in divided doses for 5–7 days. Mix powder in water or other liquid.

5. Sedatives–Use of sedatives is especially valuable in the older child with vomiting, when it is best given by rectal route. Do not overlook the possibility of a surgical condition.

6. Vitamin K–Infants with prolonged severe diarrhea may require supplemental vitamin K.

F. Gastric Lavage: In patients with toxic vomiting, give sodium bicarbonate, 1 teaspoon in 4 oz of warm water. If lavage is not available, encourage emesis by pharyngeal stimulation after giving sodium bicarbonate solution to drink.

G. Rectal Fluid Therapy: Use 5% glucose in saline, as for parenteral route. For use at home, prepare a glucose-saline solution. Give 2–4 oz every 2–4 hours. Use a rubber bulb type of syringe (ear syringe). Do not give plain water.

CONSTIPATION

Constipation refers to the character of the stool rather than to the frequency of defecation. Constipated stools are hard, dry, and small. In infants, they may occur 1–3 times per day. The normal breast-fed infant may go as long as 7 days without a bowel movement and not be constipated. Older children, especially boys, are loath to report failure of evacuation each day and may become severely constipated without the parents' knowledge.

Etiology

A. Diet: In infants, constipation may result from too little carbohydrate or fat in formula, inadequate bulk from fruits and vegetables, or insufficient fluid intake or, more rarely, exclusive milk intake. In older children, daily water intake may be too low.

B. Toilet-Training Faults: Constipation may result from too early stress on toilet training (usually little training is necessary) or too frequent use of suppositories, enemas, and cathartics. In older children, it may be due to failure to develop a regular toilet habit, failure to heed the desire to defecate while engaged in play, or embarrassment in the presence of strangers. Many healthy children produce a normal bowel movement at 2- to 4-day intervals.

C. Disease States: Hypothyroidism, marked anemia, congenital megacolon, and any disease causing fever and dehydration may cause constipation.

D. Mechanical Obstruction: Constipation may be due to mechanical obstruction.

E. Rectal Conditions: These conditions include anal fissure, causing pain on attempted evacuation, and anal or rectal stenosis (especially in infants), requiring excess effort for evacuation.

F. Drugs: Calcium salts, narcotics, and aluminum hydroxide gels tend to produce constipation in children.

Treatment

A. Acute Constipation: When evacuation is desired immediately, use mineral oil, tap water, or normal saline solution, 2–4 oz as retention enema, and await spontaneous evacuation; avoid repeated use. Suppositories of glycerin or soap are valuable in infants but are emotionally traumatic in some children.

B. Chronic Constipation: Dietary measures may be necessary.

1. Young infants–

a. Fluids–Offer plain water or water with approximately 5% carbohydrate 1–3 times daily between feedings.

b. Sugar–Increase sugar content of formula.

c. Molasses–Replace 1 tablespoon of the usual carbohydrate in the formula with 1 tablespoon of molasses.

d. Prune juice–Give 15 mL daily.

e. Stool softeners–Proprietary solutions of dioctyl sodium sulfosuccinate (Colace), 10–20 mg/d, may be employed.

2. Older infants–

a. Fluids–Attempt to increase fluid intake.

b. Fruits–Increase amounts of puréed fruits in the diet, especially prunes and plums. The amount needed will vary with individual infants.

c. Stool softeners–Solutions may be employed (see above).

3. Older children–

a. Fluids–Attempt to increase fluid intake.

b. Fruits–Add prunes, apricots, and figs to the daily diet.

c. Bulk–High-residue substances such as bran, whole wheat, oatmeal, and green leafy vegetables should be a major part of the daily diet.

d. Senokot syrup–Give 1–2 teaspoons twice daily for 2–5 days.

e. Methylcellulose–Giving 0.5 g at bedtime for a few nights may be helpful.

C. Rectal Conditions: Anal or rectal stenosis in infants may be stretched by the physician by means of daily insertion of a well-lubricated rubber-sheathed finger. One such treatment usually suffices. In a patient with anal fissure, a diagnostic rectal examination usually produces temporary relaxation of the anal sphincter sufficient to permit healing. Rarely, silver nitrate cauterization and local anesthetic ointments may be necessary.

COLIC

Colic in small infants is characterized by recurrent abdominal pain and paroxysms of crying. It usually occurs in the firstborn infant, starting at around 10 days of age and lasting through the third month. It is a source of great anxiety for the parents.

Etiology

The causes of colic are probably multiple. The following may be of varying importance in each case:

A. Air: The passage of large bubbles of swallowed air through the intestines of the infant is associated with discomfort. Excess amounts of air may be swallowed if nipple holes are too small (with leakage of air around nipple during sucking) or too big (with gulping of milk and air). When the infant cries, a cyclic pattern may be established: Cry → Swallowed air → Colic → Cry, etc. Air may also be swallowed when the hungry infant sucks on the hands and fingers.

B. Food: Overdistention of the bowel with ingested food will cause pain. This may occur through overfeeding with large volumes of formula as a result of efforts to quiet the infant by giving the infant something to eat. Paradoxically, genuine hunger may initiate this cycle of events.

C. Emotional Factors: Colic occurs most often in a firstborn infant during the first week at home. The hyperactive, tense infant is likely to have colic. Family tension and parental anxiety may be aggravating factors.

D. Allergy: Intestinal allergy to cow's milk, especially in families with a history of clinical allergy in other members, may cause colic. (See symptoms under Allergy in Table 16–2.)

Treatment

In treating colic, the physician must first deal with the acute attack; steps should then be taken to prevent recurrences.

A. Treatment of the Acute Attack:

1. Remove swallowed air from the stomach by holding the infant over the shoulder and "burping" the infant with gentle pats on the back and pressure on the lower abdomen.

2. Soothe the infant to prevent crying and further swallowing of air. "Burp" the infant and try rhythmic movement (rocking, walking, etc). Apply warmth to the abdomen, using a rubber hot water bottle wrapped in soft cloth.

3. Reassure the parents, by examination of the infant, that no serious condition exists.

4. Facilitate passage of air through the bowel by use of a suppository or enema. A small suppository will stimulate bowel movement and

expulsion of air. An enema of 1–2 oz of warm water to produce the same result may be indicated if the suppository fails.

B. Prevention of Further Attacks:

1. Examine the bottle nipples, enlarge any holes that are too small, and discard any with holes that are too large.

2. Evaluate food intake; the infant's needs should be met, and there should be no hunger periods. If the child is not being overfed, more foods may be introduced, such as solids.

3. Adjustment of the formula seldom is successful, and repeated unsuccessful changes of the ingredients usually do not reassure anxious parents. However, elimination of cow's milk may be necessary. Reduction of fat content through use of skimmed milk may be of help. In the breast-fed infant, the mother's supply may not be adequate for the moment and should be supplemented.

4. A pacifier may be of value in some children.

5. Environmental factors should be examined, especially parental attitudes and anxieties, and psychologic assistance for the parents should be given if necessary. Further attacks in the infant may be prevented by reduction of excitement to a minimum, prevention of chilling or overheating, and placement of the infant near repetitive noise (eg, by the vacuum cleaner, running water, radio).

ULCERATIVE COLITIS

Clinical Findings

A. Symptoms and Signs: Onset is most commonly between 10 and 20 years of age but may occur in a child under the age of 2 years. There is a history of insidious onset of recurrent bouts of diarrhea, often bloody and accompanied by cramping abdominal pain. Low-grade fever, anemia, weakness, and weight loss are present. Growth retardation may occur and may be manifest for years prior to the onset of bowel symptoms. A distinctive perirectal ulcerated skin lesion or arthritis may be associated. Proctoscopic examination shows mucosa to be diffusely inflamed, edematous, and often bleeding.

Differentiate from regional enteritis, irritable bowel syndrome, amebiasis, and intestinal allergic disease.

B. Laboratory Findings: Stools show mucus and blood.

C. X-Ray Findings: Barium enema demonstrates loss of normal haustral markings, together with narrowing of the colon. Twenty percent of patients may show normal findings on x-ray.

Treatment

A. General Measures: Institute a high-protein, high-carbohydrate, normal fat, low-residue diet.

B. Specific Measures: Salicylazosulfapyridine (Azulfidine), 0.5–1 g orally 3 times daily with meals, may be given. Sulfapyridine is absorbed and must be excreted through the kidney. Toxicity may occur with dehydration and dosage above 4 g/d. Corticotropin and the cortisones may be of temporary value. Rectal instillation of hydrocortisone, 50 mg in 1 dL of saline, may also produce relief.

C. Surgical Measures: Ileostomy or colectomy is indicated in protracted or severe cases.

D. Psychiatric Evaluation: Evaluation of emotional factors associated with attacks may be indicated.

Prognosis

Over half of reported patients have shown either great improvement or eventual cure of the disease. Carcinoma of the colon is found with increasing frequency after 10 years of symptomatic disease.

REGIONAL ENTERITIS
(Crohn's Disease)

Regional enteritis is a chronic inflammatory disease that most commonly involves the terminal ileum but may affect any portion of the intestinal tract from esophagus to rectum. Ulcerative colitis and regional enteritis may occur in the same family. Although regional enteritis is most commonly found after puberty, it has been reported in the first year of life.

Pathologically there is marked thickening of the intestinal submucosa, with lymphoid hyperplasia and ulceration over nonspecific granulomas.

The differential diagnosis includes acute appendicitis, intestinal tuberculosis, ulcerative colitis, amebic colitis, and lymphoma.

Clinical Findings

A. Symptoms and Signs: Cramping abdominal pain, especially in the right lower quadrant, is the most common early symptom, usually stimulated by ingestion of food. Accompanying diarrhea is common. Later in the course of disease, an abdominal mass will be found representing the thickened lower intestine and the adhesive masses of the intestinal loops. Weight loss, fever, and anemia are usually present and may precede the onset of abdominal symptoms. Sigmoidoscopy may show lesions similar to those of ulcerative colitis.

B. Laboratory Findings: Occult blood in the stool, hypochromic anemia, and lowered serum albumin levels are found early.

C. X-Ray Findings: X-ray of the small bowel shows irregular mucosa with ulceration and narrowing of the intestinal lumen.

Treatment

A. General Measures: Give a high-calorie, high-vitamin, low-residue diet, with treatment for hypochromic anemia and dehydration.

B. Specific Measures: Salicylazosulfapyridine (Azulfidine), 0.5–1 g orally 3 times daily with meals, may be helpful. Adrenocortical hormones administered in full dosage on alternate days will be useful in acute exacerbations of the disease.

C. Surgical Measures: Surgery may be necessary to manage perforation of the bowel. Resection of the small bowel may be necessary.

Prognosis

Regional enteritis is chronic and progressive, but the overall mortality rate is low. Intestinal obstruction, perforation, and fistula formation are common complications that impose a surgical risk. With bowel resection, impaired bowel function must be treated.

DISEASES OF THE LIVER

Some of the more important causes of liver disease of childhood are outlined here; reference will be made to other chapters for more detailed discussions.

HEPATOMEGALY
(Enlargement of Liver)

(See Appendix.)

JAUNDICE

(See also Chapter 9 for Jaundice of the Newborn.)

Etiology

A. Regurgitation Types: These types include bile duct obstruction, congenital biliary atresia, parasitic infestation, cirrhosis resulting from late effects of erythroblastosis, liver abscess (pressure on bile duct), and obstruction due to diseases in liver parenchyma. This latter form of obstruction may be due to poisons (including carbon tetrachloride, chloroform, mushrooms, and phosphorus) or infections (viral hepatitis, infectious mononucleosis). (See Chapter 24.)

B. Retention Types: These types include hemolytic diseases (congenital hemolytic anemia, erythroblastosis, Mediterranean anemias, sickle cell anemia, transfusion reaction following use of incompatible blood); septicemia, especially during the newborn period; hepatocellular disease such as viral hepatitis (see Chapter 24); and hepatic immaturity (physiologic jaundice of the newborn).

Laboratory Findings

A. Regurgitation Types: Urine shows absent or normal urobilinogen and increased bilirubin levels (bile foam test). Stool shows decreased or absent urobilinogen levels. Blood shows increased direct bilirubin levels.

B. Retention Types: Urine shows increased urobilinogen or absent bilirubin levels (bile). Stool shows increased urobilinogen levels. Blood shows increased indirect bilirubin levels.

PLASMA CELL HEPATITIS

Plasma cell hepatitis is a syndrome occurring mostly in young girls and characterized by severe, prolonged hepatitis, obesity, amenorrhea, generalized vascular disease, and arthralgia. The serum gamma globulin level is usually elevated. Cortisone may be effective for treatment.

MALABSORPTION DISEASES

"CELIAC SYNDROME"

A number of specific disease entities and some unknown causes can result in the syndrome once referred to as "celiac disease." The principal symptoms are acute crises with severe diarrhea; frequent pale, bulky, foul-smelling stools; failure to gain weight, along with wasting and stunting of growth; and abdominal distention.

The principal malabsorption syndromes are cystic fibrosis, gluten-induced enteropathy, disaccharidase deficiencies, idiopathic steatorrhea, and cow's milk allergy or intolerance.

1. CYSTIC FIBROSIS

Clinical Findings

A. Symptoms and Signs: Meconium ileus may be the initial manifestation in the newborn period, with signs of intestinal obstruction due to thick, claylike meconium. Chronic respiratory disease leading to bronchiectasis and pulmonary fibrosis, with few, if any, gastrointestinal symptoms, may be present. Additional symptoms of cystic fibrosis include prolapse of rectum, a peculiar form of hepatic fibrosis, heat shock due to sodium loss with excessive sweating, and retarded growth. Concentrations of essential fatty acids in the serum are abnormally low in cystic fibrosis, and a metabolic defect in prostaglandins has been postulated.

B. Laboratory Findings: A marked increase in the chloride content of sweat (above 60 mEq/L) is a striking and diagnostic feature of cystic fibrosis and may occur in the absence of any other elements of this disease. Pancreatic enzyme in duodenal juice is obtained by intubation and assayed. In cystic fibrosis, only small amounts may be obtained, and amylase, lipase, and trypsin contents are decreased. Decreased arterial oxygen tension and pulmonary function tests indicating decreased airway are early findings.

C. X-Ray Findings: Chest x-ray findings are normal early but later may show scattered areas of obstructive emphysema, increased density, lung abscesses, bronchiectasis, and bronchial pneumonia. Gastrointestinal series may show delayed emptying time of the stomach and clumping of barium in the ileum and colon. Cor pulmonale may produce characteristic cardiac changes.

Treatment

A long-term treatment regimen must be contemplated, and follow-up is extremely important. Treatment consists of 3 parts:

A. Treatment and Prophylaxis of Pulmonary Infections: The morbidity and mortality due to cystic fibrosis are essentially the result of the pulmonary defect, ie, the excessive, abnormally viscid mucus that impairs the patient's defenses against bacterial infection and causes bronchial obstruction, emphysema, and atelectasis.

1. Antibiotics–Initially, antibiotics in full therapeutic dosage (see Chapter 6) are given for at least 4 weeks. The specific drug is preferably chosen on the basis of sputum culture and sensitivity tests. The most common organisms are *Haemophilus influenzae*, *Staphylococcus aureus*, and *Pseudomonas aeruginosa*.

2. Aerosols–Aerosol therapy by mask 3 or 4 times a day, using a Mistogette mask with air compressor, may be of some value. Use 2 mL of the following solution per treatment:

℞ Propylene glycol		
Phenylephrine hydrochloride (Neo-Synephrine), 1%	āā	60 mL
Distilled water, qs ad		500 mL

Add appropriate antibiotic: neomycin, 100 mg/mL; polymyxin, 10 mg/mL; bacitracin, 10,000 units/mL; or streptomycin, 50 mg/mL.

3. Drainage and percussion–Postural drainage with chest percussion should be performed daily by parents who have been adequately instructed.

B. Treatment of Dietary Deficiencies:

1. Pancreatic extract preparations–Give pancreatin powder or granules, 5–10 g 3 times daily with meals; Viokase, 1.5 g 3 times daily with meals; or Cotazym, 2000–4000 units with each meal. These agents may be mixed with some form of solid food (bananas for small infants), Dose varies with age and with the child's need as established by trial.

2. Diet–Stress proteins and give a minimum of fat. Skimmed milk may be used in place of whole milk. Otherwise, with the use of pancreatin, no special diet is needed.

3. Diet during intestinal crisis–Treatment is as for severe diarrhea; give liquid diet, then soft diet. Supplemental salt should be added to the diet during periods when salt loss may occur.

C. Continuous Prophylaxis: When pulmonary infection becomes more severe, as indicated by increased coughing, fever, and dyspnea, antibiotic and aerosol therapy should be reintroduced. Patients should be protected from respiratory tract infection if possible. Immunizations and booster inoculations against pertussis, pneumococci, influenza, and rubeola should be given.

For excessive loss of sodium chloride in sweat in hot weather, with fever, and in patients with hyponatremia, salt should be added to the daily diet: 1 g daily in children up to 2 years of age or 2 g daily in children over 2 years of age.

Intravenous infusions of essential fatty acids (Intralipid) have been reported to produce very good results. Dosages of 20 mL/kg of 10% solution intravenously every 3 weeks have been used.

Prognosis

Owing to the present stage of development of techniques in treatment, the prognosis is unknown. It is at best guarded. Adult cases are increasingly recognized. Recovery, if it takes place, occurs at some time during adolescence. Parents of a child with congenital fibrocystic disease should be informed of the genetic etiology of the disease; they have approximately one chance in 4, with each pregnancy, of giving birth to another child with the disease.

2. GLUTEN-INDUCED ENTEROPATHY
("Celiac Disease")

A defect in enzyme activity or metabolism is possibly precipitated by an allergic reaction to the gliadin fraction of gluten.

Clinical Findings

A. Symptoms and Signs: "Celiac syndrome" (see p 355) is present in most cases. During crisis, dehydration and electrolyte deficiency problems predominate. A rare case may present with vomiting, abdominal pain, and constipation.

B. Laboratory Findings: Anemia—occasionally megaloblastic—that is resistant to iron treatment may be present. Levels of stool fat may be high; most patients demonstrate more than 4–5 g/d of fecal fat. The oral glucose tolerance curve is low. Biopsy carried out perorally gives definitive diagnosis. The pathologic features are characteristic.

C. X-Ray Findings: Upper gastrointestinal tract shows clumping of barium.

Treatment

If dehydration and electrolyte depletion crisis occur, stop all oral intake and treat as outlined in Chapter 5.

With the resumption of oral feedings, give a high-protein, low-fat diet, free of starch, with vitamin supplements and iron. Maintain a restricted diet for 3–4 months.

A diet free of wheat, oat, and rye gluten will probably be necessary for life. Fats should be introduced with care and close observation. Parents must be instructed about the wide variety of commercial products containing wheat. Examples include ice cream, frankfurters, some types of candy bars, and commercially produced fried chicken or fish.

The gluten-free diet allows dairy products, eggs, meats, vegetables, fruits, and corn and rice products. Gluten-free cereal is commercially available.

Dietary control should be dependent upon the overall appearance and change in the child rather than upon the character of the stools. Growth and weight gain are the primary measures of success.

Prognosis

Intermittent recurrence of symptoms can persist over many years. Improvement can be promised, but relapse with exposure to gluten should be expected during adulthood.

3. DISACCHARIDASE DEFICIENCIES

The basic defect in this condition is a congenital absence or an acquired deficiency of the disaccharidase enzyme required for the absorption of starch, sucrose, or lactose.

Clinical Findings

The onset is during early infancy. Explosive, foamy, watery

diarrhea occurs after ingestion of lactose in infants with congenital lactose deficiency or after ingestion of sucrose in infants with congenital sucrose or isomaltase deficiency. The glucose tolerance curve is flat following lactose or sucrose loading. Excess lactose in the stool may be demonstrated by laboratory tests.

Treatment

Treatment is the elimination of either lactose or sucrose from the diet.

A. Lactose-Free Diet: Bottle formulas containing soybean or puréed lamb are common substitutes. Nutramigen or other lactose-free, commercial products are useful. In older children, foods containing dry milk solids must be avoided. Parents must learn to read labels for lactose content and avoid the use of products containing lactose. Most dairy products and cheeses contain lactose.

B. Sucrose-Free Diet: Many commercial food preparations such as carbonated beverages, jam, honey, candy, and breakfast cereal contain sucrose. Vegetables such as peas and beans contain excessive amounts of sucrose and should be avoided. The sucrose-free diet can include dairy products, eggs, meat, and fish. So-called sugar-free beverages can be used. Green vegetables such as spinach, lettuce, broccoli, and asparagus are allowed.

Prognosis

The deficiency will persist throughout life, but tolerance to the offending carbohydrates may increase during adolescence.

4. IDIOPATHIC STEATORRHEA

Idiopathic steatorrhea is differentiated from gluten-induced enteropathy by failure of response to the withdrawal of gluten from the diet and is differentiated from disaccharidase deficiency by failure of response to manipulation of the sugar intake. Treatment includes elimination of all starches and reduction in the fat intake. Since this syndrome is of such obscure origin, it is impossible to state how long the treatment regimen should continue. Each case is a very special challenge.

5. COW'S MILK ALLERGY OR INTOLERANCE

Cow's milk allergy or intolerance is often diagnosed but not always proved. The onset is usually in patients under 3 months of age, and the symptoms are diarrhea, vomiting, and sometimes the complete "celiac syndrome." Chronic diarrhea persisting after an acute episode of vomiting and diarrhea suggests milk intolerance. Laboratory findings include eosinophilia demonstrated in a smear of rectal mucus and characteristic pathologic findings on biopsy of the small intestine perorally.

Diagnosis must be confirmed by a response to elimination of cow's milk followed by recurrence of symptoms after reintroduction of milk.

Treatment depends upon the elimination of cow's milk and cow's milk products from the diet for 6 months to 1 year. Soybean milk and "meat base formula" prepared from puréed lamb are popular substitutes. Soybean allergy has been reported, but only rarely.

Infants with cow's milk allergy eventually become able to tolerate cow's milk, usually after 6 months to 1 year.

SURGICAL DISORDERS OF THE DIGESTIVE SYSTEM

The accurate diagnosis and efficient management of surgical disorders of the gastrointestinal tract require awareness of the most common conditions that may be encountered as well as recognition of the relative emergency nature of each. (See Chapter 5 for preoperative and postoperative fluid and electrolyte therapy and the fluid management of intestinal obstruction.)

ESOPHAGEAL ATRESIA WITH OR WITHOUT TRACHEOESOPHAGEAL FISTULA

Pathology

In 88% of cases, the upper esophageal pouch ends blindly, and the lower pouch communicates directly with the back of the trachea. In about 5% of cases, there is esophageal atresia without an associated tracheal fistula.

Over 30% of children with this condition have associated anomalies; the most common of these are congenital heart disease and malformations of other portions of the intestinal tract, chiefly anorectal malformations.

Clinical Findings

A. Symptoms: This disorder can be diagnosed in the nursery shortly after the infant is born. Characteristic findings are excess salivation ("blowing bubbles"); coughing and gagging when feedings are attempted; and respiratory distress, which may lead to cyanosis.

B. Signs: Depending on the amount of feeding that has been attempted, aspiration pneumonia may not develop until 2 or 3 days after feeding was begun. Pneumonitis from reflux of gastric juice through the lower esophageal segment may be present. Diagnosis of esophageal atresia can be made by x-ray following placement of a radiopaque catheter in the esophageal pouch. A safe alternative to this is the aspiration of 1–2 mL of gastric mucus, which rules out esophageal atresia.

C. X-Ray Findings: As soon as the diagnosis is suspected, attempt to pass a 10F radiopaque catheter into the stomach so that the position can be checked on x-ray.

1. Plain x-ray–Demonstration of the large, air-filled esophageal pouch, extending down to the level of the T2 vertebral body, is sometimes possible on anteroposterior and lateral chest x-rays. A radiopaque catheter will pass only to the T2 level. Aspiration pneumonitis may be present. Air in the stomach and intestine, in association with a blind upper pouch, indicates connection between the tracheal and lower segment of the esophagus.

2. Contrast examination–Instill only 0.5 mL of contrast material directly into the upper pouch through a catheter under fluoroscopic control, with the infant held upright and laterally. All contrast material must then be aspirated from the upper pouch. Overfilling of the upper pouch leads to aspiration of contrast material into the lungs.

Treatment

A. Preoperative Care:

1. Place a sump (Replogle) catheter in the upper pouch and attach it to suction.
2. Place the infant in an incubator with the infant's head elevated at least 30 degrees to minimize aspiration of gastric juice through the distal fistula.
3. Give antibiotics if pneumonitis is present.
4. Give oxygen as necessary to prevent cyanosis.
5. Administer maintenance fluids intravenously. Give no fluids by mouth.

B. Surgical Measures:

1. If the infant has moderate or severe pneumonitis, gastrostomy should be performed.
2. Primary repair of the esophagus should be performed when the infant is clinically stable. The extrapleural approach is preferred. A premature infant or an infant with pneumonitis may tolerate only division of the fistula from the trachea, with esophageal repair postponed until the lungs clear.
3. Maintain body temperature during transport and operation.
4. Monitor blood gases and correct acidosis or hypoxia if present.

C. Postoperative Care:

1. Return the infant to an incubator, where oxygen can be given and nebulized water added to the atmosphere, for several days.
2. Administer maintenance fluids intravenously and replace gastric losses.
3. Keep the stomach deflated initially. Feedings through the gastrostomy should be started no sooner than the third postoperative day and then should be given with caution. Fifteen milliliters of a milk formula can be given in frequent feedings.
4. Begin oral feedings when the general condition of the child is good and after an esophagogram shows good healing (about the tenth postoperative day). The oral feedings are gradually increased, and the gastrostomy tube is elevated. The gastrostomy tube is usually withdrawn after 6 weeks and the gastric opening allowed to close spontaneously.

Course & Prognosis

In general, the earlier the diagnosis is made and the less the insult to the lung, the better the child's chances are of surviving the surgical procedure. Prematurity is an added risk, as is the presence of other anomalies such as congenital heart disease. Postoperative esophageal dilatations for strictures are necessary in many patients.

TRACHEOESOPHAGEAL FISTULA WITHOUT ESOPHAGEAL ATRESIA (H TYPE)

Diagnosis of this anomaly is often difficult and is made late. The connection between the esophagus and the trachea is usually small and situated in the lower cervical esophagus. Most infants with fistula have had repeated pneumonia and intermittent, marked abdominal distention because of air forced through the fistula by crying.

Clinical Findings

A. Symptoms: Symptoms include choking, coughing, or cyanosis with feedings; persistent or recurrent pneumonitis; and abdominal distention with gas.

B. Signs: There may be difficulty with feedings. Signs of pneumonitis may be present. Endoscopy is usually necessary to reveal the fistula. Results of barium studies are often normal.

Treatment

A. Preoperative Care: Give appropriate antibiotics for pneumonia and fluid replacement as necessary.

B. Surgical Measures: Division of the fistula is accomplished through a cervical incision.

C. Postoperative Care: Oral feedings may be initiated 3 days after surgery, depending on the infant's condition.

Course & Prognosis

In most cases, the prognosis is extremely favorable.

ESOPHAGEAL STRICTURE OR STENOSIS

Partial obstructions of the esophagus cause a variety of feeding problems during infancy or childhood. They may be caused by vascular ring or other congenital malformations; may be of postsurgical origin following correction of tracheoesophageal fistula; may result from ingestion of corrosive chemicals (eg, lye); or may follow peptic erosion of the lower esophagus (eg, from reflux of gastric acids through a relaxed cardia, hiatal hernia, or aberrant gastric mucosa in the lower esophagus).

The principal complications are malnutrition and aspiration pneumonia.

Clinical Findings

A. Symptoms: Regurgitation of food is the most common symptom. With vascular ring, there is usually some dysphagia during the neonatal period, but there may be no significant symptoms until the infant starts on solid food. Vomiting is not forceful; regurgitated material is usually undigested, contains saliva, and does not smell sour. Respiratory distress is suggestive of compression of the trachea by a bolus of food lodged in the esophagus or is suggestive of tracheal aspiration. Dysphagia may be the presenting symptom. Bleeding from the gastrointestinal tract is not frequent.

B. Signs: Often there are no signs, or there may be varying degrees of malnutrition, depending on the duration of symptoms. After repair of the tracheoesophageal fistula, there may be esophageal dyskinesia without significant stricture.

C. X-Ray Findings: The obstruction can be seen with the fluoroscope when the esophagus is outlined with swallowed barium. Ciné studies should include the pharynx to evaluate the swallowing mechanism and rule out dyskinesia.

The length of the obstruction varies with the disease process causing the stenosis. Congenital lesions may involve only a short segment. In hiatal hernia with reflux of gastric secretion, the stenosis may involve a short segment adjacent to the herniated stomach or may be rather extensive, involving a large portion of the lower esophagus. In strictures due to caustic chemicals, the ingestion of the chemicals usually causes extensive involvement of the esophagus.

D. Esophagoscopy: Details of the nature of the obstruction are determined by esophagoscopy.

Treatment

A. Reflux Esophagitis With or Without Hiatal Hernia:

1. Give small, frequent, thickened feedings, and keep the infant upright (60 degrees) after feedings.

2. Dilatations are of no value if reflux is not controlled.

3. Surgical control of reflux is often required to control stricture formation. The indications are failure to thrive, repeated bouts of pneumonitis, and evidence of esophagitis with developing stricture.

B. Postoperative Stricture:

1. Dilate as necessary.

2. Obtain esophagograms to rule out reflux.

3. Correct reflux if present.

C. Stricture Due to Ingestion of Corrosives: Ammonia rarely causes esophageal burns. Lye solutions usually cause stricture.

1. Esophagoscopic examination is indicated if the history reveals the possibility of a burn. Visualize the burn, but do not pass the instrument through it.

2. Give systemic antibiotics to control mediastinitis, which often complicates esophageal damage.

3. Systemic corticosteroids may or may not minimize stricture formation.

4. Gastrostomy is often necessary for nutrition and to facilitate dilatation.

5. Dilate if the esophagogram demonstrates a stricture. Dilatation may be accomplished by passing a string at esophagoscopy or by having the child swallow a string, which is then attached to rubber dilators of increasing sizes. These are drawn upward through a gastrostomy opening and then through the stenosed area.

6. Resection or esophageal replacement is usually not considered until repeated dilatation has proved unsuccessful.

INGUINAL HERNIA & HYDROCELE

The testis forms cephalad to the kidney and descends into the scrotum during the last trimester. As it descends, the peritoneum descends with it to form the tunica vaginalis. The peritoneal connection between the abdominal cavity and the scrotum (the processus vaginalis) is normally obliterated. All hernias, hydroceles, and ectopic testes relate to abnormalities in this process.

Hernia

A hernia is an intermittent bulge lateral to the pubic tubercle; the bulge appears when the patient is crying, straining, or standing and usually reduces spontaneously when the patient is relaxed or supine.

Treatment in children usually consists of elective surgery performed when the child is in good health.

The incidence of hernia in the general population is 1% and in premature infants, 5%. Males are affected most commonly (85% of cases). One-half of cases of inguinal hernia during childhood occur in infants under 6 months of age. Right-sided hernias are more frequent than those on the left (2:1). Irrespective of side, about 25% of patients have contralateral hernias. In females, hernias are often bilateral.

Incarcerated hernias do not reduce when the child is relaxed. Incarceration occurs in about 10% of cases, most often in children under 1 year of age. Strangulation follows incarceration, and the hernia becomes tender and erythematous. The abdomen becomes distended, with vomiting and signs of bowel obstruction. Pressure on testicular vessels in the inguinal canal by an incarcerated hernia can cause testicular infarction.

Incarcerated hernia can often be reduced by gently squeezing the bowel back into the abdomen along the axis of the inguinal canal. Sedation (pentobarbital, 4 mg/kg, and meperidine, 1 mg/kg) is necessary in most cases.

Strangulation is managed by nasogastric suction, rehydration, correction of electrolyte deficiencies, and surgery when the patient's condition is stable. (Stabilization should not take more than 2–3 hours.) Attempted reduction may rupture ischemic bowel or return necrotic bowel into the abdomen.

The ovary is often incarcerated in females. Strangulation is rare, and hernias may usually be repaired electively.

Hydrocele

Hydrocele is very common in newborns. Spontaneous regression by age 6 months is the rule. Frequent and rapid change in size of the hydrocele indicates a patent processus vaginalis with communication to the peritoneal cavity. Hernia often develops, and communicating hydroceles should be repaired.

Acute hydrocele may develop about the testis or in the spermatic cord and may be difficult to differentiate from incarcerated hernia. Examination at the internal ring level, with one finger in the upper rectum and another feeling the abdomen from the outside, may aid in differentiation. Acute hydrocele in the canal of Nuck presents as an oblong, firm swelling in the groin of a female infant and may be confused with a groin node. Exploration is required in doubtful cases.

ACHALASIA
(Cardiospasm)

Achalasia results from failure of the normal relaxation of the cardioesophageal junction. The resulting functional obstruction causes intermittent dysphagia and frequent regurgitation of undigested food. It is encountered more often in older children presenting with poor feeding, with failure to grow normally, and occasionally, with respiratory infections resulting from aspiration of regurgitated food. Barium swallow demonstrates the widened esophagus with a gradual narrowing at the cardioesophageal junction.

Surgical division of muscle layers over the narrowed cardioesophageal junction (Heller procedure) is necessary, since hydrostatic dilatation is usually ineffective in children.

CHALASIA
(Cardioesophageal Relaxation)

Chalasia occurs in young infants. Vomiting, usually not bile-stained and occasionally projectile, occurs when the infant is supine. Dehydration and malnutrition may result. Aspiration pneumonia may occur.

Barium examination shows free reflux from the stomach into the esophagus with absent or uncoordinated esophageal peristalsis.

Treatment consists of keeping the child upright in a small padded chair during feedings and for at least 1 hour afterward. Small, frequent, thickened feedings are administered. Most infants will stop vomiting within several months.

HIATAL HERNIA & REFLUX

Esophageal hiatal hernia is a congenital defect permitting reflux of gastric contents with vomiting (sometimes projectile), aspiration, and failure to thrive. In many cases, the esophagitis leads to stricture formation and occult bleeding. Most cases of "congenital short esophagus" are not congenital but the result of prolonged, undetected esophageal reflux with esophagitis and scarring.

An infant with reflux may have only aspiration pneumonitis, poor weight gain, or iron deficiency anemia as the presenting symptom. Symptomatic reflux often occurs in infants after tracheoesophageal fistula repair, in children with severe scoliosis, and in brain-damaged infants.

Treatment consists of maintaining the child upright (60-degree angle or more) as much as possible for several months and giving small frequent feedings of a thickened formula. If the condition does not improve with treatment or if there is esophagitis or frequent aspiration, the hernia should be repaired.

CONGENITAL HERNIA OF THE DIAPHRAGM

The most common area of herniation is in the left posterolateral portion, the foramen of Bochdalek. Foramen of Morgagni hernias rarely present during the newborn period and rarely cause significant respiratory symptoms.

Clinical Findings

A. Symptoms: Cyanosis and dyspnea in a newborn infant should suggest the diagnosis. Respiratory distress is usually constant and severe.

B. Signs: Cyanosis is usually present. Chest movements are asymmetric, and dullness is noted on the affected side. Breath sounds may be absent. The abdomen is strikingly scaphoid and will feel less full on palpation than usual. The mediastinum shifts away from the affected side.

C. X-Ray Findings: Chest x-ray (required for all infants with respiratory distress) usually shows a portion of the gastrointestinal tract in the thorax and marked displacement of the mediastinum. Avoid introducing contrast media into the gastrointestinal tract.

Treatment

A. Preoperative Care: All infants who are symptomatic in the first hours of life have severe respiratory and metabolic acidosis. As soon as the diagnosis is suspected, a nasogastric tube should be passed and attached to suction. This prevents further distention of the gastrointestinal tract with air or fluid and makes aspiration less likely. Endotracheal intubation should be performed early. This facilitates oxygenation and lowering P_{CO_2}. If P_{CO_2} rises above 85 mm Hg, the infant becomes severely obtunded. Ventilation pressures must be less than 30 mm Hg to prevent alveolar rupture and pneumothorax, an impending complication due to the associated hypoplastic lungs. Thoracic decompression is carried out on an emergency basis.

B. Surgical Measures: Diaphragmatic hernia is a surgical emergency. The viscera are reduced from the thorax through a subcostal incision. The diaphragm is closed and a chest tube left in place to water-seal drainage. The infant must be kept warm. If abdominal closure requires tension, close only the skin to prevent undue pressure on the diaphragm or inferior vena cava.

C. Postoperative Care: An endotracheal tube is left in place and attached to a T piece, CPAP (continuous positive airway pressure) equipment, or respirator as indicated. Maintain a fluid intake of 1 dL/kg/d of 10% dextrose in 0.25 N saline solution. Add potassium, 2–3 mEq/kg/d, beginning on the second day. Give antibiotics as indicated. P_{O_2} levels in the ductus arteriosus should be monitored postoperatively to detect a reversal in fetal circulation that occurs when pulmonary vasoconstriction and hypertension force the ductus arteriosus to open, thus creating a right-to-left shunt. The infant will show clinical signs of sudden illness and will require ventilation and infusion of tolazoline (Priscoline) in an initial dose of 0.25 mg/kg/min for 4 minutes. If P_{O_2} increases by 15 mm Hg or more, infuse 1–2 mg/kg/h. Keep the blood pressure over 40 mm Hg.

Course & Prognosis

Survival depends on the degree of pulmonary hypoplasia; survival rate is about 50%. Lung weights of infants who do not survive are about half those of normal infants of the same gestational age and birth weight. The morphology of the lung on the side of the hernia is that of a 28- to 30-week-old fetus. Long-term survivors have normal lung weights, although they have some degree of emphysema and decreased blood flow.

PYLORIC STENOSIS
(Congenital Hypertrophic Pyloric Stenosis)

Pyloric stenosis is more apt to occur in firstborn infants and is more common in males than in females (4:1 ratio). In most cases, the diagnosis is made between 3 and 4 weeks of age. It is important to differentiate this condition from adrenal insufficiency and subdural hematoma because all 3 conditions can produce projectile vomiting and poor weight gain.

There is a marked increase in the size of the circular musculature of the pylorus, causing obstruction of the lumen. In the average case, the enlargement is the size and shape of an olive.

Clinical Findings

A. Symptoms:

1. Vomiting–Vomiting begins in most cases after the 14th day of life. It is usually mild at first and becomes progressively more forceful and eventually projectile. Vomiting occurs within one-half hour of feeding and does not contain bile. The infant is hungry and will refeed immediately.

2. Hunger–The child is always hungry because very little food can pass into the duodenum. Appetite may be lost in the later stages when metabolic derangements are marked.

3. Bowel movements–The infant may develop loose green "starvation" stools.

4. Weight–The failure to gain weight or the loss of weight with decrease in subcutaneous fat is a sign of starvation.

5. Gastrointestinal bleeding–Gastritis due to stasis in the obstructed stomach will occasionally result in bleeding.

6. Jaundice–Jaundice develops in 2–5% of infants with pyloric stenosis. Bilirubin is mainly unconjugated and clears promptly when stenosis is relieved.

B. Signs: Dehydration, with decrease in skin turgor, may be present. There may be distention of the epigastrium; frequently, the outline of the distended stomach can be seen. Gastric waves passing from left to right may be evident during and after feeding. Palpation of the upper right quadrant frequently reveals the olive-shaped mass. If the tumor cannot be palpated during feeding, it is best to aspirate the stomach. Palpation is usually successful when the stomach is empty; with experience, the mass can be palpated in 75–90% of patients. Inguinal hernias occur in 10% of patients with pyloric stenosis.

C. Laboratory Findings: Findings include metabolic alkalosis, hypokalemia, and variable hyponatremia. Urinalysis usually reveals a markedly alkaline urine of high specific gravity. If potassium depletion is present, the infant may have an acid urine but still suffer from alkalosis. Hemoconcentration may be manifested by increased hemoglobin and hematocrit values.

D. X-Ray Findings: If the typical mass in the right upper quadrant is not palpable, a barium study will demonstrate an enlarged stomach, with increased intensity of peristaltic waves, and marked narrowing and elongation of the pylorus, with abnormal retention of the barium in the stomach. Relatively little food passes beyond the pylorus even after 6 or 7 hours. A barium swallow is unnecessary in at least two-thirds of the cases; nevertheless, if it is employed, the barium should be aspirated and the stomach lavaged with saline after the procedure.

Complications

Tetanic seizures due to metabolic alkalosis and a reduction of free serum calcium may occur.

Treatment

A. General Measures: If adequate surgical and anesthetic facilities and nursing care are not available, give methscopolamine, 0.1 mg orally or subcutaneously every 4 hours before feeding. The head should be elevated at least 30 degrees for 1–2 hours after feeding.

B. Preoperative Care:

1. Rehydration–In about three-fourths of patients, electrolyte solutions can be given by the oral route. Give 2 oz of appropriate replacement solution every 3 hours with the infant in an infant's chair and burped frequently. Rehydration can often be accomplished in this manner, and the infant will be ready for operation in 24–48 hours.

In cases of severe fluid and electrolyte deficiencies, rehydration by the intravenous route is preferred. Give 250 mL of 5% dextrose in 0.5 N saline solution to which 10 mEq of potassium chloride has been added. The rate of infusion will depend on the severity of dehydration.

Rarely, the patient will be cachectic and will require total parenteral nutrition.

2. Nasogastric intubation–One hour before operation, an 8F nasogastric tube may be inserted to preclude regurgitation and aspiration of stomach contents during anesthesia.

C. Surgical Measures: Ramstedt pyloromyotomy divides the hypertrophied muscle bundles that obstruct the pylorus. Surgery should not be performed until rehydration and correction of alkalosis are complete.

D. Postoperative Care: Begin feedings 3–4 hours after surgery. Give 5% glucose in water, 15 mL orally every hour, and gradually increase the volume to 30–60 mL every 2 hours. When this volume is tolerated, substitute 30–60 mL of formula every 3 hours, and continue with gradual increases as they are tolerated. Full tolerance is usually reached at the end of the second postoperative day. Vomiting, often in small amounts, is not unusual after the first postoperative feedings; progress is slower if vomiting occurs.

Intravenous administration of fluids may be necessary in some cases, but this is the exception rather than the rule.

Follow-up surgery for incomplete myotomy or recurrence of pyloric hypertrophy is rarely indicated. Persistent vomiting or regurgitation of feedings may be due to incompetence of the gastroesophageal sphincter. Do not perform surgery again before 2 weeks after the myotomy.

Prognosis

Complete relief is to be expected following adequate surgical repair, but children who have experienced starvation may have poorer learning abilities. Mortality rate is low.

MECONIUM ILEUS
(Obstruction of the Intestines)

Meconium ileus represents the earliest known manifestation of fibrocystic disease, which affects all the mucus-secreting glands of the respiratory and alimentary tracts (see p 355). It is characterized by marked reduction in the production of trypsin by the pancreatic glands. It is this latter disability, operating in utero, that leads to the presence of inspissated meconium, causing intestinal obstruction in the newborn. About 10–20 cm of intestine in the region of the lower ileum is obstructed. The ileocecal valve and the entire colon are normal, but there may be associated atresia of small bowel.

Clinical Findings

A. Symptoms: Intestinal obstruction in the newborn is characterized by progressively more severe vomiting, beginning within the first day or 2 of life. The vomitus contains bile. The family history may reveal a relative with known fibrocystic disease.

B. Signs: The abdomen is markedly distended, and distended loops of bowel may be seen through the abdominal wall. Firm masses within the loops strongly suggest meconium ileus. In most cases, no meconium will have been passed.

C. Laboratory Findings: If meconium appears in stools, it can be shown to contain no trypsin. The sweat test shows an increase in the chloride concentration of sweat (> 60 mEq/L) (see p 356).

D. X-Ray Findings: On upright x-ray, marked intestinal dilatation may be seen, with characteristically low or no air-fluid levels in the loops of bowel (owing to the presence of inspissated meconium). Despite the fact that their location and appearance may suggest colon, these loops are dilated small bowel. A granular, mottled appearance within a loop, due to bubbles of gas and meconium, should suggest the presence of meconium ileus. Microcolon may be seen on barium enema. Free air seen in the peritoneal cavity, or fluid between the loops of bowel, indicates perforation. Calcification of the peritoneum, when present, represents antenatal perforation and meconium peritonitis.

Treatment

A. Preoperative Care: Provide continuous gastric suction through nasogastric tube. Administer gastrografin enemas. The hypertonic contrast medium draws water into the bowel and "floats out" the inspissated meconium. This procedure, which is often successful, must be done under fluoroscopy by a radiologist familiar with newborn infants. It will not relieve associated atresia, volvulus, or peritonitis.

B. Surgical Measures: Several choices are available. The portion of the distal ileum that contains the greatest amount of meconium may be resectioned. The ends are brought out and sutured to the skin. Postoperatively, the terminal ileum and colon are cleansed with pancreatic enzyme suspension. Closure of the enterostomy is performed 2–3 weeks later.

Excision of the portion of the dilated distal ileum and end-to-side anastomosis, with creation of an exteriorized "chimney," may be indicated. The chimney is used for instillation of pancreatic enzyme, acetylcysteine (Mucomyst), and mineral oil; subsequently, it is closed electively in 6–9 months.

C. Postoperative Care: Many surgeons prefer inserting a gastrostomy tube during surgery, since use of a gastrostomy tube is associated with fewer pulmonary complications in the postoperative period than is use of a nasogastric tube. After the immediate obstruction is relieved, therapy for the prevention of pulmonary and nutritional disturbance of fibrocystic disease becomes necessary (see Cystic Fibrosis, above).

Prognosis

There is no definite relationship between meconium ileus and the severity of the symptoms of cystic fibrosis.

CONGENITAL ATRESIA OR STENOSIS OF INTESTINES & COLON

Congenital atresia and stenosis are thought to result from vascular obstruction in the mesenteric vessels during the fetal period of development. Atresia designates a complete block, while stenosis indicates narrowing of the intestinal lumen. Atresia or stenosis of the duodenum is frequently associated with Down's syndrome.

Meconium ileus must be considered in any child with intestinal atresia (see above).

Clinical Findings

A. Symptoms: Atresia of the intestinal tract or colon causes vomiting on the first day of life. Intestinal stenosis may not come to the physician's attention for weeks or months. The vomitus contains bile.

B. Signs: Depending on the level of involvement, abdominal distention is often present and becomes progressively worse. Peristaltic waves are often seen. Intestinal loops may be outlined on the abdominal wall. Dehydration is common because of persistent vomiting. Meconium may be dry and gray-green rather than black and viscous.

C. X-Ray Findings: Upright abdominal x-ray shows air and fluid levels and reveals marked dilatation of the duodenum and distention of the proximal loops of small bowel, which may contain fluid levels. The distal loops will be free of gas if the obstruction is complete. In partial obstruction, there may be gas without distention distal to the point of obstruction. Presence of free air in the abdominal cavity means that perforation has already occurred. A granular, mottled appearance in the small bowel due to gas and meconium suggests meconium ileus.

Barium enema is an important part of the preoperative x-ray study. In low intestinal atresia, it will often demonstrate the markedly decreased caliber characteristic of the unused portion of the gastrointestinal tract—the so-called microcolon. The chief indication for barium enema is to rule out Hirschsprung's disease and malrotation with volvulus, which can present with symptoms identical to those of intestinal atresia.

Treatment

A. Preoperative Care: For decompression, institute constant gastric sump suction. Give parenteral fluids and electrolytes. Prophylactic antibiotic therapy is indicated.

B. Surgical Measures: Resection of the dilated, hypertrophic intestine proximal to the atresia and end-to-end anastomosis, where possible, are usually preferred for the surgical correction of atresia or stenosis. In all cases of atresia and marked stenosis, early intervention is essential to prevent perforation. If the infant is debilitated or if perforation has occurred, ileostomy is safest for lower atresias. Duodenal and jejunal atresias should be corrected by anastomosis, because of severe fluid losses from a jejunostomy. Colonic atresias of the right side can be corrected by anastomosis; those of the left side, by colostomy and delayed anastomosis.

C. Postoperative Care: Provide fluids and antibiotics as required. Gastrostomy, if done during surgery, will simplify care in the immediate postoperative period and will prevent many pulmonary complications. Total parenteral nutrition may be necessary in selected cases.

Course & Prognosis

The mortality rate in infants with atresia or marked stenosis is increased by delay in diagnosis.

When surgical treatment is instituted early, mortality rates should be less than 10%.

MALROTATION OF INTESTINES & COLON

Malrotation, a congenital condition, is due to incomplete rotation of the gut and lack of attachment of the mesentery of the small intestine. It may result in a volvulus of the midgut or obstruction of the second part of the duodenum by peritoneal bands.

Clinical Findings

A. Symptoms and Signs: In newborns, bilious vomiting occurs most frequently at the end of the first week of life. If malrotation is accompanied by an intrinsic obstruction of the second portion of the duodenum (eg, atresia, defect in the diaphragm, stenosis), vomiting occurs within 48 hours of birth. In the early stages of midgut volvulus, the general condition is good; failure to diagnose and treat at this point will lead to rapid clinical deterioration indicative of widespread intestinal gangrene.

In older infants and children, there may be intermittent attacks of vomiting without significant abdominal distention.

The presence of blood in the stools indicates ischemic mucosal changes in the entire midgut and constitutes a surgical emergency.

B. Laboratory Findings: Hematocrit and red blood cell counts are elevated owing to dehydration. Slight leukocytosis is usually present. Marked leukocytosis suggests impending or actual gangrene of the bowel.

C. X-Ray Findings: Plain films of the abdomen may or may not show dilatation of the stomach and duodenum. Barium examination may show that the cecum and ascending colon are displaced to the left.

Treatment

A. General Measures: Gastric suction with aspiration of fluid and gas should be instituted before and maintained during and after surgery. A gastrostomy is helpful in the postoperative period. Fluid and electrolyte therapy should be rapid and adequate before early surgery is attempted. Postoperative fluid therapy is discussed in Chapter 5.

B. Surgical Measures: The goal of surgery is to relieve extrinsic compression in the duodenum by dividing the bands that bind the second and third portions to the retroperitoneum and by straightening the duodenojejunal junction. The midgut always twists in a clockwise fashion; thus, the mass of bowel loops must be unwound in a counterclockwise direction. The small bowel is then placed in the right side of the abdomen and the colon to the left.

Course & Prognosis

Recurrences after surgical correction are uncommon.

MECKEL'S DIVERTICULUM

Meckel's diverticulum may be asymptomatic throughout life or may be associated with any of the following: hemorrhage (45% of cases); Meckel's diverticulitis (20%), with symptoms identical to those of acute appendicitis; perforation (3%); intussusception (20%), with the diverticulum as the leading point; patent omphalomesenteric duct (2%), with a diverticulum opening at the umbilicus; and intestinal obstruction (10%) from a vestigial band connecting the diverticulum to the umbilicus.

Clinical Findings

Symptoms and signs depend upon the nature of the complication caused by Meckel's diverticulum. X-ray examinations are generally of no value in attempting to demonstrate Meckel's diverticulum. Recently, radioactive technetium perchlorate has been used to demonstrate ectopic gastric mucosa in the diverticulum.

Bleeding is usually massive, and the child passes tarry or bright-red blood through the rectum. The bleeding is from ulceration in the diverticulum or from the normal ileum adjacent to it. Bleeding, perforation, and diverticulitis occur only in the diverticuli that contain ectopic gastric mucosa and therefore secrete acid. Foreign bodies lodged in the diverticulum can cause any of these symptoms.

Treatment

Treatment consists of operative excision as soon as the patient can be made ready. In cases of gastrointestinal hemorrhage in which Meckel's diverticulum is suspected but unproved, operation may be deferred until the diagnosis is established or until bleeding occurs a second time. In the asymptomatic patient, elective excision or removal incidental to another surgical procedure is debatable.

Course & Prognosis

The prognosis is excellent following surgery. If perforation through a gangrenous diverticulum has occurred, massive peritonitis may follow and is a serious threat to life.

DUPLICATIONS OF THE GASTROINTESTINAL TRACT

Cysts of enteric origin are associated with and often communicating with various levels of the gastrointestinal tract. They may occur anywhere from the upper esophagus to the anus and are often intimately associated with the adjacent area of the gastrointestinal tract, usually sharing a common muscular wall. The nature of the mucosal lining varies considerably and may not necessarily correspond to the level of the gastrointestinal tract to which the cyst is adjacent. There is considerable variation in the size and shape of these cysts.

A duplication may present as an asymptomatic mass with gastrointestinal bleeding, as an intestinal obstruction resulting from volvulus or intussusception, or with evidence of localized peritonitis. Special types of duplications include neurenteric cysts and hindgut duplications. Neurenteric cysts usually arise from the proximal small bowel and extend toward the vertebral column; they are associated with a bony defect in the vertebral column and extension through the diaphragm and into the chest. Hindgut duplications actually represent a double colon and are often associated with doubling of the anus and the perineal structures.

Diagnosis may often be made by radioactive technetium perchlorate to demonstrate ectopic gastric mucosa in the duplication.

Treatment consists of resection of the duplication and, in most cases, of the adjacent bowel also. The prognosis is good.

BILIARY ATRESIA

Biliary atresia is a progressive extrahepatic biliary obstruction in the newborn. If untreated, it eventually compromises the intrahepatic biliary system and results in cirrhosis, portal hypertension, ascites, and liver insufficiency.

Biliary atresia may be classified as "correctable" or "noncorrectable" on the basis of cholangiographic findings. If the proximal and distal extrahepatic ducts are macroscopically patent (8% of cases), the atresia is correctable. If the proximal extrahepatic ducts are macroscopically nonpatent (80% of cases), it is noncorrectable. Findings show that 22% of patients with noncorrectable biliary atresia have patency of the gallbladder and distal bile ducts; in the other 78%, the entire biliary duct system is occluded. Inspissated bile syndrome and biliary hypoplasia may also be seen on cholangiogram.

Clinical Findings

Symptoms and signs include progressive or intermittent jaundice, most often becoming apparent after the second week of life; failure to thrive; hepatomegaly; and splenomegaly.

Neonatal hepatitis is the condition most often confused with biliary atresia. This and other causes of jaundice (hemolytic conditions, syphilis, cytomegalovirus, toxoplasmosis, sepsis, rubella, mucoviscidosis) must be ruled out. Iminodiacetic acid (IDA) radioactive hepatobiliary scans will usually differentiate biliary atresia from neonatal hepatitis.

Treatment

In infants with biliary atresia, bilioenteric drainage procedures are performed preferably between the first and second months of life. The disease is too far advanced after the fourth month of life.

A. Laparotomy: Laparotomy should be performed early.

B. Operative Cholangiogram: Findings indicate whether the atresia is correctable or noncorrectable (see above).

C. Wedge Liver Biopsy: The liver biopsy performed during surgery gives an indication of long-term prognosis, based upon the degree of hepatic cirrhosis.

D. Bilioenteric Drainage: Several modifications of the original hepatic portojejunostomy (Kasai procedure) have been developed during the past decade, primarily in an effort to prevent postoperative intrahepatic cholangitis. If distal extrahepatic ducts of the gallbladder are patent, cholecystoenterostomy (Kasai gallbladder procedure) is the procedure of choice. Double enterotomy of the bilioenteric conduit is most often used for other noncorrectable atresias.

E. Liver Transplant: This is now increasingly used.

Course & Prognosis

Two percent of patients with untreated biliary atresia survive for 4 years. Of treated patients with correctable atresia, 14.6% die in 1–10 years. Of treated patients with noncorrectable atresia, 52% die in 1–10 years; those with good bile drainage have an early postoperative survival rate of 71% and a 1- to 10-year survival rate of 41%. Transplant survival rates are not yet fully known.

CHOLEDOCHAL CYST

Choledochal cyst is less common than biliary atresia. The manifestations consist of intermittent jaundice, fever and chills (when infection is present), and a mass in the right upper quadrant. X-ray examination shows a mass on a plain film and indentation of the duodenum on an upper gastrointestinal series. The cyst may be excised or it may be drained into the gastrointestinal tract by means of a Roux-en-Y procedure. The overall prognosis is excellent, but some patients develop cholangitis or biliary tract stones.

INTUSSUSCEPTION

Intussusception is potentially one of the most dangerous surgical emergencies in early childhood. It is characterized by the telescoping of one portion of the intestine into a more distal portion, resulting in impairment of the blood supply and leading to necrosis of the involved segment of bowel.

In 95% of cases, no specific cause of intussusception can be found, but viral infections have been implicated. The condition is most common in infants between the ages of 5 months and 1 year. Telescoping occasionally occurs around a Meckel's diverticulum.

Pathology

Intussusception most commonly involves the telescoping of the ileum into the colon (ileocolic type). Gangrene of the intussusception occurs if the incarcerated bowel loses its blood supply.

Clinical Findings

A. Symptoms: A sudden onset of recurrent, paroxysmal, sharp abdominal pain in a healthy child suggests intussusception. The child perspires and draws up the legs to ease the pain. The child may appear well in the pain-free intervals. Vomiting frequently occurs after the onset of the abdominal pain but is not universally present. Fifteen percent of patients do not have pain.

B. Signs: The extent and severity of abnormal physical findings will depend on the duration of the symptoms.

1. Shock, dehydration, and fever–After 1 or 2 hours of recurrent pain, evidence of shock occurs with each episode and frequently persists into the intervals between attacks. It is characterized by pallor, sweating, and lassitude. After 5 or more hours, dehydration and listlessness are noted, and the eyes are sunken and soft. A low-grade fever is usually found as a result of dehydration and obstruction.

2. Mass–Careful palpation usually reveals a mass in the abdomen. It is sausage-shaped or ovoid and in most cases is quite firm and not tender. Its location varies, but it frequently is in the upper mid abdomen. The right lower quadrant is characteristically less full than usual. If the leading point of the intussusception has reached the rectum, it may be possible to palpate a mass of the shape and consistency of the cervix of the uterus by rectal examination. Blood frequently is found on the examining finger after examination, and this confirms the diagnosis.

3. Blood clot–A "currant jelly" blood clot may be evacuated in a bowel movement.

C. Laboratory Findings: Depending on the duration of symptoms, concentrations of blood and urine may be found. These findings are partial guides for replacement fluid and electrolyte therapy.

D. X-Ray Findings: A plain film of the abdomen will frequently reveal an absence of bowel gas in the right lower quadrant. Dilated loops of small bowel, when present, suggest obstruction of the small intestine. When barium enema examination is performed, the intussusception is outlined as an inverted cap, and an obstruction to the further progression of the barium is noted. There is frequently a "coiled spring" appearance to the barium column in the region of the intussusception. Barium enema may also be used to reduce the intussusception (see Treatment, below).

Treatment

A. General Measures: Nonoperative reduction by barium enema administered by a skilled radiologist under fluoroscopic control will reduce intussusception safely in two-thirds of cases. The enema must reflux through the ileocecal valve, and unless the ileum is filled, it may be impossible to tell if complete reduction has occurred. Subsequent laparotomy is necessary if reduction has not been accomplished. Perforation can occur from the pressure of the enema if the bowel wall has been weakened owing to impairment of its vascular supply.

Hydrostatic reduction (barium enema) should *not* be attempted if there are physical findings of peritonitis.

Surgical reduction is the method of choice if enema is not successful.

B. Preoperative Care: One to 2 hours of intensive fluid and electrolyte therapy are usually necessary before the child can be considered a good risk for surgery. Parenteral fluids should be started, and blood should be typed and cross-matched before the patient is sent to x-ray for hydrostatic reduction. Deflation of the stomach by constant gastric suction is essential before, during, and after surgery.

C. Surgical Measures: Surgical reduction may be indicated. The bowel is usually found to be viable. If not, resection and anastomosis should be the next step.

D. Postoperative Care: Parenteral feedings and nasogastric suction should be continued until the infant passes feces normally, since postoperative ileus may be prolonged. Fever may persist for 2 or 3 days. Antibiotics are rarely indicated unless the bowel has perforated preoperatively.

Course & Prognosis

With early diagnosis and treatment, the mortality rate is extremely low. The longer the delay before treatment, the higher the mortality rate.

With adequate early treatment, the prognosis is excellent and recurrences are uncommon. For this reason, no attempt is made to do anything more than reduce the intussusception unless some condition that caused the obstruction, such as a polyp or Meckel's diverticulum, is discovered at surgery.

Children over 4 years of age who have intussusception frequently have a small bowel lymphosarcoma, polyp, or other leading point for the intussusception.

POLYPS OF THE INTESTINAL TRACT

Most polyps are located in the rectum, but they may be found anywhere in the intestine. They may be single or multiple. They are usually soft, and they may show ulceration of the surface. Intussusception may occur when the polyp acts as the initiating focus.

Clinical Findings

A. Symptoms: Severity of rectal bleeding depends on the degree and severity of surface erosion of the polyp. Bleeding may be severe for a brief period if the polyp sloughs. The blood is bright red when the polyp is in the rectum or sigmoid, whereas blood from other areas may be dark or occult. Abdominal cramps occasionally occur, or the sharp pain typical of intussusception may be present.

B. Signs: Pallor of anemia may be present owing to chronic bleeding from a polyp. Prolapse of the rectum occasionally occurs. The polyp may be palpable on rectal examination.

C. Laboratory Findings: Anemia may be confirmed by laboratory evaluation.

D. Proctoscopy: The polyp may be visualized if within reach of the proctoscope.

E. X-Ray Findings: A barium enema should be performed to determine the presence of polyps in the colon, particularly those beyond the reach of the proctoscope; filling defects should be looked for by enema and double contrast enemas. It is difficult to demonstrate rectal polyps by barium enema.

Treatment

In most cases, removal of the polyp from the lower intestine is possible through a proctoscope or sigmoidoscope. General anesthesia is usually employed. Blood transfusion may be given preoperatively to correct anemia.

Course & Prognosis

Polyps found in children under 10 years of age are invariably juvenile polyps and have no malignant potential. Laparotomy is never indicated in this age group unless bleeding causes persistent anemia or intussusception develops. Juvenile polyps will slough in time.

Multiple polyps in the older child raise the question of Peutz-Jeghers syndrome, Gardner's syndrome, or multiple polyposis. Family history, excisional biopsy of the lowest polyp, and examination for cutaneous manifestations will rule out these rare causes of polyps. All children with Gardner's syndrome and multiple polyposis should have total or subtotal colectomy with ileoproctostomy.

CONGENITAL MEGACOLON
(Hirschsprung's Disease)

Infants with Hirschsprung's disease lack normal development of Meissner's and Auerbach's plexuses in the distal bowel. The defect always begins at the anorectal junction and may involve all or most of the large bowel. Normally, an 0.5- to 1.5-cm segment of the distal rectum is hypoganglionic or aganglionic. In most cases, only the rectosigmoid is involved. The disease is 5 times more common in males and usually causes symptoms soon after birth.

Clinical Findings

A. Symptoms: Obstipation, abdominal distention, and vomiting may begin in the first few days of life. Ninety percent of patients with aganglionosis fail to pass meconium during the first 24 hours of life. Obstipation may alternate with watery diarrhea. Complete obstruction, perforation, or acute enterocolitis may develop at any time. Poor weight gain and specific nutritional deficiencies are common.

B. Signs: The abdomen is distended, often with palpable loops of bowel and wasted extremities. Rectal examination shows no stool in the ampulla. There may be an explosive release of feces and flatus when the examining finger is withdrawn.

C. X-Ray Findings: An upright abdominal x-ray may show massive distention of the colon with gas and feces. In advanced cases, there may be air-fluid levels. Look carefully for air in the wall of the bowel, which indicates enterocolitis.

Barium enema should be performed *without* the usual bowel preparation. Use only sufficient barium to study the colon up to the junction of the collapsed bowel and that distended with stool. A positive finding reveals that the involved segment is spastic, with an irregular, sawtoothed outline. This may be best seen on a lateral view. In the newborn, this may not be striking, and the only positive finding may be retention of barium in the proximal bowel for more than 24 hours after the examination.

D. Rectal Biopsy: This should be performed after the barium enema has been completed if there is doubt in the diagnosis. A biopsy specimen shows absence of ganglion cells in both Meissner's and Auerbach's plexuses. In Hirschsprung's disease, there is often marked hypertrophy of nerve fibers in Meissner's plexus but no ganglion cells.

Treatment

Only in rare cases should the patient be managed without surgery. Symptoms may be controlled with stool softeners and enemas, but enterocolitis is a constant threat to life.

A. General Measures: Measures include rehydration, correction of electrolyte depletion, and replacement of albumin or blood as necessary. Give antibiotics if there is evidence of enterocolitis or perforation.

B. Surgical Measures: Colostomy is usually necessary and must be done as an emergency procedure if perforation or enterocolitis is suspected.

Resection of the aganglionic segment, with reestablishment of continuity (Swenson, Duhamel, or Soave procedures), may be performed when the patient is 6 months or older. Waiting allows the patient to resume normal growth and allows the distended proximal colon to resume its normal size.

Anorectal myectomy may be all that is required for a patient with a very short involved segment.

Course & Prognosis

At least 90% of patients are symptom-free after surgical treatment. Fecal incontinence or damage to the sacral nerves is rare if the procedures are properly performed.

ANORECTAL MALFORMATIONS

Most males with an anorectal malformation have a fistula to the membranous urethra and no connection between the hindgut and the perineal skin. Most females have a fistula to the perineum at the posterior junction of the labia (posterior fourchette). In the female, communication between the rectum and the urinary tract is extremely rare.

Clinical Findings

A. Males: There is no opening where the anus should be. The intergluteal fold may be well developed, with good sphincter response to perineal stimulation. Look for a fistula along the median raphe. Watch for meconium in urine. There is a significant incidence of associated atresias in the gastrointestinal tract, especially tracheoesophageal fistula. Absence of a perineal fistula means that the patient probably has a communication to the urethra and requires a colostomy. In doubtful cases, injection of contrast medium is occasionally of value.

B. Females: Look for a fistula in the posterior fourchette and perineum. Gentle dilatation of the fistula with a sound will often relieve obstipation temporarily. A high vaginal fistula cannot be handled by dilatation; the patient should have a colostomy.

C. General Findings: Since there is a high incidence of absence of kidneys and strictures of the ureteropelvic and ureterovesical structures, all infants with imperforate anus require intravenous urograms.

Treatment

A. Conservative Measures: Pass a nasogastric tube if no fistula is found or if the abdomen is distended. Perforation can occur if the bowel is allowed to become massively distended. Time should not be wasted waiting for air to distend the rectum for x-ray confirmation.

B. Surgical Measures: Perineal fistulas in males or females require only dilatation during the newborn period; anoplasty can be done later. Pull-through operations for patients with a high imperforate anus should be done after the age of 6 months. The best results are reported following a transcoccygeal approach. The results are poor if the child has myelomeningocele or a significant malformation of the lumbosacral spine.

Prognosis

All infants with perineal fistulas should be continent because bowel passes normally through the levators. Infants with a high pouch have only a fair chance for complete rectal continence. Fecal impaction is a frequent problem, and infants may require stool softeners, suppositories, or anal dilatation.

APPENDICITIS

Appendicitis is the most common pathologic lesion of the intestinal tract requiring surgery in childhood. Most cases are seen in children between the ages of 4 and 12 years and may be associated with other illnesses, especially measles. The cause is not clear, although some cases seem to result from impaction of a fecalith in the lumen of the appendix with resultant congestion of the distal appendix and bacterial invasion by organisms residing in the intestinal tract. Pinworms may occasionally cause appendicitis.

Clinical Findings

A. Symptoms: Acute periumbilical or generalized abdominal pain is usually constant. After 1–5 hours, the pain becomes localized in the right lower quadrant. Urinary pain or frequency may be present if the appendix lies near the bladder or ureters. When vomiting occurs, it is usually only after prolonged pain. Constipation occurs frequently, but diarrhea is only occasionally seen.

B. Signs:

1. Fever–Fever is low-grade, varying from 37.8 to 38.7 °C (100 to 101.6 °F), or may be absent early in the course. Very high fevers are suggestive of appendiceal perforation, with peritonitis, or of the simultaneous presence of bacterial enteritis, especially if accompanied by diarrhea. **Note:** Appendicitis may complicate enteritis.

2. Appearance–The child usually is anxious and may be "doubled up" (with hips flexed) or walk bent over, often holding the right side.

3. Palpation–Palpation may reveal a difference in muscular tension between the 2 sides of the abdomen. The hand should be warm and palpation gentle. Localization of tenderness may be difficult, but an opinion about whether the pain is greatest on the right or left side may be formed by observing the child's expression while palpating each area and noting the involuntary spasm of the abdominal musculature.

4. Psoas sign–Most children tend to flex the right thigh in an effort to decrease the spasm of the psoas muscle. However, the elicitation of a positive psoas sign on hyperextension of the leg, revealing spasm and pain, is generally of doubtful value in small children.

5. Rectal tenderness or mass–There may be rectal tenderness, a mass consisting of peritoneal fluid, or an indurated omentum wrapped around an inflamed appendix.

C. Laboratory Findings: Two or 3 consecutive determinations of white blood cells will frequently show a rise in the total white blood cell count, with an accompanying shift to the left in the neutrophilic series. It is imperative that a careful urinalysis be made in order to rule out inflammation of the kidney or bladder. **Note:** Irritation of the ureter may occur, and a few white or red blood cells may appear in the urine. A neglected abscess behind the bladder may lead to hematuria and urgency.

D. X-Ray Findings: In uncomplicated appendicitis, plain films of the abdomen (rarely necessary) may show a fecalith, scoliosis, or an abnormal gas pattern. When exudate has formed, evidence of peritoneal inflammation may be established by noting disappearance of the peritoneal line and preperitoneal fat line along the right wall of the abdomen or by noting obliteration of the psoas shadow.

The judicious use of a barium enema is valuable in special situations. Normal filling of the appendix tends to exclude the diagnosis of appendicitis. In well-established cases of appendicitis, persistent pressure defects and other abnormalities of the cecum may be noted.

In the presence of perforation, fluid may accumulate between loops of the bowel. However, free intra-abdominal air is rare except in children under 2 years of age. With abscess formation, there may be evidence of a soft tissue mass in the region of the perforation. In atypical cases, a plain film of the chest is of value to rule out reflex pain and abdominal spasm of an undiagnosed pneumonitis.

Differential Diagnosis

A. Mesenteric Lymphadenitis: Abdominal rigidity is generalized, and the pain in the right lower quadrant results from swelling of mesenteric nodes. A respiratory infection or streptococcal sore throat generally precedes the abdominal pain. Tenderness is minimal, vomiting absent, and the white blood cell count normal or elevated. Fever tends to be higher with lymphadenitis than with appendicitis.

B. Pyelitis.

C. Pneumonia: Cough and increased respiratory rate usually are present. The fever commonly is very high, 40–40.6 °C (104–105 °F), and the white blood cell count may be over 20,000/μL. Rales frequently are heard, and abdominal spasms are likely to be temporary and to decrease gradually during gentle palpation.

D. Gastroenteritis: In viral or bacterial gastroenteritis, diarrhea frequently accompanies the vomiting and abdominal pain. Localizing tenderness is absent. A history of similar illness in other members of the family is helpful in making the diagnosis.

E. Pneumococcal Peritonitis: Pneumococcal peritonitis is most frequently seen in children with nephrosis. Tenderness is general, and fever is quite high, 40–40.6 °C (104–105 °F). The white blood cell count is markedly elevated.

F. Constipation: Abdominal pain occurs without fever. Feces can usually be felt through the abdominal wall and by rectal examination. A gentle enema may bring prompt relief of symptoms.

G. Pinworms.

H. Meckel's Diverticulitis.

Complications

Complications include appendiceal perforation and abscess formation, paralytic ileus, and obstruction (if adhesions are formed following surgery or perforation).

Treatment

A. Preoperative Care:

1. Use nasogastric suction preoperatively to deflate the stomach and prevent vomiting.

2. Rehydrate with 0.5 N saline solution. Add potassium chloride as necessary after the child has voided. Defer surgery until the urine specific gravity is 1.020 or less.

3. Administration of plasma depends on the degree of toxicity but is usually indicated in cases of peritonitis.

4. Temperature must be brought below 38.9 °C (102 °F) with hydration and rectal aspirin.

B. Surgical Measures: Appendectomy should be done as soon as the child has been prepared by adequate fluid and electrolyte administration. If there is doubt as to diagnosis, an exploratory laparotomy, with removal of the appendix and culture of peritoneal fluid, should be performed. Intravenous antibiotic therapy may be indicated if peritoneal contamination has occurred. Penrose drains are indicated for localized abscesses.

C. Postoperative Care: Patients with simple appendectomy do not require a nasogastric tube. Intravenous fluids are usually required for 24 hours.

For patients with ruptured appendix, give nothing by mouth until the ileus is terminated. Continuous gastric suction should be employed until intestinal peristalsis is normal. Fowler's position (semi-sitting) should be maintained in order to permit drainage into the pelvic region. Parenteral fluid therapy is administered as indicated (see Chapter 5). Antibiotics are given as needed (see Chapter 6).

D. Treatment of Complications:

1. Appendiceal perforation–Antibiotic therapy is required and should be begun before surgery. Perforation is relatively uncommon (10% of cases) in the first 24 hours of the disease but increases to about 80% during the second to fourth days.

2. Paralytic ileus–This results from peritoneal infection or electrolyte imbalance. When peritonitis causes paralytic ileus, drugs to increase intestinal tone and to stimulate peristalsis are contraindicated. Gastric suction should be continued.

3. Obstruction–This results from the formation of adhesions. It is best treated conservatively by passage of a Miller-Abbot or Harris tube until the obstruction is relieved. If intestinal obstruction occurs late, reexploration may be required to remove obstruction adhesions and bands.

Prognosis

Prognosis is excellent with early diagnosis and surgical removal.

FOREIGN BODIES IN THE GASTROINTESTINAL TRACT

The incidence of foreign bodies in the gastrointestinal tract is highest in children 1–3 years of age. Coins, toys, and marbles may lodge in the esophagus. If passed into the stomach, they usually pass through the entire gastrointestinal tract without incident. If x-rays are taken for presumed ingestion, be sure to include the esophagus and pharynx if the foreign body is not in the abdomen.

Pointed foreign bodies (eg, pins, nails, screws) usually pass without incident. Explore only for pain, fever, vomiting, or local tenderness. Only 2–4% of such cases require surgery. X-ray examination is required only if the foreign body has not passed in 4 or 5 days. If a pin or other sharp object remains in the same location for 4 or 5 days, the point may have penetrated the bowel, and surgery is then indicated.

Blood* | 17

CHILDHOOD ANEMIAS

Anemias in children differ from those in adults in that they may be more pronounced and develop much more rapidly. This is due in part to the fact that growth in childhood is associated with an increased need for blood-building substances. Furthermore, infections, which are so common in childhood, have a more profound effect on blood formation in early life than in adulthood.

Etiologic Classification of Anemias

A. Hypochromic Microcytic Anemias: Anemia may result from iron deficiency due to inadequate storage (prematurity), deficient intake (dietary deficiency), poor absorption, chronic blood loss, poor utilization of iron (infections and inflammation), or milk sensitivity with intestinal dysfunction and blood loss. Other hypochromic microcytic anemias include thalassemia (Mediterranean anemia), copper deficiency, pyridoxine deficiency, and lead poisoning.

B. Normochromic Normocytic Anemias: Anemia may be due to sudden hemorrhage, decreased blood formation (eg, leukemia, hypothyroidism), inflammation (eg, juvenile rheumatoid arthritis, inflammatory bowel disease), some infections, and many hypersplenic states.

C. Macrocytic Anemias: These anemias include folate or vitamin B_{12} deficiency, megaloblastic anemia of infancy, malabsorption syndrome (occasionally seen), hypothyroidism (rarely seen), and early anemia of prematurity. Anemia may occur with some conditions in which the bone marrow is very active.

PHYSIOLOGIC "ANEMIA" OF THE NEWBORN

A gradual drop in red cells and hemoglobin occurs normally during the first 10–12 weeks of life, owing to shortened red cell survival time, expanded intravascular volume, and decreased erythropoietin produc-

*Revised with the assistance of Raleigh Bowden, MD.

tion during this period. The red blood count is reduced to 3.5–4.5 million/μL, and the hemoglobin level may reach a low of 10–12 g/dL in full-term infants and 7 g/dL in premature infants. This is followed by a gradual increase in the number of red cells, with a correspondingly slower rise in hemoglobin level (which results in a relative hypochromic microcytic blood picture). Early changes occur even if the nutritional status of the mother during pregnancy was adequate.

In the full-term infant, the initial drop is not altered by early treatment with iron, but supplemental iron after the second or third month prevents a further reduction and results in a gradual rise of hemoglobin levels.

ANEMIA OF PREMATURITY

Although at birth the red cell count and hemoglobin level of a premature infant are only slightly lower than those of a full-term one, the subsequent reduction that occurs is greater in premature infants. The magnitude of the drop of red cell count and hemoglobin level is inversely proportionate to the size of the infant. In very small infants (< 1 kg at birth), a reduction of hemoglobin to 7–8 g/dL and a reduction of red cells to 2.5–3 million/μL may occur. Lowest levels are reached at about the end of the second month of life. More severe anemia occurs in premature infants than in full-term infants, because there is a greater growth in body size and a correspondingly greater increase in blood volume in premature infants. Furthermore, the total stores of blood-building substances that may be utilized for hemoglobin production are smaller in the premature infant, since most of a newborn's iron is acquired during the last 3 months of gestation; in addition, the hematopoietic system may be less active.

Pallor is the principal manifestation. The anemia generally is normochromic and poikilocytic early in the course of disease and hypochromic and microcytic late in the course.

The initial drop in hemoglobin level or red blood cell count cannot be prevented by early treatment with iron. After the second month of life, supplemental iron should be made available; transfusions seldom are necessary.

IRON DEFICIENCY ANEMIA

Because expansion of blood volume is part of the growth process, the need for iron in children is greater than that in adults. In the average full-term infant, the stores of iron available at birth are adequate for 3–6 months. In the premature infant, twin, or child born of a mother with iron deficiency, the iron reserves will be expended earlier, placing these children at increased risk of developing iron deficiency anemia.

Iron deficiency anemia may result from inadequate storage, deficient intake, chronic blood loss, poor utilization of iron, or milk protein sensitivity. The latter may be associated with chronic respiratory disease and diarrhea. Iron deficiency anemia is uncommon in breast-fed infants.

Clinical Findings

A. Symptoms and Signs: Pallor may be the only early finding. Easy fatigability, weakness, listlessness, and irritability appear later. Interference with growth may occur in long-standing cases, and delayed development (reversible) may occur in anemia of short duration. In more marked cases, heart murmurs, splenomegaly, and hepatomegaly may also be found. Congestive heart failure occurs occasionally; generalized edema, rarely. Pica, especially of ice, occasionally occurs.

B. Laboratory Findings: In hypochromic microcytic anemia, hemoglobin values are decreased, and there is relatively less reduction in red cells. Anisocytosis, poikilocytosis, and polychromatophilia may be marked. The reticulocyte count may be low, normal, or slightly elevated. The serum ferritin concentration is reduced; serum iron level is low; iron-binding capacity is increased; transferrin saturation is reduced; and the level of free erythrocyte protoporphyrin is elevated. Blood may be present in stools. Precipitins to milk are found in some cases. Histologic abnormalities of the bowel may be present. In severe iron deficiency, there may be associated copper deficiency, a decreased serum albumin level, and thrombocytosis.

Treatment

Iron is specific therapy. Other blood-building elements are not necessary.

A. Medicinal Iron: Iron should be given as the ferrous salt. Elemental iron, 4.5–6 mg/kg/d in 3 divided doses, should be given before meals. Adequate vitamin C should be given to ensure optimal iron absorption. Therapy should be continued for several months after the concentration of hemoglobin returns to normal in order to build up some reserve of iron.

Intramuscular iron (iron dextran injection [Imferon]) should be used only when treatment with oral iron is not feasible. The dosage should be determined according to the following formula:

$$\text{Dose} = \frac{\text{Normal hemoglobin} - \text{Initial hemoglobin}}{100} \times 5.1 \times \text{Blood volume}$$

The first injection should consist of a test dose, with subsequent injections being given daily until the total dose is administered.

B. Dietary Iron: Food contains insufficient iron for effective therapy of iron deficiency anemia. Absorption of iron from most foods is generally good; phytates (oatmeal, brown bread) may inhibit absorption. Good sources of iron include liver; dried fruits such as apricots, prunes, and raisins; and pinto beans. Fair food sources of iron include beef, veal, carrots, beans, spinach, peas, sweet potatoes, and peaches.

C. Transfusions: Transfusions of packed red cells are reserved for patients with severe symptomatic anemia for whom a rapid rise in hemoglobin concentration is desired. If evidence of heart failure is present, transfuse very slowly. Parenteral diuretics, partial (isovolumetric) exchange transfusion, and packed red cells may be of value.

Course & Prognosis

Progressive anemia will result unless medicinal or dietary therapy is instituted and the underlying abnormality, if any, corrected. Improvement is then prompt, with a rise in the reticulocyte count appearing in 4–7 days and a rise in the hemoglobin concentration of approximately 0.1–0.2 g/dL/d. Simple iron deficiency anemia due to a low intake of iron should clear rapidly, but the presence of other deficiencies, hematologic abnormalities, congenital malformation, infection, or poor compliance with therapy may alter this favorable outcome.

Administration of iron, 2 mg/kg/d for full-term infants and 4 mg/kg/d for prematures during the first year, in infant formulas or in a medicinal form, has been recommended to prevent iron deficiency.

ANEMIA OF CHRONIC INFECTION & INFLAMMATION

Chronic infection or inflammatory disease is often accompanied by anemia. These chronic conditions may inhibit iron exchange by blocking the release of catabolized iron from the red cells to the reticuloendothelial system. This form of anemia is often confused with iron deficiency anemia, because the red cells may be slightly hypochromic (although they are often normal) and the reticulocyte count is low. However, in anemia of chronic infection, the serum ferritin level is normal, and the anemia does not respond to iron therapy. Anemia may be an important clue to an underlying inflammatory condition and resolves when the primary disease process is controlled or resolves.

HYPOPLASTIC & APLASTIC ANEMIAS

Congenital hypoplastic anemia (Diamond-Blackfan anemia, aregenerative pure red blood cell anemia) is associated with decreased hemoglobin concentration and reticulocyte counts. Erythroid precursors are decreased or absent from the marrow. Patients usually respond well to corticosteroids; transfusions may be necessary. There are no skeletal anomalies.

Children may develop transient erythroblastopenia, with a temporary halt in red cell production manifested by normochromic normocytic anemia, reticulocytopenia, and the absence of red cell precursors in otherwise normal bone marrow. Erythroblastopenia is usually preceded by viral or bacterial infection and can be differentiated from congenital hypoplastic anemia (Diamond-Blackfan anemia) by the presence of normal hemoglobin F, low mean corpuscular volume (< 80 fL), and a normal quantity of i antigen. Recovery is spontaneous without treatment, often within a few weeks.

Hypoplastic anemia, often with pancytopenia, presenting after the age of 2 years may occur as an autosomal recessive disorder in association with abnormal pigmentation, skeletal anomalies (eg, absent, hypoplastic, or supernumerary thumb; hypoplastic or absent radius), retarded growth, hypogonadism, small head, renal anomalies, microphthalmos, strabismus, and abnormalities of the reproductive tract (Fanconi's syndrome). The condition may respond to testosterone; some reports suggest also using corticosteroids.

Aplastic anemia, characterized by pancytopenia and hypoplasia of the bone marrow, is rare in childhood. The peak incidence is 3–5 years of age. Acquired aplastic anemia may occur as a toxic reaction to drugs or chemicals (chloramphenicol, phenylbutazone, sulfonamides, solvents, insecticides), as a complication of infection, or in association with early manifestations of leukemia. Although anemia appears to be acquired in most cases, no causative agent can be identified in as many as 50% of patients (idiopathic or constitutional aplastic anemia). Children with aplastic anemia present with pallor, fatigue, fever, and increased bleeding tendencies. Hepatosplenomegaly and adenopathy do not result. The prognosis of aplastic anemia is extremely poor; fewer than 10% of patients recover fully within 5 years, and 50% of patients die from hemorrhage or infection within the first 6 months. Bone marrow transplant from a sibling with HLA-compatible marrow may increase survival to 50–70% and is presently the treatment of choice. When bone marrow transplant is not feasible, the use of corticosteroids or androgens may be of value.

Caution: Most children given large doses of chloramphenicol temporarily develop some degree of bone marrow depression; in some instances, permanent and potentially fatal aplastic anemia may occur even after small doses. A rise in serum iron level and a decrease in reticulocyte count may be premonitory findings. Hepatocellular carcinoma has been noted in association with androgen therapy for the treatment of aplastic and hypoplastic anemias.

HEMOLYTIC ANEMIAS

General Considerations

Hemolytic anemias of childhood may be due to congenital defects in the production of red cells or hemoglobin or both (hereditary spherocytosis, congenital nonspherocytic hemolytic anemia, congenital elliptocytosis, thalassemia, congenital hemoglobinopathies, and congenital deficiencies of erythrocyte enzymes [eg, glucose-6-phosphate dehydrogenase]); or they may result from acquired defects in the red cells or their environment (hemolytic anemia due to toxic substances, infections, radiation, thermal injury, specific antigen-antibody reactions, idiosyncratic reactions to certain organic substances, hypersplenism, and incompatible blood transfusions). The principal feature of the hemolytic anemias is a reduction of the life span of the erythrocytes.

Symptoms and signs of hemolytic anemia may include easy fatigability, jaundice, and splenomegaly. Gallstones may develop after many episodes of hemolysis.

The peripheral blood usually shows reticulocytosis, nucleated red blood cells, hyperbilirubinemia, and markedly diminished levels of haptoglobin. The urine and feces contain increased amounts of urobilinogen. Erythroid hyperplasia of the bone marrow often results in widening of the marrow spaces. In long-standing cases, hemosiderosis may occur.

AUTOIMMUNE HEMOLYTIC ANEMIA

In autoimmune hemolytic anemia, hemolysis occurs when IgG or IgM antibodies are directed against and cause damage to the red cell membranes. IgG-mediated disease is primarily an extravascular process, with hemolysis occurring in spleen cells or other reticuloendothelial cells, while IgM-mediated disease is generally intravascular. The cause of anemia cannot be identified in about half of affected patients (idiopathic autoimmune hemolytic anemia). Anemia in other patients may be associated with immunoproliferative disorders (subacute lupus erythematosus, Hodgkin's disease, and other malignant diseases), infection (especially tuberculosis, cytomegalovirus, and other viral infections), and chronic inflammatory conditions (ulcerative colitis).

The clinical presentation may be indolent or fulminant, with symptoms of anemia (pallor, malaise, and congestive heart failure); jaundice (common), with increased amounts of urobilinogen in the urine; and splenomegaly, which is more common with the IgG-mediated form of the disease. Laboratory findings include reticulocytosis and the presence of microspherocytes. Results of direct Coombs tests are positive for IgG antibody in sera from patients with IgG-mediated anemia, negative for IgG antibody in sera from those with IgM-mediated anemia, and usually positive for complement fixation in both groups.

If hemolysis is mild, treatment may not be necessary. Most patients respond to prednisone administered for 7–10 days; an initial larger dose is decreased over the next few days. Splenectomy is reserved for patients with severe hemolysis that is unresponsive to an adequate trial of steroids. Transfusions are given if signs of congestive heart failure are present. ***Caution:*** Care should be taken to avoid further overloading of the circulatory system.

ISOIMMUNE HEMOLYTIC ANEMIA

Isoimmune hemolytic anemia is seen primarily in the newborn and is due to incompatibility with maternal Rh, ABO, or other antibodies. It may also occur with transfusion reactions in patients of all ages. Findings are similar to those of autoimmune hemolytic anemia. After the source of exogenous antibody has been discontinued, the anemia is usually self-limited. However, exchange transfusion may be required, especially in patients with Rh incompatibility.

CONGENITAL (HEREDITARY) SPHEROCYTOSIS

Congenital spherocytosis is a hereditary (dominant) disease due to excessive destruction of abnormally shaped cells (spherocytes). The disease may be discovered during a ''hypoplastic'' crisis, when the reticulocyte count may be very low and the degree of anemia more profound than usual. Crises may occur at periodic intervals.

Other members of the family may have overt or subclinical disease with slight spherocytosis and increased osmotic fragility of red blood cells (demonstrated in hypotonic saline solution). In a small percentage of cases, no family involvement can be determined.

Findings include spherocytosis, increased osmotic fragility, and reticulocytosis. The osmotic fragility test will show abnormal findings if the blood is incubated (at 37 °C for 24 hours) prior to testing. The autohemolysis test results are also abnormal. Maturation arrest of all elements in the marrow may be present at times of crises. Neonates may show early and exaggerated jaundice, often requiring exchange transfusion. Cholelithiasis may develop in the second or third decade.

Treatment is by splenectomy, ideally performed in patients after the age of 3–4 years. Because of the increased risk of sepsis in splenectomized individuals, prophylactic penicillin should be given until the patient is at least 4 or 5 years of age. Until the time of splenectomy, folic acid, 1 mg/d, should be given. Pneumococcal vaccine provides additional protection.

Following removal of the spleen, the underlying defect of the red cells persists, but most patients will have a complete remission from hemolysis and anemia.

NONSPHEROCYTIC HEMOLYTIC ANEMIA ASSOCIATED WITH DEFICIENCIES OF VARIOUS ENZYMES

See also General Considerations, p 392.

Approximately 10% of black males, a small percentage of whites, and varying percentages of Orientals have a deficiency of erythrocyte glucose-6-phosphate dehydrogenase. The deficiency may predispose them to increased hemolysis upon exposure to primaquine, naphthalene, sulfonamides, synthetic vitamin K, fava beans, aspirin, acetanilid, phenacetin, or acetaminophen. Hemolysis is occasionally precipitated by certain infections. The disorder is inherited as an X-linked recessive trait.

In addition, other patients may have other intrinsic defects of the red blood cells, with clinical manifestations that appear during the neonatal period. They may have a deficiency of pyruvate kinase or an unstable hemoglobin. These conditions are inherited by autosomal recessive transmission.

There may be macrocytosis, increased mean corpuscular volume, reticulocytosis, and basophilic stippling of the red cells. Serum iron levels may be normal or low. Osmotic fragility is normal or increased. The autohemolysis test, when done with and without glucose and ATP, is useful in classifying this group of anemias. Precise diagnosis usually requires highly specialized laboratory facilities.

Transfusions should be given for severe anemia. Splenectomy benefits a few patients.

HEMOLYTIC-UREMIC SYNDROME
(Syndrome of Hemolytic Anemia, Thrombocytopenic Purpura, & Nephropathy; Thrombotic Microangiopathy)

Hemolytic-uremic syndrome, occurring mainly in children between the ages of 6 months and 6 years, is characterized by (1) a sudden onset of hemolytic anemia (with pallor, mild jaundice in some cases, and, usually, a negative Coombs test result); (2) thrombocytopenic purpura (with petechiae, ecchymoses, and adequate megakaryocytes in the bone marrow); (3) nephropathy (with renal insufficiency, azotemia, and acute renal necrosis); and (4) central nervous system involvement (with drowsiness and convulsions). Clinical manifestations of the syndrome are frequently preceded by diarrhea (commonly due to enterovirus infection) or, less often, by an upper respiratory tract infection, with an intervening symptom-free period of 1–10 days. Other findings that may be present include hepatosplenomegaly, severe abdominal pain, hypertension, and cardiac failure. The red blood cells may be fragmented and helmet-shaped or burr-shaped. The mortality rate is high (> 25%). Disseminated intravascular coagulation and pathologic consumption of platelets may be factors in the progressive pathologic changes.

Packed red blood cell transfusions and peritoneal dialysis are often required as supportive measures. Therapy with heparin, inhibitors of platelet function, or activators of fibrinolysin, or a combination of aspirin, dipyridamole, and heparin is of value in some cases. Complete recovery from hematologic manifestations usually occurs, but permanent impairment of renal function is not uncommon.

Partial forms of the disease may occur. The patient's siblings may also be affected.

HEREDITARY ELLIPTOCYTOSIS
(Ovalocytosis)

See also General Considerations, p 392.

Hereditary elliptocytosis is a congenital disease characterized by numerous elongated or oval cells. It is usually asymptomatic, but some patients may have mild to severe hemolysis. In the latter, splenectomy may be of value.

• • •

HEREDITARY HEMOGLOBINOPATHIES

BETA-THALASSEMIA

Beta-thalassemia is a relatively common anemia that is due to an inherited defect in the synthesis of the beta chains of hemoglobin. It may occur in a severe homozygous form, characterized by pronounced changes in the blood and in various organ systems; or it may occur as the "trait," with little or no anemia and no systemic changes. It is most common in Italians and Greeks but occurs occasionally in Southeast Asians and other persons of non-Mediterranean background.

Table 17–1. Summary of findings in abnormal hemoglobin diseases and thalassemia.

	Hemoglobin Type	Anemia	Spleno-megaly	Arthralgia	Increased Blood Destruction	Target Cells	Sickling	Microcytosis	Hypochromia
Normal adult	A(A_2,F*)	0	0	0	No	0	0	0	0
Normal newborn	A,F†	0	0	0	No	0	0	0	0
Iron deficiency anemia	A(A_2,F*)	+ to ++++	±	0	No	±	0	+ to ++++	+ to ++++
Some acquired anemias	A,F†	+ to ++++	+ to ++++	±		±	0	0	0
β-Thalassemia major	A,F†	++++	++++	0	Yes	++	0	++++	++++
β-Thalassemia minor	A,A_2(F†)	±	0 to +	0	±	+	0	0 to +	0 to +
β-Thalassemia–hemoglobin C disease	C,A	+	0		Yes	+++	0	+	±
β-Thalassemia–hemoglobin E disease	E,F†	+++	++		Yes	++	0	+	+
β-Thalassemia–hemoglobin G disease (?)	G,F†		++			++	+	+	0
Sickle cell trait	A,S	0	0	0	No	+	+	0	0
Sickle cell anemia	S,S(F†)	+++	±	++	Yes	++	+++	0	0 to +
Sickle cell–hereditary spherocytosis	S,A	++	++			++	+	+	0
Sickle cell–β-thalassemia disease	S,F†,A,A_2	++	+++	++	Yes	++	++	++	++
Sickle cell–$β^o$-thalassemia disease	S,F†,A_2	++	+++	++	Yes	++	++	++	++
Sickle cell–hemoglobin C disease	S,C(F†)	+	++	±	Yes	+++	++	±	+
Sickle cell–hemoglobin D disease	S,D(F†)	+	++		Yes	±	+	+	+
Sickle cell–hemoglobin G disease	S,G	0	0		No	0	+	0	0
Hemoglobin C trait	A,C	0	0	0	No	0 to +++	0	0	+
Homologous hemoglobin C disease	C,C	+	+++	+	Yes	++++	0	±	+
Hemoglobin D trait	A,D	0	0		No	?	0	0	0
Hemoglobin E trait	A,E	0	0	0	No	±	0	0	0
Homologous hemoglobin E disease	E,E(F†)	++	±		Yes	+++	0	++	0
Hemoglobin G trait	A,G	0	0	0	No	0	0	0	0
Homologous hemoglobin G disease	G,G	0	0		No	0	0	0	0
Hemoglobin H trait (?)	A,H	+	++		Yes	+	0	+	+
Hemoglobin I trait	A,I	0	0		No	0	0	0	0

*A_2 and F are usually < 5% of the total hemoglobin. †Elevated levels.

Thalassemia Major (Homozygous Form; Mediterranean Anemia, Cooley's Anemia)

The homozygous form is a severe hypochromic microcytic anemia that starts in the first year of life. Both parents will be carriers of the "trait." Symptoms are secondary to the anemia and include pallor, characteristic facies due to widening of the tabular bones of the skull, jaundice of varying degrees, enlargement of liver and spleen, and pathologic fractures. Laboratory findings (see Table 17–1) include hypochromic microcytic anemia, anisocytosis, poikilocytosis, basophilic stippling, and decreased fragility of the red cells, with the presence of target cells, nucleated erythrocytes, and an increased number of reticulocytes in the peripheral blood. (Reticulocyte count may fall in association with a drop in hematocrit.) Levels of hemoglobin F are elevated. Findings on x-ray include changes in the bones due to extreme marrow hyperplasia. These changes include widening of the medulla, thinning of the cortex, and coarsening of trabeculation (the so-called hair-on-end appearance).

Thalassemia Minor (Heterozygous Form; Thalassemia Trait, Cooley's Carrier State)

In the heterozygous form, evidence of mild anemia and splenomegaly may be present. Blood smears show hypochromic microcytosis, target cells, anisocytosis, and poikilocytosis. The diagnosis may be confirmed by finding elevated levels of fetal or A_2 hemoglobin on hemoglobin electrophoresis.

Treatment

Transfusions are the only effective means of temporarily overcoming the anemia in severe cases, but they do not alter the underlying disease. Other hematopoietic agents are entirely ineffective and should not be used. Recent reports suggest that iron chelation with deferoxamine and vitamin C combined with hypertransfusion (maintaining hemoglobin at high levels [> 11 g/dL]) may be beneficial. Chronic hypoxia and iron loading are the significant factors in the production of myocardial and hepatic damage.

Splenectomy may be necessary when the spleen is so large as to produce discomfort or if an acquired hemolytic component is superimposed on the primary disease. However, the risk of infection in splenectomized children with thalassemia is great, and prophylactic penicillin should be given.

Course & Prognosis

In spite of repeated transfusions, children with thalassemia major generally die within the first 2 decades from intercurrent infections or from hemochromatosis. Gallbladder stones frequently develop in patients surviving to the early teens. Thalassemia trait is associated with a normal life span.

The more severe the anemia and the earlier its onset, the more rapidly the disease progresses to a fatal outcome. Maintaining the hemoglobin level above 10 g/dL may be effective in improving the condition of children with abnormal cardiac symptoms.

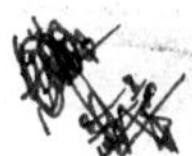

SICKLE CELL ANEMIA

Sickle cell anemia is an inherited abnormality of hemoglobin (hemoglobin S) limited mainly to blacks. In hemoglobin S, the amino acid valine replaces the normally occurring glutamic acid in the beta chain. Although the sickle trait occurs in about 8% of the black population, the disease with anemia occurs only in homozygotes.

Clinical Findings

A. Symptoms and Signs: Onset of clinical manifestations may be at any time in the first decade. Findings include fever, headache, joint involvement (pain and swelling), osteopathy (particularly of metacarpals and phalanges), abdominal pain and tenderness, pallor, jaundice, splenomegaly (in the very young), hepatomegaly, cardiomegaly, and hemic heart murmurs. Ulceration of the skin over the lower extremities is unusual during childhood but may occur in teenagers. The spleen ceases to function normally early in childhood, and "autosplenectomy" occurs as a result of repeated thromboses. There may be episodes of vascular occlusion and infarction. Enuresis and nocturia may be present. Patients with sickle cell anemia have an increased resistance to malarial infection; an increased susceptibility to bacterial sepsis, osteomyelitis, pneumonia, and meningitis; and an increased risk of anesthetic complications. They may have an increased appetite for salt. In the severe form, the general picture is of poor health, development, and nutrition. Folic acid deficiency is common. During a painful "crisis," the picture may be that of acute rheumatic fever, acute surgical abdomen, or infection of the central nervous system. "Aplastic" crises may occur, with diminished red cell production superimposed on rapid destruction.

B. Laboratory Findings: Sickle-shaped red blood cells are seen in peripheral blood smears. Other findings include normochromic anemia, reticulocytosis, nucleated red blood cells in the peripheral blood, leukocytosis, hyperbilirubinemia, increased excretion of urobilinogen, increased lactate dehydrogenase levels, increased resistance of red blood cells to osmotic lysis, and an abnormal electrophoretic pattern, with 50–100% hemoglobin S and increased amounts of fetal hemoglobin. There is excretion of excessive quantities of urine of low specific gravity. Severe hyponatremia may occur during a crisis. Zinc deficiency may be an attribute of short stature and delayed onset of puberty.

Heterozygotes (carriers of sickle trait) may be identified by use of a screening test (Sickledex test; sodium metabisulfite test) and hemoglobin electrophoresis. Characteristically, 35–45% hemoglobin S is found. Heterozygotes are not anemic and—except for conditions with extreme hypoxia—are asymptomatic.

Treatment

Parenteral fluid therapy, analgesics, and transfusion for severe anemia and crises are the only consistently effective methods of treatment. Placing the patient in oxygen during the crisis and giving bicarbonate have been recommended.

Adequate hydration of the patient at the onset of a crisis sometimes obviates the need for transfusions. Because infection exacerbates sickling of the patient's red blood cells, all infections should be treated promptly and vigorously.

Folic acid, 1 mg/d, should be given. The routine administration of aspirin and prophylactic penicillin has been advocated.

Course & Prognosis

The course is determined by the severity of the sickling tendency and resulting hemolysis, the frequency and duration of crises, and the age of the patient. Interference with growth, nutrition, and general activity is common, although many patients lead active lives with persistent hemoglobin levels of 7–9 g/dL.

The use of repeated transfusions in conjunction with deferoxamine chelation, designed to maintain hemoglobin levels above 11 g/dL and thus decrease bone marrow production of S hemoglobin, may delay or reverse some of these changes.

BLEEDING DISEASES IN CHILDHOOD

GENERAL CONSIDERATIONS

Family History

A family history of easy bruising and excessive bleeding is valuable in the following disorders: (1) hemophilia (males only), (2) hemophilialike disease in which either sex may be affected, (3) congenital thrombocytopenia or platelet dysfunction syndromes, (4) hereditary hemorrhagic telangiectasia, and (5) deficiencies of factor V, VII, X, or XI (Table 17–2), which may be hereditary and not X-linked.

Table 17–2. Blood clotting factors and deficiency diseases.

	Clotting Factor*	Deficiency Disease
I	Fibrinogen.	Afibrinogenemia, factor I deficiency disease.
II	Prothrombin.	Prothrombin deficiency disease, factor II deficiency disease.
III	Tissue thromboplastin.	
IV	Calcium (Ca^{2+}).	
V	Proaccelerin; labile factor.	Proaccelerin deficiency disease, plasma and serum accelerator globulin (AcG) deficiency disease, factor V deficiency disease.
VII	Proconvertin; stable factor.	Proconvertin deficiency disease, stable factor deficiency disease, serum prothrombin conversion accelerator (SPCA) deficiency disease, cothromboplastin deficiency disease, factor VII deficiency disease.
VIII	Antihemophilic globulin (AHG); antihemophilic factor (AHF).	Hemophilia A, AHF deficiency disease, factor VIII deficiency disease.
IX	Plasmin thromboplastin component (PTC); Christmas factor.	Hemophilia B, PTC deficiency disease, Christmas disease, factor IX deficiency disease.
X	Stuart factor; Stuart-Prower factor.	Stuart-Prower factor deficiency disease, factor X deficiency disease.
XI	Plasma thromboplastin antecedent (PTA).	Hemophilia C, PTA deficiency disease, factor XI deficiency disease.
XII	Hageman factor.	
XIII	Fibrin-stabilizing factor.	Fibrin-stabilizing factor deficiency disease, factor XIII deficiency disease.

*Factor VI is not considered a separate entity.

Physical Examination

Bleeding disorder should be considered in patients with abrupt changes in the pattern or severity of bruising and bleeding, unexplained bleeding from a circumcision, or excessive bleeding at the site of surgery.

Bruises on the extremities are found in many normal children following trauma and usually have no clinical significance. Generalized lymphadenopathy and petechiae are not produced by any of the diseases resulting from a defect of the clotting mechanism. In infants and young children, petechiae frequently occur in the head and neck areas in association with crying, vomiting, or coughing. In other circumstances, the presence of petechiae may indicate an abnormality in the number or function of the platelets or a defect of the blood vessels. Hemarthrosis is uncommon except in patients with hemophilia.

Laboratory Examination

"Routine" preoperative bleeding and clotting time determinations are essentially valueless without an adequate history and careful physical examination.

HEMOPHILIA

Hemophilia is an X-linked bleeding disorder transmitted by females to their male offspring. Hemophilia A (factor VIII deficiency, or classic hemophilia) comprises 75% of hemophilia. It occurs with an incidence of 7 per 100,000 population. Affected family members generally have equally severe disease. Hemophilia B (factor IX deficiency, or Christmas disease) is much less common. It may demonstrate the same levels of severity.

Clinical Findings

A. Symptoms and Signs: Symptoms vary greatly in severity; many cases are mild. Severely affected patients are usually identified at circumcision or in the first year of life and show signs of increased bruising and hemarthrosis (most commonly of the knees, ankles, or hips) as they begin to walk. In older patients, bleeding may occur in the large muscle groups, the genitourinary tract, or the skin. Mucous membrane bleeding, usually of the mouth, is also a problem after even a minor laceration or contusion. Mildly affected patients rarely have bleeding into the joint and may present with hemophilia only at the time of a surgical procedure.

B. Laboratory Findings: (See Table 17–3.) Results of routine bleeding and clotting tests are often normal in patients with mild hemophilia. The kaolin partial thromboplastin time (PTT) test and the thromboplastin generation test should be performed in any suspected case of hemophilia. If the PTT is prolonged, a specific-factor assay should be carried out to confirm the diagnosis. The carrier state may be detectable by appropriate specific-factor assays.

Treatment

A. Specific Measures: The specific treatment of hemophilia consists of replacing missing clotting factors. In hemophilia A, only fresh frozen plasma, lyophilized fresh plasma, factor VIII concentrates, or cryoprecipitates of fresh plasma should be used. In younger children, this can be achieved with cryoprecipitates (100 units of factor VIII per plastic pack); for dosage, see Therapeutic Blood Fraction Products, p 404. Older children with hemophilia A may be given factor VIII concentrates (250 units per vial). The dosage for concentrates is lower than that for cryoprecipitates, but use of concentrates carries a higher risk of hepatitis than does use of cryoprecipitates. In hemophilia B, use of stored or fresh blood, fresh frozen plasma (200–250 units per plastic

Table 17–3. Differentiation of coagulation defects.

Disease*	Coagulation Time	Bleeding Time	Platelet Count	One-Stage Prothrombin Time	Partial Thrombo-plastin Time	Thrombin Time
Factor I deficiency disease	No clot	N	N	↑	N	↑
Factor II deficiency disease	N (↑)	V†	N	↑	N	N
Factor V deficiency disease	↑	N	N	↑	↑	N
Factor VII deficiency disease	N	N	N	↑	N	N
Factor VIII deficiency disease	↑	N	N	N	↑	N
Factor IX deficiency disease	↑	N	N	N	↑	N
Factor X deficiency disease	N (↑)	N	N	↑	↑	N
Factor XI deficiency disease	N (↑)	N	N	N	↑	N
Factor XIII deficiency disease	N	N	N	N	N‡	N
Thrombasthenia (Glanzmann's syndrome)	N	↑	N	N	N	N
Thrombocytopenia	N	↑	↓	N	N	N
Von Willebrand's disease‡§	N (↑)	↑	N	N	↑	N

*See Table 17–2 for synonyms of factor deficiency diseases.

†Variable.

‡Diagnosis should be suspected in a congenital bleeding state when results of all screening tests are normal. Findings on thromboelastograph may be abnormal; diagnosis is confirmed by showing instability of fibrin clot in urea.

§Associated with factor VIII deficiency in most cases.

pack), or a concentrate of factor IX (Konyne; 550 units of factor IX per vial) is effective; for dosage, see Therapeutic Blood Fraction Products, p 404. Because of the danger of hepatitis, whole blood or frozen plasma should be used instead of pooled plasma when possible. Dosage is determined by the severity of the bleeding to be treated. Hypervolemia may be avoided by the use of antihemophilic factor (AHF) or factor VIII concentrates in smaller doses. Therapy in some patients may be complicated by the development of platelet dysfunction, probably related to the relatively large amounts of fibrin degradation products contained in the AHF concentrates or in stored plasma.

B. Special Problems:

1. Head injuries–Head injuries can be life-threatening in severe hemophiliacs. Raise the factor VIII level to over 50% as soon as possible. Patients with head injuries often require repeated factor replacement initially and, if intracranial hemorrhage is documented, for several weeks.

2. Hemarthroses–In patients with bleeding into the joints or muscles, raise the factor VIII levels to 20–40% every day until the pain becomes less severe. Bed rest and a short period of immobilization (usually for no longer than 24 hours) are indicated. This is followed by a slow increase in the level of physical therapy, with an active range of motion to regain full use of the joint. Acetaminophen is usually sufficient for analgesia if the patient is transfused early. Aspirin should not be used. Subsequent therapy includes diathermy, passive and then active exercises, and prevention of ankylosis in the unphysiologic position. Repeated episodes of joint effusion as well as hematuria may be treated by corticosteroids.

3. Sutures–If suturing is necessary, raise the factor VIII levels to 20–40% every other day until the sutures are removed, including the day of removal.

4. Hematuria–Patients with hematuria may be treated with a short course of corticosteroids.

5. Open wounds–In patients with bleeding from open wounds (skin, tooth socket), follow the measures outlined above, as indicated. Do *not* cauterize the wounds. Avoid suturing if possible. Use pressure bandage and application of cold to accessible areas. Thrombin is the hemostatic agent of choice. Gelatin foam or fibrin may be used as a vehicle for the thrombin.

Prognosis

The prognosis has been much improved since home care programs of prophylactic therapy have been used. Many of the problems of chronic joint disease have been avoided. Major problems of repeated administration of blood products include the increased risk of hepatitis and the development of inhibitors (IgG antibody) to factor VIII or IX in 10–15%

of patients. With home transfusion programs, most patients are successful in leading independent and nearly normal life-styles.

VON WILLEBRAND'S DISEASE

Von Willebrand's disease is a mild to severe familial bleeding disorder characterized by abnormalities of the factor VIII molecule. In severe classic von Willebrand's disease, the factor VIII procoagulant activity (VIIIc), the portion of the molecule that corrects the bleeding time defect and supports ristocetin-induced aggregation of platelets (VIIIvWd), and the factor VIII measured by heterologous antibodies (VIII antigen) are reduced or absent. Variants of the disorder are seen in which combinations of the above attributes of the factor VIII molecule are defective.

Patients with von Willebrand's disease show skin and mucous membrane bleeding (epistaxis, menorrhagia). The disorder is usually inherited as an autosomal dominant trait. The bleeding time is usually prolonged, as is the partial thromboplastin time, although in mild cases, measurements of VIIIc, VIII antigen, and VIIIvWd must be made to establish the diagnosis.

Treatment consists of infusions of fresh frozen plasma (10–15 mL/kg) or cryoprecipitate (one plastic pack per 6 kg).

THERAPEUTIC BLOOD FRACTION PRODUCTS

When therapeutic blood fractions are given, there is a risk of transmitting the virus of serum hepatitis; this risk is greater when pooled blood fraction products are given than when single donor products are used. There appears to be an increased risk of AIDS syndrome with the usc of factor VIII concentrates or other blood components.

AHF or Factor VIII Concentrates (Cryoprecipitates)

Cryoprecipitates are a blood bank product made from fresh frozen plasma. One pack of cryoprecipitate contains 100 units.*

A. Indications: For therapy of factor VIII deficiency (hemophilia A or von Willebrand's disease).

B. Dosage and Administration: Reconstitute lyophilized material (stored at 4 °C) and inject by intravenous push. Dose is calculated as follows:

Units* of factor VIII = Desired in vivo level in percent × 0.5 × Weight (kg)

*A unit of a clotting factor is that contained in the equivalent of 1 mL of fresh plasma with 100% clotting activity.

A dosage of one pack per 5 kg usually gives a factor VIII level of 40%. The usual level desired is 40%; however, 20% is the minimal hemostatic level.

Factor IX Complex

Factor IX complex (Konyne) is a lyophilized product containing factors IX, II, VII, and X in vials of 500 units.*

A. Indications: For therapy of congenital factor IX deficiency (hemophilia B, or Christmas disease) or severe liver disease.

B. Dosage and Administration: Dosage is calculated as for factor VIII (see above) except that twice the calculated dose is given initially (for tissue diffusion).

Normal Human Plasma

Products contain a 5% solution of heat-treated human plasma protein fraction (Plasmanate).

A. Indications: For treatment of shock due to dehydration and infection.

B. Dosage and Administration: Give 10 mL/kg (15 mL/lb) intravenously no faster than 5–10 mL/min.

Normal Human Serum Albumin

Products contain 5 g of normal serum albumin (salt-poor) and 20 mL of buffer diluent, or a 5% solution (12.5 g in 250 mL or 25 g in 500 mL; Albumisol).

A. Indications: As replacement therapy for deficiency diseases and as treatment for hypoproteinemia, hyperbilirubinemia, shock due to hemorrhage (if no whole blood is available), and peripheral vasomotor collapse from other causes.

B. Dosage and Administration: Give intravenously; 5 g of albumin is therapeutically equivalent to 100 mL of citrated plasma.

OTHER BLEEDING DISEASES

DISSEMINATED INTRAVASCULAR COAGULATION

Disseminated intravascular coagulation (DIC) is characterized by intravascular consumption of plasma clotting factors (factors I, II, V, and VIII) and platelets; fibrinolysis, with production of fibrin split products; widespread deposition of fibrin thrombi that produce tissue

*A unit of a clotting factor is that contained in the equivalent of 1 mL of fresh plasma with 100% clotting activity.

ischemia and necrosis in various organs (principally the lungs, kidneys, gastrointestinal tract, adrenals, brain, liver, pancreas, and skin); generalized hemorrhagic diathesis; microangiopathic hemolytic anemia, with fragmented, burred, and helmet-shaped erythrocytes; and shock and death. The disorder has been found in association with infections, surgical procedures, burns, neonatal conditions (especially sepsis and respiratory distress syndrome), malignant neoplastic disease, severe hypoxia and acidosis, other metabolic disorders, and a variety of miscellaneous causes (eg, hemangioma, transfusion reactions, drugs, hemolytic-uremic syndrome). The clinical manifestations depend on the systems involved. Laboratory findings include prolonged prothrombin and partial thromboplastin time, elevated levels of monomers and fibrin split products, decreased levels of fibrinogen, and decreased platelet counts.

Therapy consists of treating the underlying cause (sepsis, acidosis, hypoxia) and replacing clotting factors with fresh frozen plasma, 10 mL/kg, or platelet transfusions. In the newborn with severe disseminated coagulation, exchange transfusion may be of value. Indications for use of heparin include severe meningococcemia (to prevent necrotic lesions), associated large vessel thrombosis, purpura fulminans, and promyelocytic or monocytic leukemia.

PURPURAS

Purpuras are bleeding diseases that may be due to a reduced number or abnormal function of platelets or to a defect in or abnormality of the vascular system.

CLASSIFICATION OF PURPURAS

Purpuras are differentiated by the clinical picture, the number and type of platelets in the peripheral blood, and the number and type of megakaryocytes in the bone marrow.

Purpuras With Low Platelet Counts & Normal or Increased Numbers of Megakaryocytes

(1) Immunologic purpura, including (a) postinfectious purpura; (b) drug-induced purpura; (c) certain collagen diseases (eg, lupus erythematosus); and (d) congenital purpura due to isoimmunization resulting from maternal sensitization to some drugs, with passive transfer of maternal antiplatelet antibody.

(2) Infectious mononucleosis.

(3) Hypersplenic states (eg, Banti's syndrome, Gaucher's disease, postinfectious states, cirrhosis).

(4) Thrombotic thrombocytopenia.

(5) Hemolytic-uremic syndrome.

(6) Purpura associated with large hemangiomas.

(7) Wiskott-Aldrich syndrome.

Purpuras With Normal Platelet Counts & Abnormalities of the Vascular System

(1) Anaphylactoid or ''vascular'' (Henoch-Schönlein) purpura.

(2) Scurvy.

(3) Nonthrombocytopenic purpura associated with infection (eg, meningococcemia, subacute infective endocarditis) or chemical and animal agents (eg, penicillin, snake venoms).

(4) Hereditary hemorrhagic telangiectasia.

(5) Traumatic or mechanical purpuras, including those associated with certain skin diseases (eg, Ehlers-Danlos syndrome, telangiectatic purpura).

(6) Purpura associated with chronic disease (eg, hypertension, cardiac disease, Cushing's syndrome).

(7) Psychogenic purpura.

(8) Toxic purpura.

Purpuras With Normal Platelet Counts, Normal Megakaryocytes, & Defective Function of Platelets

(1) Thrombasthenia.

(2) Congenital thrombocytopathy.

(3) Uremia.

(4) Cirrhosis of the liver.

(5) Von Willebrand's disease.

(6) Purpura following aspirin ingestion.

Purpuras With Low Platelet Counts & Decreased Numbers of Megakaryocytes

(1) Toxic purpura following exposure to various poisons and drugs.

(2) Purpura due to severe infections.

(3) Uremia.

(4) Purpura associated with hypoplastic and aplastic anemias.

(5) Leukemia and other malignant neoplastic diseases.

(6) Purpura resulting from ionizing irradiation.

(7) Purpura associated with megaloblastic anemia.

(8) Congenital purpura, which may be associated with absence of the radius.

IDIOPATHIC THROMBOCYTOPENIC PURPURA (Immunologic Thrombocytopenic Purpura)

Idiopathic thrombocytopenic purpura of childhood is a relatively common bleeding disorder most likely mediated by antiplatelet antibodies. It usually occurs in patients between 2 and 10 years of age and commonly follows an infection (viral, upper respiratory tract, or gastrointestinal tract infection or, sometimes, urinary tract or dental infection) by 2–3 weeks. In the neonatal period, thrombocytopenic purpura may follow infection or exchange transfusion or may be due to maternal isoantibodies to the infant's platelets.

Clinical Findings

A. Symptoms and Signs: Bleeding into the skin or from the nose, gums, and urinary tract is the most common symptom. Bleeding into joints or from the bowel is uncommon. Central nervous system bleeding occurs rarely but may be fatal. Petechiae usually are present. Fever, pallor, lymphadenopathy, and hepatomegaly are usually absent. Splenomegaly is rare.

B. Laboratory Findings: The platelet count is low, and the bleeding time is prolonged. Large immature platelets are occasionally seen. Red and white blood cell counts are normal unless severe hemorrhage has occurred. Megakaryocytes in the bone marrow are normal or increased in number. Antiplatelet antibodies may be demonstrated. Results of other hematologic tests are normal.

In the congenital form, the mother may also exhibit thrombocytopenia at the time; or she may have specific platelet antibodies.

Treatment

A. Specific Measures: Transfusion of platelet concentrates (and corticosteroids) may be given when there is central nervous system bleeding. Usually the effect of transfused platelets is short-lived (less than 24 hours). Infusion of compatible platelets from the mother or exchange transfusion has been recommended for neonatal isoimmune thrombocytopenia.

B. General Measures: Eradicate infection, if present. In the presence of active infection, antibiotics and chemotherapeutic agents are not contraindicated unless the thrombocytopenia is the result of the administration of these drugs, in which case therapy with other agents is indicated. All medications should be given either orally or intravenously. The value of corticosteroids is not proved; some investigators advise short courses (2–4 weeks) for patients with severe thrombocytopenia (platelet counts of $< 10,000/\mu L$) and patients at increased risk of central nervous system bleeding. In the treatment of chronic idiopathic thrombocytopenic purpura not responding to conventional therapy, the value of immunosuppressive agents has not been proved.

Other measures include transfusions to maintain hemoglobin levels, prevention of trauma, institution or maintenance of regular diet with vitamins, and avoidance of aspirin. Watchful waiting for 6–8 months is appropriate for many cases.

C. Surgical Measures: Splenectomy is indicated (preferably after age 8 years) if conservative therapy has been carried out for 6–12 months without improvement, if the disease process is very severe, if the patient is becoming steadily worse in spite of other therapy, if the patient develops a sudden intracranial hemorrhage, or if the patient is having recurrent bouts of severe thrombocytopenic purpura for which no definite cause can be determined. Splenectomy is also indicated in an adolescent girl with severe menorrhagia. Splenectomy should be avoided, if possible, in children under 8 years of age, and the procedure is contraindicated if the number of megakaryocytes in the bone marrow is decreased.

Course & Prognosis

Clinical activity may continue to be evident for 2 weeks to several months, but significant improvement usually occurs within 4–6 weeks. At least 75% of children who have thrombocytopenic purpura with normal or elevated numbers of megakaryocytes in the bone marrow will have a spontaneous and complete recovery within 6 months even without therapy, but spontaneous recovery may occur after a period of as long as 3½ years. A few will need splenectomy, and very occasionally a child will die in spite of all forms of therapy.

Adolescents tend to have a more chronic course, often associated with the presence of other antibodies, proteinuria, or abnormal renal function. Idiopathic thrombocytopenic purpura during adolescence may be associated with subsequent development of subacute lupus erythematosus.

ANAPHYLACTOID OR "VASCULAR" PURPURA (Henoch-Schönlein Purpura)

Anaphylactoid purpura is a disease of unknown cause. Many patients have a history of allergic manifestations. Some cases of anaphylactoid purpura follow infections; a causal relationship with group A streptococcal infections has been suspected. The disease tends to recur, and it may persist over a span of many years.

Clinical Findings

A. Symptoms and Signs: Abdominal and joint pains are present in most children, but the pain may occur only in the abdomen (Henoch type) or only at the joints (Schönlein type). The pain may precede the development of skin lesions. Either small or large joints may be involved. The joints are painful and swollen. Ecchymoses, petechiae, or bullous hematomas (or a combination of these findings) may be present. The initial lesions may resemble urticaria, but these soon become hemorrhagic. They often appear first around the elbows and ankles and over the buttocks. Gastrointestinal hemorrhage is common in children. Nephritis may occur early or after the acute phase in over one-third of cases. Intussusception may develop. Associated group A β-hemolytic streptococcal infections are frequent.

B. Laboratory Findings: Platelet counts and most hematologic test results are normal; the partial thromboplastin time may be short. Eosinophilia may be present in some cases. Serum IgA levels may be elevated.

Treatment

In many cases, treatment is either unnecessary or ineffective.

A. Specific Measures: Therapy includes eradication of infection, using appropriate antibiotics, and elimination of allergens (if known). Antihistamines may be given if allergy is suspected.

B. General Measures: Corticosteroids may relieve joint and abdominal symptoms. They do not appear to benefit patients with renal complications.

C. Prevention of Recurrences: Give prophylactic penicillin if a streptococcal cause can be established. Remove other known allergens.

Course & Prognosis

The disease may vary in degree from mild to quite severe. Complete recovery eventually occurs in most cases, but recurrences are not infrequent and nephritis occasionally persists and may become chronic. Death during the acute phase of the disease is rare.

HYPERCOAGULABILITY

Hypercoagulability describes an increased tendency toward thrombosis in patients with certain underlying conditions. Patients at risk include those with antithrombin III deficiency, a hereditary disorder that presents with deep venous thrombosis or strokes at an early age; newborns and older children with central plastic catheters or prosthetic heart valves; postsurgical patients who required prolonged periods of bed rest and thus are susceptible to venous stasis; and patients with vasculitic processes (eg, systemic lupus erythematosus, nephritis, hemolytic-uremic syndrome) in which damaged endothelium provides a nidus for clot formation and occasionally for progression to a more generalized disease process.

The patient may present with pain and swelling of the involved extremity or with symptoms of a stroke. The diagnosis of thrombosis is made by physical examination. Supporting laboratory findings may include decreased levels of fibrinogen or antithrombin III, decreased platelet counts, or elevated levels of fibrin split products or monomers; these findings, however, may be normal even in the face of significant thrombosis.

Treatment involves interruption of the triggering process. Heparinization should be instituted at once, with the goal of increasing the partial thromboplastin time to 1½ times that of normal. Give a loading dose of heparin, 100 units/kg, followed by a continuous intravenous infusion of 15–20 units/kg/h. Newborn infants may require an increased dosage. Prolonged anticoagulation for 4–6 months with warfarin (Coumadin) may be indicated once the initial thrombosis is controlled. Antiplatelet agents (aspirin, sulfinpyrazone, dipyridamole) may be indicated in cases in which a prosthetic heart valve or arterial malformation is the inciting agent for thrombosis. The use of fibrinolytic agents (streptokinase, urokinase) is still experimental, and doses have not been defined for children.

CHRONIC CONGESTIVE SPLENOMEGALY (Banti's Syndrome)

Chronic congestive splenomegaly is characterized by splenomegaly, moderate hepatic enlargement in early cases, moderate anemia, leukopenia, thrombocytopenia, and varices and hemorrhages of the upper gastrointestinal tract. It may result from a congenital abnormality of the splenic vessels or may follow hepatic disease with obstruction of the splenoportal circulation, thrombophlebitis of splenic vessels, or pressure of enlarged lymph nodes on the veins. In some instances, the underlying pathology may lie in the spleen itself.

Therapy is with transfusions when necessary and treatment of the underlying disease whenever possible. Splenectomy and bypass operations to improve collateral circulation have been of value in cases where the underlying defect appears to be in or around the spleen.

ABSENCE OF THE SPLEEN

Absence of the spleen, whether the absence is congenital, postsurgical, or functional (secondary to an underlying disease such as sickle cell anemia), places the child at significant risk for infection with encapsulated bacteria. The overall incidence of infection is 5–10%, with the fatality rate of 30–50%. Those at greatest risk are children under 2 years of age and children with recent splenectomy (ie, for the first 2 years following splenectomy). The classic hematologic finding is the presence of Howell-Jolly bodies on the peripheral blood smear.

The tendency to develop life-threatening infections is markedly decreased in older children when the spleen is removed for trauma, idiopathic thrombocytopenic purpura, portal vein thrombosis, local tumors, or hereditary spherocytosis. The risk is significant in those with histiocytosis, inborn errors of metabolism, hepatitis with portal hypertension, thalassemia, and Wiskott-Aldrich syndrome.

The use of prophylactic antibiotics remains controversial. Some physicians use continuous penicillin prophylaxis in the younger child, while others treat at the first sign of fever. Pneumovax (which protects against infection with many of the common pneumococci) may be given to all splenectomized children and repeated in early childhood if given to infants under 2 years of age. Prompt therapy with antibiotics in any child with fever has been recommended.

SPLENOMEGALY

Splenomegaly is generally an indicator of systemic disease. The tip of the spleen may normally be felt in 30% of newborn infants and occasionally in young children. Splenomegaly may be associated with other signs of systemic disease, particularly adenopathy, hepatomegaly, petechiae, ecchymoses, and jaundice. Less common causes of splenomegaly include acute viral infections (particularly infectious mononucleosis and cytomegalovirus), hematologic disorders (eg, congenital or acquired hemolytic anemias, red cell membrane defects, disorders of hemoglobin synthesis), metabolic diseases (eg, Gaucher's disease, Niemann-Pick disease), vascular abnormalities (eg, portal hypertension), and, rarely, cysts (eg, splenic cysts). When leukemia or other malignant neoplastic disease presents with splenomegaly, it is usually accompanied by adenopathy, pallor, and other signs of systemic illness.

Evaluation of patients with splenomegaly should include an assessment of the complete blood count, platelet count, peripheral blood smear, and reticulocyte count. Other studies may include tests for viral titers, liver-spleen scan, a hemolytic evaluation, bone marrow examination, and culture of fibroblasts.

NEUTROPENIA

Neutropenia, a total granulocyte count below 1500/μL, may result from poor release of granulocytes from the bone marrow, decreased survival of granulocytes in the circulation, or abnormalities of granulocyte production and development. With counts below 1000/μL, skin and mouth infections may occur. Counts below 500/μL are often associated with cellulitis, pneumonia, and sepsis; the usual causative microorganisms are *Staphylococcus aureus*, fungi, and enteric bacteria. The forms of neutropenia include: (1) cyclic neutropenia, occurring at 2- to 4-week intervals in association with mucous membrane ulcers, cervical lymphadenopathy, and stomatitis; (2) benign chronic neutropenia, which may be genetically transmitted (as a dominant or recessive trait), with manifestations of mild infection; (3) severe congenital neutropenia, transmitted as a recessive trait, with life-threatening infection in early infancy; (4) Schwachman-Diamond syndrome, with metaphyseal chondrodysplasia, dwarfism, pancreatic exocrine insufficiency, anemia, and thrombocytopenia; (5) cartilage-hair hypoplasia, with short limb dwarfism, abnormally fine hair, and T cell deficiencies; (6) Chédiak-Higashi syndrome; and (7) acquired neutropenia. Acquired neutropenia may occur with marrow replacement by malignant cells or fibrosis; with systemic complement activation; or with isoimmune maternal sensitization to neutrophil-specific antigens that cross the placenta, destroy the infant's polymorphonuclear leukocytes, and predispose the infant to life-threatening infections. Acquired neutropenia may be induced by drugs or toxins or an autoimmune mechanism.

Benign forms of neutropenia may not require therapy. In other forms, infections should be treated with appropriate antibiotics. In patients with severe neutropenia, HLA-MLC-compatible marrow transplant from a sibling may be indicated. Corticosteroids may be of value in some cases of cyclic and immune forms of neutropenia. Patients with neutropenia associated with acute suppression of the bone marrow from cytotoxic drugs should be treated with broad-spectrum antibiotics; leukocyte transfusions may be of value.

• • •

IMMUNOLOGIC DEFICIENCY SYNDROMES
(Antibody Deficiency Syndromes, Hypogammaglobulinemias)

Immunologic deficiency diseases are characterized by (1) increased susceptibility to bacterial, viral, fungal, and protozoal infections; (2) a generalized or selective deficiency in the serum immunoglobulins; (3) a diminished capacity (in varying degrees) to form circulating antibodies or to develop cellular immunity (delayed hypersensitivity) after an appropriate antigenic stimulus; and (4) clinical and immunologic variability. Several broad categories are definable based upon whether the defect originates with a disturbance of antibody-producing lymphoid cells (B cells) or with thymus-derived cells that mediate cellular immunity (T cells).

Classification of Immunologic Disorders

A. Immunoglobulin Deficiencies:

1. Infantile X-linked agammaglobulinemia (IgG, IgA, IgM deficiency).

2. Selective immunoglobulin deficiency (dysgammaglobulinemia).

3. Acquired hypogammaglobulinemia–

a. Primary–In patients of all ages; various immunoglobulin defects; associated autoimmune disorders, sporadic and familial.

b. Secondary–In diseases with loss of serum proteins (nephrosis, protein-losing enteropathy) or in lymphoid neoplasms.

4. Transient hypogammaglobulinemia of infancy.

B. Cellular Immunity Deficiency With "Normal" Immunoglobulins:

1. Thymic dysplasia (Nezelof type).

2. DiGeorge's syndrome (congenital absence of thymus and parathyroids; third and fourth pharyngeal pouch syndrome).

C. Combined Immunoglobulin and Cellular Immunity Deficiencies:

1. Congenital–

a. Severe combined immunodeficiency (Swiss type agammaglobulinemia, thymic dysplasia).

b. Wiskott-Aldrich syndrome (dysgammaglobulinemia and progressive cellular immunity deficiency).

2. Acquired–

a. Hodgkin's disease (advanced).

b. Iatrogenic conditions (steroid or antimetabolite therapy).

c. Acquired immune deficiency syndrome (AIDS).

Clinical Findings

In patients with immunoglobulin deficiency disease, recurrent pyogenic bacterial infections predominate, and chronic otitis media, sinusitis, and bronchiectasis are especially common. In agammaglobulinemia, viral infections (such as measles, varicella, and mumps) are weathered without incident. In individuals with cellular immunity defects, progressive vaccinia has been a frequent complication, and vaccination should be avoided. Candidal infections are not uncommon in such patients, and unusually severe infections with cytomegalovirus, herpesvirus, and *Pneumocystis* occur as well. In the acquired forms, malignant disorders of the lymphoreticular system occur with increased frequency. AIDS, which has been reported in children with hemophilia and in Haitian children, is often difficult to distinguish from congenital deficiency disease.

Laboratory Findings

Diagnosis is based on results of the following:

(1) Quantitative immunochemical determination of the serum levels of IgG, IgM, and IgA.

(2) Isohemagglutinin determination. These antibodies to the blood group substance belong for the most part to the IgM class. They are normally present after about 1 year of age in all individuals of blood groups A, B, and O. Therefore, their absence is presumptive evidence of IgM deficiency.

(3) Absolute lymphocyte count. The count is 4000–6000/μL in normal children but reduced in patients with cellular immunity deficiency (especially in patients with severe combined immunodeficiency).

(4) Examination of bone marrow for plasma cells.

Confirmatory tests include the following:

(1) Results of immunization with well-characterized antigens (eg, diphtheria toxoid, tetanus toxoid) in terms of specific antibody produced and plasma cell development.

(2) Presence of germinal center formation, plasma cells, and small lymphocytes in a biopsy of the regional lymph node taken 1 week after antigenic stimulation.

(3) Reaction to *Candida* and mumps skin tests.

(4) Induction of contact dermal hypersensitivity with dinitrochlorobenzene.

(5) Results of in vitro tests of lymphocyte function (phytohemagglutinin [PHA], antigens, allogeneic cells).

Treatment

Treatment for patients with immunoglobulin deficiency consists of replacement therapy with immune globulin, which is chiefly IgG. Give 200 mg/kg (intramuscularly only) and then 100 mg/kg every 3 or 4 weeks. Preparations consisting solely of IgM and IgA are not yet available.

Each individual has genetically determined differences in gamma globulins, and isoimmunization can occur as a result of giving genetically foreign gamma globulin. Since isoimmunization may have some deleterious effects, injudicious administration of immune globulin should be avoided.

Therapy of cellular immunity deficiencies is still experimental.

18 | Urogenital System*

CLINICAL FINDINGS

Frequent clinical and laboratory manifestations of diseases of the urinary tract include abnormalities of urination (frequency, urgency, incontinence, dysuria, straining or dribbling, enuresis); dehydration; acidosis; edema; ascites; fever; costovertebral angle pain; lower abdominal pain; anemia; hypertension; pyuria, proteinuria,† hematuria,‡ and other abnormal cellular urinary elements; and fixation of the specific gravity of the urine or inability to concentrate above 1.020.

The unspun sediment from a fresh, clean specimen of urine should be stained with Gram's stain and examined for organisms. The finding of more than one or 2 organisms per high dry field in the stained sediment from a clean-catch midstream specimen correlates well with a positive culture. Organisms may be present even though pyuria is absent. Avoid routine catheterization, if possible. The most reliable means of collecting urine for culture is suprapubic needle aspiration of the bladder (see Chapter 32). Any organisms obtained by this means probably signify a urinary tract infection. Culture of a clean-voided midstream urine specimen (discarding the first few milliliters of urine) often gives helpful information, especially in males. Bacterial colony counts greater than 100,000/mL, if in a pure culture of known pathogens, usually indicate infection but should be repeated in the symptomatic patient. Those between 10,000/mL and 100,000/mL are suspect and should be repeated in any patient. Those less than 10,000/mL are usually due to urethral contamination and frequently indicate the need for examination of a urine specimen obtained by suprapubic aspiration.

*Revised with the assistance of Gary M. Lum, MD.

†Surveys have shown that approximately 5% of children will exhibit proteinuria, but only 20% of those with proteinuria will exhibit it on retesting. There is a greater prevalence of proteinuria between 10 and 16 years of age than at other ages. Mass screening for hematuria and proteinuria may be unrewarding in asymptomatic children.

‡Hematuria occurring after any type of trauma requires a careful examination of the urinary tract. Findings on intravenous urography are abnormal in one-third of such cases.

In cases with renal parenchymal disease, chemical studies may show depressed creatinine clearance, elevated blood urea nitrogen, altered serum protein, lowered calcium, and elevated phosphorus levels and evidence of chronic acidosis or anemia.

Vague signs and symptoms such as the following should always arouse suspicion of disease of the urinary tract: failure of adequate gain in weight and height; unexplained fever; abdominal pain; a mass in the region of the bladder, ureter, or kidney; convulsions; rickets after infancy; and any change in urinary habits.

In newborn infants, congenital absence of the abdominal musculature or the presence of a single umbilical artery, abdominal masses, unexplained dehydration, acidosis, anemia, abnormalities of the spinal cord and lower extremities, myelodysplasia, sacral agenesis, chromosomal disorders, imperforate anus, aniridia, hemihypertrophy, cystic disease of the liver, hepatic fibrosis, congenital ascites, positive family history of renal disease, oligohydramnios, bilateral pulmonary hypoplasia, or abnormalities of the ears or external genitalia is often associated with abnormalities of the urogenital tract and other anomalies.

SPECIAL DIAGNOSTIC STUDIES

Obstruction may occur at any level of the urinary tract. Symptoms may be absent even if infection exists. The symptoms of obstruction are seldom diagnostic of the site of obstruction; special tests may be necessary for diagnosis.

Voiding cystourethrogram and cinefluoroscopy may give information about vesicoureteral reflux, bladder outlet function, and the presence of residual urine.

Observe the size, regularity of flow, and force of urinary stream.

Intravenous urography to visualize the kidneys and upper urinary tract may also reveal important information about renal development and anatomy. (Better x-ray films may be obtained through the gas-distended stomach; distention will result after the ingestion of 150–240 mL [5–8 oz] of a carbonated drink.)

Cystoscopic inspection will demonstrate trabeculation, diverticula, and the integrity and location of the ureteral orifices. At this time, retrograde visualization of the upper tract may be carried out to permit examination of the upper urinary tract and give information regarding sites of obstruction and the state of the renal pelves and calices.

Less invasive studies such as ultrasonography and CT scan can be very helpful.

Renal arteriography is required to visualize tumors, blood vessels, etc, and to disclose the presence of kidneys, which may not be visualized by other radiographic techniques. Radioisotope renal scans may be of value. In cases of renal parenchymal disease, a renal biopsy may be performed for diagnostic and prognostic purposes.

NONOBSTRUCTIVE CONGENITAL MALFORMATIONS

CYSTIC KIDNEYS

Classification

A. Polycystic Kidneys (Infantile Type; Often Autosomal Recessive): The renal tissue is filled with multiple small cysts. The kidneys are generally very enlarged. Polycystic disease is often present in the liver, pancreas, or lungs.

B. Polycystic Kidneys (Adult Type; Often Autosomal Dominant): Numerous cysts involve all portions of both kidneys and, occasionally, other organs.

C. Multicystic Kidneys: Multicystic disease usually affects only one kidney, which is moderately enlarged with large cysts; the renal parenchyma is hypoplastic or absent. The calices and pelvis are malformed, hypoplastic, or absent and the ureter is atretic. The other kidney is often dysplastic.

D. Other Cystic Kidneys: Other varieties of cystic kidneys include medullary cystic disease (juvenile nephronophthisis), dysplastic kidney, solitary renal cyst, and hamartomatous cystic or multilocular kidney.

Clinical Findings

A. Symptoms and Signs: In addition to enlargement of the kidney, cystic diseases may be manifested by evidences of increasing renal insufficiency such as hypertension, anemia, explained dehydration, azotemia, tubular dysfunctions, and rickets; acid-base imbalance; and disturbances of growth in long-standing cases.

B. Laboratory Findings: Findings include hematuria, inability to concentrate the urine, elevated blood urea nitrogen levels, acidosis, hypocalcemia, hyperphosphatemia, and osteodystrophy. Occasionally, recurrent bacteriuria and proteinuria are seen.

C. Urologic Studies: Urograms show marked enlargement of the kidneys and deformity of the calices and pelves to varying degrees (sometimes resembling "spider pelvis") due to pressure of the cysts. Excretion of dye is usually delayed.

Treatment

Treatment is supportive and palliative. Combat renal acidosis and insufficiency. Administer vitamin D, prevent infection, regulate diet, and treat hypertension. Dialysis and transplantation may be of value in some cases.

Prognosis

Infants with polycystic kidneys of the infantile type often die within the first few days of life. With other forms, there is occasionally variable decrease in renal function, which may not become evident for several years.

EXSTROPHY OF THE BLADDER

In exstrophy of the bladder, a split in the anterior walls of the abdomen and bladder permits a direct passage of urine to the outside. There is usually an associated separation of the pubic rami, as well as epispadias, undescended testes, inguinal hernia, and occasionally, defects of the bowel. The exposed bladder mucosa and trigone form parts of the external abdominal wall.

Constant dribbling of urine excoriates the skin. Ulceration of the bladder mucosa may occur. Children walk with a waddling and unstable gait.

Renal function and intravenous urograms are generally normal for a few (3–10) years, after which hydronephrosis and pyelonephritis usually occur. The disease may be compatible with a normal life span in some patients.

The results of plastic reconstruction are generally poor, but urinary diversion (eg, ureteroileostomy) may preserve kidney function.

PATENT URACHUS

Patent urachus is due to persistence of the embryonic connection of the bladder with the umbilicus. The connection normally is obliterated by the time of delivery. The urachus may be open at either end; may be closed at both ends, with a cyst between (most common type); or may be open throughout its course, permitting urine to dribble from the umbilicus. Treatment is by surgical correction, preceded by antibacterial therapy if infection is present.

OBSTRUCTIVE CONGENITAL MALFORMATIONS

URINARY TRACT OBSTRUCTION

Uncorrected lower urinary tract obstruction is often accompanied by bilateral hydronephrosis with infection, azotemia, or both. In males, it may be produced by urethral "valves" or other urethral constriction. Neuromuscular bladder dysfunction produces similar end results.

The bladder dilates, hypertrophies, becomes trabeculated, and may develop diverticula. Residual urine is present. The ureters may dilate and become elongated and tortuous. The pelvis of the kidney enlarges; kidney tissue is eventually destroyed as a result of obstruction, infection, or both, until only a thin shell of cortex remains.

Abnormalities of urination include difficulty in starting the stream, dribbling, straining during urination (bowel movement may occur each time urine is passed), weak or thin stream, or abrupt cessation during urination. Dilatation of the bladder, ureter, or kidney may be variable and may be palpable. Infection is frequent and may be persistent or intermittent, acute or chronic. Pyelonephritis is the usual result, but chronic pyelonephritis may be completely silent and asymptomatic.

Treatment is usually both medical and surgical (see below).

Renal insufficiency or hypertension may be the outcome in progressive and untreated cases. High surgical drainage is usually beneficial in spite of considerably lowered renal function. Marked improvement often results, and life may be prolonged for many years, allowing nearly normal growth and development until such time as renal transplantation becomes necessary.

UPPER URINARY TRACT OBSTRUCTION

Most cases of upper urinary tract obstruction are produced by obstruction of the ureter as it passes through the bladder wall or joins the pelvis of the kidney (ureteropelvic junction obstruction), duplication of the ureter to one kidney (with ectopia of the ureteral orifice), stricture or diverticulosis of the ureter, pressure of an aberrant blood vessel, or calculi.

ACQUIRED ABNORMALITIES OF THE URINARY TRACT

URINARY TRACT INFECTION

Acute urinary tract infection may be limited to the lower urinary tract, but persistent or recurrent cases often progress to involve the renal pelvis and parenchyma, producing pyelonephritis. Newborns of both sexes and females of all ages seem at highest risk of developing urinary tract infections.

Infection may be caused by a variety of organisms, particularly *Escherichia coli* and other organisms commonly found in the intestinal tract. Kidney involvement often results from ascending infection. Congenital abnormalities associated with obstruction and ureterovesical reflux may be important predisposing factors. Meatal stenosis or distal urethral obstruction, as diagnosed by currently available techniques, does not appear to be a factor of importance in most cases.

Urethral catheterization is a significant predisposing factor.

In children, reinfection with a different organism usually implies cystitis; relapse due to the same organism is more commonly associated with pyelonephritis.

The value of treating asymptomatic bacteriuria found on random examination in children who do not have disease is not yet proved.

Clinical Findings

Urinary tract infections may occur in combination with other infections.

A. Symptoms: Symptoms may be absent, particularly in the chronic form of the disease. Onset may be gradual or abrupt. Fever may be as high as 40.3 °C (104.5 °F), accompanied by chills. Urinary frequency, urgency, incontinence, dysuria, prostration, anorexia, and pallor may occur. Vomiting may be projectile. There may be irritability and sometimes convulsions. Any of the findings listed on p 416 may be present. Asymptomatic bacteriuria occurs in 1% of schoolgirls. Newborn infants may manifest temperature instability, poor feeding, and lethargy. Allergy may be a factor in recurrent genitourinary tract infections.

B. Signs: Signs include dull or sharp pain and tenderness in the kidney area or abdomen. Hypertension and evidence of chronic renal failure may be present in long-standing and severe cases. Jaundice may occur, particularly during early infancy.

C. Laboratory Findings: Pyuria is characteristic, but it may be absent in the majority of patients during some phase of the disease. Slight or moderate hematuria occasionally occurs. There may be slight proteinuria. Pathogenic organisms and casts of all types may be present in the urine, but the urine may be normal for long periods of time. Anemia is found in cases of long-standing infection. Leukocytosis is usually in the range of 15,000–35,000/μL. The diagnosis of urinary tract infection should be suspect if it is based on examination of a single voided urine specimen. Renal biopsy is of no value.

D. Urologic Studies: The performance of intravenous urograms and voiding cystourethrograms is recommended by many investigators for all children after the initial infection. Others feel that these procedures should be performed after the first urinary tract infection for newborn infants, boys of all ages, and girls with symptoms suggestive of pyelonephritis or after second infections. The need for further urologic evaluation depends on the nature and severity of any abnormalities noted.

Treatment

A. Specific Measures: Eradicate infection with appropriate chemotherapeutic or antibiotic therapy (see Chapter 6), usually for at least 10 days and particularly with drugs to which the patient has not recently been exposed. A prolonged course of urinary tract antisepsis (2–6 months or longer) may be indicated, especially for repeated infections. Repeat urinalysis and culture 48 hours after starting treatment and at intervals of 1 or 2 months for at least a year.

B. General Measures: Force fluids during the acute stage. If possible, have the patient shower instead of bathing. Discontinue "bubble baths." Avoid constipation.

C. Surgical Measures: There is no clear evidence that routine surgical correction—by either bladder neck revision, dilatation, urethrotomy, or meatotomy—alters the course of recurrent urinary tract infections to any significant degree, but repair of clearly obstructive lesions is probably indicated.

D. Prophylactic Measures: After control of the infection, a prophylactic regimen using nitrofurantoin, sulfisoxazole, or methenamine mandelate may be of value depending on the organism; if methenamine is used, the urine should be kept acid. Nalidixic acid may be an effective substitute for methenamine. Frequent urine cultures are indicated. The dipstick nitrite test is a useful adjunct to home screening for infection.

In some cases, it is not sufficient to institute treatment only for clinical exacerbations, since subclinical infection may persist and be associated with progressive severe renal damage.

Reinfection in children without obstructive malformation is not uncommon and is usually due to a different organism. Recurrences with the same organism are most likely to occur when there is an underlying urologic abnormality and pyelonephritis exists. Children should be checked periodically for at least 5 years.

VULVOVAGINITIS

Vulvovaginitis may occur in patients of all ages. It is most commonly nonspecific (75% of cases) and is sometimes related to improper hygiene, local irritation, infections, or relative estrogen lack in prepubertal girls. Vulvovaginitis may also be an early sign of diabetes mellitus. Specific vulvovaginitis may be due to bacteria (eg, gonococci), fungi *(Candida),* viruses (herpes simplex, etc), trichomonads, pinworms, allergy, or foreign body.

Clinical Findings

A. Symptoms and Signs: There are often no symptoms, but the child may have any of the findings listed on p 416. The child may be irritable and have pruritus and local irritation. The vaginal discharge may be white and mucoid, cottage cheese-like, yellow, yellow-green, purulent, thin, or thick. A blood-tinged discharge suggests a foreign body. In the pubescent female, a benign cottage cheese-like discharge confined to the vulva may be present. Vaginal washings show abundant desquamated, cornified epithelial cells.

B. Laboratory Findings: Bacterial, fungal, vaginal cytologic, viral, and special studies may be indicated (see Special Diagnostic Studies, above). Nonspecific vulvovaginitis causes contaminated urine culture if urine is collected by the clean-catch method.

Treatment

Nonspecific vulvovaginitis should be treated by correcting local hygiene and treating infection elsewhere, if present. Treat locally with estrogen cream; lactic acid solution, 1 teaspoon to 1 pint of water; or nitrofurazone (Furacin) urethral inserts placed in the vagina, one daily for 10–14 days. Antibiotics may be necessary for secondary infection.

Specific vulvovaginitis should be treated with specific therapy.

ACUTE GLOMERULONEPHRITIS
(Acute Nephritis)

There are many forms of acute glomerulonephritic syndromes. One of these, acute postinfectious glomerulonephritis, appears to be due to an immunologically mediated reaction associated most frequently with an antecedent β-hemolytic streptococcal infection. Generally, the acute symptoms of the primary infection have cleared when the nephritis appears.

The disease may occur in epidemic form following infection of the throat or skin with a type-specific *Streptococcus* (especially types 4, 12, 25, and 49), and under such circumstances, the majority of patients have abnormalities of the urine but no clinical manifestations. Acute glomerulonephritis is rare in children under 3 years of age.

A progressive form of acute nephritis is membranoproliferative glomerulonephritis. It may present with findings ranging from microscopic hematuria and slight proteinuria to severe acute nephritis. Although the condition may be associated with streptococcal infections, the course does not appear to be that of acute poststreptococcal disease. There are several types of membranoproliferative diseases, the most common of which are types I and II. Hypocomplimentemia occurs in both types I and II, but it is persistent in type II (the more severe form) and often results in end-stage disease.

Nephritis may also be associated with syphilis, toxins (lead, trimethadione, mercury, hydrocarbons), amyloid disease, renal vein thrombosis, anaphylactoid purpura, lupus erythematosus, various virus infections, dysproteinemias, and malignant neoplastic diseases. Recurrent gross hematuria over periods of several years may be part of a syndrome associated with minimal physical and laboratory findings. In these cases, the episodes are frequently preceded by upper respiratory tract infections not related to group A streptococcal infections. Berger's disease (IgA glomerulonephritis), nephropathy with focal segmental nephritis, and a benign course may occur.

Clinical Findings

A. Symptoms and Signs:

1. Uncomplicated acute poststreptococcal nephritis–The intensity of the disease varies, but most patients are not markedly ill. Hematuria is generally the first symptom. There may be oliguria, slight to moderate edema (rapid weight gain may be the only indication of developing edema), hypertension, slight cardiac enlargement in first 2 weeks, slight headache and malaise, gastrointestinal disturbances, and fever of variable degree.

2. Acute nephritis with hypertensive encephalopathy–In addition to the signs and symptoms of uncomplicated cases, there may also be restlessness, stupor, convulsions, vomiting, and visual disturbances. Headache may be severe. Hypertensive encephalopathy may be the presenting or only clinical finding of acute nephritis. Seizures appear to be related to the rate of rise of the blood pressure.

3. Acute nephritis with cardiac involvement–This form of the disease is characterized by cardiac enlargement and gallop rhythm, electrocardiographic changes, or attacks of pulmonary edema, peripheral edema, increasing venous pressure, and hypervolemia. Cardiac failure can be a cause of death in acute nephritis and is usually due to persistent hypertension.

4. Acute nephritis with uremia–There may be no specific signs or symptoms, or there may be evidences of acidosis and decreased renal function (drowsiness, coma, stupor, muscular twitchings, and convulsions) as well as respiratory and gastrointestinal disturbances.

B. Laboratory Findings:

1. Urine–The urinary output is decreased. Microscopic or gross hematuria is present but may be very slight during the initial phase of the disease. When hematuria is present, the urine is usually brown or smoky in appearance. Specific gravity is high, although fixed specific gravity (around 1.010–1.012) may occur temporarily early in the disease. Moderate to severe proteinuria is present, and there are moderate numbers of white cells and hyaline, granular, and cellular casts. Red cell casts establish the renal origin of the hematuria.

2. Blood–The blood urea nitrogen level is usually increased, sedimentation rate is elevated, and serum albumin level is often slightly depressed. Acidosis occurs in some patients. Serum complement (C3) is usually decreased.

Antistreptolysin levels are usually elevated within 1 or 2 weeks of onset. Serum antistreptolysin O (ASO) titers will not rise if the preceding streptococcal disease involved only the skin or if eradication of streptococci was accomplished by early treatment with antibiotics. Antistreptococcal DNase, antihyaluronidase nicotine deaminase, and antistreptococcal M protein levels may be elevated in some patients in whom ASO titers are normal. The streptozyme test and the streptococcal DNase B test are useful screening tests.

3. Renal function tests–Results of these tests are normal in 50% of patients, with varying degrees of elevation of blood urea nitrogen and serum creatinine levels in others.

Treatment

There is no specific therapy that influences healing of the glomerular lesions in most cases of poststreptococcal glomerulonephritis.

A. Specific Measures: Mild hypertension may be corrected by limiting fluid and sodium intake and maintaining sedation. Moderate or severe hypertension may require diazoxide (preferred) or reserpine or propranolol with hydralazine, given until the hypertension has been controlled. In refractory cases, the addition of a ganglionic blocking agent in combination with reserpine and hydralazine may be necessary. In cases resulting in renal failure, dialysis may be necessary.

B. General Measures: The patient should be at bed rest until hypertension is well controlled. Give a regular diet appropriate for the age and as tolerated, with sodium restriction if the patient is hypertensive. In treatment of the uncomplicated form, fluids may be taken as desired. Penicillin may be given during the acute phase of the disease. Any coexisting infection should be eradicated with appropriate antibiotic or chemotherapeutic agents (see Chapter 6).

Treatment of Complications

A. Hypertensive Encephalopathy: Correct hypertension and give oxygen.

B. Cardiac Failure: Correct hypertension and give oxygen, morphine, and digitalis. Venesection may be of value if pulmonary edema is present. Restrict sodium intake.

C. Acute Oliguria: Correct hypertension and treat anuria. Severe oliguria should be treated in the same way as acute renal failure. Avoid administration of sodium. Maintain adequate nutrition. During the acute phase and with elevated blood urea nitrogen levels, protein catabolism should be reduced to a minimum to reduce the rate of accumulation of toxic end products. Give a high-calorie diet rich in carbohydrate and fat and low in protein and potassium. Transfusion should be avoided unless anemia is profound. Administer antibiotics as indicated.

Course & Prognosis

Symptoms and physical signs of uncomplicated poststreptococcal glomerulonephritis disappear in 2 or 3 weeks. Blood chemistry returns to normal during the second week. Microscopic hematuria and traces of protein in the urine may persist for months or even years. The glomerular filtration rate, degree of hypertension, and serum complement level may assist in assessing progression.

It has been commonly believed that approximately 95% of patients recover completely, 2% die during the acute phase of the disease, and 2% go on to have chronic nephritis. Recent evidence, however, suggests a higher incidence of chronicity appearing after many years.

CHRONIC GLOMERULONEPHRITIS
(Chronic Nephritis)

Chronic glomerulonephritis may present with persistent hematuria and proteinuria or may appear as acute glomerulonephritis. With primary chronic glomerulonephritis, there are usually no known predisposing causes. In some cases, exacerbations are preceded by acute upper respiratory tract infections. The primary form of chronic nephritis is membranoproliferative glomerulonephritis.

An inherited (dominant) familial progressive form of nephritis, often associated with nerve deafness and sometimes with ocular lesions (Alport's syndrome), may occur; involvement is commonly severe in males and mild in females.

Other forms of chronic disease may occur with disseminated lupus erythematosus, Henoch-Schönlein purpura, and other diseases.

Clinical Findings

A. Symptoms: There are often no symptoms until renal failure develops. Symptoms then include weakness and easy fatigability, vomiting, headache and restlessness, muscular cramps and twitchings, drowsiness, and coma and convulsions in the terminal phases.

B. Signs: Edema of variable degree may occur. Other signs are hypertension, renal insufficiency, retinal abnormalities (hemorrhages, exudates, and arteriolosclerosis), poor growth and nutrition, and anemia.

C. Laboratory Findings:

1. Urine–Findings include hematuria and proteinuria of variable degrees and casts of various types. Broad casts ("renal failure casts") occur in late stages. Fixed specific gravity is 1.008–1.012.

2. Blood–After onset of renal failure, levels of blood urea nitrogen and other nitrogenous substances are elevated, serum phosphorus is elevated, and serum calcium is decreased. Serum sodium and chloride may be decreased late, and serum potassium may be elevated terminally. Resistant anemia is present.

3. Renal function tests–Results of tests, especially the creatinine clearance, show progressive renal impairment.

Treatment

No specific treatment is favored for the basic disease process in primary idiopathic chronic glomerulonephritis, although a favorable response occasionally has been associated with the use of agents such as azathioprine, cyclophosphamide, corticosteroids, and anticoagulants. Immunosuppressants may only be beneficial prior to the stage of terminal renal failure. Efforts should be directed toward the alleviation of symptoms and the correction of chemical imbalance or the causative agent or mechanism when known.

Permit activity as tolerated. Provide a normal diet appropriate for age, although restriction of proteins may be of some value. Treatment for progressive renal failure should include correction of fluid and electrolyte imbalance and oliguria and control of hypertension with methyldopa or hydralazine and propranolol. Antihypertensive agents that lower cardiac output (such as guanethidine) should be avoided.

Aluminum hydroxide, calcium lactate, and vitamin D are valuable as means of reducing the phosphate absorption and increasing calcium absorption from the intestinal tract. Chronic dialysis (both peritoneal and extracorporeal) and homotransplantation may offer effective methods of prolonging life.

Corticosteroid therapy may be of value for treatment of patients with membranoproliferative glomerulonephritis.

Course & Prognosis

In spite of markedly reduced renal function, the patient may appear to do quite well until puberty, when the growth spurt and other physiologic changes may impose a final burden upon the kidneys sufficient to cause death. Progression may be interrupted for indefinite periods of clinical well-being. A nephrotic stage is not infrequent during the course of the disease; minimal lesion nephrosis may have to be differentiated by renal biopsy. Dialysis and renal transplantation may be initiated when end-stage disease is present.

IDIOPATHIC NEPHROTIC SYNDROME OF CHILDHOOD

Idiopathic nephrotic syndrome of childhood (“nil” lesion, minimal change disease, lipoid nephrosis) consists of generalized edema, marked proteinuria, hypercholesterolemia, and hypoproteinemia. It occurs chiefly in children between 18 months and 6 years of age. The course is usually insidious, with a tendency to remissions and exacerbations, but in most instances nephrosis appears as the first manifestation of renal disease in an apparently healthy child.

The cause of nephrosis is obscure. Renal biopsy usually reveals no significant glomerular abnormalities. Electron microscopy reveals fusion of the foot processes of the epithelial cells, but basement membrane thickness is normal. Immunofluorescent studies yield negative results.

Nephrotic syndrome may complicate many glomerulonephritides, in which case lesion is excluded. The presence of significant hypertension, azotemia (especially hypercreatinemia), hematuria, or hypocomplementemia suggests a more serious and inflammatory glomerular lesion. The syndrome may also occur in association with systemic lupus erythematosus, syphilis, renal vein thrombosis, trimethadione and other types of drug toxicity, bee stings, poison oak dermatitis, Henoch-Schönlein purpura, and focal glomerulosclerosis. Rarely, a severe, sometimes familial form presents in early infancy and is often refractory to treatment and invariably fatal, although maintenance of nutrition, control of infection, and transplantation have been of value.

Clinical Findings

A. Symptoms: Symptoms include anorexia, with diminished food intake and malnutrition; gastrointestinal disturbances; severe infections; and irritability and depression.

B. Signs: Insidious onset of edema is usually the first sign. Edema, usually periorbital in the morning, is sometimes accompanied by ascites; it eventually becomes very marked and may persist for weeks or months. Oliguria is present during periods of edema. Retinopathy and persistent hypertension are usually not present.

C. Laboratory Findings:

1. Urine–Findings include marked selective proteinuria and many casts (granular, hyaline, fatty, hyaline containing doubly refractile bodies, and Maltese crosses [detected by use of polaroid filters]).

Hematuria is absent or transient. When hematuria is present, the urine is usually red with a yellow supernatant, and 70–90% of red cells are well preserved.

2. Blood–Total serum protein is reduced, serum albumin is reduced, and total serum globulin is normal or increased (albumin/globulin ratio is reversed), with an increase in α_2-globulin, β-globulin, and IgE and a reduction in the gamma fraction. The amino acid level is low. Anemia is absent or slight. The sedimentation rate is markedly accelerated. Lipid (cholesterol, etc) and lipoprotein levels are increased. The serum calcium level may be depressed, owing chiefly to a deficit in the nondiffusible fraction bound to protein. Serum sodium, carbon dioxide, and pH levels may be normal or reduced. The blood urea nitrogen level is usually normal. The urinary sodium level is typically low, owing to secondary hyperaldosteronism.

3. Renal function tests–The glomerular filtration rate is typically normal or elevated in minimal lesion nephrosis but may be depressed if severe glomerulodestructive disease exists.

Treatment

Approximately 85% of children under 6 years of age (except those with the congenital form) respond to treatment with adrenocortical steroids. Those showing steroid dependency or resistance should be biopsied; if confirmed to have idiopathic nephrotic syndrome of childhood, they are likely to respond to a short course of another immunosuppressive drug such as chlorambucil or cyclophosphamide. These children should be permitted to lead as normal lives as possible, with activity as tolerated and an adequate diet with liberal protein intake as tolerated. Infections must be treated vigorously as they occur.

Sodium restriction helps limit edema formation, but no method is consistently successful in reducing edema. No salt should be added to the diet unless it is required to maintain the child's appetite. Furosemide, especially with slowly administered sodium-poor albumin, may give striking (though transient) benefit; however, hypochloremia and alkalosis may result.

The aim of therapy is elimination of the urinary protein loss.

Thoracentesis is occasionally required for life-threatening respiratory distress due to extensive pleural effusion. Abdominal paracentesis should be avoided except to ease respiratory difficulty. Diuresis produced with albumin and furosemide is generally safer.

Corticotropin, the corticosteroids (see Chapter 22), spironolactone, and the thiazides are of value in precipitating diuresis. Steroids should be continued for 6 months, although occasionally a single intensive course of corticosteroid therapy may be adequate. Prednisone appears to be a satisfactory steroid. During the initial period of daily therapy, give 2 mg/kg (maximum of 60 mg) and continue this dosage until the urine is protein-free; thereafter, give the same dose on alternate days for a total course of 4 months. Taper the course to withdrawal over a period of 2–3 weeks.

If relapses occur after adequate courses of therapy or if the patient becomes steroid-resistant or steroid-dependent, perform a biopsy to establish the diagnosis of minimal lesion nephrosis and to rule out glomerulonephritis. Then give chlorambucil (preferred) or cyclophosphamide and administer prednisone daily through the period of diuresis and then every other day. No salt should be added to the diet until diuresis ensues. (***Caution:*** Toxicity of cyclophosphamide includes impaired fertility, hair loss, and leukopenia. Chlorambucil may also affect the gonads.)

In some children, corticosteroid administration may produce a significant increase in proteinuria independent of a change in the status of the disease. Posterior subcapsular cataract is not uncommon in children treated with corticosteroids; its severity seems to be related to dosage.

Course & Prognosis

About two-thirds of patients tend to have more than one episode of edema interspersed with normal periods that may persist for months or years. Evidence of progressive renal failure may develop in children who appeared clinically to have a pure lipoid nephrosis at onset but will be shown to have another lesion (most often focal glomerulosclerosis, which may progress to end-stage disease) at biopsy. Proteinuria may be used as an index of improvement.

There is increased susceptibility to infections, especially pneumococcal infections, with a predisposition to peritonitis. Skin infections, often erysipeloid in nature, may occur. There is an increased tendency for intravascular thrombosis, especially in those receiving corticosteroids.

Recovery can occur even though the condition has recurred for many years. Relapses may occur months or even years after control of the disease. Recovery is most likely in patients in whom renal biopsy revealed only minimal pathologic changes.

ACUTE RENAL FAILURE
(Oliguria, Acute Tubular Necrosis)

Oliguria may be due to any of several causes, including poisonings, transfusion reactions, burns, crush injuries, glomerulonephritis, severe dehydration, and drugs (sulfonamides, ampicillin, bismuth, carbon tetrachloride). Many cases are due to unknown causes. Spontaneous recovery can occur after more than 4 weeks of oliguria or even anuria (suspect obstruction with complete anuria). A diuretic phase commonly follows an initial oliguric phase.

Treatment

The treatment of persistent marked oliguria or anuria is as follows:

A. Specific Measures: (Do not delay.) Treat the underlying disease if possible. Rule out total obstructive uropathy as a cause. Reverse the mechanism responsible for anuria by (1) giving blood and plasma transfusions for extensive thermal burns, blood loss, or trauma and to alleviate any prerenal components, (2) alkalinizing the urine in cases of transfusion reaction, and (3) catheterizing the ureters in cases of sulfonamide toxicity to determine whether crystals may be obstructing the ureters.

If oliguria is not alleviated, prepare for central venous pressure readings and install an indwelling catheter in the urinary bladder. Give mannitol, 0.5–1 g/kg of 25% solution (maximum of 25 g) over 30 minutes, and furosemide, 1–5 mg/kg intravenously initially. Whenever the positive effect has worn off, repeat the dose that produces a response. If improvement does not occur, begin a regimen that includes careful control of potassium and sodium intake, electrolyte balance, acidosis, and fluid balance. To avoid circulatory overload, use of furosemide without mannitol may be safer in cases where prerenal factor is not obvious. Avoid overhydration.

B. General Measures: Control of the fluid and electrolyte balance and caloric intake is the most promising means of therapy (Table 18–1).

Administer just enough water (by mouth, vein, or intestinal tube) to balance sensible and insensible water losses minus water of oxidation plus replacement of nasogastric losses if present. Excessive administration of water is injurious. Sodium may be replaced in an amount equivalent to urinary losses.

The daily water requirement of the anuric child (Table 18–1) will vary with the numerous factors that affect water balance (eg, activity, sweating, body temperature, metabolic rate, vomiting, diarrhea, and the

Table 18–1. Approximate daily water and glucose requirements in patients with anuria.*

Age (Yr)	Glucose	Water
< 1	10 g/kg	30 mL/kg
1–2	90 g	325 mL
2–4	110 g	375 mL
4–8	140 g	457 mL
8–12	150 g	525 mL
Adult	200 g	700 mL

*Adapted from Pratt.

environmental temperature and humidity). **Note:** Weigh the child daily so that a gain in weight indicative of excessive fluid administration will be detected. Small amounts of weight should be lost each day.

Determine plasma concentrations of sodium, chloride, bicarbonate, potassium, blood urea nitrogen, and serum and urine osmolality at frequent intervals. Exchange transfusion, peritoneal dialysis, or hemodialysis will be helpful in those cases that cannot be managed medically (1) if hyperkalemia is intractable and severe enough to produce changes in the ECG (or is > 8 mEq/L); (2) if uremia with restlessness, lethargy, or coma is present in spite of the use of glucose, insulin, potassium exchange resins, and intravenous calcium; or (3) if significant bleeding due to some anticlotting factor occurs.

Other measures include cation resins for hyperkalemia, calcium gluconate for hypocalcemia, aluminum hydroxide gel to prevent phosphate absorption, fresh packed red blood cells for anemia, and hydralazine plus propranolol or reserpine for hypertension.

ORTHOSTATIC PROTEINURIA
(Lordotic Albuminuria, Postural Proteinuria)

In children with orthostatic proteinuria, protein appears intermittently in the urine when the child is in the erect position; protein is decreased in the reclining position, but levels of protein may still be greater than those in normal children. Orthostatic proteinuria may occur in children with apparently normal kidneys but is usually not present in the morning, and it may occur in children with certain stages (particularly early) of acute and chronic glomerulonephritis.

To obtain a specimen of urine for testing, have the patient void 1–2 hours after assuming the recumbent position. Discard this urine. Then collect a timed urine specimen before the patient gets out of bed and assumes the erect position. The test should be repeated on several occasions. Protein excretion should be less than 0.03 mg/min.

Note: Orthostatic proteinuria may be an early sign of progressive or healing nephritis, but it does not occur as the only finding in the nephrotic syndrome.

RENAL TUBULAR DEFECTS

Hereditary diseases may occur with disturbances of one or a combination of several renal functions (renal glycosuria, cystinuria, renal tubular acidosis, diabetes insipidus, hyperphosphaturia, or vitamin D-resistant rickets), possibly as the result of an absence or deficiency of an essential enzyme system in the renal tubules and perhaps elsewhere.

DE TONI-FANCONI-DEBRÉ SYNDROME

De Toni-Fanconi-Debré syndrome is characterized by vitamin D-resistant hypophosphatemic rickets, hyperchloremia, acidosis with alkaline urine, renal glycosuria, hyperaminoaciduria, and organic aciduria, and it is sometimes associated with cystinosis. The renal abnormality consists of deficient proximal tubular reabsorption of phosphorus, amino acids, and glucose along with a deficiency in the tubular mechanism for reabsorbing base without acid.

Therapy, which is often ineffective, is with large doses of vitamin D and sufficient sodium bicarbonate to correct the acid-base disturbance.

RENAL TUBULAR ACIDOSIS

Hyperchloremic renal acidosis may occur as an idiopathic disease, usually during early infancy, or it may occur in several diseases (eg, chronic renal diseases, hereditary fructose intolerance, hypergammaglobulinemic states). There may be failure to thrive, muscular hypotonia, anorexia, vomiting, and constipation starting in early infancy. There may also be polyuria and polydipsia. An alkaline urine is excreted despite metabolic acidosis. In one form of the disease, late findings include nephrocalcinosis, renal stones, osteoporosis, osteomalacia, and rickets.

The 2 best-known forms of renal tubular acidosis are the "classic" or distal (type I) form and the proximal (type II) form. The type II form most commonly occurs during infancy and often resolves spontaneously. Diagnosis requires simultaneous determinations of serum and urine pH. The varied metabolic consequences that may occur in these conditions are directly related to the renal loss of alkali or inability to excrete normal acid loads. This may be associated with inability to reabsorb filtered phosphate and potassium; calcium wasting occurs as a consequence of the acidosis. Thus, severe electrolyte disturbances, bone disease, and nephrocalcinosis can become significant complications.

Alkali therapy is indicated and is aimed at restoring normal pH and normal electrolyte balance, with resultant promotion of more normal growth and development.

HEMOLYTIC-UREMIC SYNDROME
(Syndrome of Nephropathy, Hemolytic Anemia, & Thrombocytopenic Purpura)

(See Chapter 17.)

19 | Eye*

Examination of the eye, including visualization of the retina, is an integral part of the complete physical examination. Dilatation of the pupil in the infant eye to facilitate ophthalmoscopic examination can be accomplished by instilling drops containing a combination of 1% tropicamide (Mydriacyl) with 2.5% phenylephrine or 0.2% cyclopentolate with 1% phenylephrine (Cyclomydril) 2–3 times at intervals of 10–15 minutes. In children 2 years of age and older, 1% cyclopentolate (Cyclogyl) or 5% homatropine instilled twice at 5- to 10-minute intervals provides good pupillary dilatation, usually within 30–45 minutes. The 10% solution of phenylephrine should not be used in infants and should be avoided in small children because of possible absorption into the bloodstream and systemic toxicity.

While poor vision is an occasional cause of failure to do well in school, parents and school nurses frequently blame impaired eyesight when other conditions are responsible. In such cases, the physician (utilizing a test chart) must demonstrate the normality of eyesight to the satisfaction of the parents. It may be necessary to give sedation or generalized anesthesia to infants before the examination is performed, especially if a neoplasm is suspected.

DISORDERS OF THE EYELIDS

EPICANTHUS

Epicanthus is a congenital malformation characterized by a concave bilateral lidfold at the inner angle of the lids. It is normal in the Mongolian race, is found in children with Down's syndrome, and may be observed also in otherwise normal Caucasian children, usually as a family trait.

If epicanthus is marked, it may give the appearance of a convergent squint, since the pupil is closer to the lidfold at the inner angle than at the outer angle. No therapy is indicated.

*Revised with the assistance of Philip P. Ellis, MD.

STY
(External Hordeolum)

A sty is a purulent infection of a sebaceous gland in the lid, usually caused by *Staphylococcus aureus*. There is localized edema, swelling, redness near the lid edge, and pain, with the point of maximum tenderness over the affected gland.

Treatment

A. Local Measures: Hot moist compresses constitute the most effective treatment. Topical antibiotics may prevent complicating conjunctivitis, hasten resolution, and prevent recurrences and involvement of other glands. Use sulfacetamide sodium (10% ointment) or an antibiotic ophthalmic ointment. Never squeeze the sty.

B. Systemic Antibiotics: Systemic antibiotics should be given in severe cases, especially if there is a surrounding cellulitis.

Prognosis

The acute inflammation usually resolves in 4–10 days, but recurrences are frequent. Continued therapy at night with an antibiotic ointment may prevent recurrence.

INTERNAL HORDEOLUM

Internal hordeolum is an infection of a meibomian gland or duct and is caused by a pyogenic organism, usually *Staphylococcus aureus*. Pain, tenderness, redness, and swelling on the inner side of the eyelid occur. There may be marked edema of the skin of the entire lid.

Internal hordeolum is an acute form of chalazion (see below).

Treatment

A. Local Measures: Warm moist compresses may be used. Local antibiotic therapy with bacitracin, neomycin, polymyxin, or sodium sulfacetamide ophthalmic ointment may be indicated. Occasionally, use of systemic antibiotics is required.

B. Surgical Measures: Make an incision at the right angle to the lid margin, and drain from the conjunctival side when the lesion is well localized. Avoid the lid margin. If incision is necessary, it should not be done when the infection is in the acute phase.

Course & Prognosis

Cure usually follows spontaneous evacuation of pus or incision and drainage.

CHALAZION

Chalazion is a relatively painless mass that may result from obstruction, retention, and chronic granulomatous inflammation of one of the meibomian glands in the upper or lower lid.

The irregularity of the lid may be cosmetically disturbing. A slight feeling of irritation of the eye may also be present.

Treatment

A. Local Measures: When the area is chronically infected or the condition is recurrent, antibacterial ointments may be used.

B. Surgical Measures: Give local anesthesia, and open the chalazion by conjunctival incision and curettage.

Complete excision for biopsy is suggested in recurrent or unusual cases.

Prognosis

Prognosis for eradication is good with incision and curettage or excision. Without such definitive treatment, recurrent infection and irritation are to be expected. In the absence of repeated infections, chalazion is a cosmetic problem that in itself may make surgery desirable. A large chalazion can produce astigmatism through pressure on the globe.

BLEPHARITIS
(Granulated Lids)

Chronic inflammation of the lid margins is caused by infection with pyogenic bacteria (usually *Staphylococcus aureus*). *Pityrosporum ovale* is associated with the seborrheic type of blepharitis in adolescents. Seborrheic dermatitis and dandruff are often associated. Refractive errors may aggravate this condition, probably because patients with refractive errors rub their eyes frequently.

Blepharitis is characterized by chronic purulent discharge, with matting of the eyelashes, chronic reddening and thickening of the lid margins, and frequent rubbing and irritation of the eye. Fine scales may be seen along the base of the eyelashes, and ulceration and bleeding occur at the base of the lash in severe cases.

Treatment

Depending on the causative agent, local antibiotic or chemotherapeutic medication is indicated, together with warm water soaks of lid margins. The lid margins should be cleansed with a cotton applicator moistened with a weak baby shampoo. Treat dandruff and seborrheic dermatitis. Refractive errors should be corrected.

Examine and treat siblings and parents.

Prognosis

There is a marked tendency to chronicity. Treatment usually controls the condition, but complete cures are difficult to obtain. Spontaneous cures are common in staphylococcal infections. Permanent loss of the eyelashes may result from severe blepharitis.

PTOSIS
(Drooping of the Upper Eyelids)

Ptosis is characterized by drooping lids and backward tilting of the head in an attempt to see below the upper lids. It is due to paresis or paralysis of the levator muscle of the upper lid, which is supplied by a branch of the oculomotor nerve. There may be associated weakness of the superior rectus muscle.

Practical note: When ptosis is acquired, myasthenia gravis should be suspected and ruled out by specific tests.

Ptosis may be congenital (sometimes accompanied by a marked epicanthus) or acquired. It is generally bilateral but frequently asymmetric. Acquired ptosis is seen less often in children than in adults and suggests neurologic disease. Slight ptosis results from interruption of cervical sympathetics (Horner's syndrome).

Treatment

To prevent visual loss, early plastic surgery is indicated when ptosis is moderate or severe and interferes with vision. In patients with milder forms of ptosis, no surgical treatment is required except for cosmetic reasons.

Prognosis

Prognosis is excellent for surgical cure when levator paralysis is partial. Good results are usually obtained when the paralysis is complete.

TICS OF THE EYELIDS
(Blepharospasm)

Frequent blinking may be due to refractive errors, chronic blepharitis, or conjunctivitis, but it usually suggests emotional tension. Correction of the physical cause may lead to rapid improvement. Blepharospasm due to tension states may disappear spontaneously or with psychotherapy or use of tranquilizers. The patient's parents should be reassured of the good prognosis and urged to adopt a more permissive attitude toward the child. Not infrequently, however, signs of blepharospasm give way to other signs of tension states during the postadolescent period.

• • •

OBSTRUCTION OF THE LACRIMAL APPARATUS
(Dacryostenosis)

Dacryostenosis is one of the most common congenital abnormalities of the eye. It may also be acquired. Trauma concomitant to silver nitrate or penicillin instillation, as well as chronic conjunctivitis, may predispose to the development of this disorder.

Tearing and conjunctivitis may be noted. Mucopurulent discharge is often present or may be expressed from the lacrimal sac. The condition may be unilateral or bilateral.

Treatment & Prognosis

A. Local Measures: The lacrimal sac should be gently massaged, using a pumping action with a small finger in the lacrimal fossa. If infection is present, local chemotherapy with sodium sulfacetamide ophthalmic drops is advised. In 95% of cases, correction occurs spontaneously or following massage.

B. Surgical Measures: Probing is easily and safely performed in patients after 6–9 months of age. It is seldom performed earlier because the condition usually resolves spontaneously. Probing is successful in most cases; if it fails, however, dacryocystorhinostomy may be indicated.

CONJUNCTIVITIS OF THE NEWBORN
(Ophthalmia Neonatorum)

Etiology

There are 3 main causes of conjunctivitis in the newborn:

A. Silver Nitrate: This is by far the most common cause. Onset is in the first 2 days of life, usually the first.

B. Gonococci or Staphylococci: The onset is at any time after birth, usually between the second and fifth days.

C. Chlamydiae: The onset of inclusion blennorrhea is between the third and 14th days.

Clinical Findings

A. Symptoms and Signs:

1. Silver nitrate conjunctivitis–The mucopurulent discharge may become purulent if secondary infection occurs.

2. Gonococcal or staphylococcal conjunctivitis–The discharge is frankly purulent and very profuse.

3. Inclusion blennorrhea–The discharge is moderately profuse. Characteristically, the conjunctiva in the lower fornix is hypertrophied.

B. Laboratory Findings:

1. Silver nitrate conjunctivitis–Smears of pus reveal cellular debris but few, if any, bacteria. Bacteriologic cultures yield negative results early in the course.

2. Gonococcal or staphylococcal conjunctivitis–Gram-stained smears of discharge will reveal gram-negative intracellular diplococci (gonococci) or gram-positive cocci in clusters (staphylococci). Blood agar plate cultures in duplicate are indicated, one plate being placed under low oxygen tension for incubation. This will favor the growth of gonococci.

3. Inclusion blennorrhea–The demonstration of inclusion bodies (by smear of conjunctival scrapings) and a monocytic cell response confirm the diagnosis. Giemsa's stain or hematoxylin-eosin stains are required for isolation of *Chlamydia*.

Treatment

Silver nitrate conjunctivitis responds well to saline irrigation and is usually self-limited. Bacterial conjunctivitis requires prompt therapy with chemotherapeutic agents such as sodium sulfacetamide, bacitracin, or tetracycline ointment 4 times daily for 4–6 days. Topical and systemic chemotherapy is advisable for treatment of patients with gonococcal conjunctivitis. Patients with inclusion blennorrhea should be treated with 10% sodium sulfacetamide drops or ointment or 1% tetracycline ointment or solution instilled every 2–4 hours. Cure results in 2–4 days.

Prophylaxis

Replacement of silver nitrate with an antibiotic ophthalmic ointment has been advocated to prevent silver nitrate conjunctivitis.

Prepartum therapy of gonorrhea-infected mothers may prevent gonococcal conjunctivitis, but instillation of silver nitrate or an antibiotic affords an additional safeguard.

Inclusion blennorrhea originates from an asymptomatic subclinical infection of the mother's cervix with the specific chlamydial organism. No method of prevention is available.

Prognosis

The prognosis with treatment is generally very good, and cure should result within 2–4 days. If bacterial conjunctivitis is untreated, permanent scarring of the cornea and partial or complete loss of vision may result, depending on the severity and duration of the untreated condition.

CONJUNCTIVITIS

Conjunctivitis is most often caused by local bacterial, viral, or fungal infections (secondary to other mycotic infections) or by systemic diseases.

A. Bacterial Conjunctivitis: *Staphylococcus aureus, Streptococcus pneumoniae,* β-hemolytic streptococci, *Moraxella lacunata,* and *Haemophilus influenzae* are the agents usually responsible for "pink-eye." Inclusion blennorrhea and trachoma are due to chlamydial infection. *Actinomyces* infection of canaliculi is an occasional cause of unilateral canaliculitis and medial conjunctivitis.

B. Viral Conjunctivitis: Viruses of epidemic keratoconjunctivitis (adenovirus type 8 or 19), pharyngoconjunctival fever (usually adenovirus type 3), and herpes simplex may occur.

C. Fungal Conjunctivitis: A variety of fungal organisms (often secondary to other mycotic infections) may rarely produce conjunctivitis.

D. Allergic Conjunctivitis: Conjunctivitis may be due to seasonal allergy (eg, vernal conjunctivitis). It may also be due to bacterial allergy to tuberculoprotein, giving rise to the characteristic phlyctenular keratoconjunctivitis. In the continental USA, many patients with phlyctenular disease do not have hypersensitivity to tuberculoprotein but are probably sensitive to other bacterial or fungal proteins.

E. Systemic Disease: Systemic diseases may cause conjunctivitis, eg, vitamin A deficiency (xerophthalmia), measles, and erythema mul tiforme (Stevens-Johnson disease).

Clinical Findings

A. Symptoms and Signs: Symptoms and signs include photophobia, itching, and burning; feeling of roughness underneath the lids; congestion of the conjunctiva; mucoid or mucopurulent discharge (in bacterial forms); watery discharge or no discharge (in viral and allergic forms); small subconjunctival hemorrhages; edema of the lids; and preauricular adenopathy.

B. Laboratory Findings:

1. Bacterial conjunctivitis–Bacterial pathogens may be demonstrated by stained smear and culture. Many polymorphonuclear leukocytes may be present. Inclusion bodies may be demonstrated in conjunctival scrapings (in trachoma and inclusion blennorrhea only).

2. Viral conjunctivitis–The cell response is predominantly lymphocytic and mononuclear. Adenovirus may be demonstrated by a rise in antibody titer, and a viral agent may be isolated.

3. Fungal conjunctivitis–Stained smears of conjunctival scrapings reveal causative organisms.

4. Allergic conjunctivitis–Eosinophils may be present in scrapings from the conjunctiva.

5. Systemic disease–The primary disease is diagnosed.

Treatment

A. Specific Measures:

1. Bacterial conjunctivitis–Local instillation of ophthalmic bacitracin, neomycin, or sulfacetamide is indicated. For trachoma and inclusion conjunctivitis, apply tetracycline antibiotic ointment locally 4 times daily. For active trachoma, systemic tetracycline should be added. *Actinomyces* responds to penicillin or tetracycline, but concretions in the canaliculi or tear sac must be mechanically removed.

2. Fungal conjunctivitis–Local instillation of natamycin (Natacyn) drops, 5% suspension, or amphotericin B suspension, 1.5–3 mg/mL, is indicated.

3. Allergic conjunctivitis–Instillation of 1:4000 epinephrine hydrochloride and the systemic use of antihistaminic drugs are indicated. Topical instillation of a weak corticosteroid solution such as 0.125% prednisolone (or equivalent) every 2 hours is also effective. Observe closely for complications.

4. Systemic disease–The treatment or recovery from systemic disease usually results in improvement of the eye lesion.

B. General Measures: Measures include use of cool compresses (not ice), eye irrigations, and dark glasses for treatment of older children. Never use eye patches.

Prognosis

The prognosis in all types of conjunctivitis is generally excellent if proper treatment is instituted. In untreated cases, corneal scarring and diminution or loss of vision in the affected eye may occur.

REFRACTIVE ERRORS

MYOPIA
(Nearsightedness)

In myopia, the focus of distant objects lies anterior to the retina, resulting in poor vision for distant objects. The focus of near objects lies closer to the retina (ie, nearsighted). Myopia is often hereditary and is frequently associated with prematurity.

Myopia should be suspected when the condition exists in either parent. It usually results from excessive length of the eyeball but may be caused by increased refractive power in the cornea or lens. Myopia tends to become gradually more severe during the growing period.

Clinical Findings

Myopia is manifested by poor vision for distant objects, squinting, and difficulty in reading the blackboard at school. When the patient is 3 years of age, a fundus examination should be done with a cycloplegic agent (see p 434).

Holding reading matter close up is not necessarily a sign of myopia, since children have much greater powers of accommodation than do adults.

The refractive error in either myopia or hyperopia may be estimated by use of the direct ophthalmoscope. Use of a cycloplegic agent is necessary in children. If the examiner is emmetropic or wearing corrective lenses, the subject's approximate refractive error can be read in diopters as the most plus (black numbers) in the ophthalmoscope with which retinal detail can be seen clearly. (With less plus, the examiner will accommodate to maintain a clear view.) This technique of examination has definite limitations and should not be relied on completely for the diagnosis of refractive errors.

Treatment & Prognosis

Except for patients with mild cases, proper lenses for full correction of the refractive error should be worn at all times. In general, it is the parents' distaste for eyeglasses rather than the child's lack of cooperation that interferes with early treatment. Children as young as 2 years of age usually can wear eyeglasses comfortably.

HYPEROPIA
(Farsightedness)

An emmetrope has perfect vision for distance without focusing (accommodating). The hyperope also usually has perfect distant vision but must accommodate to see clearly. Hyperopia usually results from shortness of the eyeball but may be caused by reduced refractive power of the cornea or lens. Some degree of hyperopia is normal before puberty. The condition is largely familial and should be suspected if either of the parents suffers from it.

The condition may be asymptomatic. Headache and eyestrain may be present in older children during close work. Internal strabismus (esotropia) is often related to moderate or severe hyperopia.

For diagnosis by direct ophthalmoscope, see the discussion under Myopia, above.

Treatment & Prognosis

Only in children with marked degrees of hyperopia or strabismus is optical correction required, since some improvement can be expected when the child reaches puberty.

ASTIGMATISM

Astigmatism is characterized by a difference in refractive power of one meridian of the cornea as compared with the meridian at right angles to it. The difference between the 2 is the degree of astigmatism, and the meridian in which a corrective cylinder is placed is the axis of the astigmatism. Optically, this causes the horizontal component to be out of focus with the vertical component (or vice versa, depending upon the meridian of astigmatism).

Astigmatism is largely familial and is usually caused by developmental variations in the curvature of the cornea. Lenticular astigmatism is much less common than corneal astigmatism.

Clinical Findings

Astigmatism is usually seen in children who also have either myopia or hyperopia. Common findings are headache, fatigue, eye pain, reading difficulties, and a tendency to frown.

Treatment & Prognosis

Eyeglasses or contact lenses may be required, at least for reading and for watching television or movies. The degree of farsightedness or nearsightedness determines whether eyeglasses must be worn constantly. No spontaneous improvement may be expected. A contact lens will correct corneal astigmatism. The usual contact lens will not correct lenticular astigmatism; special lenses may be made to correct moderate degrees of this condition.

CONTACT LENSES

Contact lenses can be fitted satisfactorily on any patient who is sufficiently motivated to undergo the discomforts of adaptation, but the child should be old enough to remove and insert the lenses without help. Contact lenses may be useful in infants who have undergone unilateral cataract surgery, provided that the parents are understanding and cooperative and learn the techniques of contact lens care. Since corneal damage may result from improper fitting or handling, contact lenses should be prescribed and fitted only by persons qualified to give critical follow-up care and to treat injury or infection early.

The recently developed soft contact lenses may be used for therapeutic purposes—protection of the cornea, bandaging of corneal injury, and treatment of corneal edema. Some patients who cannot wear the conventional lenses may tolerate the soft lenses.

STRABISMUS
(Squint)

Strabismus is characterized by ocular deviations or failure of the eyes to maintain parallelism. Squinting in infants under 6 months of age may not be true strabismus. Deviations after 6 months are true strabismus, often requiring treatment.

Because the eyes fail to maintain parallelism, the image of the deviating eye is suppressed, with consequent progressive diminution of vision on that side leading to loss of sight (amblyopia), which may be permanent if not recognized and treated. All patients with strabismus should be examined by an ophthalmologist.

Etiology

The exact cause of strabismus cannot be determined in most cases. Congenital or hereditary strabismus is more common than the acquired form.

A. Paralytic Strabismus: Paralytic strabismus is due to a congenital or acquired anomaly of a particular extraocular muscle or paresis of its nerve supply.

B. Concomitant (Nonparalytic) Strabismus: There are 4 types of concomitant strabismus.

1. The accommodative type is due to hyperopia and has its onset in patients at 2–4 years of age.

2. The congenital (muscular, innervational) form has its onset at or near birth.

3. Anisometropia is characterized by a marked difference in refractive error of the 2 eyes.

4. In the visual form of concomitant strabismus, there is poor vision in one eye, due to a developmental anomaly or malignant tumor of the retina, or there are opacities of the media, interfering with fixation and fusion.

Clinical Findings

A. Symptoms: Eso (internal) deviations are most common in children; older children and adults tend to develop exo deviations. Vision may be decreased on the affected side. With alternating squint, good vision is maintained in both eyes. Personality disorders may occur and may be reflected in social maladjustment and poor school work.

B. Signs: Deviation of the eye may be in any direction and may be intermittent or constant, alternating or monocular. If strabismus is paralytic and the lesion is neurologic in nature, the angle of deviation varies with the direction of the gaze, increasing in the direction of action of the paretic muscle. If strabismus is concomitant, the angle of deviation remains unaffected by the direction of the gaze.

Treatment

Diagnosis of the usual congenital types should be possible in a patient by 6 months of age, and early therapy should be instituted. Many cases become apparent with increasing near use of the eyes, ie, in the school years (accommodative type). Ocular disease must be ruled out by ophthalmoscopic examination.

A. General Measures: A patch must be placed over the unaffected eye to force the child to use the deviated eye and prevent amblyopia. This patch must be worn all day and should cover the entire eye. The use of a patch may be required for many months. Patching is generally of little value in patients after the age of 8 years.

Correction by glasses at 12–20 months of age is imperative where marked refractive errors are found.

Orthoptic exercises have been recommended in an attempt to avoid surgery, but children under 5–7 years of age are rarely able to cooperate satisfactorily. Injudicious use of orthoptics often merely postpones definitive therapy unnecessarily.

If nonoperative procedures result in improvement, surgery may be postponed.

B. Surgical Measures: Surgery is indicated when vision is equal in both eyes and the deviation cannot be corrected by glasses; it is also indicated for cosmetic reasons when vision cannot be equalized. Surgery may be performed in a child as early as 1 year of age. Early correction is desirable if there is a good potential for fusion. Cosmetic surgery is usually done in children closer to the school years.

Prognosis

Good results are usually obtained in the treatment for strabismus associated with refractive errors. Good cosmetic results usually follow surgical treatment. Binocularity depends upon sensory mechanisms, which are usually abnormal in patients with congenital and small angle strabismus; in these patients, there is a less favorable prognosis.

MISCELLANEOUS EYE DISORDERS

INFLAMMATION OF THE CORNEA (Keratitis)

The healthy cornea possesses no blood vessels and is clear. Any blood vessels or opacities seen in it are pathologic.

Etiology

(1) Keratitis may be due to vitamin A deficiency occurring in malnourished children, in allergic children on restricted diets, and in children with biliary tract anomalies that interfere with absorption of vitamin A. (See also Chapter 4.)

(2) Bacterial ulcers usually follow trauma by a foreign body or injuries infected by bacteria, including *Streptococcus pneumoniae,* hemolytic streptococci, *Klebsiella pneumoniae, Pseudomonas aeruginosa,* and *Moraxella lacunata.* These ulcers lead to hypopyon (pus in the anterior chamber), great corneal destruction, and loss of the eye if not treated intensively. Gonococcal conjunctivitis also frequently leads to corneal ulceration, hypopyon, and ultimately perforation.

(3) Phlyctenular keratitis may be due to an allergic reaction to tuberculoprotein but also may result from sensitivity to other proteins (bacterial or fungal). Tuberculosis can also cause a deep form of keratitis.

(4) Interstitial keratitis is associated with congenital or acquired syphilis (90% of cases) or may follow infectious diseases such as herpes zoster, mumps, and tuberculosis.

(5) Mycotic ulcers are usually associated with penetration of the cornea with vegetable material, eg, a stick.

(6) Viral keratitis may be due to herpes simplex or vaccinia.

Clinical Findings

A. Symptoms and Signs: Regardless of the course, keratitis is usually characterized by pain, photophobia, tearing, and blurred vision. Defects in the epithelium will stain with fluorescein. This green stain can be seen with an ordinary flashlight but is fluorescent with a cobalt-blue filter or with a Wood's lamp. Iritis is usually associated and would be suggested by the presence of a ciliary flush (limbal injection) and of aqueous flare and cells (usually seen only with a slit lamp).

1. Xerophthalmia–Xerophthalmia is characterized by a cornea that has lost luster and appears cloudy and dry (xerosis). Typically, there is little vascular reaction. Epithelial defects and secondary infection occur. As the condition progresses, these dry areas become progressively whiter (Bitot's spots) and usually are seen at the limbus on the temporal side of the corena. The end stage is keratomalacia and obscured vision. Bitot's spots are grayish-white, foamy lesions, usually on the temporal conjunctiva adjacent to the limbus. They are associated with poor nutritional states but are not always accompanied by vitamin A deficiency.

2. Bacterial ulcers–In the early stages, there is a gray area of infiltration of the cornea associated with a dilatation of the circumcorneal blood vessels, producing the characteristic ciliary flush. There is more pain than is expected from such a small lesion, and the corneal epithelium is markedly hazy. The area enlarges and spreads very rapidly (creeping ulcer); a level of pus often appears in the anterior chamber (hypopyon).

3. Phlyctenular keratitis–The limbus is usually first affected, with the appearance of a small, vascularized, elevated nodule. Gray infiltrates with secondary vascularization may occur in the superficial layers of the corneal stroma and may progress to shallow ulcers. The ulcer extends toward the center of the cornea and results in extensive scar formation. Photophobia is most marked in phlyctenulosis.

4. Interstitial keratitis–Marked, insidious, early congestion is present, with coincident iridocyclitis and clouding of the cornea. The cornea may become so cloudy that the iris cannot be seen. Photophobia may be severe. Deep stromal vessels are present.

5. Viral keratitis–The dendrite is suggestive of herpes simplex, which may also present as stippling or as a geographic corneal ulcer. Corneal hypesthesia is usually present.

B. Laboratory Findings: Bacteriologic cultures of serpiginous ulcers reveal the presence of pathogenic bacteria; direct scrapings for Gram's stain often can give more prompt specific diagnosis. Serologic tests for syphilis and tuberculin testing with very dilute ($\geqslant$ 1:100,000) tuberculin material should be done in suspected cases. Vitamin A levels and tolerance test results are abnormal in patients with vitamin A deficiency.

Complications

Corneal involvement may give rise to iritis and clouding of the central area, which may lead to blindness. Purulent endophthalmitis may lead to loss of the eye.

Treatment

A. Specific Measures:

1. Xerophthalmia–Vitamin A therapy is specific. Parenteral therapy may be required in some cases.

2. Bacterial ulcers–Early specific local and systemic antibiotic therapy is imperative and must be based on findings obtained from scrapings and cultures from the ulcer itself. Neomycin-polymyxin-bacitracin ophthalmic ointment or gentamicin solution (2–10 mg/mL) may be used pending bacterial diagnosis. These drugs are effective against *Pseudomonas* ulcers and will also combat common cocci or rods. The pupil should be kept dilated with 1% atropine or 5% homatropine. The corticosteroids have been used locally in combination with antibiotic therapy. Results remain controversial, and caution is advised unless the organism is identified and known to be sensitive to an antibiotic. Corticosteroids are detrimental for use in some patients with viral infections, especially those with herpes simplex.

3. Phlyctenular keratitis–Use of topical corticosteroids, 1 drop every 2 hours, results in dramatic improvement. **Note:** Children with phlyctenular keratitis may be hypersensitive to tuberculin, and skin testing should be done with the greatest of caution at dilutions of 1:100,000 or greater.

4. Interstitial keratitis–Specific therapy for syphilis and tuberculosis may improve the eye lesion. Topical cortisone probably minimizes scarring. Local use of cycloplegics is imperative.

5. Viral keratitis–For treatment of patients with herpes simplex and vaccinia keratitis, use 0.1% idoxuridine (Herplex, Stoxil) topically, 1 drop each hour during the day and every 2 hours at night for 4–7 days. Idoxuridine ointment, 0.5%, instilled 5 times a day, may be equally effective. Topical application of vidarabine (Vira-A), 3% ointment, or trifluridine (Viroptic), 1% solution applied every 2 hours, is often effective in controlling herpes simplex keratitis when topical idoxuridine is unsuccessful. Corticosteroids should never be used in viral types of keratitis. They may enhance invasiveness of the virus and have in many cases caused spontaneous perforation of the cornea in patients with herpetic keratitis.

6. Mycotic ulcers–Treat with natamycin (Natacyn), 5% suspension, or topical amphotericin B, 1.5–3 mg/mL.

B. General Measures: Sedation and analgesia are most important in symptomatic care. Topical anesthetics are contraindicated because they impair corneal healing. A cycloplegic, such as 1% atropine or 5% homatropine, should be instilled, 1 drop 2–3 times a day. Hot compresses applied for 15 minutes 3 or 4 times a day may decrease pain. Dark glasses will relieve photophobia.

The routine use of systemic broad-spectrum antibiotics should be discouraged. Specific bacteriologic diagnosis should guide therapy when possible.

Course & Prognosis

A. Xerophthalmia: Even when marked clouding of the cornea has interfered with vision, complete regression frequently will occur after adequate vitamin A therapy.

B. Bacterial Ulcers: With early specific antibiotic therapy, prognosis is good. Prognosis is guarded in *Pseudomonas,* gonococcal, and hemolytic streptococcal ulcers.

C. Phlyctenular Keratitis: Recurrences are frequent and in many cases are of unknown cause. The ultimate prognosis depends on the frequency and severity of these recurrences. Prognosis for vision is much better now that attacks can be controlled with corticosteroids.

D. Interstitial Keratitis: Corneal scars may interfere with vision. In many of these, however, visual acuity is eventually excellent. Corneal transplants may be of value in selected cases.

E. Viral Keratitis: Complaints of photophobia and pain usually persist for a long time, frequently for several months, until healing has occurred. The ulcers never perforate spontaneously but may give rise to considerable scarring. (Perforation has occurred when corticosteroids have been used topically.)

ORBITAL & PERIORBITAL CELLULITIS

Cellulitis is often secondary to sinusitis and may also occur as a complication of trauma and septicemia. The most common organisms are streptococci, staphylococci, and *Haemophilus influenzae.*

Periorbital cellulitis is characterized by erythema and swelling of the eyelids. The conjunctiva and orbital tissues are not involved. Preauricular lymphadenopathy may be present.

Orbital cellulitis is marked by erythema and swelling of the eyelids, conjunctival chemosis, proptosis, limitation of ocular movements, fever, and leukocytosis. In cases of *H influenzae* infection, the skin of the eyelids has a distinct magenta discoloration.

Complications include meningitis and cavernous sinus thrombosis.

Treatment consists of use of hot packs and specific systemic antibiotic drugs. Drainage of loculated abscesses is occasionally necessary.

CATARACT

Cataract is an opacity of the lens or of its capsule and may be present at birth or may develop in childhood. Cataracts are often bilateral and symmetric.

Clinical Findings

A. Symptoms: Visual acuity is diminished. There is no pain if the cataract is uncomplicated by other diseases of the eye.

B. Signs: The lens nucleus and cortex both may be opaque. If no clear lens remains, the cataract is termed "mature." Strabismus may be the first indication of cataract. Nystagmus (searching or pendular type) develops if visual acuity is impaired to 20/100 (6/30) or worse.

On dilatation of the pupil, the opaque areas are seen to be white by direct light (leukocoria). The red reflex of the retina is not seen if the cataract is dense.

Etiology

A. Congenital Cataract: Maternal rubella occurring during the first or early in the second trimester of pregnancy may result in congenital cataracts. It is probable that other viral and systemic diseases may result in congenital cataracts. These causes, however, are less well explored.

B. Cataracts of Childhood:

1. Trauma–Traumatic cataract results from penetrating wounds or other trauma to the eyeball. The cataract may develop in a short time and progress rapidly; it frequently is followed by secondary glaucoma.

2. Systemic disease–Diabetes, hypoparathyroidism, galactosemia, Down's syndrome, and Lowe's syndrome may cause cataracts.

3. Poisoning–Cataracts may result from poisoning, chiefly from ingestion or inhalation of naphthalene or diphenyl.

4. Other eye disease–Cataracts may result as a complication of other diseases of the eye, including retinitis pigmentosa, glaucoma, uveitis, and iridocyclitis; cataracts may be a late stage of retrolental fibroplasia.

5. Corticosteroids–Cataracts may be due to long-term use of systemic or topical corticosteroids in high doses.

Treatment

A. General Measures: In the unusual case of dense central cataract, it is worthwhile to try to improve vision with 1% tropicamide (Mydriacyl), 1 drop in the involved eye twice during the day. If this is successful, surgery may be postponed until the visual status can be evaluated more completely.

B. Surgical Measures: In cases that cannot be managed temporarily with mydriatic eyedrops, surgical removal should be done early.

Prognosis

The extent of the cataract and the presence or absence of complicating ocular disease will determine whether or not useful vision can be expected. If nystagmus has developed, vision will rarely be better than 20/200 (6/60), even after successful surgery.

GLAUCOMA

Glaucoma is increased intraocular pressure involving one or both eyes, giving rise to optic nerve damage and visual field loss. Infantile congenital glaucoma (in children under 3 years of age) is an autosomal recessive trait. Most cases of congenital glaucoma are sporadic; some show a hereditary pattern. Glaucoma may also follow injury or disease of the eye. It can occur as a complication of topical corticosteroid therapy. A juvenile form of glaucoma (in persons age 6 years and older) may also occur.

Clinical Findings

A. Congenital Glaucoma: Photophobia is often the earliest symptom. The eyes may water. Persistent pain may be present, but more often there is none. Vision gradually deteriorates. Peripheral vision is affected first.

The eye may enlarge, and the corneal diameter may increase. Corneal edema may be present. The pupil is often dilated, and the sclera may be thin and bluish. The eyeball is large and firm to pressure. The optic nerve shows increased cupping. The difference between the normal and the affected eye in unilateral glaucoma is marked.

B. Juvenile Glaucoma: The signs and symptoms are similar but less pronounced.

Treatment

A. General Measures: Pilocarpine will control intraocular pressure in some cases of juvenile glaucoma but has little effect on congenital glaucoma. Attempts to relieve pain with analgesic drugs are usually unsuccessful. Acetazolamide given orally may be of value in the treatment of juvenile glaucoma; it is of little or no value in the treatment of infantile congenital glaucoma.

B. Surgical Measures: Surgery generally is required to relieve intraocular pressure. In congenital glaucoma, goniotomy or trabeculotomy may improve the function of the filtration angle. Enucleation is indicated if the eye continues to be painful and if vision has been lost.

Course & Prognosis

Generally, glaucoma is slowly progressive. Without treatment, blindness usually occurs eventually, although impairment of vision may progress gradually over a period of many months. With surgical treatment, vision frequently is saved. Prognosis is always guarded.

RETROLENTAL FIBROPLASIA

Retrolental fibroplasia is a disease of the retina that occurs almost exclusively in premature infants of low birth weight (< 1500 g) and gestational age (< 6–7 months). It is invariably bilateral—sometimes unequally so—and leads, in its severe form, to wildly disorganized retinal vascular overgrowth and permanent blindness. In the past, it was the most common cause of blindness in children in the USA. The incidence has declined with awareness of the toxic effects of oxygen on the retina. Recently, therapy employing high concentrations of oxygen to treat respiratory distress syndrome in premature infants has again been used, and retrolental fibroplasia has occurred with increasing frequency.

High oxygen tension in the bloodstream for a prolonged period is the main precipitating factor. The disease is quite rare when supplemental oxygen therapy is not used and is uncommon when oxygen concentrations in incubators are kept below 40%. If oxygen therapy is necessary, the concentration in the incubator should be controlled by direct measurement with an oximeter rather than by monitoring the rate of flow from the tank; this has recently assumed considerable medicolegal importance. Monitoring of arterial O_2 or P_{CO_2} is the best method of determining oxygen tension in the bloodstream.

All premature infants should have careful ophthalmoscopic examinations, including detailed inspection of the peripheral retina.

UVEITIS

Inflammation of the uveal tissues (iris, ciliary body, and choroid) may be granulomatous or nongranulomatous. Uveitis may be due to specific infection with bacteria, viruses, fungi, or parasites; or a nonspecific inflammatory reaction may occur, probably as a hypersensitivity or autoimmune process. Anterior uveitis (iritis and cyclitis) in children and adolescents may be associated with juvenile rheumatoid arthritis.

Anterior involvement (iridocyclitis) is characterized by inflamed eye, photophobia, blurred vision, ciliary injection, pupillary constriction, inflammatory cells in the anterior chamber, and keratic precipitates on the back of the cornea. Posterior involvement (choroiditis) is characterized by blurred vision and vitreous floaters. The vitreous is hazy on ophthalmoscopic examination. Acute choroid lesions appear as white indistinct masses; old lesions are seen as pigmented, disorganized scar tissue of the choroid and retina.

Complications consist of glaucoma, cataracts, and retinal detachment. Optic neuritis may be associated.

Patients with nonspecific anterior uveitis should be treated with topical administration of 1% atropine twice a day and topical corticosteroids (1% prednisolone or equivalent) 4–8 times a day. Patients with posterior involvement require systemic corticosteroids and salicylates.

OPTIC NEURITIS

Two types of optic neuritis are seen in childhood: (1) papillitis (anterior involvement with papilledema) and (2) retrobulbar neuritis (disks appear normal). Most cases follow viral infections or represent localized encephalomyelitis. Optic neuritis may also be due to drug toxicity or associated with neurologic disease.

The symptoms consist of loss of visual acuity, field defects (central scotomas), and, occasionally, pain on movement of the eye. Papilledema is present in the anterior form only.

Treatment is nonspecific. Systemic corticosteroids are of questionable value. The prognosis is good.

20 | Bones & Joints*

INFECTIONS OF THE BONES & JOINTS

OSTEOMYELITIS

Osteomyelitis is an infectious process that may involve all parts of a bone, although the initial focus is usually in the metaphysis of a bone. It is usually caused by staphylococci, although streptococci, salmonellae, and other organisms may be the causative agents. Infection generally occurs via hematogenous spread but may be due to local extension from an infected focus. A history of trauma, usually mild, is common in the hematogenous type.

Considerable areas of cortex may undergo necrosis and produce sequestra that cannot be readily absorbed and that usually must be removed surgically if not extruded. During repair, new bone is laid down beneath the elevated periosteum and tends to form an encasement (involucrum) of the necrotic area. Complete healing takes place only when all dead bone has been destroyed, discharged, or excised. A joint is more readily invaded when the metaphysis lies within the confines of the capsule.

Clinical Findings

A. Symptoms and Signs: Early signs are localized tenderness over the metaphysis and pain on weight-bearing. Later, there usually is localized erythema, warmth, tenderness, and swelling; fever; elevated pulse; severe, constant, throbbing pain over the end of the shaft; and limitation of joint motion.

B. Laboratory Findings: Leukocytosis may be marked. Results of blood cultures are generally positive early in the course. A smear of aspirated pus shows cocci or rods. The most useful procedure is aspiration of the metaphysis for culture and sensitivity testing. Even minimal fluid may yield positive results on culture.

C. X-Ray Findings: Spotty rarefaction is followed shortly by periosteal new bone formation (generally absent for the first 10–14 days

*Revised with the assistance of Robert E. Eilert, MD.

of the disease; range, 3–14 days). The bone is demineralized. Findings on bone scintigraphy with technetium polyphosphate may be positive before bony changes are present on the roentgenogram.

Treatment

A. Specific Measures: Culture blood and bone specimens, and give a synthetic penicillinase-resistant penicillin intravenously until results of sensitivity tests are available. Continue this therapy until all parameters (fever, white blood cell count, sedimentation rate, local tenderness, x-ray) show significant improvement; improvement usually takes place after a few days in cases detected early and in up to 3 weeks in those detected late. Give intravenous antibiotics for 10–21 days until all signs of infection, including sedimentation rate, are improving. Subsequent oral antibiotics should be monitored by serum and inhibitory concentrations and given for a minimum of 1 month.

B. General Measures: Immobilization relieves pain and decreases lymphatic spread of infection.

C. Surgical Measures: Incision and drainage are indicated for treatment of late infection with gross pus in the bone and of early infection that does not show improvement within 24 hours. This procedure reduces the ischemia caused by pressure of the pus on the dilated blood vessels.

PYOGENIC ARTHRITIS

Pyogenic arthritis is an infection of one or more joints by hematogenous spread (most common) or by direct extension of pathogenic bacteria. The most common organisms are *Staphylococcus aureus,* gonococci, meningococci, pneumococci, and *Haemophilus influenzae*.

Initially, there is an effusion that rapidly becomes purulent. Destruction of cartilage occurs at areas of joint contact. Bone is not affected in the early stages, but the femoral and humeral heads, if involved, may undergo necrosis, subsequent fragmentation, and pathologic dislocation. Epiphyses whose synchondroses are located within the joint capsule are particularly apt to be involved by infection and necrosis.

During the chronic phase of the disease and the phase of repair, there is an organization of the exudate present in the joint, and granulation tissue appears and becomes fibrous. This may bind the joint surfaces together with a fibrous ankylosis. When motion is present, the synovial fluid tends to regenerate, but limitation of motion and associated pain generally remain as a result of the production of residual strong intrasynovial adhesions.

Clinical Findings

A. Symptoms and Signs: In the newborn or young infant, symptoms and signs include poor feeding, irritability, and low or normal temperature. In the older child, fever and malaise may occur, and the child may refuse to walk. Pain may be severe, motion is limited, and the joint is splinted by muscular spasm; in infants, this may produce a pseudoparalysis. Effusion may not be palpable in deep joints such as the hip. The overlying tissues become swollen, tender, and warm. Contractures and muscular atrophy may result.

B. X-Ray Findings: Distention of the joint capsule is the first change. Narrowing of the cartilage space, erosion of the subchondral bone, irregularity and fuzziness of the bone surfaces, bone destruction, and diffuse osteoporosis occur subsequently.

Treatment

A. Specific Measures: Aspiration for diagnosis should be performed promptly. Surgical drainage is almost always indicated when pus can be aspirated from the joint. Appropriate parenteral antibiotics should be given in large doses.

B. General Measures: Measures include immobilization and traction during the acute phase and physical therapy when the infectious process has subsided.

SKELETAL DISORDERS

Congenital and idiopathic disorders of the bone are shown in Table 20–1.

INFANTILE CORTICAL HYPEROSTOSIS (Caffey-Smyth-Roske Syndrome)

Infantile cortical hyperostosis is a sometimes familial, usually benign disease of unknown cause, starting before the sixth month of life. The disease produces irritability, fever, and nonsuppurating, tender, painful, hard swellings. Swellings may involve almost any bone of the body, but they are seen most frequently in the mandible (100% of cases), clavicle (50%), ulna, humerus, and ribs. The disease is limited to the shaft, does not involve the subcutaneous tissues or joints, and persists for weeks or months. Pallor, pseudoparalysis, and pleurisy may occur. Anemia, leukocytosis, increased sedimentation rate, and elevated alkaline phosphatase levels are usually present. Cortical hyperostosis is demonstrable by x-ray and may be evident prenatally.

Cortisone is effective and should be used, especially for treatment of severe cases. The prognosis is generally good; the disease usually terminates without deformity but may occasionally recur. Death may occur without treatment.

Periosteal new bone may develop in one-third of normal infants after the first month of life. The cause is not known.

HYPERVITAMINOSIS A

Hypervitaminosis A is caused by excessive ingestion of vitamin A (100,000 IU or more daily) for prolonged periods of time and is manifested by irritability; anorexia; firm, painful, subcutaneous masses in the skull and extremities; fissuring of the lips; dry skin that is often pruritic; alopecia; jaundice; hepatomegaly; and increased cerebrospinal fluid pressure. There is cortical thickening of bone similar to that seen in infantile cortical hyperostosis (see above), but children with hypervitaminosis A are generally older and the mandible is not involved. The blood vitamin A level is very high. Fever is absent.

The only therapy necessary is discontinuation of excessive doses of vitamin A. Clinical improvement begins within a few days, but a return of the bones to normal may not occur for several months.

CONGENITAL DYSPLASIA OF THE HIP JOINT (Congenital Dislocation of the Hip)

Congenital dysplasia of the hip joint is an abnormality of the hip, often hereditary and occurring more commonly in females and in breech presentations. The acetabulum is shallow; the ossification center for the femoral head, which normally appears in infants at 3–5 months of age, is delayed in its appearance; and the joint capsule is stretched. The head of the femur becomes dislocated superiorly and laterally and comes to lie on the dorsal aspect of the ilium, where constant pressure may result in the formation of a false acetabulum.

All newborn infants should be routinely tested for instability of the hip (Ortolani's sign—a jerking of the hip as the head reduces into place over the posterior acetabular rim).

Clinical Findings

A. Symptoms and Signs: During the first weeks of life, there may be diminished spontaneous movement, partial flexion of the thigh, inability to abduct the hip fully, and asymmetry of the gluteal and thigh folds. The key signs are those of instability (Ortolani's and Barlow's signs). Barlow's sign is used to demonstrate instability of the hip (ie, that the hip subluxates with adduction and applied pressure). In some cases, patients who develop subluxation have no abnormal signs initially.

Table 20–1. Characteristics, treatment, and prognosis of congenital and idiopathic disorders of the bone.

Disease	Family History	Clinical Findings	X-Ray Findings	Treatment and Prognosis
Osteogenesis imperfecta (fragilitas osseum, osteopsathyrosis), congenital and tarda types	Familial in congenital type. Absent in tarda type.	Increased bone fragility and fractures. Normal healing. Blue sclerae. Flaccidity of ligaments and muscles. Deafness (due to otosclerosis and labyrinthine changes). Elevated levels of pyrophosphate.	Bones slender with thin cortices, bulbous ends, and areas of demineralization. Multiple fractures and healed fractures. Exuberant callus formation.	Magnesium oxide may be of value. May die at any age or may have fewer fractures at puberty.
Osteopetrosis (osteitis condensans generalisata, marble bone disease, Albers-Schönberg disease)	Familial and hereditary.	Bony deformities due to pathologic fractures. Myelophthisic anemia. Splenomegaly. Visual and auditory manifestations. Square head. Facial paralysis sometimes. Pigeon breast. Dwarfing. May appear at any age.	Bones show increased density, transverse bands in shaft, clubbing of ends, and vertical striations (long bones). Thickening about cranial foramina. May have heterotopic calcification of soft tissues.	No treatment. Prognosis fair.
Chondrodystrophies				
Achondroplasia (classic chondrodystrophy)	Often present.	Short arms and legs. Upper arm and thigh proportionately shorter than forearm and leg. Bowing of extremities. Waddling gait. Limitation of motion sometimes. Relaxation of ligaments sometimes. Short, stubby fingers of almost equal length. Prominent forehead. May have moderate hydrocephaly. Depressed bridge of nose. Lumbar lordosis. Mentality and sexual function normal.	Tubular bones are short and thick. Epiphyseal plates generally irregular. Ends of bone are thick, broad, knoblike, and cupped. Epiphyseal centers may be delayed and small in early childhood. Skull dysplasia and shortening; premature fusion of tribasilar bone. Calvarium enlarged. Fibula relatively long compared to tibia.	No treatment. Prognosis good. Deformities do not increase after puberty.
Chondroectodermal dysplasia (Ellis–van Creveld syndrome)	Familial.	Ectodermal dysplasia. Congenital heart disease. Polydactyly and frequently syndactyly. Teeth poorly formed. Some or all of teeth may be absent. Mental retardation.	May show changes of chondrodystrophy. Shortening and bowing of tibiae and fibulae. Hypoplastic, eccentric proximal tibial epiphyses. Fusion of carpal bones.	No treatment. Prognosis depends on type of heart disease.

Gargoylism (dysostosis multiplex, Hurler's syndrome, lipochondrodystrophy)	Often present.	Mental retardation. Coarse, grotesque facies. Flat nose, thickened lips, and big tongue. Corneal opacities. Deafness. Orange peel–like skin. Hepatosplenomegaly. Kyphosis. Limited extension at joints. Hirsutism. Short neck, broad "clawlike" hands, and slow growth. Reilly cells in blood and inflammatory sites. Increased urinary chondroitin sulfate B and heparan sulfate.*	Elongated sella turcica. Shortened vertebral bodies with concave anterior and superior surfaces. Thickening of tubular bones and metacarpals with tapering of ends. Arms more involved than legs. May show other changes of chondrodystrophy.	No treatment. The value of corticosteroids remains to be determined. Prognosis poor.
Hereditary multiple exostoses (dyschondroplasia, diaphyseal aclasis, osteochondroma)	Present.	Slow-growing masses, usually near joints or in spine. Generally asymptomatic but may cause pain, interference with joint function, or pressure disturbance. Deformity and shortening of long bones may occur.	Bilaterally symmetric osteocartilaginous masses at metaphyseal ends of long bones assume bizarre shapes; may be long and tapering, resembling spurs. Osteochondromatosis may develop from exostoses.	Excision when symptomatic. Prognosis good. May undergo malignant degeneration in adulthood.
Multiple enchondromas (Ollier's disease)	Absent.	May have hemiatrophy. May have pathologic fractures and resultant deformities. Large lesions have tendency to recur. Growing tumors in adults may be malignant.	Islands of cartilage lie in the metaphyseal ends of the shaft along the long axis of the bone. End of bone thickened. Lesions are asymmetric and multiple and usually limited to one extremity or one side of the body.	No treatment may be needed. Remove growing tumors in adults. Prognosis good for nongrowing tumors.
Osteochondritis dissecans	Absent.	Pain, synovial effusion, and atrophy of muscles. Joints may lock or "give way." Occurs in boys during late adolescence.	Synovial effusion. Fragment of bone in joint. Usually involves knee.	Immobilization. Remove bone fragments. May heal spontaneously.

*May be due to a deficiency of hexosaminidase (β-galactosaminidase) activity with accumulation of mono- and disialogangliosides and glycolipids in tissues.

Table 20–1 (cont'd). Characteristics, treatment, and prognosis of congenital and idiopathic disorders of the bone.

Disease	Family History	Clinical Findings	X-Ray Findings	Treatment and Prognosis
Chondrodystrophies (cont'd)				
Osteochondrodystrophy (Morquio's disease)	Often present.	Normal intelligence. Spine shows shortening, kyphosis, and scoliosis. Moderate shortening of extremities. Sternum protrudes. Prominent abdomen. Hepatosplenomegaly, minimal involvement of skull. Waddling gait due to genu valgum and flexion and limitation of motion of hip joint. Appears after age 1 yr.	Findings similar to those of achondroplasia. Wedged, flattened vertebral bodies. Abnormality of metacarpals. Irregularity of epiphyses. Lower extremities tend to be involved more than upper.	No treatment. Prognosis fair.
Osteochondrosis deformans tibiae (Blount's disease)	Absent.	Extreme bowing of the legs. Waddling gait or limp.	Proximal tibia or distal metaphysis of femur (or both) shows faulty growth, delayed ossification, enlarged medial condyle, and a beaklike extension of metaphysis posteriorly and caudally.	Orthopedic correction if necessary. Prognosis good.
Polyostotic fibrous dysplasia (osteitis fibrosa disseminata, McCune-Bruch-Albright syndrome)	Absent.	Large brown areas of pigmentation ("café au lait" spots), predominantly unilateral. Advanced bone age and short stature. Local pain or tenderness may occur. More common in males. Precocious puberty in females.	Fibrous replacement of bone (predominantly unilateral). Thinning and expansion of cortex associated with multiple radiolucent areas having sclerotic margins. Base of skull may be dense.	No treatment. Prognosis good.

After 3 months, the signs of instability are replaced by those of contracture, and the following occur: more marked asymmetry of gluteal, inguinal, and knee folds; external rotation of the leg; shortening of the affected leg; telescoping of the involved extremity; limitation of full abduction; bulge of the femoral head; positive Trendelenburg sign; and delay in learning to walk. With bilateral dislocations, lordosis and waddling gait may be marked.

B. X-Ray Findings: Findings include deformity of the normally symmetric obturator-femoral curve on the deformed side (Shenton's line); delayed appearance of the femoral epiphyseal center, which is often hypoplastic; absence of the upper lip of the acetabulum; shallow acetabulum; increase of the angle formed by the acetabular shelf with the horizontal plane; and lateral and superior displacement of the femur.

Treatment

In younger children, closed reduction and maintenance of the affected hip in the position of maximum stability may be indicated. In older children, open reduction may be necessary. To avoid avascular necrosis, the position should not be extreme.

Open reduction is indicated if closed reduction is unsatisfactory.

COXA VARA

Coxa vara is a disorder in which the angle between the neck and shaft of the femur is decreased toward or below a right angle. The disorder may be congenital or may result from epiphyseal separation, fractures, osteochondrosis, chondrodysplasia, or hypothyroidism. Debilitating disease, rickets, and obesity may be contributing factors. The congenital form is due to maldevelopment of the femoral neck and to disordered enchondral ossification of that region and is accompanied by a disordered epiphyseal growth with premature fusion.

Symptoms include shortening of the leg, pain (often referred to the knee on the affected side), limp, muscle spasm, limited abduction and internal rotation of the hip, and upward tilting of the pelvis on the affected side with shortening of the leg.

Treatment

Osteotomy is often necessary to restore normal bone alignment. The underlying cause should be treated.

Table 20–2. Characteristics, treatment, and prognosis of osteochondrosis.

Site	Clinical Findings	X-Ray Findings	Treatment and Prognosis
Head of femur (Legg-Perthes disease)	Tenderness in hip. Pain in hip or knee (or both). Limp. Appears at age 3–10 yr.	Flattened, fragmented femoral head with widening of neck and increase in the joint space.	Ambulation without weight-bearing. Shoe lift or crutches. Surgery occasionally indicated. Usually lasts 2–5 yr. Better prognosis with onset at early age.
Head of second metatarsal (Freiberg's infraction)	Pain and tenderness.	Fragmentation. Increased density.	Rest. Shoe support. Prognosis excellent. May produce stiff, painful metatarsophalangeal joint.
Lunate (Kienböck's disease)	Pain or weakness (or both) in wrist. Later, limitation of motion. Appears at age 4–10 yr.	Early, cysts of semilunar. Later, irregularity, fragmentation, and increased density.	Immobilization. May require fusion of wrist. Healing in 1–3 yr. Symptoms may persist.
Os calcis (Sever's disease)	Heel pain and tenderness. Limp.	Fragmentation or flattening. Increased density.	Rest. Prognosis good.
Primary epiphyses of vertebral body (Calvé's disease, vertebra plana)	Usually asymptomatic. May have weakness of back. May be due to eosinophilic granuloma of vertebral body.	Destruction or collapse of vertebra with "waferlike" appearance.	Immobilization. May need no treatment. Prognosis excellent.
Secondary epiphyses of vertebral body (Scheuermann's disease)	Usually asymptomatic. Dorsal kyphosis. May have hamstring "tightness."	Wedged deformity of vertebral bodies. Irregularity of superior and inferior bodies.	Exercise. Brace, if severe. Prognosis good. May have residual deformity.
Tarsal navicular (Köhler's disease)	Pain in foot. Limp. May have local swelling, redness, and heat.	Irregularity and flattening or fragmentation. Delayed maturation of ossification center.	Treatment conservative, with rest and support as required. Complete healing in 5–8 yr.
Tibial tubercle (Osgood-Schlatter disease)	Pain, swelling, and tenderness. Weak knee extension. Slight limp. Frequently bilateral. More common in boys than in girls.	Fragmentation and enlargement of tibial tubercle. Swelling of infrapatellar ligament.	Treatment symptomatic. Immobilization in severe cases. Prognosis good.

SLIPPED FEMORAL EPIPHYSIS

Slipped femoral epiphysis is a nontraumatic separation of the femoral head through the epiphyseal plate. It is more common in males and in thin and tall or overweight children. Slipped femoral epiphysis occurs at adolescence and may present with sudden posteromedial displacement of the epiphyses following minor trauma or with slowly progressive displacement and pain, loss of internal rotation, limp, and shortening of the leg. It may be bilateral. X-ray reveals thickening and irregularity of the epiphyseal plate (early) followed by posteromedial displacement of the head of the femur, relative to the neck.

Treatment & Prognosis

Internal fixation of epiphysis in situ is indicated for treatment of an early slip. For complete separation, closed reduction and pin fixation should be attempted, but osteotomy of the proximal femur after closure of the epiphysis may be necessary.

Patients with slight slipping have a favorable prognosis when treated early. Late treatment of patients with severe displacement often results in permanent disability regardless of the form of therapy.

OSTEOCHONDROSIS

Osteochondrosis is a disease of unknown cause that produces aseptic necrosis of the epiphyses as a result of impairment or blockage of the blood supply to the affected bone (Table 20–2).

TRANSIENT SYNOVITIS OF THE HIP

Transient synovitis of the hip is the most common cause of painful hip in children in the USA. It is a self-limiting disease of unknown cause lasting days (usually) to weeks; it affects children between the ages of 3 and 10 years (boys more than girls). The disease is characterized by a sudden onset of unilateral mild or severe pain in the hip, thigh, or knee, especially with movement or weight-bearing. There is tenderness over the hip joint anteriorly and, occasionally, palpable swelling and limp. The hip is usually held in flexion, abduction, and external rotation. Motion is usually limited. Fever is variable and often absent. X-rays usually show normal findings but may show capsular swelling. Treatment is symptomatic. Traction may be necessary in severe cases. In some patients, osteonecrosis of the proximal femoral epiphysis has developed several months later.

COMBINED DEFECTS

Acrocephalosyndactyly

Acrocephaly (tower skull) may occur in combination with fused or webbed fingers or toes.

Marfan's Syndrome

Marfan's syndrome is an autosomal dominant disease due to a defect in the metabolism of acid mucopolysaccharides. Manifestations include abnormal length of fingers, toes, and extremities (arachnodactyly), sometimes associated with hypermobility of the joints, subluxation of the lens, other abnormalities of the eyes (cataract, coloboma, enlarged cornea, strabismus, nystagmus), high palate, defects of the spine and chest (pigeon breast), and congenital heart disease (particularly weakness of the media of the aorta). Serum mucoproteins may be decreased, and urinary excretion of hydroxyproline may be increased. There may be an altered ratio of chondroitin sulfate to keratosulfate in the costal cartilage.

Some of the findings of Marfan's syndrome may occur in patients with homocystinuria.

Cleidocranial Dysostosis

Cleidocranial dysostosis is an absence of part or all of the clavicle, often associated with delay of ossification of the skull. The facial bones may be underdeveloped, the sinuses absent, the palate highly arched, the dentition defective, the skull enlarged (especially in the parietal and frontal regions), and other bones defective.

Craniofacial Dysostosis (Crouzon's Disease)

Craniofacial dysostosis consists of acrocephaly (tower skull), hypoplastic maxilla, beaked nose, protrusion of the lower lip, exophthalmos, external strabismus, and hypertelorism. The syndrome may be familial.

Klippel-Feil Syndrome

Klippel-Feil syndrome is characterized by failure of segmentation of some or all of the cervical vertebrae. The neck is short and limited in motion, and the hairline is low. Other defects, including scoliosis, cervical rib, spina bifida, torticollis, webbed neck, congenital high position of the scapula, deafness, and renal anomalies, may be present also.

Mandibulofacial Dysostosis (Treacher-Collins Disease, Franceschetti's Syndrome)

Mandibulofacial dysostosis is a hereditary disease characterized by hypoplasia of the facial bones (especially the malar bones and mandible), antimongoloid slant to the eyes, coloboma of the eyelids, malformation of the external ear, abnormal hearing, groove extending from the mouth to the ear, hair growing down over the cheeks, and other anomalies (defects of palate, lip, heart, etc).

Laurence-Moon-Biedl Syndrome

Laurence-Moon-Biedl syndrome consists of retinitis pigmentosa, polydactyly, obesity, hypogenitalism, and mental retardation. The syndrome may be incomplete or associated with other abnormalities.

Pterygium Colli (Congenital Webbed Neck)

In pterygium colli, there is the formation of a thick fold of loose skin on the lateral aspect of the neck. It may occur alone or may be associated with gonadal dysgenesis, ie, Bonnevie-Ullrich-Turner syndrome. This syndrome is characterized by congenital lymphedema of the hands and feet, shortness of stature, cubitus valgus, shield chest, cardiac anomalies, sexual infantilism, deep-set nails (particularly on the feet), numerous moles on the skin, telangiectasia of the bowel, short tubular bones of the hands and feet, elevated excretion of urinary gonadotropins, and an XO configuration of chromosomes and negative chromatin pattern in the majority of females. Estrogen therapy is indicated in puberty. (See Appendix.)

Absence of the Radii

Absence of the radii may occur with absent or hypoplastic thumb, congenital amegakaryocytic thrombocytopenia, leukemoid peripheral blood, and heart anomalies.

Pierre Robin Syndrome

Pierre Robin syndrome consists of micrognathia and partial cleft palate. The tongue may fall back and cause respiratory distress. There may be congenital glaucoma and retinal detachment.

Marchesani's Syndrome

Manifestations of Marchesani's syndrome include brachydactyly, shortness of stature, stocky chest, thick spherical lens, and retardation in carpal ossification.

MISCELLANEOUS DEFECTS*

ARTHROGRYPOSIS MULTIPLEX CONGENITA (Amyoplasia Congenita)

Arthrogryposis multiplex congenita is a congenital and usually symmetric limitation of motion of many or all of the joints. There may be contractures in either flexion or extension. The joints appear enlarged in relation to the atrophic limbs and spindle-shaped. The periarticular tissues fail to develop normally, and the joint volume is decreased. There may be numerous other congenital anomalies. The condition is probably due to abnormal development of muscle or nerve.

SPRENGEL'S DEFORMITY

Sprengel's deformity is a congenital condition in which one or both scapulae are elevated and small. The child with this deformity cannot raise the arms completely on the affected side, and there may be torticollis. There is asymmetry of the shoulders.

OTHER DEFECTS

Brachydactyly (abnormal shortness), clinodactyly (deviation of the distal phalanx, usually of the fifth digit), syndactyly (webbing), and symphalangia (joint absence) may involve the fingers and toes.

COMMON FOOT PROBLEMS

When a child begins to stand and walk, there is a natural tendency for the long arches to seem flattened and the feet to be mildly pronated. Genu varum (bowleg) is present before 2 years of age, and genu valgum (knock-knee) is present up to 8 years of age. As the child grows, the limbs straighten, and the arches become more evident, with increasing strength and decreasing ligamentous laxity.

*Craniosynostosis is discussed in Chapter 21.

FLAT FOOT
(Weak Foot, Flexible Foot, Strained Foot, Static Foot)

Flat foot occurs in most normal infants but clears spontaneously in the majority by the time walking is well established; it is characterized by a relaxed longitudinal arch, which the child is unable to elevate. Flat foot in an older child may be one manifestation of a generalized state of muscular and ligamentous weakness, or it may be an inherited abnormality.

Treatment

For patients with severe and painful flat foot, use of supportive shoes will help maintain the position of the feet during growth. The shoes should be sturdy and have longitudinal arch supports and Thomas heels with small (3/16- to 1/4-inch) medial wedges.

TALIPES CALCANEOVALGUS

Talipes calcaneovalgus is a disorder in which there is excessive dorsal flexion at the ankle and eversion of the foot. It is often present at birth but corrects itself spontaneously in the majority of cases.

Treatment & Prognosis

Treatment consists of passive exercise or casting prior to the age of walking. In older children, scaphoid pads and 1/8-inch or 3/16-inch inner heel and inner sole wedges are used.

CAVUS FOOT

Cavus foot may be due to heredity, poliomyelitis, short heel cord, congenital syphilis, or neurologic conditions affecting the posterior and lateral columns of the spinal cord. It is manifested by an excessively high longitudinal arch and overactive long toe extensor tendons, which produce hyperextension at the metatarsophalangeal joint and flexion at the interphalangeal joints.

Early (conservative) treatment consists of metatarsal pads and bars and stretching exercises. Surgical transplantation of the long toe extensor tendons, together with arthrodesis, if indicated, need not be undertaken until later.

HAMMER TOE

Hammer toe is a flexion deformity, usually congenital, of either or both interphalangeal joints of any toe. It is generally asymptomatic and requires no treatment except for cosmetic reasons or if a callus forms.

METATARSUS VARUS
(Pigeon Toe)

Metatarsus varus is a common disorder of infants, characterized by adduction of the forefoot on the hindfoot.

Treatment

A. Postural Type: The postural type of deformity is flexible. If the problem is discovered early (before the child begins to walk), treatment consists of mild overcorrection by passive manipulation or reversal of shoes. If the problem is not discovered until later, the same treatment as for the structural type may be required.

B. Structural Type: In the structural type of metatarsus varus, the deformity is fixed and cannot be corrected by passive manipulation. Treatment consists of manipulation and plaster casts so that the forefoot is forced into a position of overcorrection and held there for 6 weeks. If this treatment fails or the older child has been untreated, surgery may be indicated.

Prognosis

The prognosis for the postural type of metatarsus varus is excellent. For the structural type, the prognosis is good if treatment is started early.

TALIPES EQUINOVARUS
(Clubfoot)

Talipes equinovarus is a congenital fixed deformity in which the inner border of the forefoot is turned up, the anterior half of the foot is adducted, the calcaneal tendon is shortened, the heel is drawn up, and the foot is held in inversion and plantar flexion. Clubfoot may be associated with spina bifida with paralytic changes in the lower extremities.

Treatment & Prognosis

Treatment should be started in the infant at birth and consists of manipulation and plaster casts (early) and surgery as indicated (later) for residual deformity.

Prognosis is good if there is no associated neurologic defect.

• • •

SHOES

Shoes are not necessary for children with normal feet until walking is well established. Any covering for an infant's foot should be soft enough to allow the maximum in foot freedom for muscle development. The main purpose of shoes is protection.

A tennis shoe or sandal may offer an adequate covering for the normal foot.

21 | Neuromuscular Disorders*

DEVELOPMENTAL DISORDERS OF THE NERVOUS SYSTEM

Developmental disorders of the nervous system may be due to genetic factors; toxicity during pregnancy; uterine anoxia; infection with rubella virus, cytomegalovirus, or toxoplasmosis; or, possibly, overexposure to x-ray in the pelvic area during pregnancy. Many disorders classed as developmental are of unknown cause.

HYDROCEPHALUS

Hydrocephalus is usually due to obstruction of the circulation of the cerebrospinal fluid anywhere along its course. The obstruction results from the defective development of the ventricular foramina; the presence of neoplasm, infection, or hemorrhage; or an unknown cause. A nonobstructive or oversecretion type of hydrocephalus is due to choroid plexus papilloma. Hydrocephalus often accompanies myelodysplasia.

Clinical Findings

A. Symptoms and Signs: There may be a history of central nervous system infection, bacterial or viral. The head may appear normal at birth, but within 2 or 3 months, an abnormal rate of enlargement may be noted (see Inside Front Cover). Fontanelles and sutures may be palpably widened. In congenital aqueductal atresia (Arnold-Chiari syndrome), the infant may show macrocephaly at birth. Lethargy, irritability, vomiting, and disturbances of vital signs are late signs.

B. X-Ray Findings: Plain film of the skull may show, in addition to widening of fontanelles and sutures, cranial abnormalities or intracranial calcification due to toxoplasmosis or cytomegalic inclusion disease. CT scan is the most effective noninvasive method of demonstrating ventricular enlargement and following the course of disease.

C. Special Examinations: Transillumination of the skull may be of

*Revised with the assistance of Gerhard Nellhaus, MD, and Charlotte E. Thompson, MD.

value, especially in subdural hematoma in infants. Ultrasonography is sometimes comparable to the CT scan in diagnostic value. Ventriculography is employed if CT scan and ultrasonography are not available.

Treatment

Several operative procedures have been devised to establish artificial channels for reducing the pressure in the ventricles. Nonshunting operations such as ventriculostomy and choroid plexectomy may be effective. Slowly developing hydrocephalus may be controlled with diuretics such as acetazolamide.

Prognosis

The prognosis for a normal life and fair to normal intelligence has improved recently, as shunt procedures and control of postoperative infection have improved. With surgical intervention, if successful, only about one-fourth of survivors have normal intelligence. Without surgery, about one-fourth of children will survive, almost all requiring supportive nursing care. Common sequelae are severe mental retardation, visual defects, cerebellar ataxia, spastic diplegia, and convulsions.

MYELODYSPLASIA
(Spina Bifida, Spinal Dysraphism)

Myelodysplasia is a malformation of the spinal cord and vertebrae resulting in varying degrees of failure of alar plate closure: vertebral, neural, meningeal, or cutaneous. It occurs most frequently in the lumbosacral region of the spine.

Myelodysplasias are the most common developmental defects of the central nervous system, occurring about once in 1000 births.

Classification

A. Spina Bifida Occulta: In spina bifida occulta, the most common type of myelodysplasia, there is no externally visible sac. Vertebrae are defective, usually with no damage to the spinal cord (an incidental finding by x-ray in 5% of the population).

B. Meningocele: The sac is composed only of meninges, with cord and nerve roots not grossly apparent. Microscopic examination reveals cord and root structures.

C. Meningomyelocele: Meningomyelocele occurs once in 800 births. There is a soft, round, cystlike mass, the wall of which contains neural tissue of the usually imperfectly developed and damaged cord.

D. Encephalocele: This form consists of a defect at any point of the skull; the defect may be associated with a meningocele or an encephalomeningocele. The most common sites are at the midline in the occipital and parietal areas, but the frontal bone, orbit, or nose may be involved.

E. Diastematomyelia: Findings include a projection of bony, cartilaginous, or fibrous septum from the posterior surface of the vertebral body and a segmental division of the cord and meninges.

F. Other: Dermal or pilonidal sinuses anywhere along the cerebrospinal axis should be investigated by x-ray to rule out a communication with the subarachnoid space.

Clinical Findings

A. Spina Bifida Occulta: Most cases are asymptomatic. There may be gradual development of cavus deformities of the feet, as well as loss of bladder and bowel control, as the child grows. This is due to stretching of the spinal cord, and surgical intervention may be necessary. X-ray studies may give little evidence of the nature of the problem. CT scan of the spine or myelography may be necessary to further define the problem.

B. Meningocele: Rarely, there is evidence of motor weakness or sphincter disturbance. The lesion transilluminates easily. Electromyography may demonstrate subclinical asymmetric muscle denervation.

C. Meningomyelocele: Meningomyelocele transilluminates less easily than does meningocele. There may be flaccid paralysis, absent sensation, and deformities of the legs. In cervical lesions, there may be spasticity and hyperactive reflexes in the lower extremities.

D. Encephalocele: Symptoms depend on the location of the lesion and the extent of involvement of the nervous tissue.

E. Diastematomyelia: Symptoms depend on the location and extent of the malformation but usually involve the lower extremities, with progressive weakening and sensory loss. Localized hypertrichosis, dermal sinus, and defects of the skin frequently occur.

Treatment

A. Surgical Measures: The correction of meningomyeloceles probably should be done as quickly as possible after the infant is delivered. Gross hydrocephalus or extensive paralysis contraindicates surgery. Spina bifida occulta is usually not treated unless there is an underlying lesion such as a lipoma, in which case surgical intervention is required. The head size should be charted daily and x-ray studies undertaken if the circumference increases.

B. General Measures: The infant should be kept on his or her abdomen and the sac covered with sterile dressings. Fluid intake should not exceed minimum daily requirements.

Prognosis

The prognosis is guarded at best and depends principally upon the extent of spinal cord involvement. If there is associated hydrocephalus, the prognosis is generally poor but varies with the severity and treatability of the disease. Spina bifida occulta without other symptoms may be associated with loss of sphincter control later in childhood.

CRANIOSYNOSTOSIS

Craniosynostosis is a developmental disorder of the skull bones that results in closure of one or more cranial sutures in utero. Diagnosis is based on distortion of the normal skull shape: elongation, narrowing, or broadening and shortening. X-rays confirm the diagnosis and define the sutures involved.

Head measurements should be done frequently and carefully during the first 2 years of the infant's life to determine if normal increase in skull size has been interrupted.

Treatment is by surgical incision of sutures when normal increase in skull size is not taking place or for cosmetic improvement. When several sutures are involved, especially the coronal, reoperation is sometimes necessary.

Prognosis is usually good, but mental retardation may be apparent in 5% of children despite surgical intervention.

DEGENERATIVE DISORDERS OF THE NERVOUS SYSTEM

The degenerative disorders of the central nervous system are almost all due to genetically transmitted enzyme defects resulting in either toxic accumulations of metabolic products or deposition of such products in the central nervous system tissue. The disease entities usually have a variable but insidious onset in a child considered normal at birth. Once apparent, the symptoms progress steadily.

Some of the more common of these diseases will be briefly reviewed.

Schilder's Disease

Schilder's disease is an eponymic term for a variety of disorders of myelin formation or myelin breakdown. It includes familial sudanophilic leukodystrophy, X-linked recessive adrenoleukodystrophy, diffuse sclerosis (which may be a variant of multiple sclerosis), and the rubeola-associated subacute sclerosing panencephalitis (SSPE).

Motor disturbances, incoordination, visual loss, mental deterioration, and loss of speech are found in patients with any of these disorders. Convulsions may occur late. Other symptoms, laboratory findings, and the course of disease will vary, depending upon the disorder and the patient.

No treatment is available. The course of disease may be rapid (death within months) or slow (death within a few years of onset). In patients with diffuse sclerosis, corticosteroid therapy has been reported to occasionally produce a remission.

Tay-Sachs Disease

Tay-Sachs disease is a familial disorder found in east European Jewish families and transmitted as a recessive condition. It is due to a deficiency in hexosaminidase A. Onset is usually at age 3–6 months, with symptoms of spasms and a shrill characteristic cry. Blindness occurs early, with the finding of a characteristic cherry-red spot on the macula. Decerebrate posture develops rapidly, and death occurs usually by age 2–3 years.

Genetic screening of adults can offer the possibility of prevention. Laboratory studies of an affected infant will show the enzymatic defect and also typical vacuolated lymphocytes.

Subacute Necrotizing Encephalomyelopathy (Leigh's Syndrome)

Subacute necrotizing encephalomyelopathy is probably due to a thiamine pyrophosphate-adenosine triphosphate inhibitor. It is transmitted as a recessive trait, and symptoms may appear from infancy through late childhood. Blindness occurs early, and motor paralysis progresses to spasticity. The course of the disease is usually rapid, with death in several months to 1 year.

The urine can be assayed for the inhibitor system. Blood levels of lactate and pyruvate are high.

Neuronal Ceroid Lipofuscinosis (Cerebromacular Degenerations)

Neuronal ceroid lipofuscinosis is a recessive condition probably due to an enzyme deficiency (defect unknown).

The infantile type, also known as Bielschowsky-Jansky disease, has an onset in children between ages 2 and 5 years, with ataxia and visual difficulty and eventually total blindness. The ataxia progresses to decerebrate posture, and seizures may occur. Death occurs within about 5 years of onset. The blood shows vacuolated lymphocytes with azurophilic hypergranulation of the polymorphonuclear cells. Rectal biopsy will reveal ballooned ganglion cells.

Onset of the juvenile form (Spielmeyer-Vogt disease) is in children between ages 5 and 15 years. Progressive visual difficulty, which leads to blindness, is usually the first symptom. Ataxia occurs and slowly develops into spasticity. Death occurs 10–15 years after onset. Laboratory findings are similar to those in the infantile form.

The adult form of this disorder (Kufs' disease) has its onset in persons over age 15 years, with psychotic behavior and ataxia as the principal symptoms. These symptoms progress very slowly, and the patient may live to old age.

Glucosylceramide Lipidosis (Gaucher's Disease)

Gaucher's disease is a rare familial disorder that is considered to result from a deficiency of glucocerebrosidase in brain and other organs, giving rise to a blocked degradation of gangliosides and accumulation of glucocerebrosides. The disorder is more common among Jews and appears at any age. It is characterized by splenomegaly; wedged pingueculae (light yellowish-brown discolorations of the conjunctiva on either side of the cornea); pigmentation of the skin; hemorrhages, especially from the nose and mouth; pain in the extremities; and bone lesions (including thinning of the cortex and widening of the bone). Neurologic symptoms are similar to those of cerebromacular degeneration. Mental retardation is prominent when the disease starts in early childhood. Anemia, leukopenia, and thrombocytopenia may occur. Blood levels of total fats, cholesterol, and lecithin are usually normal. Typical Gaucher's cells containing abnormal amounts of kerasin can often be demonstrated by splenic or bone marrow puncture or biopsy. Leukocytes demonstrate the enzyme deficiency.

Treatment is symptomatic. Removal of the spleen is indicated only because of its excessive size. Patients may live many years, but progressive neurologic involvement leading to death is the rule in the infantile form.

Niemann-Pick Disease

Niemann-Pick disease occurs in Jewish infants in 50% of cases. It is due to a sphingomyelinase deficiency, with accumulation of sphingomyelin in the brain and other organs, and is characterized by hepatosplenomegaly, lymphadenopathy, abdominal distention, weight loss, and mental retardation. Infants appear normal at birth and for the first few weeks or months of life. A cherry-red spot is found in the region of the macula in about half the cases. The symptoms of central nervous system involvement are similar to those of cerebromacular degeneration. There is moderate anemia and leukopenia or leukocytosis. Foamy Niemann-Pick cells may be found in the bone marrow, lymph nodes, or spleen and occasionally in the blood. X-rays of the lungs may reveal disseminated nodules that resemble miliary tubercles.

No treatment is effective, and death usually occurs in 2 years although chronic forms of the disease have been reported.

Metachromatic Leukodystrophy

Metachromatic leukodystrophy is a sulfatide lipidosis transmitted as a recessive trait and due to the lack of arylsulfatase. The accumulated material is found in the white matter of the brain, peripheral nerves, and renal epithelium. Onset is usually in the second year of life, with occasional infantile or juvenile cases; it is characterized by the development of ataxia, spasticity, mental deterioration, and peripheral neuropathy. Diagnosis is based on decreased enzyme levels in urine, leukocytes, or cultured skin fibroblasts. Nerve biopsy shows metachromasia. Urinary sediment, when stained with cresyl violet or toluidine blue, may show cytoplasmic metachromatic granules. No treatment is known. Death occurs early in the infantile forms and more slowly in the later forms.

Hepatolenticular Degeneration (Wilson's Disease)

Wilson's disease is a recessively inherited disorder due to a defect in copper-containing enzymes or an abnormality in copper-binding proteins in the respiratory chain, resulting in accumulation of copper within the body.

Onset is in late childhood, with symptoms of anemia and cirrhosis of the liver, including hepatomegaly and jaundice. Neurologic signs, including dysarthria, tremors, emotional lability, and eventually extensive muscular rigidity, may be intermittent in early stages and then persist. Pericorneal pigmentation with a narrow, gray-green zone overlying the outer margin of the iris (Kayser-Fleischer ring) is a diagnostic finding seen best by slit lamp examination.

Treatment is with penicillamine (Cuprimine) given orally until urinary copper levels reach normal.

The prognosis is poor, with death usually occurring in 3–5 years.

SPINOCEREBELLAR DEGENERATIVE DISEASE (Hereditary Ataxias)

Spinocerebellar degenerative diseases are characterized by degeneration of various parts of the central nervous system, including the ascending and descending tracts of the spinal cord, the cerebellum, and the optic nerves. In a number of these diseases, disorders of carbohydrate metabolism are found. Several clinical entities are recognized.

Friedreich's Ataxia

Friedreich's ataxia is the most common type of spinocerebellar degenerative disease. It is a familial hereditary disease with onset in children 5–15 years of age. Early symptoms affect the lower limbs, with ataxic gait. Feet may be characteristically high-arched with hammer toes. Scoliosis is common. Nystagmus is usually present. Speech is jerky, explosive, and indistinct. The disease progresses to the upper limbs and spinal muscles. Diabetes mellitus occurs in about 40% of cases, and cardiomyopathy is also common. Death usually occurs from cardiac failure during the third or fourth decade of life.

Charcot-Marie-Tooth Disease

Charcot-Marie-Tooth disease, a variant of Friedreich's ataxia seen in children as well as adolescents, is a disorder of peripheral nerves with slowly progressive muscle weakness. It is characterized by distal weakness with involvement of the muscles innervated by the peroneal nerves. The symptoms include high arches, "stork-leg" appearance with thinning of the calf, loss of deep tendon reflexes, decreased vibratory sense, and a decrease in nerve conduction time. This disease is familial, transmitted as a dominant trait.

DYSTONIA MUSCULORUM DEFORMANS

Dystonia musculorum deformans, a genetic degenerative disease of the basal ganglia, is transmitted as a dominant trait with a very slow course or, in Jewish children, as an autosomal recessive trait with a very rapid course after onset in childhood. The disease begins in the form of hypertonia of leg muscles and spreads progressively to the trunk, the back, and, eventually, the arms. Spasticity and involuntary movement are accentuated by emotional and physical activity. Characteristically, spasticity and involuntary movement disappear during sleep; strength, coordination, and reflexes are normal if relaxation is maintained. Pallidectomy or thalamotomy may afford relief for several years.

CEREBRAL PALSY

Cerebral palsy is a term applied to the neuromotor components resulting from various types of brain damage and is characterized by paralysis, weakness, incoordination, or ataxia. Convulsions, mental retardation, visual defects, hearing defects, and emotional disturbances may also be present. Cerebral palsy is the largest cause of congenital crippling disease in children in the USA. Of those affected, about one-fourth are mentally retarded, one-third are capable of considerable improvement, and one-sixth are so mildly affected that treatment is not necessary. One-sixth are so severely affected as to be bedridden.

Etiology

A. Prenatal Factors: These include radiation to the mother, intrauterine hypoxia or bleeding, Rh or ABO incompatibility, maternal rubella infection, toxoplasmosis, and cytomegalic inclusion disease. The incidence is high in low-birth-weight infants.

B. Natal Factors: These include hypoxia due to anesthetic or to analgesic drugs, cerebral trauma during delivery, and hyperbilirubinemia due to blood incompatibility.

C. Postnatal Factors: These include brain contusion or hemorrhage, infection, and poisoning.

Clinical Symptoms

Infants are frequently hypotonic at birth and then gradually develop one of the following syndromes:

A. Spastic Type With Pyramidal Tract Involvement: Hyperactive stretch reflex is seen. Topographic classification of spastic cerebral palsy includes hemiplegia, diplegia, and quadriplegia.

B. Extrapyramidal Involvement and Basal Ganglia: There is involuntary and uncoordinated movement of the muscle groups.

C. Dystonias: Rigid postural attitude, with resistance to passive motion, is characteristic.

D. Ataxias: Involvement of the cerebellum and loss of balance occur.

Treatment

Treatment in all types of cerebral palsy is difficult and must be planned individually over a period of years. Physical therapy to establish automatic motion and eliminate unwanted motions is most important. Speech training requires much time and the use of special skills on the part of the trainer. Vision and hearing defects may be present and should be corrected if possible. Diazepam (Valium) may reduce uncontrollable motions. Occupational therapy will be most useful in teaching the activities of daily living.

Orthopedic surgery offers much improvement and the possibility of a more normal life in spastic cases. Bracing, splinting, and reconstructive procedures (eg, muscle and tendon transfers, joint arthrodesis, and denervations) are all potentially valuable.

TRAUMATIC DISORDERS OF THE NERVOUS SYSTEM*

SUBARACHNOID HEMORRHAGE

Bleeding into the spinal fluid of the subarachnoid space from blood vessels on the surface of the brain may be the result of trauma or vascular malformation. Bleeding can also occur with blood dyscrasias, leukemia, hypertension, or intracranial tumor.

Clinical Findings

A. Symptoms and Signs: Onset may be sudden or gradual up to 48 hours after trauma. Increasing lethargy, headache, nausea, and vomiting appear first. Following trauma, these symptoms may develop during sleeping hours. The child should be aroused every 1–2 hours up to 72 hours after trauma to detect the first symptoms. Late symptoms include delirium and coma. Signs of meningeal irritation (see p 643) or fever up to 38.3 °C (101 °F) may be present. Onset is sudden with rupture of congenital aneurysm or with hypertensive hemorrhage.

There may be no symptoms in cases where bleeding is slight and occurs for only a short period of time. A small linear skull fracture in a young child may be followed months or years later by the development of a leptomeningeal cyst, with a resultant significant cranial defect and irreversible neurologic deficit. Diagnosis may be made by skull x-ray 4–6 months following injury.

B. Laboratory Findings: Spinal fluid contains blood, which does not diminish in concentration with continued flow of fluid. Samples of cerebrospinal fluid taken at 5-minute intervals show no change in the red cell count or in the gross color. Xanthochromia is noted on centrifugation. Microscopic examination early shows crenated red cells and few white cells.

Treatment

The underlying hemorrhagic disease should be treated if present. Measures to combat cerebral edema are most important. Restrict fluids, elevate the head, and give corticosteroids, urea, or mannitol. Further lumbar puncture is contraindicated unless infection or renewed bleeding is suspected.

Surgical correction of blood vessel abnormalities or removal of tumor may be possible following demonstration by CT scan or angiography.

*Child abuse and neglect are discussed in Chapter 10.

Prognosis

If the hemorrhage is not massive and is self-limited, the prognosis is excellent. With massive hemorrhage, large areas of the brain may be permanently damaged, with resultant sequelae such as cerebral palsy or convulsive disorders.

SUBDURAL HEMATOMA

Subdural hematoma is a unilateral or bilateral collection of blood between the dura and the piarachnoid, resulting from physical trauma at any age, including birth trauma. In infants, especially if the history is inconsistent, consider child abuse (see Chapter 10).

Clinical Findings

Subdural hematoma is suggested by abnormal enlargement of the head in association with any of the symptoms listed below. In older children, a history of trauma to the head may be elicited, preceding onset of symptoms by 2–4 weeks.

A. Symptoms and Signs: Insidious onset of signs and symptoms apparently unrelated to the central nervous system makes the diagnosis difficult. In infants, early symptoms may be regarded as a "feeding problem," with irritability, anorexia, vomiting, and failure to gain weight. The head size increases, and the anterior fontanelle may bulge and pulsate. Retarded motor development, retinal hemorrhages, and hyperactive reflexes are also found. In older children, symptoms of increasing intracranial pressure such as lethargy, anorexia, headache, and vomiting become apparent slowly. Convulsions and coma may occur early in infants but later in older children.

B. Special Diagnostic Procedures: Diagnosis may be established by bilateral subdural tap in infants. In older children, it is necessary to make bur holes through the skull before a needle is introduced. The findings on EEG are frequently abnormal. Carotid angiography shows a filling defect. Echoencephalography and CT scan are simple, efficient diagnostic techniques that may be of value.

Treatment

Treatment usually consists of subdural taps, with removal of 10–20 mL of fluid daily until the quantity and the protein content of the withdrawn fluid remain constant over a period of 3 or 4 days. With bilateral hematomas, tap one side every other day. If the quantity of fluid obtainable decreases steadily, surgical removal may not be necessary. If after 10 days there is no decrease in fluid, a surgical shunt may be put in place. Remnants of the clot and the surrounding membrane may require surgical removal. Hemoglobin and total protein levels should be determined frequently.

Prognosis

The prognosis is generally excellent with the above treatment, although mental retardation, convulsions, ocular abnormalities, or paralysis may become apparent, depending upon the damage to the underlying brain suffered with the initial insult.

EXTRADURAL HEMATOMA

In extradural hematoma, the bleeding from dural or emissary veins or from middle meningeal vessels is usually a complication of a closed head injury.

Clinical Findings

A. Symptoms and Signs: There may be local evidence of head trauma and a history of momentary unconsciousness followed by a lucid interval of 30 minutes to several hours and then increasing drowsiness. The child with extradural hematoma should be observed in the same manner as the child with subarachnoid hemorrhage (see above). Hemiparesis, unequal pupils, hyperactive deep tendon reflexes, and positive Babinski signs may be found. Weak, rapid pulse, low blood pressure, and respiratory irregularity are ominous signs. Drowsiness may rapidly progress to stupor, coma, and convulsions.

B. Laboratory Findings: Lumbar puncture is not necessary, since the findings will not change the management of the case. Skull x-ray may show a fracture across the middle meningeal artery groove. Cerebral angiography and CT scan will establish the diagnosis.

Treatment

Surgical intervention may be an emergency procedure but should not be done until intravenous infusion has been started and blood for transfusion is available.

TOXIC DISORDERS OF THE NERVOUS SYSTEM

LEAD POISONING
(Lead Encephalopathy)

Lead poisoning in children—especially those under 5 years of age—produces an encephalopathy. The onset is insidious. Early manifestations include weakness, irritability, personality change, loss of weight, and vomiting, which may eventually become projectile. Developmental regression, with generalized convulsions and coma, is a late sign of increased intracranial pressure.

Symptoms may be precipitated by infection or acidosis. A history of pica involving flaking paint in older homes, lead toys, yellow and orange crayons, artists' paints, leaded gasoline, or fruit tree sprays can often be obtained.

An increased urine lead level is the definitive laboratory finding. Screening tests depend upon the determination of elevated levels of urinary coproporphyrins (> 500 μg/L), blood lead (> 80 μg/dL), and urinary aminolevulinic acid (> 13 mg/L). Red blood cell aminolevulinic acid dehydratase levels and red blood cell stippling are satisfactory screening tests. Blood lead levels exceeding 40 μg/dL on 2 or more occasions require further investigation. Cerebrospinal fluid shows an elevated white blood cell count, usually exceeding 100 cells/μL. Lumbar puncture should be performed with extreme caution, because of the increased pressure.

X-rays may demonstrate increased density in the metaphyses of the long bones, and lead may be seen in the gastrointestinal tract.

Treatment

A. Specific Measures:

1. Combination therapy with dimercaprol (BAL) and calcium disodium edathamil (EDTA) is indicated. This treatment should not be initiated until urine flow is established. Start with BAL, 4 mg/kg given intramuscularly every 4 hours (maximum, 75 mg/kg/d). With the second dose of BAL, give EDTA, 12.5 mg/kg intravenously or intramuscularly. The treatment should be continued every 4 hours for 3–5 days, at which time the blood lead level will usually be reduced to normal range.

If blood lead concentration exceeds 100 μg/dL of whole blood on the 14th or 25th day, give a second 5-day course of BAL and EDTA.

When the patient can tolerate oral medication, start penicillamine, 100 mg/kg/d (maximum, 1 g).

Do not administer medicinal iron while BAL is being given.

2. For initial control of seizures, diazepam (Valium) in frequent doses is preferred whenever there is significant increase in muscle tone or muscle twitching. Phenobarbital or phenytoin sodium may be necessary.

3. Avoid overhydration during therapy. Renal toxicity due to EDTA treatment is indicated by increasing hematuria and proteinuria. Daily urinalyses should be performed and the dosage of EDTA reduced if signs of toxicity appear.

4. Surgical decompression, hypothermia, urea, or mannitol (see p 487) may be necessary in severe cases with markedly increased intracranial pressure.

5. Oral penicillamine may be of value in asymptomatic children with chronic lead poisoning.

B. General Measures: *Prevent reexposure to lead,* and give anticonvulsants (see Table 21–4). High-calcium, high-phosphorus diet (milk) and large doses of vitamin D assist in removing lead from the blood by depositing it in the bones.

Prognosis

The prognosis is poor in the child under 2 years of age; the mortality rate in this age group is 25%. In the older child—and in cases of peripheral neuritis without encephalopathy—the prognosis for recovery is excellent.

BENIGN INTRACRANIAL HYPERTENSION
(Pseudotumor Cerebri, Otitic Hydrocephalus)

Benign intracranial hypertension is a clinical syndrome of elevated intracranial pressure, otherwise normal cerebrospinal fluid findings, and a midline ventricular system of normal or small size.

The condition may occur 1–2 weeks after various infections, particularly of the middle ear; withdrawal of corticosteroid therapy; or trauma to the jugular vein. In some cases, no apparent cause can be discovered. It may occur with hypoparathyroidism, exposure to some insecticides, Addison's disease, vitamin A overdosage, and the administration of tetracycline or nalidixic acid.

Clinical findings include sudden onset of headache, vomiting, papilledema, and sixth nerve paresis, together with ataxia, drowsiness, or stupor. Convulsions and focal neurologic abnormalities are uncommon. The findings on EEG may be abnormal.

Serial spinal punctures, corticosteroids, fluid restriction, hypertonic solutions, and the administration of diuretics have all been used for treatment. Surgical decompression may occasionally be necessary. An increased incidence in obese prepubertal females has been described. The prognosis is excellent, although long-standing emotional disturbances may develop.

ACRODYNIA
(Pink Disease)

Acrodynia (rare in the USA) is a disease of early childhood characterized by marked irritability, restlessness, or apathy; symmetric swelling and marked erythema of the hands, feet, and the tip of the nose; pa[illegible] and desquamation of the hands and feet, which may go on to loss of n[illegible] and portions of the digits; photophobia; inflammation in the mouth; excessive perspiration; hypertension; and profuse salivation. The child has marked hypotonia, often assumes a "penknife" position, and squirms constantly in an attempt to allay the intense itching. Chronic mercurial poisoning is the cause of many cases, and treatment with dimercaprol (BAL) is indicated.

CHOREA
(Sydenham's Chorea, St. Vitus' Dance)

Chorea is an encephalopathy characterized by quick, twitching, involuntary, incoordinate movements of the face, trunk, and extremities. It is more common in girls than boys and in the age group from 6 to 10 years. It often follows group A streptococcal infection or rheumatic fever. Tests for precise muscle control, such as finger-to-nose or buttoning clothes, will demonstrate involuntary actions in mild cases. Gait and speech may be markedly impaired. Muscle strength is diminished. Emotional instability, confusion, irritability, and insomnia are common.

Treatment includes bed rest, sedation with chlorpromazine or phenobarbital, and penicillin prophylaxis as for rheumatic fever.

The prognosis is good for eventual recovery. Recurrent episodes are not uncommon. Associated rheumatic fever or rheumatic heart disease may complicate the situation.

ENCEPHALITIS IN CHILDREN

Infectious encephalitis results from direct invasion of brain tissue by an infectious agent (Table 21–1). Evidence of a chronic viral encephalitis has been demonstrated in western equine encephalitis, Japanese B encephalitis, and herpes encephalitis. Chronic, continuing viral activity might be extremely important in explaining some of the serious and slowly developing sequelae of infectious encephalitis in children.

Parainfectious encephalitis, as the name implies, is associated with an infection but is not due to direct invasion of the nervous system by the infecting agent. These cases are of 2 basic types: (1) those probably due to an antigen-antibody reaction associated with a systemic infection and (2) those due to the direct effect of a toxin that is the by-product of bacterial or viral proliferation in a systemic infection (Table 21–2). Postvaccinal encephalitis is included in this category because it is clearly related to an infectious agent and because the pathologic process is similar to encephalopathy that follows or accompanies an acute infection such as rubeola or varicella. The en-

Table 21–1. Infectious encephalitis in the USA.

Source	Infection
Arboviruses (arthropod-borne)	Eastern equine encephalitis St. Louis encephalitis Western equine encephalitis
Enteroviruses	Coxsackievirus Echovirus Poliovirus
Other viruses	Adenovirus Herpes simplex Lymphocytic choriomeningitis Mumps Rabies
Other agents	
Cryptococcus neoformans	Cryptococcosis
Mycoplasma pneumoniae	Primary atypical pneumonia
Toxoplasma gondii	Toxoplasmosis
Unknown	Cat-scratch disease

cephalopathy that follows inoculation of killed pertussis vaccine is unique in that the pathologic process is entirely similar to that associated with a systemic infection.

Clinical Findings

A. Symptoms and Signs: The essential clinical feature of encephalitis is impairment of brain function, affecting the state of consciousness

Table 21–2. Parainfectious encephalitis in the USA.

Type	Infection
Antigen-antibody	Accompanying or following: Herpes zoster (?) Infectious mononucleosis Roseola infantum (?) Rubella Rubeola Varicella
Antigen-antibody	Following: Pertussis vaccine Rabies vaccine Smallpox vaccine* Yellow fever vaccine
Toxic	Influenza Salmonellosis Scarlet fever Shigellosis

*Now extremely rare.

and the activity of the cerebral cortex. Hence the symptoms are usually those of lethargy, coma, and convulsions. The earliest signs are headache, nausea, and vomiting and are related to the cerebral edema accompanying the inflammatory process. In very early childhood, headache may be manifested by irritability. Anorexia, nausea, and vomiting may be the first symptoms noted by the mother. An inflammatory reaction of the meninges produces the classic stiffness of neck and back together with varying degrees of impairment of straight leg raising. Severe encephalitis can produce a confusing array of neurologic phenomena. Cerebral edema alters brain function in various areas at random. A wide variety of signs may be elicited such as the Babinski sign, hypo- or hyperreflexia of the deep tendons, tremors of the extremities, and even sensory changes. Findings may vary from hour to hour as small changes occur in the degree of cerebral edema.

B. Laboratory Findings: See Table 21–3.

Table 21–3. Laboratory and clinical clues to causes of encephalitis.

Infection*	Cerebrospinal Fluid: Usual White Blood Cell Count (per mL)	Cerebrospinal Fluid: Glucose Level	Routine Clinical or Laboratory Findings Suggest Cause
Infectious encephalitis			
Adenovirus	100–1000	Normal	No
Cat-scratch disease	100–200	Normal	Yes (lymphadenopathy)
Coxsackievirus	< 400	Normal	Yes (pleurodynia and herpangina syndromes)
Cryptococcosis†	10–150	Low	Yes (cerebrospinal fluid)
Echovirus‡	200–1000	Normal	Yes (morbilliform rash)
Encephalitis (eastern equine, St. Louis, western equine)	< 200	Normal	No
Herpes simplex†	< 200	Normal	Yes (eruption)
Lymphocytic choriomeningitis†	200–3000	Normal	Yes (cerebrospinal fluid)
Mumps†	200–3000	Normal	Yes (cerebrospinal fluid)
Poliovirus†	< 200		Yes (asymmetric, flaccid paralysis)
Rabies†	< 100	Normal	
Toxoplasmosis†	50–200	Normal	Yes (?)
Parainfectious encephalitis			
Antigen-antibody type‡	< 150	Normal	Yes (primary disease symptoms, history, and routine blood count)
Toxic type†	< 50	Normal	Yes (clinical and culture)

*Sources and types of infection are listed in Tables 21–1 and 21–2.
†Serologic tests and culture techniques often available.
‡Serologic tests and culture techniques available only under special conditions.

Treatment

A. Specific Measures: No specific measures are known.

B. General Measures:

1. Give initial treatment as for bacterial meningitis of unknown type until viral cause is clear (see p 645).

2. Increased intracranial pressure may be relieved as a temporary measure for periods up to 4 hours by hypertonic intravenous infusions of mannitol. Give 1.5–2 g/kg as a 20% solution in water intravenously over 10–15 minutes. Monitor the patient carefully to avoid impairment of urinary flow due to marked dehydration or electrolyte imbalance.

3. Convulsions should be controlled with phenobarbital (see Table 21–4) or phenytoin, 10 mg/kg intravenously at a rate not to exceed 50 mg/min. The maintenance dose of phenytoin is 7–8 mg/kg/d, given every 4–6 hours.

4. Maintenance of airway is the most important consideration, and tracheostomy may be required if usual techniques are not effective.

5. General hygiene includes care to avoid bedsores and to keep the skin well cleansed. The patient should be isolated to prevent other infections.

Prognosis

The prognosis following encephalitis should always be guarded. The severity of the damage apparent in convalescents is not a guide to long-term prognosis. Subtle impairment of central nervous system function can become increasingly apparent with increasing age. In contrast, children with apparently serious damage have occasionally shown remarkable improvement with the passage of time.

REYE'S SYNDROME

Reye's syndrome is a fulminant encephalopathy of unknown cause that may be associated with influenza, influenzalike illnesses, or varicella viruses. Toxic factors, particularly salicylate ingestion, have been incriminated. The onset is abrupt, with rapidly deepening coma. The cerebrospinal fluid may occasionally show a pleocytosis of fewer than 30 white cells. Hepatic involvement is characteristic, with elevated serum ammonia and transaminase levels and fatty degeneration of the liver demonstrable on biopsy or autopsy. Cerebral edema is severe. Hypoglycemia occurs.

Intensive supportive care is needed as for other types of encephalitis (see above) and for hepatic failure. Peritoneal dialysis and exchange transfusion have been recommended, but their value is not proved. Hypoglycemia should be corrected. Intracranial pressure must be monitored.

The prognosis is poor. Mortality rates in reported series are over 75%.

CONVULSIVE DISORDERS

(See also Fig 30–2.)

Convulsive seizures are relatively common in children. They may be of unknown cause, genetic, or related to the following: (1) central nervous system and other infections (meningitis, encephalitis, brain abscess, tetanus); (2) fever; (3) trauma to and vascular accidents in the brain; (4) tumors of the central nervous system; (5) disturbances in physiology of the brain (hypoxia, hypoglycemia, water intoxication, changes in CO_2 tension, hypocalcemia); (6) drugs and poisonings (Metrazol, lead, tranquilizers, strychnine); (7) defective development and vascular anomalies of the brain; (8) hypertensive encephalopathy; (9) progressive degenerative diseases (Tay-Sachs disease, Niemann-Pick disease, Gaucher's disease, tuberous sclerosis, Schilder's disease, and others); and (10) rarely, pyridoxine deficiency and dependency.

FEBRILE CONVULSIONS

Generalized ("simple") convulsive seizures may occur in children between infancy and age 5 years and are associated with sudden high fever to levels above 40 °C (104 °F). There may be a family history of similar seizures. The episode usually lasts less than 5 minutes but may continue for up to 15 minutes. Focal ("complex") febrile convulsions may last longer than 15 minutes or recur several times in a 24-hour period.

Differential Diagnosis

If the child has an obvious source of infection, such as in the ear, pharynx, nose, or lungs, treat the infection as a source of the fever, observe the child carefully, and perform follow-up examinations. If lumbar puncture is not done to rule out central nervous system infection accompanying infection found in the ear, larynx, nose, or lungs, observe and examine the child frequently until the success of any treatment program is assured.

In the absence of signs of infection, studies to determine a source of the fever include complete blood count, examination of the cerebrospinal fluid, and, especially in girls, careful urinalysis for asymptomatic urinary tract infection. In the small infant, meningitis may present as a seizure, with fever and few other signs of central nervous system irritation.

Treatment

Maintain the airway, turning the child on the abdomen to avoid possible aspiration of vomitus. Lower the body temperature by applying cool but not cold wet cloths or by holding the child in a tub of water at about 38 °C (100.4 °F).

When the seizure subsides, give antipyretics as follows: aspirin, 130 mg per year of age per dose, every 2–4 hours for 6 doses; or acetaminophen, 60 mg per dose for children under age 1 year, 60–120 mg per dose for age 1–3 years, or 120 mg per dose for age 3–6 years.

If convulsions persist or recur, treat as for status epilepticus (see p 492).

Prophylaxis

Controversy continues on the issue of prophylaxis. Prolonged administration of phenobarbital has been recommended for all children who have had a febrile seizure. Parents' compliance with administration of such drugs for a long time when there are no symptoms is always doubtful.

Two schools of thought, however, have developed at present. One school (Rabe) recommends that phenobarbital or valproic acid (Table 21–4) be given to maintain a blood level of 15–20 μg/mL for 2 seizure-free years if the child meets *one* of the following criteria: (1) the child is under age 18 months; (2) findings on ECG are positive 7 or more days after the seizure; (3) seizures lasted longer than 15 minutes, recurred in 24 hours, or were focal in origin; (4) there is a family history of seizures; or (5) evidence of neurologic or developmental abnormalities was present prior to the febrile seizure. The other school (Gellis) recommends that phenobarbital or valproic acid (as above) be given only after a second febrile seizure episode.

Prognosis

Long-term studies have indicated that about 65% of children having a febrile seizure will have no subsequent seizures; 32% will have one or more further episodes associated with fever but none without fever; and 2% had epilepsy by age 7 years.

Table 21–4. Anticonvulsant drugs for children.

Drug	Average Daily Dosage (mg/kg)*	Usual Therapeutic Blood Level (μg/mL)	Indications	Toxic Reactions and Precautions
Carbamazepine (Tegretol)	20	4–8	Generalized tonic-clonic and focal seizures.	Leukopenia, agranulocytosis, liver dysfunction, dizziness, diplopia.
Clonazepam (Clonopin)	0.1	20–60	Minor motor seizures, infantile spasms, petit mal; as alternative to ethosuximide.	Ataxia, slurred speech, liver dysfunction.
Ethosuximide (Zarontin)	15	40–100	Drug of choice for petit mal. If grand mal seizures accompany and are increased, use with phenobarbital.	Leukopenia, liver dysfunction, nausea and vomiting, headache, drowsiness.
Mephobarbital (Mebaral)	5	15–40	Stronger but otherwise similar to phenobarbital.	As in phenobarbital.
Methsuximide (Celontin)	20	10–40	May be used with phenobarbital when latter is not completely effective.	Ataxia, headache, diplopia, morbilliform rash.
Phenobarbital	5	15–40	One of the safest drugs for all epilepsies, especially as adjunct. Drug of choice for initial trial.	Toxicity is rare. Drowsiness, increased excitability, morbilliform rash may occur.
Phenytoin (Dilantin)	6	10–20	Often used with phenobarbital in the management of grand mal and many cases of psychomotor epilepsy.	May accentuate petit mal. With prolonged use, gum hypertrophy, nervousness, ataxia, nystagmus, nausea and vomiting.
Primidone (Mysoline)	15	5–12	Second choice to phenobarbital for grand mal and otherwise uncontrolled major seizures. Useful in psychomotor seizures.	Urticaria, diarrhea, nausea and vomiting.
Trimethadione (Tridione)	30	Up to 20	As alternative to ethosuximide; with aggravation of grand mal, give phenobarbital.	Leukopenia, agranulocytosis, nephrosis.
Valproic acid (Depakene)	25	40–100	Absence seizures and prophylaxis in febrile convulsions when phenobarbital is not tolerated.	Liver dysfunction.

*Usually divided into 3 equal doses given every 8 hours.

EPILEPSY
(Idiopathic Convulsive State, Paroxysmal Cerebral Dysrhythmia)

Epilepsy refers to recurrent seizures that usually involve involuntary movements of muscles and impairment of consciousness, memory, or vegetative function, either singly or in various combinations.

Clinical Findings (See also Fig 30–2.)

A family history can be elicited in one-third of cases. Attack may be precipitated by overhydration, vasomotor reactions, illness, fatigue, emotional tension, hyperventilation, or autonomic disturbances.

A. Types of Seizures and Manifestations:

1. Generalized convulsions–Generalized tonic-clonic (grand mal) convulsions are the most common type and are frequently preceded by a motor or sensory aura, staring or deviation of the eyes, loss of consciousness, and a short tonic convulsion. The child may salivate, bite the tongue, and have urinary or fecal incontinence. Seizures may be followed by headache, confusion, or deep sleep.

2. Absence seizures–In patients with absence (petit mal) seizures, staring and loss of consciousness occur for a few seconds. There may be slight rhythmic motor disturbances (head nodding, eye blinking). The child may be unaware of the attacks, and there is no aura or drowsiness.

3. Akinetic seizures–There is a brief loss of consciousness and muscle tone. There are no tonic or clonic movements. Postconvulsion somnolence may occur.

4. Myoclonic seizures–Brief involuntary contractions of limbs or groups of muscles, sometimes localized to one side of the body, occur. These may result in falling or injury, but there may or may not be brief loss of consciousness.

5. Psychomotor seizures–In patients with psychomotor ("epileptic equivalent," "psychic variant") seizures, there is a brief period of increased muscular tonicity preceded by an aura and visceral symptoms (nausea, vomiting, epigastric sensation) and followed by movements of the mouth and integrated but confused, semipurposeful movements during a period of impaired awareness or amnesia. A history of birth trauma or "complex" febrile convulsions is frequently present. Seizures may progress to a generalized convulsion. Personality disturbances, especially an overactive, aggressive type, may be present between seizures.

6. Jacksonian seizures–Motor or sensory disturbances begin locally (focal seizures) in one part of the body and spread or extend according to a fixed pattern. The seizure may eventually involve the entire body and become indistinguishable from a generalized (grand mal) seizure.

B. Electroencephalographic Findings: Although abnormal patterns may be found on EEG in apparently normal individuals, and although individuals with idiopathic convulsive state may have a normal pattern, there is usually a characteristically abnormal tracing. With the exception of petit mal, there are no specific abnormalities characteristic of a specific clinical syndrome. Hyperventilation tends to bring out and accentuate the abnormality.

C. Other Studies: Spinal tap should be done after the first seizure or in the presence of fever to rule out infection. Skull x-ray or CT scan will be useful; pneumoencephalography or cerebral angiography may be done if CT scan is not available. Serum electrolyte and calcium levels may be useful. The pattern of seizures may indicate a relationship to hypoglycemia (fasting blood glucose level is low).

Treatment

The goal of treatment is the prevention of seizures. The type of convulsion determines to some extent the drug used (see Table 21–4), but the response of the patient is the most important criterion. Prolonged use of sedative drugs does not cause mental retardation.

A. Management of Individual Seizures: Except in status epilepticus (see below), give no treatment. Institute procedures to protect the patient from injury.

B. Management of Status Epilepticus: Diazepam (Valium), 0.2 mg/kg intravenously and repeated in 10–20 minutes as necessary, is the treatment of choice. After the emergency is controlled, start phenytoin (Dilantin) intramuscularly every 3 hours or phenobarbital intramuscularly every 6–8 hours. It is often necessary to establish an airway and give oxygen and intravenous fluids.

C. General Measures: The family and the child must be impressed with the necessity for faithful adherence to the treatment regimen. The patient should avoid excessive fatigue and keep in optimal physical condition. Acetazolamide (Diamox) may be useful in addition to other anticonvulsant drugs, especially in absence seizures. The suggested daily dose is 8–30 mg/kg orally in divided doses to a maximum of 1 g/d.

Prognosis

Although death may occur during status epilepticus or as a result of accidents, the outlook for life is generally good. The majority of patients can be controlled with drug therapy. With control, in spite of long-continued drug administration, the mental status remains unchanged. If deterioration occurs, it is generally due to the underlying process causing the seizures. Therapy may need to be continued for several years until long-continued freedom from attacks and eventual disappearance of the abnormal pattern on EEG suggest that drugs may be gradually discontinued.

BREATH-HOLDING SPELLS
(Infantile Syncope)

Breath-holding spells may occur in some children when they are frightened, hurt, or angered; they cry vigorously for a short time and then "hold their breath." After a few seconds, they may become slightly cyanotic or pallid, lose consciousness, and become limp. This may be followed by a few jerks of the limbs, a short period of increased tonus, or even opisthotonos. Micturition occasionally occurs. There is no postictal confusion. The spells occur most commonly in children between 6 months and 2 years of age and usually stop by 5 years of age. In contrast to an epileptic seizure, cyanosis precedes the seizure rather than follows it. Findings on EEG are normal.

Treatment with drugs or psychotherapy is not indicated.

MIGRAINE

Headaches in young children require more careful study than do headaches in older children and young adults. Tension headaches become more common in the latter age group. Migraine is not uncommon in young children, and onset at age 2 years has been reported. It is said to affect about 5% of the general population.

The headache is believed to result from an initial cerebral arterial vasoconstriction followed by a dilatation of these blood vessels.

Clinical Findings

A family history of migraine or convulsive seizures will be found in 30% of cases. Headache attacks have a sudden onset, with severe throbbing or pulsing pain, often unilateral. A small child distraught with pain may have difficulty localizing the source to the head. The pain is often preceded by visual disturbances, flashing lights, vertigo, nausea, vomiting, or sensory phenomena.

Basilar artery migraine, as a variant, occurs mainly in adolescent girls. Symptoms include cyclic vomiting, vertigo, ataxia, dysarthria, and tinnitus. Headache is not always present. Attacks are consistent, clearing rapidly without residua.

Treatment

Aspirin or acetaminophen is often effective in young children. In adolescents, aspirin with butalbital (Fiorinal) given every 4 hours may be useful.

Vasoconstrictors are used especially in adolescents and young adults. Give ergotamine tartrate (Cafergot), 1 tablet with premonitory symptoms, repeated every 30 minutes for a total of 4 tablets. Suppositories can be used if the patient is vomiting.

In patients with severe, frequently recurrent episodes, use of phenytoin (Dilantin) daily or tranquilizers such as diazepam (Valium) or chlordiazepoxide hydrochloride (Librium) may be helpful. Propranolol may also be useful.

Prophylaxis

The role of food allergy as a cause of headache has been discussed for many years. Food allergy as one cause of migraine headaches seems well established. Frequent offenders are eggs, milk, chocolate, onion, wheat, potato, beef, beans, nuts, citrus fruits, chicken, and artificial food coloring. A diet eliminating these items should be tried. Reintroduction with recurrence of headache will establish the causative role.

Hypoglycemia, a cause of migraine headaches in adults, should be ruled out for children by glucose tolerance test.

Prognosis

The prognosis for early relief is guarded. If allergy is the cause, a successful elimination program commonly brings relief. Emotional factors may be important, and symptoms may be relieved by their resolution.

• • •

MENTAL RETARDATION

Etiology

A. Prenatal: Prenatal factors include biochemical disorders such as those described under Degenerative Disorders of the Nervous System, above; other metabolic disorders (Table 21–5); isoimmunization; and chromosomal disorders such as trisomy 21 (Down's) syndrome, trisomy 8 (mosaicism) syndrome, partial deletion of the long arm of chromosomes 18, 13, or 4, and Duchenne's muscular dystrophy (X-linked recessive) (see p 502). Maternal infections affecting the fetus or newborn include acute bacterial infections, tuberculosis, specific viral infections (rubella, influenza, poliomyelitis, herpes simplex, chickenpox, mumps, measles, cytomegalic inclusion disease), nonspecific viral infections, and those due to spirochetes and protozoa (eg, toxoplasmosis).

B. Natal: Natal factors include maternal or placental hypoxia; hypoxia due to respiratory obstruction; breech delivery with delay in delivery of the head; and cerebral hemorrhage (traumatic [obstetric], cephalopelvic disproportion, precipitate delivery, prematurity).

C. Postnatal: Postnatal factors include central nervous system infection, brain trauma, cerebral degenerative disease (Tay-Sachs), hypoxia (recurrent severe convulsions or hypoglycemia), toxic encephalopathy (lead poisoning), and neonatal hypothyroidism.

D. Other Causes: Cretinism and "primary amentia" are other factors.

Classification

The classic terms moron (IQ 51–75), imbecile (IQ 21–50), and idiot (IQ 0–20) have been abandoned in favor of a less pejorative terminology. A child with an IQ of 70–85 is now classified as dull normal, one with an IQ of 50–69 is considered borderline mentally retarded, and one with an IQ of below 20 is considered severely mentally retarded.

Clinical Findings

Familiarity with the potential causes of mental retardation should enable the physician to recognize mental deficiency at an early age and to plan with the family for future care and therapy.

In the absence of clinical evidence of disease associated with mental deficiency, mental retardation usually becomes apparent to the family and physician in a slow and insidious manner.

Psychometric and audiologic testing is necessary to clearly establish the diagnosis and avoid tragic misdiagnosis.

A. Developmental: Neuromuscular coordination does not develop consistently at a normal rate (see Fig 3–2).

B. Educational: There is failure to profit from experience and instruction.

C. Social: The failure to achieve social standards of maturation at successive age levels is best noted by comparison with children of similar age and manifested by lack of reliance, unacceptable conduct, and inability to "get along with others."

Treatment & Prognosis

Except for severely retarded children (IQ below 20), most of the mentally retarded can be taught to take a place in society (see Chapter 10). Care within the family requires emotional adjustment. Institutional care is indicated when the child has a serious behavior or personality disorder or when there are no community facilities to aid the family in management and education.

Many communities have established special parent groups and special classes for the mentally retarded. Treatment is possible in many types of chemical disorders (see Table 21–5).

Table 21–5. Biochemical disorders often associated with central nervous system symptoms and mental retardation (MR).*

Syndrome	Amino Acids Increased in Plasma	Amino Acids or Organic Acids Increased in Urine	Biochemistry	Clinical Features and Treatment
Histidine metabolism				
Formiminoglutamic-aciduria				
Type A	Normal.	N-Formiminoglutamic acid (FIGLU) after histidine load.	Formiminotransferase deficiency.	Somatic and intellectual retardation, round face, obesity, hypersegmentation of PMNs.
Type B	Normal.	FIGLU before and after histidine load.	Folic acid transport defect (?).	Ataxia, megaloblastic anemia, MR, convulsions.
Phenylalanine metabolism				
Oasthouse syndrome	Not reported.	Phenylalanine, methionine, tyrosine.†	Not known.	Infantile spasms with interim flaccidity and unresponsiveness, sparse hair, MR, general unawareness.
Phenylketonuria	Phenylalanine.		Phenylalanine hydroxylase deficiency.	Usually severe MR, convulsions, eczema, fair hair and complexion. Urine smells musty. Prevent classic phenylketonuria by detection in neonatal period and institution of a phenylalanine-free diet. Mild or transient phenylketonuria also requires diet therapy. Defects in biopterin biosynthesis and dihydropteridine reductase deficiency will prevent successful diet therapy, and retardation continues.
Tyrosinosis (several clinical types)	Tyrosine, methionine.	Normal for age.	Transient *p*-hydroxyphenylpyruvic acid oxidase deficiency.	General failure to thrive, convulsions. Temporary response to low-phenylalanine diet.

Proline metabolism				
Hydroxyprolinemia	Hydroxyproline.	Hydroxyproline, 1-methylhistidine.	Hydroxyproline oxidase deficiency.	MR, moderate hematuria and pyuria.
Hyperprolinemia				
Type A	Proline.	Proline, hydroxyproline, glycine.	Proline oxidase deficiency.	Familial nephritis, deafness, renal hypoplasia, epilepsy, abnormal EEG.
Type B	Proline.	Proline, hydroxyproline, glycine.	Δ^1-Pyrroline-5-carboxylic acid dehydrogenase.	Convulsions, coma, MR.
Sulfur-containing amino acids				
Cystathioninuria		Cystathionine.	Cystathionine cleavage enzyme deficiency.	Congenital malformation, talipes, deafness, abnormal ears and sensation. One case with high phenylalanine, one with thrombocytopenia and renal calculi. Treat with large doses of pyridoxine.
Homocystinuria	Methionine.	Homocystine.	Cystathionine synthetase deficiency.	MR, spastic paraplegia, occasional convulsions, cataracts, lenticular dislocation, friable hair, malar flush, thromboembolic disease, bone changes. Treat with low-methionine, cystine-supplemented diet or with large doses of pyridoxine.
Methionine malabsorption syndrome		α-Hydroxybutyric acid in excess in urine and feces.	Methionine, leucine, isoleucine, and valine are rejected by bowel wall.	Convulsions, episodic diarrhea, hyperventilation, MR, and odor as in oasthouse syndrome.
Tryptophan metabolism				
Congenital tryptophanuria	Tryptophan after oral load.	Tryptophan.	Possible tryptophan oxygenase deficiency.	MR, photosensitivity, rough hyperpigmented skin, telangiectasia of conjunctiva. Treat with nicotinic acid.

*Modified from O'Brien D: *Rare Inborn Errors of Metabolism in Children with Mental Retardation,* 2nd ed. US Department of Health, Education, and Welfare, Children's Bureau, 1968.

†Perhaps also leucine, isoleucine, α-hydroxybutyric acid.

Table 21–5 (cont'd). Biochemical disorders often associated with central nervous system symptoms and mental retardation (MR).*

Syndrome	Amino Acids Increased in Plasma	Amino Acids or Organic Acids Increased in Urine	Biochemistry	Clinical Features and Treatment
Tryptophan metabolism (cont'd)				
Hartnup disease		All neutral amino acids.	Tryptophan rejection by bowel and renal tubular epithelium.	MR in some, pellagralike skin rash, ataxia, and other cerebellar signs. Treat with nicotinic acid and low-protein diet.
Urea synthesis cycle				
Argininosuccinicaciduria		Argininosuccinic acid, citrulline.	Argininosuccinate lyase deficiency.	MR, ataxia, convulsions, friable hair, rough skin, coma due to ammonia intoxication. Treat with low-protein diet.
Citrullinuria	Citrulline, methionine.	Citrulline, alanine, aspartic acid, glycine, glutamic acid, histidine.	Argininosuccinate synthetase deficiency.	MR, episodes of severe vomiting and coma due to ammonia intoxication. Treat with low-protein diet.
Congenital lysine intolerance	Lysine.	Lysine, ornithine, arginine, cystine, GABA, ethanolamine.	Not known exactly, but excess lysine inhibits arginase.	Vomiting, convulsions, MR. Responds to low-protein intake.
Ornithine transcarbamoylase deficiency		Generalized aminoaciduria.	Ornithine carbamoyltransferase deficiency.	Episodes of vomiting, restlessness, ataxia, and coma in early life from ammonia intoxication. Treat with low-protein diet.
Miscellaneous				
β-Alaninemia	β-Alanine.	β-Alanine, BAIB, taurine, GABA.	Possible β-alanine-α-ketoglutarate transaminase deficiency.	Lethargy, somnolence, hypotonia, hyporeflexia, grand mal seizures.

Hyperglycinemia Ketotic	Glycine.		Methylmalonyl-CoA isomerase or propionyl-CoA carboxylase deficiency.	Vomiting, acidosis, ketosis, infections, somatic and mental retardation.
Nonketotic	Glycine.		Defect in conversion of glycine to serine.	Seizures, MR.
Hypervalinemia	Valine.		Not known.	Failure to thrive, hypotonia, unresponsiveness, nystagmus, loss of vision, MR. Low-valine diet may prevent retardation.
Isovalericacidemia	Isovaleric acid after protein-rich meal.	Isovaleric acid much increased.	Isovaleric acid dehydrogenase deficiency.	Intellectual and motor retardation. Odor of "sweaty feet" on breath and skin. Leucine load precipitates coma. Dietary treatment.
Maple syrup urine disease	Leucine, isoleucine, valine, and their keto acids.		Defective onward metabolism of branched-chain keto acids.	Hypoglycemia, acidosis, convulsions; if untreated, death usually occurs in the newborn period. Urine smells like maple syrup. Dietary treatment.
Sarcosinemia	Sarcosine (methylglycine).		Sarcosine oxidase deficiency.	Hypotonia, mental and physical retardation.

*Modified from O'Brien D: *Rare Inborn Errors of Metabolism in Children with Mental Retardation,* 2nd ed. US Department of Health, Education, and Welfare, Children's Bureau, 1968.

DOWN'S SYNDROME
(Mongolism, Trisomy 21)

Down's syndrome occurs in about 1 of every 600 live births in all races. It is associated with trisomy of chromosome 21 and is most common among firstborn infants of women over 35 years of age. Clinical findings include mental retardation and a characteristic facies, with slanted palpebral fissures, prominent epicanthic folds, and a small brachycephalic head. The hands are broad, with a short, incurved fifth finger and a rudimentary second phalanx. The space between the first and second toes is wide, and there is increased mobility of the joints. Other findings present in most patients with Down's syndrome include small or absent ear lobes, constantly open mouth, red cheeks, irregular alignment of teeth, high-arched palate, raucous voice, Brushfield's spots (circle of silver-gray spots near the periphery of the iris) in young infants, flat nipples, delayed development of frontal sinuses, hypoplasia of the base of the skull, and reduced acetabular angles of the hip joint. Leukemia occurs more frequently in these patients than in the general population. Interatrial septal defect of the primum type is common.

Down's syndrome must be differentiated from congenital hypothyroidism, which it resembles in some ways.

The child with Down's syndrome may be quite adaptable to living at home and can be taught socially acceptable behavior in the family and community. The average maximum mental age attained is about 8 years.

MINIMAL BRAIN DYSFUNCTION SYNDROME
(Attention Deficit Syndrome)

Minimal brain dysfunction syndrome does not produce gross motor or sensory deficits or generalized impairment of the intellect. There are, however, demonstrable limited alterations of behavior or intellectual functioning. These alterations may be combinations of impaired perception, conceptualization, language, memory, impulse, or motor function. The child is described by parents and teachers as overactive, excitable, and with a very short attention span. Learning disabilities in reading and arithmetic are obviously apparent early. The incidence is estimated at from 2% to 5% of elementary school children. The term "hyperactive child" is often applied to children with this syndrome. Minimal brain damage, chemical toxicity from heavy metals, premature birth, and psychosocial and genetic factors have all been considered causative factors of this syndrome.

Diagnostic Evaluation*

Diagnostic evaluation should include the following:

A. Medical Evaluation:

1. Histories–

a. Medical–Include pre-, peri-, and postnatal information. Details of all childhood illnesses should be obtained, including age of child at time of illness, symptoms, severity, course, and care (such as physician in attendance, hospitalization).

b. Developmental–Include details of motor, language, adaptive, and personal-social development.

c. Family and social–Include information regarding acculturation factors, interpersonal family dynamics, and interpersonal family stresses.

2. Physical examinations–

a. General–Give special attention to possible systemic disease affecting learning and behavior.

b. Neurologic–Look for possible specific disorders of the nervous system, and evaluate integrated motor acts as opposed to simple reflexes. "Neurologic soft signs" may be significant; hyperactive deep tendon reflexes, moderate difficulty with coordination, and tight heel cords are examples.

3. Special examinations–

a. Ophthalmologic–Include visual acuity and fields examinations, as well as funduscopy.

b. Otologic–Include audiometric and otoscopic examinations.

4. Routine laboratory tests–Include complete blood count, urinalysis, and serology.

5. Special laboratory tests–Perform only when specifically indicated.

a. Electroencephalography–Include waking, sleeping, and serial tracings. Dysrhythmias are found in about half of cases studied.

b. CT scan–Findings are abnormal in nearly 40% of cases.

c. Pneumoencephalography and cerebral angiography–These are rarely indicated.

d. Biochemistry–Include determinations of urine and serum amino acid levels. Perform hair analysis for heavy metals.

e. Genetic assessment–Analyze chromosomes.

B. Behavioral Assessment:

1. Academic history–Include teachers' and principal's observations regarding the child's school behavior as well as academic progress and achievement. The child's school records, including samples of schoolwork and test results, should be available to the diagnostic team.

*Report of National Institute of Neurological Diseases and Blindness, US Department of Health, Education, and Welfare, NINDB Monograph No. 3, 1966.

2. Psychologic evaluation–Include the core items of psychologic evaluation: individual comprehensive assessment of intellectual functioning, measures of complex visual-motor-perceptual functioning, behavioral obvservations in a variety of settings, and additional indices of learning and behavior as indicated.

3. Language evaluation–Include detailed assessment of speech and language behavior: audiometric screening; assessment of articulation, voice quality, and rate; and the expressive and receptive aspects of language.

4. Educational evaluation–An educational diagnostician should conduct detailed analyses of academic abilities, including achievement assessment for details of levels and methods of skill acquisition, eg, reading, number concepts, spelling, and writing.

Treatment

Any treatment program must involve parents, teachers, and a clinical psychologist or psychiatrist. Great emphasis must be placed upon acceptable behavior. Tutoring under the direction of school authorities can be most valuable. Drug therapy with dextroamphetamine or methylphenidate (Ritalin) may be useful but has become a controversial issue through overenthusiastic application.

Prognosis is always guarded. Strenuous effort must be maintained over a period of several years to effect the best outcome.

DISORDERS AFFECTING THE MUSCLES

Disorders affecting the muscles are universally characterized by weakness. This symptom is also characteristic of a number of disorders of the nervous system such as spinal cord disease, motor neuron dysfunction, and peripheral nerve damage. In the approach to a possible muscular disease, the neuroanatomic site of dysfunction must be determined first. Table 21–6 outlines this approach.

THE MUSCULAR DYSTROPHIES

The muscular dystrophies are genetically determined diseases of skeletal muscle. These diseases are X-linked genetic disorders and are classified into 6 groups: (1) X-linked muscular dystrophy (Duchenne type progressive pseudohypertrophic muscular dystrophy), (2) facioscapulohumeral (FSH) muscular dystrophy, (3) limb-girdle muscular dystrophy, (4) distal myopathy, (5) ocular myopathy, and (6) "oculocraniosomatic syndrome."

Table 21–6. Evaluation of muscle weakness by anatomic area.*

Anatomic Area	Manifestations
Corticospinal pathways	Hyperactive stretch reflexes. Spasticity. Abnormal reflexes. Weakness usually greater than atrophy.
Lower motor neuron	
Anterior horn cell	Fasciculation. Hypoactive or absent reflexes. Usually proximal in children. Atrophy usually in proportion to weakness.
Peripheral nerve	Above plus sensory changes.
Myoneural junction (myasthenia gravis)	Extraocular musculature usually involved. Fatigues easily following contraction. Strength increases following rest. Variable and fluctuating course.
Muscle fiber	Hypoactive or absent reflexes. Atrophy usually in proportion to weakness. Usually proximal distribution.
Functional	Cogwheel response. Inconsistencies. Hoover's sign. Bizarre gait. Slowness of motion. Overflow of activity.

*Reproduced, with permission, from Fowler WM Jr: Muscle weakness and atrophy: Clinical and laboratory evaluation. *Calif Med* 1968;108:25.

The X-linked, or Duchenne, type of muscular dystrophy is the most common, with onset in early childhood. Boys are affected almost exclusively and are noted to have difficulty keeping up with children their own age in walking and running. Trunk and pelvic girdle weakness produces the classic Gowers' sign (ie, when rising from the supine position, the child climbs up on his or her legs). Enlargement of the calves or pseudohypertrophy occurs in about 80% of patients.

Laboratory findings include markedly elevated serum enzyme levels (creatine phosphokinase, SGOT, lactate dehydrogenase, and aldolase). Electrocardiographic abnormalities are present in about 70% of cases. Electromyographic abnormalities are present in all cases. Muscle biopsy should be done on frozen tissue with histochemical stains. A moderately severely involved muscle should be used, but not the gastrocnemius.

Treatment is palliative. Physical therapy, night splints, and surgery to release contractures, when done at the appropriate time, can prolong walking for 2–4 years. Careful pulmonary care in the late stages, with postural drainage and the use of portable breathing machines, may also prolong life and make the patient more comfortable. Vigorous antibiotic therapy for even simple respiratory tract infections is indicated in the late stages. Digitalis is necessary for treatment of patients with cardiac involvement.

The prognosis is for progression to immobility before age 12 years and death some time between age 15 and 30 years.

The facioscapulohumeral type is an autosomal dominant condition with onset generally between age 7 and 20 years. It is rarely found at birth. Facial and shoulder girdle muscles are generally involved at the same time. Pelvic girdle weakness and bilateral foot drop will develop later. The course is progressive, and the laboratory findings are similar to those of the Duchenne type.

The limb-girdle dystrophies are a group of disorders that probably have several different genetic causes. Proximal shoulder and pelvic girdle weakness occurs gradually over a period of years. The serum enzyme levels may be elevated, and muscle biopsy may show split fibers.

Distal myopathy is not found in childhood, and it is considered an autosomal dominant trait.

"Oculocraniosomatic syndrome" occurs principally in adults over 40 years of age. However, it may have its onset during infancy or childhood, with eye muscle involvement, visual loss, intellectual deterioration, and cerebellar disturbances.

WERDNIG-HOFFMANN DISEASE (Infantile Progressive Spinal Muscular Atrophy)

Werdnig-Hoffmann disease is a disease of the lower motor neurons with resultant effects upon the muscle. Hypotonicity is usually apparent during early infancy. The muscles of the lower extremities are affected first and most severely. Deep reflexes are absent, and there is no response to faradic or galvanic stimulation of the affected muscles. A less severe form of the disease may appear in children over 6 months of age and is nonprogressive.

Serum enzyme levels are normal. Electromyography will show lower motor neuron damage. Biopsy is necessary for diagnosis.

There is no specific treatment, and the disease is usually fatal. In mild forms, braces for the back and neck may be of some help.

KUGELBERG-WELANDER DISEASE

Kugelberg-Welander disease is first noted in children between 5 and 15 years of age and is slowly progressive to the late 20s. It is a disease of proximal musculature that may mimic Duchenne type muscular dystrophy. Fasciculations of the muscles of the chest wall may be noted, and a fine tremor on extension of the hands is also common. Serum enzyme levels are normal or slightly elevated. Muscle biopsy is diagnostic of neurogenic disease.

MYOTONIC DYSTROPHY
(Steinert's Disease)

Myotonic dystrophy is a hereditary disease transmitted as an autosomal dominant trait and characterized by inability to relax the muscles after contractions and by fatigability.

In infants, the disease is characterized by floppiness, with facial diplegia, difficulty in sucking, and hyporeflexia. In older children and adolescents, there is inability to relax the muscles (such as with hand grasp), which is more severe during cold weather or emotional upset. The muscles of the face may waste, producing a characteristic appearance. Mild to moderate mental retardation is not uncommon. Endocrine, cardiac, and immunologic dysfunction occurs often. Cataracts develop in nearly 80% of cases.

Electromyographic findings are distinctly myotonic. Results of muscle biopsy are distinctive and diagnostic.

Procainamide or phenytoin may reduce the symptoms.

Most patients are confined to a wheelchair during late adult life, but life expectancy is usually normal.

MYASTHENIA GRAVIS

Myasthenia gravis, an uncommon disease in childhood, involves striated muscles; there is weakness with rapid fatigue but no atrophy. Transient myasthenia gravis (present for about 6 weeks) often occurs in infants born to women with myasthenia gravis.

Clinical Findings

Onset may be at any age but usually is not until after puberty. Muscles supplied by the cranial nerves are usually first and most severely affected, with ptosis of the eyelids, diplopia, and dysphagia.

A therapeutic test with edrophonium chloride (Tensilon), 0.1 mg intramuscularly in infants or 1–9 mg in children, depending on age, will cause a temporary disappearance of symptoms and signs within minutes. Neostigmine bromide (Prostigmin), 0.02 μg/kg subcutaneously, may also be used for this purpose.

Treatment

A. Specific Measures:

1. Pyridostigmine (Mestinon), 15–45 mg orally every 4 hours, depending on the size of the child, may be used.

2. Neostigmine bromide, 5–15 mg orally in 2–4 doses daily, should be regulated according to the response.

3. Neostigmine methylsulfate, 0.5–1.5 mg subcutaneously 2–4 times per day, may be used if tablets are ineffective.

4. Ephedrine sulfate, sometimes recommended for adults, is of little value in children.

5. Atropine may be added to control side effects such as abdominal cramps, nausea, and vomiting.

B. General Measures: Surgical removal of the thymus may produce improvement.

Prognosis

With treatment, the prognosis is usually good. Despite treatment, death may occur from respiratory failure in progressive disease.

FAMILIAL PERIODIC PARALYSIS

Familial periodic paralysis is a rare autosomal dominant disease that usually appears first during adolescence. It is characterized by recurrent attacks of flaccid paralysis, with normal musculature and no apparent weakness between attacks, and is most commonly accompanied by an intermittent increase in the secretion of aldosterone, with retention of sodium and lowering of serum potassium levels. Tumors of the adrenal glands may be present.

Treatment

Treatment of acute attack consists of potassium chloride, 2–10 g by mouth. Administration of potassium chloride intravenously as a 2% solution is a very dangerous procedure and should be undertaken only by experienced individuals. Adrenal tumors must be removed.

Prophylaxis

Potassium chloride, 2–4 g/d orally with meals, may be given for prophylaxis. Acetazolamide (Diamox), 5–30 mg/kg/d orally, may prevent attacks.

Prognosis

The prognosis is excellent with treatment. Death due to cardiac or respiratory failure may occur during an attack. Paralytic episodes may become less frequent and less severe in adult life.

FAMILIAL DYSAUTONOMIA
(Riley-Day Syndrome)

Familial autonomic dysfunction is a recessive disease of unknown cause occurring chiefly in Jewish children and characterized in almost all cases by defective lacrimation, skin blotching, excessive perspiration, drooling, emotional instability, motor incoordination, hyporeflexia, and relative indifference to pain. Most children also exhibit hypertension, urinary frequency, breath-holding spells during infancy, frequent pulmonary infections, frequent unexplained fever, cyclic vomiting, mental retardation, short stature, and convulsions.

Treatment is symptomatic. Bethanechol (Urecholine) may reduce difficulties in swallowing as well as abdominal distention. Psychotherapy for the patient and family may be very important. Chlorpromazine may control cyclic vomiting.

TORTICOLLIS
(Wryneck)

Torticollis is malposition of the head due to spasm or shortening of the cervical or sternocleidomastoid muscles. A congenital type noted in the neonatal period is usually due to a hematoma in the sternocleidomastoid muscle, especially following a breech delivery.

Acquired torticollis may develop at any age and is secondary to atrophy of the cervical or sternocleidomastoid muscles following nerve injury or poliomyelitis. It may also follow viral respiratory tract infection or mild neck trauma. Stretching of the infant's affected muscle by the mother 4–6 times daily for several months may be successful. If not, surgery after the age of 1 year is usually necessary. Diazepam (Valium) may reduce muscle spasm.

22 | Endocrine & Metabolic Disorders*

DISTURBANCES OF GROWTH & DEVELOPMENT

It is estimated that over 1 million children in the USA have abnormally short stature and that there are at least 10 million children whose growth is potentially abnormal.

Failure to thrive is a term usually reserved for infants who fail to gain weight and is most often due to undernutrition.

Tall stature is a much less frequent presenting complaint than short stature and is usually a matter of concern only to adolescent girls. The recent trend toward acceptance of tall stature in women has decreased the number of young people evaluated and treated for this condition.

SHORT STATURE

In most instances, abnormally short stature is due to a normal variation from the usual pattern of growth. The possible roles of such factors as sex, race, size of parents and other family members, intrauterine factors, nutrition, pubertal maturation, and emotional status must all be evaluated in the total assessment of the child (see Table 22–1). The causes of unusually short stature can usually be differentiated on the basis of significant findings in the history, physical examination, and radiographic estimation of skeletal maturation ("bone age").

1. CONSTITUTIONAL DELAYED GROWTH & ADOLESCENCE

Many normal children have a delay in the onset of skeletal maturation that is considered to be "constitutional." Puberty progresses normally after a delayed onset. In other respects, they appear entirely

*Revised with the assistance of Ronald Gotlin, MD.

normal. There is often a history of a similar pattern of growth in one of the parents or other members of the family. These children usually reach normal adult height although at an age later than average.

2. PITUITARY DWARFISM
(Growth Hormone Deficiency)

Growth hormone (GH) deficiency is an uncommon cause of short stature; approximately half of cases are idiopathic (rarely familial), and the remainder are secondary to pituitary, central nervous system, or hypothalamic disease (craniopharyngioma, infections, tuberculosis, sarcoidosis, toxoplasmosis, syphilis, trauma, reticuloendotheliosis, vascular anomalies, and other tumors such as gliomas). GH deficiency may be an isolated defect or may occur in combination with other pituitary hormone deficiencies.

At birth, affected infants may be small. Growth retardation is evident during infancy, and there may be infantile fat distribution, youthful facial features, small hands and feet, and delayed sexual maturation. Excessive wrinkling of the skin is present in older individuals. Hypoglycemia and microphallus may occur. Dental development and epiphyseal maturation ("bone age") are delayed to an equal degree or more so than height age (median age for patient's height). Headaches, visual field defects, abnormal skull x-rays, and symptoms of posterior pituitary insufficiency (polyuria and polydipsia) may precede or accompany the GH deficiency in cases resulting from central nervous system disease.

GH deficiency is associated with low levels of somatomedin C and GH in the serum and a failure of the GH level to rise in response to arginine, oral levodopa, exercise, or insulin-induced hypoglycemia or during normal physiologic sleep. Laron type dwarfism is a rare condition in which there is an inability to generate somatomedin in response to GH. Other children may have an immunoreactive GH with reduced bioactivity.

Treatment is with human pituitary growth hormone. Protein anabolic agents (testosterone, fluoxymesterone, oxandrolone, etc) may be effective in promoting linear growth, but these drugs may cause acceleration of epiphyseal closure with decrease in eventual height. Cyproheptadine in conjunction with human growth hormone (hGH) is said to enhance growth.

3. HYPOTHYROIDISM

(See p 523.)

Table 22–1. Causes of short stature.

Familial, racial, or genetic factors

Constitutional short stature with delayed adolescence

Endocrine disturbances
- Adrenal insufficiency
- Cushing's disease and syndrome (including iatrogenic causes)
- Diabetes insipidus
- Diabetes mellitus (poorly controlled)
- Hyperaldosteronism
- Hypopituitarism
- Hyposomatotropinism (isolated or with other pituitary deficiencies)
- Hypothyroidism
- Sexual precocity

Primordial short stature (intrauterine growth retardation)
- Primordial dwarfism with premature aging
  - Progeria (Hutchinson-Gilford syndrome)
  - Progeroid syndrome (Cockayne's syndrome, Werner's syndrome)
- With associated anomalies (eg, Bloom's syndrome, Cornelia de Lange syndrome, Hallerman-Streiff syndrome, leprechaunism, Seckel's bird-headed dwarfism, Silver's syndrome)
- Without associated anomalies

Inborn errors of metabolism
- Altered metabolism of calcium or phosphorus (eg, hypophosphatasia, hypophosphatemic rickets, infantile hypercalcemia, pseudohypoparathyroidism)
- Aminoacidemias and aminoacidurias
- Body defense disorders (eg, Bruton's agammaglobulinemia, chronic granulomatous disease, thymic aplasia)
- Disorders of mineral metabolism (eg, magnesium malabsorption syndrome, Wilson's disease)
- Epithelial transport disorders (eg, Bartter's syndrome, cystic fibrosis, pseudohypoparathyroidism, renal tubular acidosis, vasopressin-resistant diabetes insipidus)
- Metabolic anemias (eg, pyruvate kinase deficiency, sickle cell disease, thalassemia)
- Organic acidemias and acidurias (eg, isovaleric acidemia, maple syrup urine disease, methylmalonic aciduria, orotic aciduria)
- Storage disease
  - Mucolipidoses (eg, fucosidosis, generalized gangliosidosis, mannosidosis)
  - Mucopolysaccharidoses (eg, Hunter's syndrome, Hurler's syndrome)
  - Sphingolipidoses (eg, Gaucher's disease, Niemann-Pick disease, Tay-Sachs disease)
  - Miscellaneous (eg, cystinosis)

Constitutional (intrinsic) diseases of bone
- Abnormalities of density of cortical diaphyseal structure or metaphyseal modeling (eg, osteogenesis imperfecta congenita, osteopetrosis, tubular stenosis)
- Defects of growth of tubular bones or spine (eg, achondroplasia, metatropic dwarfism, diastrophic dwarfism, metaphyseal chondrodysplasia)
- Disorganized development of cartilage and fibrous components of the skeleton (eg, fibrous dysplasia with skin pigmentation, multiple cartilaginous exostoses, precocious puberty of McCune-Albright)

Table 22–1 (cont'd). Causes of short stature.

Chromosomal defect association
Autosomal (eg, cri du chat syndrome, Down's syndrome, trisomy 18)
Sex chromosomal (eg, penta X, XXXY, Turner's syndrome-XO)

Chronic systemic diseases, congenital defects, and malignant neoplasms (eg, cardiovascular disease, central nervous system disease, chronic infection and infestation, collagen vascular disease, hematologic disease, hepatic disease, inflammatory bowel disease, malignant neoplastic disease, malnutrition, pulmonary disease, renal disease)

Nutritional deficiency
Zinc deficiency

Psychosocial dwarfism (maternal deprivation)

Miscellaneous syndromes (eg, arthrogryposis multiplex congenita, cerebrohepatorenal syndrome, Noonan's syndrome, Prader-Willi syndrome, Riley-Day syndrome)

4. PRIMORDIAL SHORT STATURE (Intrauterine Growth Retardation)

Primordial short stature may occur in a number of disorders, including craniofacial disproportion (see Table 22–1), or may occur in individuals with no accompanying significant physical abnormalities. Children with primordial short stature have birth weight and length below normal for gestational age. Head circumference may be normal or reduced. Thereafter, they grow parallel to but below the third percentile. Plasma GH levels are usually normal but may be elevated. In some instances, somatomedin levels are subnormal. There is an increased incidence of functional fasting hypoglycemia. In most instances, skeletal maturation ("bone age") corresponds to chronologic age or is only mildly delayed, in contrast to the more marked delay often present in children with GH and thyroid deficiency.

There is no satisfactory treatment for primordial short stature, although there may be an increase in growth rate in response to large doses of hGH.

5. SHORT STATURE DUE TO EMOTIONAL FACTORS (Psychosocial Short Stature, Deprivation Dwarfism)

Psychologic and emotional deprivation with disturbances in motor and personality development may be associated with short stature. Growth retardation in some of these children is the result of undernutrition; in others, undernutrition does not seem to be a factor. In some instances, in addition to being small, the child may have increased (often voracious) appetite and a marked delay in skeletal maturation. Polydipsia and polyuria are sometimes present. These children are of normal size at birth and grow normally for a variable period before growth stops. A history of feeding problems during early infancy is common. Emotional disturbances in the family are the rule.

Placement in a foster home or a significant change in the psychologic and emotional environment at home usually results in significantly improved growth, a decrease of appetite and dietary intake to more normal levels, and personality improvement. Treatment with growth-promoting agents is not indicated.

LABORATORY STUDIES IN DIAGNOSIS OF SHORT STATURE

When the cause of short stature is not apparent from the history and physical examination, the following laboratory studies, in addition to determining "bone age," are useful in detecting or categorizing the common causes of short stature: (1) complete blood count; (2) erythrocyte sedimentation rate; (3) urinalysis; (4) stool examination for occult blood, parasites, and parasite ova; (5) serum electrolyte level; (6) blood urea nitrogen level; (7) buccal smear and karyotyping, which should be performed in all short girls with delayed sexual maturation with or without clinical features of Turner's syndrome; (8) thyroid function tests, including determinations of thyroxine (T_4) and thyroid-stimulating hormone (TSH); and (9) GH concentration.

FAILURE TO THRIVE

There are many reasons for failure to thrive, although a specific cause often cannot be established.

Classification & Etiologic Diagnosis

The diagnosis of failure to thrive is usually apparent on the basis of the history and physical examination. In failure to thrive, it is useful to compare the patient's chronologic age with the height age (median age for the patient's height), weight age, and head circumference. On the basis of these measurements, 3 principal patterns can be defined and will provide a starting point in the diagnostic approach.

Group 1. This group is the most common type. The head circumference is normal, and the weight is reduced out of proportion to height. In the majority of cases of failure to thrive, undernutrition is present as a result of deficient caloric intake, malabsorption, or impaired caloric utilization.

Group 2. The head circumference is normal or enlarged for age, and the weight is only moderately reduced, usually in proportion to height. Failure to thrive is due to structural dystrophies, constitutional dwarfism, or endocrinopathies.

Group 3. Although the head circumference is normal, the weight is reduced in proportion to height, owing to a primary central nervous system deficit or intrauterine growth retardation (see Primordial Short Stature, above).

An initial period of observed nutritional rehabilitation, usually in a hospital setting, is often helpful in the diagnosis. The child should be placed on a regular diet for age, and the caloric intake and weight should be carefully plotted for 1–2 weeks. During this period, evidence of lactose intolerance is sought by checking pH and reducing substances in the stool. If stools are abnormal, the child should be placed on a lactose-free diet and further observed. Caloric intake should be increased if weight gain does not occur but intake is well tolerated. The following 3 patterns are often noted during the rehabilitation period. Pattern 1 is by far the most common.

Pattern 1. In this most common type, the intake is adequate and the weight gain is satisfactory, but the feeding technique is at fault. A disturbed infant-mother relationship leads to the decreased caloric intake.

Pattern 2. The intake is adequate, but there is no weight gain. If weight gain is unsatisfactory after increasing the calories to an adequate level (based on the infant's ideal weight for his or her height), malabsorption is a likely diagnosis. If malabsorption is present, it is usually necessary to differentiate pancreatic exocrine insufficiency (cystic fibrosis) from abnormalities of intestinal mucosa (celiac disease). In cystic fibrosis, growth velocity commonly declines from the time of birth, and appetite usually is voracious. In celiac disease, growth velocity is usually not reduced until 6–12 months of age, and inadequate caloric intake may be a prominent feature.

Pattern 3. The intake is inadequate, owing to the following: (1) Sucking or swallowing difficulties due to central nervous system or neuromuscular disease or to esophageal or oropharyngeal malformations may result in inadequate intake. (2) Inability to eat large amounts is common in patients with cardiopulmonary disease or in anorexic children suffering from chronic infections, inflammatory bowel disease, and endocrine problems (eg, hypothyroidism). Patients with celiac disease often have inadequate caloric intake in addition to malabsorption. (3) Inadequate intake may be due to vomiting, spitting up, or rumination in patients with upper intestinal tract obstruction (eg, pyloric stenosis, hiatal hernia, chalasia), chronic metabolic aberrations and acidosis (eg, renal insufficiency, diabetes mellitus and insipidus, methylmalonic acidemia), adrenogenital syndrome, increased intracranial pressure, or psychosocial abnormalities.

TALL STATURE

Although there are several conditions (Table 22–2) that may produce tall stature, by far the most common cause is a constitutional variation from normal. Tall stature is usually of concern only to adolescent and preadolescent girls.

Table 22–2. Causes of tall stature.

Constitutional (familial, genetic) factors	**Genetic causes**
Endocrine causes	Klinefelter's syndrome
Androgen deficiency (normal height as children, tall as adults)	Syndromes of XYY, XXYY (tall as adults)
Anorchidism (infection, trauma, idiopathic)	Testicular feminization
Klinefelter's syndrome	**Miscellaneous syndromes and entities**
Androgen excess (tall as children, short as adults)	Cerebral gigantism (Soto's syndrome)
Pseudosexual precocity	Diencephalic syndrome
True sexual precocity	Homocystinuria
Hyperthyroidism	Marfan's syndrome
Somatotropin excess (pituitary gigantism)	Total lipodystrophy

On the basis of family history, previous pattern of growth, state of physiologic development, assessment of epiphyseal development ("bone age"), and standard growth data, the physician should make a tentative estimate of the patient's eventual height. Hormonal therapy with conjugated estrogenic substances (eg, Premarin), 1.25–5 mg daily orally (continuously or cyclically), has been recommended by some in cases in which the patient's predicted height is considered to be excessive and the physiologic age as determined by stage of sexual maturity and epiphyseal development has not reached the 12-year-old level. Because of known and unknown long-term effects of estrogen administration in children and variable effects of therapy, treatment with estrogen should seldom be recommended and should be used with caution.

Testosterone in high doses has been used to decrease height in excessively tall boys. The results are variable (average reduction in adult height is approximately 5 cm). Testicular function may be altered for a prolonged period after treatment.

DIABETES INSIPIDUS

Diabetes insipidus may result from deficient secretion of vasopressin (ADH), lack of response of the kidney to ADH, or failure of osmoreceptors to respond to elevations of osmolality. Hypofunction of the posterior lobe of the pituitary with ADH deficiency may be idiopathic or may be associated with lesions of the posterior pituitary or hypothalamus (trauma, infections, suprasellar cysts, tumors, reticuloendotheliosis, or some developmental abnormality). Congenital ADH deficiency may be transmitted as an autosomal dominant trait. In nephrogenic diabetes insipidus, a hereditary (dominant) disease affecting both sexes but more severe in males, the renal tubules fail to respond normally to ADH, and no lesion of the pituitary or hypothalamus can be demonstrated.

Clinical Findings

The onset is often sudden, with polyuria, intense thirst, constipation, and evidences of dehydration. High fever, circulatory collapse, and secondary brain damage may occur in young infants on an ordinary feeding regimen. Serum osmolality may be elevated (above 305 mosm/L), but urine osmolality remains below 280 mosm/L (specific gravity approximately 1.010) even after a 7-hour test period of thirsting. Rate of growth, sexual maturation, and general body metabolism may be impaired, and hydroureter and bladder distention may develop.

Diabetes insipidus may be differentiated from psychogenic polydipsia and polyuria by permitting the usual intake of fluid and then withholding water for 7 hours or until weight loss (3% or more) demonstrates adequate dehydration. With neurogenic or nephrogenic diabetes insipidus, the urine osmolality does not increase above 300 mosm/L even after the period of dehydration. Normal children and those with psychogenic polydipsia will respond to the dehydration with a urinary osmolality above 450 mosm/L. Patients with long-standing psychogenic polydipsia may be unable to concentrate urine initially, and the test may have to be repeated on several successive days. Eventually, dehydration will increase urine osmolality well above plasma osmolality. The ADH and hypertonic saline tests may be employed to distinguish between the various forms of diabetes insipidus. The administration of carbamazepine (Tegretol), clofibrate (Atromid-S), or nicotine, which are direct stimuli of ADH release, or chlorpropamide, which augments the action of ADH, may be of value in differentiating cases of osmoreceptor failure from those with hypothalamic and pituitary lesions.

Treatment

The treatment of choice for central diabetes insipidus is intranasal desmopressin acetate (1-desamino-8-D-arginine vasopressin; DDAVP).

The dosage must be adjusted, but the duration of action is generally 12 hours and eliminates troublesome nocturia. Replacement with lypressin (as Syntopressin Spray, Diapid), vasopressin tannate (Pitressin Tannate), or posterior pituitary powder for nasal insufflation is of less value because of short duration of action, impurities, less uniform activity, or need for injection.

Chlorpropamide, 150–400 mg/d orally before breakfast, may be effective in controlling symptoms in mild cases. If hypoglycemia occurs, reduce the dose. The cautious use of chlorothiazide and ethacrynic acid may be of value in nephrogenic diabetes insipidus. (Check levels of serum electrolytes, uric acid, and blood glucose periodically.) For nephrogenic diabetes insipidus, also administer abundant quantities of water at short intervals and feedings containing limited electrolytes and minimal (but nutritionally adequate) amounts of protein. X-ray therapy and drug therapy are used for some cases of tumor (eg, reticuloendotheliosis). When no specific cause can be found, the search for an underlying lesion should be continued for many years.

• • •

SEXUAL PRECOCITY

(See also p 842.)

In sexual precocity, the onset of secondary sexual development is earlier than anticipated by chronologic age, body mass, and family history. Sexual precocity is generally divided into 2 major types, true precocity and pseudoprecocity. True (complete) precocity is the result of premature increases in gonadotropin either from stimulation of the hypothalamic-pituitary mechanism (eg, in children with no abnormality or in those with tumor, infection, trauma, etc) or from gonadotropin-producing tumors (eg, hepatoma, choriocarcinoma). Pseudoprecocity is initiated by nongonadotropin-producing conditions (eg, adrenal, ovarian, and testicular tumors and other lesions) or by administration of sex steroids.

In the past, true sexual precocity was considered to be idiopathic in approximately 80% of girls and 50% of boys. Currently, through the use of CT scans, small abnormalities in the region of the hypothalamus are more commonly recognized.

Sexual precocity has been arbitrarily defined as the development of secondary sex characteristics beginning before age 8 in girls and age 9½ in boys. Breast development is usually the first sign in girls, but the pattern of development is variable. Height may be normal initially, but it is often increased; osseous maturation ("bone age") may be even more advanced than height age, particularly in pseudoprecocious patients.

Psychologic development tends to correspond to chronologic age. Ovarian luteal cysts of the ovaries may be present; their role in production of the precocity is not clear. When sensitive assays are employed, urinary and serum gonadotropin levels are elevated for age, and adrenal androgen levels may be elevated to the pubertal range. Findings on EEG are frequently abnormal, particularly in boys.

Adrenal lesions (see pp 534–544) are the most common causes of pseudoprecocity. Gonadal tumors are uncommon causes; the granulosa cell and theca lutein cell tumors of the ovary are the most common, are generally unilateral and of low malignant potential, and produce excessive amounts of estrogen. In almost all instances, the tumor can be palpated transabdominally or rectally, but it is advisable to examine females with pelvic ultrasonography.

When possible, treatment is directed at the underlying cause. In the idiopathic variety, treatment with conventional agents (eg, medroxyprogesterone acetate [Depo-Provera] and cyproterone) is often unsatisfactory. Recently, promising results employing agonists and antagonists of gonadotropin-releasing hormone have been reported. Psychologic management of the patient and family is important. Children who initially have no definable causative lesion should be examined at periodic intervals for evidence of previously occult abdominal or central nervous system lesions.

Precocious Development of the Breast (Premature Thelarche)

Precocious development of one or both breasts may occur at any age. In most cases, the onset is in the first 2 years of life; in two-thirds of these cases, breast development is obvious in the first year. The condition is not associated with other evidence of sexual maturation. It may represent unusual sensitivity of the breasts to normal amounts of circulating estrogen or a temporarily increased secretion or ingestion of estrogen. Both breasts are usually involved, and enlargement may persist for months or years; the nipples generally do not enlarge. Rapid growth, advanced skeletal maturation, and menstruation do not occur in these patients, in contrast to patients with sexual precocity. Extensive diagnostic investigation is seldom warranted; no treatment is necessary. Puberty occurs at the normal time.

Premature Adrenarche (Premature Pubarche)

Premature development of sexual hair may occur at any age and in both sexes (more often in females than in males). About a third of cases occur in organically brain-damaged children. It appears to result from a premature slight increase in production of adrenal androgens. (Serum dehydroepiandrosterone concentrations are elevated.) Pubic hair usually develops first, but axillary hair is present in about half of cases when these patients are first seen. True virilization does not develop; children are of normal stature, and osseous development is not advanced. Urinary 17-ketosteroid and testosterone excretions are normal. Premature adrenarche requires no treatment.

Menstruation

The age at menarche ranges from 9 to 16 years; menarche is considered delayed if it has not occurred by age 17 years or within 5 years after development of the breasts. Primary amenorrhea is the result of gonadal lesions (ie, gonadal dysgenesis) in about 60% of patients, and in such cases serum and urine gonadotropin levels are elevated. In the remaining cases of primary amenorrhea, extragonadal abnormalities are present (eg, pituitary-hypothalamic hypogonadotropinism; congenital anomalies of the tubes, uterus, or vagina; androgen excess or other endocrine imbalance; and chronic systemic disease or pelvic inflammatory disease).

Once regular periods are established, amenorrhea (ie, secondary amenorrhea; see Table 22–3) during adolescence is often the result of either pregnancy or significant organic or psychiatric disease. Secondary amenorrhea should therefore be viewed as a symptom requiring prompt evaluation and, when possible, treatment.

Table 22–3. Causes of secondary amenorrhea.

I. Pregnancy.
II. Decreased ovarian function.
   A. Decreased gonadotropin level (secondary ovarian insufficiency).
      1. Due to organic and idiopathic hypothalamic disease, pituitary disease, or both.*
      2. Due to "functional abnormalities of the hypothalamic-pituitary axis" ("psychogenic").
      3. Due to hypothalamic-pituitary disease secondary to chronic systemic illness.
         a. Nutritional disorder (eg, anorexia nervosa).
         b. Chronic infection or systemic disease (eg, cancer, collagen vascular disease, inflammatory bowel disease).
      4. Secondary to endogenous hormones (eg, androgen excess, feminizing or masculinizing ovarian tumor).
      5. Secondary to exogenous drugs (eg, long-term contraceptive drugs, androgens, estrogens, tranquilizers).
   B. Increased gonadotropin level (primary ovarian insufficiency).
      1. Due to acquired diseases (destruction of ovaries by infection or tumor, "premature menopause," radiation castration, surgical removal of ovaries).
      2. Due to ovarian agenesis and dysgenesis* (eg, Turner's syndrome).
III. Congenital and acquired lesions of the uterine tubes and uterus, including cases of chromosomal intersex (eg, adhesions, congenital absence of the uterus, cryptomenorrhea, hysterectomy, synechia of the uterus, testicular feminization syndrome).

*Usually or often associated with primary amenorrhea.

THE GONAD

Deficiency of gonadal tissue or function may result from a genetic or embryologic defect; from hormone excess affecting the fetus in utero; from inflammation and destruction following infection (eg, mumps, syphilis, tuberculosis); from trauma, irradiation, autoimmune disease, or tumor; or as a consequence of surgical castration. Secondary hypogonadism may result from pituitary insufficiency (eg, destructive lesions in or about the anterior pituitary, irradiation of the pituitary, starvation), diabetes mellitus, androgen excess (eg, adrenogenital syndrome), or insufficiency of either the thyroid or adrenals.

CRYPTORCHIDISM

Cryptorchidism (undescended testes) is a common disorder in children. It may be unilateral or bilateral and may be classified as ectopic, total, or incomplete. About 3% of term male infants and 20% of premature male infants have undescended testes at birth. In over half of these cases, the testes will descend by the second month; by age 1 year, 80% of all undescended testes are in the scrotum. Further descent may occur at puberty, perhaps stimulated by endogenous gonadotropin. If cryptorchidism persists into adult life, failure of spermatogenesis is the rule, but testicular androgen production usually remains intact. The incidence of cancer (usually seminoma) is appreciably greater in testes that remain in the abdomen after puberty.

Cryptorchidism may merely represent delayed descent of the testes or may be due to prevention of normal descent by some mechanical lesion such as adhesions, short spermatic cord, fibrous bands, or endocrine disorders (ie, decreased gonadotropins). It is probable that many undescended testes are congenitally abnormal and that this abnormality in itself prevents descent.

A causal relationship between failure of spermatogenesis and an abdominal location after puberty is assumed. However, the normally descended testis of a male with unilateral cryptorchidism may not have normal spermatogenesis, and cases have been described in which persistent intra-abdominal testes have been associated with normal spermatogenesis. On occasion, the apparent abnormality of an abdominal testis may be reversible (even if the testes are histologically abnormal at the time they are placed in the scrotum).

Clinical Findings

In palpating the scrotum for the testes, the cremasteric reflex may be elicited, with a resultant ascent of the testes into the abdomen (pseudocryptorchidism). To prevent this ascent, the fingers first should be placed across the upper portion of the inguinal canal. Examination in a warm bath is also helpful.

Bilaterally undescended testes that have never been in the scrotum are often associated with a relatively flat scrotum.

Treatment

The best age for medical or surgical treatment has not been determined, but there has been a recent trend toward operation in early childhood. Some recommend surgery before age 5 years; others say during the first year. There appears to be a high incidence of azoospermia in testes operated on after age 10 years; recent evidence indicates that damage to germ and Leydig cells of intra-abdominal testes may occur by age 3–4 years, but the relationship of these changes to fertility is unproved. The risk of surgical injury to the testes must be weighed against the possible benefits. Surgical repair is indicated for cryptorchidism persisting beyond puberty, since the incidence of cancer is appreciably greater in glands that remain in the abdomen beyond the second decade of life.

A. Unilateral Cryptorchidism: Most cases are due to local mechanical lesions or a defective testis on the involved side. If pseudocryptorchidism has been ruled out and if descent has not occurred by age 5 years, many investigators recommend surgical exploration, with testicular biopsy and relocation by a surgeon skilled in this procedure. Gonadotropin therapy (chorionic gonadotropin, 1500 units intramuscularly 2–3 times a week for 5–9 weeks in prepubertal boys) is recommended by some before surgery.

B. Bilateral Cryptorchidism: Treatment with chorionic gonadotropin (see above) may be tried prior to surgery. The child with bilaterally undescended testes should be evaluated for sex chromosome abnormalities and genetic sex determined by buccal smear or chromosome analysis in the newborn period. Androgen treatment (testosterone enanthate) is indicated only as replacement therapy in the male beyond the normal age of puberty who has been shown to lack functional testes.

C. Pseudocryptorchidism: Retractile testes, ie, those that are sometimes in the scrotum but not at the time of examination, generally require no treatment.

Prognosis

Following surgery, the prognosis is guarded with respect to spermatogenesis in the involved testis.

KLINEFELTER'S SYNDROME

Klinefelter's syndrome is occasionally familial, appears during puberty, and is characterized by atrophic sclerosis of the seminiferous tubules with normal Leydig cells and normal masculinization. It is often accompanied by bilateral gynecomastia, relatively long extremities, abnormally small testes, and azoospermia or oligospermatogenesis. Gonadotropin levels (particularly luteinizing hormone levels) are usually elevated. Testosterone levels are normal or low. Many patients are mentally retarded. Some patients have histories of severe psychopathologic disorder. There is an extra X (female) chromosome (most commonly an XXY chromosome pattern) and a positive nuclear chromatin pattern. Typical histopathologic changes may occur in men whose only complaint is sterility.

Klinefelter's syndrome must be differentiated from the physiologic gynecomastia that occurs in some boys at puberty as well as from feminizing tumors of the adrenal cortex or testes.

There is no satisfactory treatment, but methyltestosterone, 20–40 mg/d orally, or testosterone enanthate, 200–400 mg intramuscularly every 3 weeks, continued for several months, may produce positive physical and behavioral changes and reduce gynecomastia. If it does not, surgical mastectomy for cosmetic purposes is indicated.

DISEASES OF THE THYROID

GOITER

Goiter is not uncommon in children and adolescents and is most commonly due to chronic lymphocytic thyroiditis (see Thyroiditis, below). It may also result from acute inflammation, iodine deficiency, infiltrative processes, neoplasms, ingestion of goitrogens, or an inborn error in thyroid metabolism (familial goiter). With the exception of hyperthyroidism (and possibly pregnancy), thyroid enlargement results from the stimulation of excess thyroid-stimulating hormone (TSH). Regardless of the cause, patients may be clinically and biochemically euthyroid, hypothyroid, or hyperthyroid.

Familial goiter results from enzymatic defects in hormonogenesis, eg, (1) iodide trapping, (2) iodide organification, (3) coupling, (4) deiodination, and (5) production of thyroglobulin and serum carrier protein. Patients with any of these defects display an autosomal recessive mode of inheritance; the organification defect may be associated with severe congenital deafness (Pendred's syndrome). The age at onset of symptoms of hypothyroidism is variable.

Substances implicated in the development of goiter include cabbage, soybeans, turnips, rutabagas, aminosalicylic acid (PAS), resorcinol, phenylbutazone, iodides (particularly in individuals who have also received corticosteroids), and drugs that interfere with iodide trapping (eg, thiocyanates).

Clinical Findings

The clinical features and physical characteristics of patients with goiters vary depending on the cause and are seldom diagnostic.

Nodular goiter may occur during childhood. The likelihood that a nodule is malignant increases when the nodule is single, hard, or associated with paratracheal lymph node enlargement or does not concentrate radioactive iodide (see Carcinoma of the Thyroid, below).

Treatment

Remove or avoid precipitating factors if possible. With the exception of hyperthyroidism and instances where specific causes can be eliminated or corrected (eg, iodide deficiency, goitrogens), treatment is with full replacement of thyroid hormone (see p 524). Surgery is occasionally necessary if cancer is a possibility.

Prophylaxis

Prophylaxis in endemic areas of iodine deficiency consists of the use of bread containing iodides or iodized salt (1 mg of iodine per 100 g of salt) or the administration of 1–2 drops of saturated solution of potassium iodide per week. Iodination of the water supply is also a satisfactory preventive measure.

NEONATAL GOITER

Neonatal goiter may result from the transplacental passage, from mother to infant, of iodides, goitrogens, antithyroid drugs, or human-specific thyroid stimulator immunoglobulin (HTSI). The latter occurs in pregnancies in which the mother has or once had Graves' disease. The offspring may temporarily be hyperthyroid, with exophthalmos. Regardless of the cause, the goiter is usually diffuse and relatively soft but may be large and firm enough to compress the trachea, esophagus, and adjacent blood vessels. Treatment varies with the cause; iodides, antithyroid drugs, or thyroid hormone (eg, levothyroxine, 0.05 mg/d) for a few weeks may be indicated. Occasionally, surgical division of the thyroid isthmus may be necessary.

HYPOTHYROIDISM

Hypothyroidism may be either congenital or acquired. Congenital hypothyroidism may be due to aplasia, hypoplasia, or maldescent of the thyroid, resulting from an embryonic defect of development; the administration of radioiodide to the mother; or, possibly, an autoimmune disease. It may be caused by defective synthesis of thyroid hormone (familial goiter; see Goiter, above). Other cases of congenital hypothyroidism may result from the maternal ingestion of medications (eg, goitrogens, propylthiouracil, methimazole, iodides), from iodide deficiency (endemic cretinism), or, rarely, from thyroid hormone unresponsiveness. Thyroid tissue in an aberrant location is present in most patients with sporadic "athyreotic" cretinism.

Acquired (juvenile) hypothyroidism is most commonly the result of chronic lymphocytic thyroiditis (see Thyroiditis, below) but may be idiopathic or the result of surgical removal, thyrotropin deficiency (usually associated with other pituitary tropic hormone deficiencies), the ingestion of medications (eg, iodides, cobalt), or a deficiency of iodides. An ectopic thyroid gland, a relatively common cause of hypothyroidism, may maintain normal function for variable periods postnatally. Breast feeding may mitigate severe hypothyroidism and perhaps prevent impaired neurologic development in the hypothyroid patient.

Clinical Findings

The findings depend on age at onset and the degree of deficiency.

A. Symptoms and Signs:

1. Functional changes–Findings include physical and mental sluggishness; pale, gray, cool skin; decreased intestinal activity (constipation); large tongue; poor muscle tone (protuberant abdomen, umbilical hernia, lumbar lordosis); hypothermia; bradycardia; diminished sweating (variable); carotenemia; decreased pulse pressure; hoarse voice or cry; slow relaxation on eliciting tendon reflexes (normal for children is 180–360 ms, as measured by photomotogram; reflex time is shorter in boys and in younger children); and transient deafness. Prolonged gestation, large size at birth, nasal obstruction and discharge, large fontanelles, hypoactivity, and persistent jaundice may also be present during the neonatal period. Even with congenital deficiency of thyroid hormone, the first findings may not appear for several days or weeks.

2. Retardation of growth and development–Findings include shortness of stature; infantile skeletal proportions, with relatively short extremities; infantile naso-orbital configuration (bridge of nose flat, broad, and undeveloped; eyes seem to be widely spaced); retarded "bone age" and epiphyseal dysgenesis; retarded dental development and enamel hypoplasia; and large fontanelles in the neonate. Slowing of mental responsiveness and retardation of development of the brain may occur. In older children and adolescents, growth failure may be the only manifestation of hypothyroidism.

3. Sexual precocity–Rarely, isosexual precocity may occur, resulting from elevated gonadotropin levels. Galactorrhea may be present, and menometrorrhagia has been reported in older girls. Testicular enlargement occurs rarely in boys.

4. Other changes–Myxedema of tissues may occur. The skin may be dry, thick, scaly, and coarse, with a yellowish tinge from excessive deposition of carotene. The hair is dry, coarse, and brittle (variable) and may be excessive. The axillary and supraclavicular pads may be prominent. Muscular hypertrophy (Debré-Sémélaigne syndrome) occasionally is present. Pseudoanorexia nervosa and psychosis secondary to myxedema have been described. An ectopic thyroid gland may produce a mass at the base of the tongue or in the midline of the neck.

B. Laboratory Findings: Thyroxine (T_4) and thyroid-stimulating hormone (TSH) levels are the most helpful aids in diagnosing congenital hypothyroidism in the first 5 days of life. Levels of T_4 and radioiodide uptake are reduced. Serum carotene and cholesterol levels are usually elevated in hypothyroid children but may be normal in some hypothyroid infants; a rise to abnormally high levels occurs 6–8 weeks after cessation of therapy. The basal metabolic rate is low (unreliable in children). TSH levels may be elevated. Urinary creatine excretion is decreased; urine creatinine is increased. Serum alkaline phosphatase levels are reduced. Erythrocyte glucose-6-phosphate dehydrogenase activity is decreased. Sweat electrolyte levels are often increased. Circulating autoantibodies to thyroid constituents may be found. Urinary hydroxyproline levels are reduced. Plasma GH levels and GH response to insulin-induced hypoglycemia and arginine stimulation may be subnormal.

C. X-Ray Findings: Epiphyseal development ("bone age") is delayed. The cardiac shadow may be increased. Epiphyseal dysgenesis, coxa vara, coxa plana, and vertebral anomalies may occur. The pituitary fossa may be enlarged.

Treatment

Levothyroxine sodium (Synthroid) is a reliable synthetic agent for thyroid replacement therapy. The dose is approximately 3.75 ± 0.6 μg/kg. Older children, adolescents, and adults require 0.15–0.2 mg daily in one dose. In hypothyroid patients, particularly myxedematous infants, low doses (0.025–0.05 mg) should be used initially and increased weekly in small increments. The therapeutic range is evaluated by clinical response (appearance, growth, development), sleeping pulses, and thyroid function tests. (T_4 levels, when a euthyroid state has been reached, may be 25% higher than accepted "normal" levels in untreated individuals.) Improvement usually occurs in 1–3 weeks. If a patient can tolerate appreciably more than the above doses, the diagnosis of hypothyroidism should be questioned, since hypothyroid individuals may be more sensitive to thyroid hormone than are normal individuals.

Course & Prognosis

In patients with congenital hypothyroidism, growth and motor development can be returned to normal with adequate replacement therapy. The prognosis for mental development is guarded if treatment is delayed beyond 3 months of life. In patients with acquired hypothyroidism, restoration of physical and mental function to the predisease level is to be expected following replacement therapy. Overtreatment with thyroid drugs may produce accelerated skeletal maturation and craniosynostosis.

HYPERTHYROIDISM

Hyperthyroidism appears to occur in individuals who demonstrate a reduced capacity to remove host-directed immunoglobulins. In addition, psychic trauma, psychologic maladjustments, disturbances in pituitary function, infectious disease, heredity, and imbalance of the endocrine system all have been incriminated in the etiology and pathogenesis of hyperthyroidism. Congenital hyperthyroidism, sometimes persisting or recurring for months or years with or without exophthalmos, may occur in infants of thyrotoxic mothers and be associated with premature synostosis, minimal brain dysfunction, accelerated "bone age," and goiter.

Hyperthyroidism (with normal T_4 levels) may result from isolated hypersecretion of triiodothyronine (T_3 toxicosis) but is uncommon during childhood except in relapse.

Clinical Findings

A. Symptoms and Signs: The disease usually develops rapidly and is much more common in girls, with the highest incidence between ages 12 and 14 years. The manifestations may include the following in any combination: "nervousness" (ie, restlessness, mood swings, hand tremors); palpitations and tachycardia, even during sleep, and systolic hypertension with increased pulse pressure; warm and moist skin and flushed face; exophthalmos; diffuse goiter, usually firm, with or without bruit and thrill; weakness and loss of weight in spite of polyphagia; accelerated growth and development; and poor school performance. Amenorrhea is common in adolescent girls. Premature craniosynostosis may occur.

B. Laboratory Findings: Levels of T_4, free thyroxine, and T_3

resin uptake are elevated. The level of radioiodide uptake is increased and suppressed less than 40% after administration of T_3 (25 μg) 3 or 4 times daily for 7 days. T_3 levels may be elevated. Serum cholesterol and TSH levels are low. Serum tyrosine levels and erythrocyte glucose-6-phosphate dehydrogenase activity are elevated. Agglutinating antithyroglobulin antibodies are found in some patients. Circulating HTSI levels are usually above normal. There is moderate leukopenia. Glycosuria may be present, and urinary hydroxyproline and creatine levels are increased. During relapse, the T_3 level may be elevated when the T_4 level is normal.

Treatment

Antithyroid drugs, radioactive iodide, and surgical methods are equally capable of eliminating the manifestations of hyperthyroidism and yield approximately equal numbers of "cured" patients.

A. General Measures:

1. Restricted physical activity–Activity should be restricted, especially in severe cases, in preparation for surgery, or at the beginning of a medical regimen.

2. Diet–The diet should be high in calories, proteins, and vitamins.

3. Sedation–Large doses of barbiturates or tranquilizers may be necessary to control nervousness.

4. Sympatholytic drugs–These drugs (eg, propranolol) decrease the peripheral conversion of T_4 to T_3 and diminish cardiovascular and some neurologic symptoms. They are helpful in preparation for thyroid surgery.

B. Specific Measures: With medical treatment, clinical response may be noted in about 2–3 weeks, and adequate control may be achieved in 2–3 months. The thyroid gland frequently increases in size after initiation of treatment, but it usually decreases in size after 3 months.

1. Propylthiouracil–This drug blocks the hormonogenesis and release of thyroid hormone as well as the peripheral conversion of T_4 to T_3. It may be used in the initial treatment of the patient with hyperthyroidism, but if the T_4 fails to return to a normal range, surgery may be necessary, although some patients may be controlled by long-continued (> 5 years) medical therapy. Relapses occur in 25–50% of patients, and severe cases may not respond. Therapy must usually be continued at least 2–3 years with the minimum drug dosage that will produce a euthyroid state.

a. Initial dosage–Give 100–800 mg/d in 3 or 4 divided doses 6 or 8 hours apart until results of thyroid function tests are normal and all signs and symptoms have subsided. Larger doses may be necessary.

b. Maintenance dosage–Give 100–150 mg/d in 1–3 divided doses. The drug may be continued at higher doses until hypothyroidism has resulted, and then a supplement of oral thyroid may be added. Thyroid hormone should also be given if the gland remains large after 1–2 months of propylthiouracil therapy.

2. Methimazole (Tapazole)–This may be used in 1/15–1/10 the dosage of propylthiouracil. Toxic reactions are slightly more common with this drug than with the thiouracils.

3. Iodide–Iodide is generally not recommended.

4. Radioactive iodide–Radioiodide therapy is currently recommended by some either as initial treatment or if medical therapy fails. Regardless of the dose or type of radioactive iodide employed, hypothyroidism generally can be anticipated at variable periods after treatment.

5. Other drugs–Antithyroid drugs, antibiotics, sedation, propranolol, reserpine, and guanethidine may be of value for the treatment of thyroid storm.

C. Surgical Measures: Subtotal thyroidectomy is considered by some to be the treatment of choice for children, especially if close follow-up is difficult or impossible. The patient should be prepared first with bed rest, diet, propranolol, and sedation (as above) and with propylthiouracil (for 2–4 weeks). Iodide (2–10 drops daily of saturated solution of potassium iodide for 10–21 days) may be of value. Continue for 1 week after surgery.

Course & Prognosis

It has been claimed that approximately one-third of adults will respond without specific therapy; the results of similar management in children are not available. Without treatment, there will be partial remissions and exacerbations for several years. With medical treatment alone, prolonged remissions may be expected in about half of cases. The actual increased risk of developing leukemia or carcinoma of the thyroid after treatment with radioactive iodide has not been determined.

CARCINOMA OF THE THYROID

(See also Chapter 23.)

Carcinoma of the thyroid is uncommon. It is most likely to occur following irradiation of the neck and chest. Findings include goiter, neck discomfort, dysphagia, and voice changes or a nodule of the thyroid that fails to regress despite therapy with a large dose of thyroid hormones for a period of 1–2 months. Surgical extirpation of the entire gland, with removal of all involved nodes, is the treatment of choice. Radical neck dissection is seldom necessary. Postoperatively, the patient may be allowed to become hypothyroid and a diagnostic scan with radioactive iodide then done; metastases, if present, can be treated with ^{131}I or removed surgically, if feasible. Subsequent thyroid replacement therapy should consist of larger than maintenance doses. Patients with papillary carcinoma have a good prognosis for prolonged (> 10 years) survival.

Medullary carcinoma may be familial and associated with multiple endocrine adenomatosis, Marfanlike body habitus, nodularities (mucosal neuromas) of the tongue and mucous membranes, and pheochromocytoma or visceral ganglioneuromas. The serum calcitonin level is elevated.

GOITROUS CRETINISM

(See Familial Goiter, p 521.)

THYROIDITIS

Acute thyroiditis produces an acute inflammatory goiter and may be due to almost any pathogenic organism (viral or bacterial) or may be nonspecific or idiopathic. Most children are euthyroid and free of symptoms, but hypothyroidism or hyperthyroidism may be present. Specific antibiotic therapy and corticosteroids may be of value.

Subacute thyroiditis (pseudotuberculosis, de Quervain's giant cell thyroiditis) is characterized by mild and transient manifestations of hypermetabolism and an enlarged, very tender, firm thyroid gland. The T_4 concentration is elevated, and ^{131}I uptake by the gland is reduced. Aspirin (mild cases) and corticosteroids and thyroid hormone (severe disease) may be of value.

Chronic thyroiditis (lymphomatous or Hashimoto's struma, autoimmune thyroiditis) is being seen with increasing frequency, particularly in pubertal patients ("adolescent goiter"). It is characterized by firm, nontender, diffuse or nodular, "pebbly" enlargement of the thyroid with variable activity. Occasionally, there are symptoms of mild tracheal compression. Definitive diagnosis can be made only by histologic examination; thyroid function tests, antithyroid antibody tests, and scanning studies provide varying results. Needle biopsy of the gland is often diagnostic but is not generally indicated. Treatment is with thyroid hormone in full replacement dosage; corticosteroids may produce symptomatic improvement. Hypothyroidism is often an end result, and lifelong treatment may be required.

DISEASES OF THE PARATHYROID GLANDS

HYPOPARATHYROIDISM

Hypoparathyroidism may be idiopathic, may result from parathyroidectomy, or may be one feature of a general autoimmune disorder associated with candidiasis, Addison's disease, pernicious anemia, diabetes mellitus, thyroiditis, ovarian failure, and alopecia. Transient hypoparathyroidism may occur in the neonate as a result of parathyroid gland immaturity; the condition is more common in the offspring of diabetic and of hyperparathyroid mothers.

Clinical Findings

A. Symptoms and Signs:

1. Tetany–Symptoms and signs include numbness, cramps and twitchings of extremities, carpopedal spasm, laryngospasm, a positive Chvostek sign (tapping of the face in front of the ear produces spasm of the facial muscles), a positive peroneal sign (tapping the fibular side of the leg over the peroneal nerve produces abduction and dorsiflexion of the foot), a positive Trousseau sign (prolonged compression of the upper arm produces carpal spasm), and a positive Erb sign (use of galvanic current to determine hyperexcitability).

2. Prolonged hypocalcemia–In addition to the findings listed above, prolonged hypocalcemia may be associated with blepharospasm and chronic conjunctivitis, cataracts, unexplained bizarre behavior, diarrhea, photophobia, irritability, loss of consciousness, convulsions, poor dentition, skin rashes, ectodermal dysplasias, fungal infections *(Candida)*, "idiopathic" epilepsy, symmetric punctate calcifications of basal ganglia, and steatorrhea. Candidiasis, Addison's disease, thyroiditis, and pernicious anemia may precede or follow the hypoparathyroidism in the familial "autoimmune" form.

B. Laboratory Findings: (See Table 22–4.) Findings in confirmatory tests are as follows:

1. Serum parathyroid levels are inappropriately low.

2. In the Ellsworth-Howard test, there is a greater than 100% increase in the excretion of urinary phosphorus following the injection of parathyroid extract (200 units) intravenously. False-negative results are common.

3. In the prolonged parathyroid extract test, results show a rise in serum calcium, fall in serum phosphate, and increase in urine phosphate levels following the injection of parathyroid extract, 5–10 mL (100 units/mL) in divided doses intramuscularly daily for 3–4 days.

4. Urinary cAMP levels normally rise 5- to 50-fold following the

Table 22–4. Laboratory findings in rickets and disorders of calcium metabolism.*

Condition	Metabolic Features: Serum Concentration Ca^{2+}	P	Alk P'tase	PTH	Urinary Excretion Ca^{2+}	P
Chronic renal insufficiency	↓ (N)	↑	↑ (N)	↑	↓ (N)	↓
Hypoparathyroid states	↓	↑	N		↓	↓
Malabsorption syndrome	↓ (N)	↓ (N)	↑ (N)	↑ (N)	↓	N (↑ ↓)
Rickets						
Familial hypophosphatemic vitamin D-resistant	N (↓)	↓	N	N (↑)	N	↑
Hereditary vitamin D-refractory	↓	↓ (N)	↑	↑		↑
Vitamin D- deficient	↓ (N)	↓	↑	↑	↑	↑
Transient tetany of the newborn	↓	↓ (N)	↓ (N)	↓ (N)	↓ (N)	↓ (N)

*Tubular reabsorption of phosphate (TRP) normally is 83–98%; the lower values are associated with higher serum levels of phosphorus. In hypoparathyroidism, TRP values vary from 40 to 70%. Low TRP values are also found in some forms of inherited renal tubular disease, eg, vitamin D-resistant rickets.

administration of parathyroid hormone. Failure to rise indicates severe renal disease or end-organ unresponsiveness to the hormone.

Treatment

The objective of treatment is to maintain serum calcium at a low normal level. A simple, practical method of regulating therapy is by Trousseau's test and Sulkowitch's (urine) test, but the latter may not always accurately reflect hypercalciuria, particularly in infants.

A. Tetany: In patients with acute or severe tetany, immediate correction of hypocalcemia is indicated. Give calcium intravenously and orally.

B. Prolonged Hypocalcemia: For maintenance therapy in patients with hypoparathyroid and chronic hypocalcemia, use calciferol (most valuable) or dihydrotachysterol (see Drug Dosages in Appendix). The diet should be high in calcium, with added calcium lactate or gluconate; should be adequate in phosphorus (except for high phosphate for patients with the vitamin D-resistant form of hypoparathyroidism); and should exclude milk, cheese, and egg yolk. Thiazide diuretics may be used to increase urinary calcium reabsorption.

PSEUDOHYPOPARATHYROIDISM
(Seabright Bantam Syndrome)

Pseudohypoparathyroidism consists of a group of disorders generally having a familial X-linked dominant syndrome in which there is no lack of parathyroid hormone but a failure of response in the end organs (eg, the renal tubule). The symptoms and signs of hypocalcemia are the same as in idiopathic hypoparathyroidism. Patients with pseudohypoparathyroidism have round, full faces, stubby fingers (shortening of the first, fourth, and fifth metacarpals), shortness of stature, delayed and defective dentition, and early closure of the epiphyses. X-rays may show dyschondroplastic changes in the bones of the hands, demineralization of the bones, thickening of the cortices, exostoses, and ectopic calcification of the basal ganglia and subcutaneous tissues. Corneal and lenticular opacities may be present.

Treatment is with vitamin D and supplementary oral calcium lactate.

Pseudohypoparathyroidism type II is the result of a cellular defect in which neither cAMP nor parathyroid hormone produces a phosphaturic effect.

HYPERPARATHYROIDISM

Hyperparathyroidism may be primary (occasionally familial) or secondary. Primary hyperparathyroidism may be due to adenoma or diffuse parathyroid hyperplasia. The most common causes of the secondary form are chronic renal disease (glomerulonephritis, pyelonephritis), congenital anomalies of the genitourinary tract, pseudohypoparathyroidism, and vitamin D-refractory rickets. Rarely, it may be found in osteogenesis imperfecta, cancer with bony metastases, and vitamin D-resistant rickets.

Clinical Findings

A. Symptoms and Signs:

1. Due to hypercalcemia*–Findings include hypotonicity and weakness of muscles; nausea, vomiting, and poor tone of the gastrointestinal tract, with constipation; loss of weight; hyperextensibility of joints; bradycardia; and shortening of the Q–T interval.

2. Due to increased calcium and phosphorus excretion– Polyuria, hyposthenuria, polydipsia, and precipitation of calcium phosphate in the renal parenchyma or as urinary calculi (ie, sand or gravel) may occur.

3. Related to changes in the skeleton–Findings include osteitis fibrosa, absence of lamina dura around the teeth, spontaneous fractures, and a "moth-eaten" appearance of the skull. If the patient drinks

*Hypercalcemia may also be secondary to immobilization, excess intake of vitamin D, sarcoidosis, milk-alkali syndrome, extensive fat necrosis of the newborn, or certain types of cancer, or it may occur as a familial disease.

Table 22–5. Laboratory findings in hypercalcemia.

Condition	Metabolic Features: Serum Concentration			Urinary Excretion		Bone Pathology
	Ca^{2+}	P	P'tase	Ca^{2+}	P	
Excessive vitamin D	↑	↑	N	↑	N (↑)	
Hyperparathyroidism	↑	↓	N (↑)	↑	↑	Generalized osteitis fibrosa
Hyperparathyroidism with impaired renal function	↑	N (↑)	↑	↑	↑	Generalized osteitis fibrosa
Hyperproteinemia	↑ (total) N (ionized)	N	N	N	N	
Idiopathic hypercalcemia	↑	N	N	↑	N	See text
Neoplasms of bone	N (↑)	N	N (↑)	↑	N (↑)	Bone destruction

adequate quantities of milk, renal stones will occur but bone disease will not.

B. Laboratory Findings: Urinary phosphorus, serum parathyroid hormone, cAMP, and hydroxyproline excretion levels are increased. (See also Table 22–5.)

C. X-Ray Findings: Bone changes usually do not occur in children with an adequate calcium intake. When bone changes occur, there is a generalized demineralization with a predilection for the subperiosteal cortical bone. The distal clavicle is usually first affected. Nephrocalcinosis is an important additional x-ray finding.

Treatment

Complete removal of tumor or subtotal removal of hyperplastic parathyroid glands is indicated. Preoperatively, fluids should be forced and the intake of calcium restricted. Postoperatively, the diet should be high in calcium, phosphorus, and vitamin D.

Treatment of secondary hyperparathyroidism is directed at the underlying disease. Diminish the intake of phosphate by use of aluminum hydroxide orally and by reduction of milk consumption.

Course & Prognosis

Although the condition may recur (particularly in patients with familial forms of hyperparathyroidism), the prognosis following subtotal parathyroidectomy or removal of an adenoma is usually quite good. The prognosis in the secondary forms depends on correcting the underlying defect. Renal function may remain abnormal.

• • •

IDIOPATHIC HYPERCALCEMIA

Idiopathic hypercalcemia is an uncommon disorder probably related to either excessive intake or increased sensitivity to vitamin D. The disease is characterized in its severe form by peculiar facies (receding mandible, depressed bridge of nose, relatively large mouth, prominent lips, hanging jowls, large low-set ears, "elfin" appearance), failure to thrive, mental and motor retardation, irritability, purposeless movements, constipation, hypotonia, polyuria, polydipsia, hypertension, and heart disease (especially supravalvular aortic stenosis). Generalized osteosclerosis is common, and there may be premature craniosynostosis and nephrocalcinosis with evidence of urinary tract disease. Hypercholesterolemia, azotemia, and serum vitamin A elevations may be present. Familial benign hypercalcemia has been reported.

Clinical manifestations may not appear for several months. Severe disease may end in death. Mild disease may occur without the typical facies and other findings and has a good prognosis.

Treatment is by rigid restriction of dietary calcium and vitamin D and, in severely involved children, the administration of corticosteroids in high doses. Other methods of treatment that have also been reported to be of value include addition of sodium sulfate to the diet, administration of thyroxine, and the use of furosemide (especially for its acute effect).

HYPOPHOSPHATASIA

Hypophosphatasia is an uncommon heritable condition characterized by rickets and a deficiency of alkaline phosphatase. The earlier the age at onset, the more severe the condition. Failure to thrive, premature loss of teeth, widening of the sutures, bulging fontanelles, convulsions, bony deformities, dwarfing, and renal lesions have been reported. Premature closure of cranial sutures may occur. Late features include osteoporosis, pseudofractures, and rachitic deformities. Signs and symptoms may be similar to those of idiopathic hypercalcemia. The serum calcium level is frequently high. The urinary hydroxyproline level is low during infancy. The plasma and urine contain phosphoethanolamine in excessive amounts. No specific treatment is available; corticosteroids may be of value.

THE ADRENALS:

DISEASES OF THE ADRENAL CORTEX

ADRENOCORTICAL INSUFFICIENCY
(Adrenal Crisis, Addison's Disease)

Adrenocortical hypofunction may be due to atrophy; autoimmune disease; destruction of the gland by a tumor, hemorrhage (Waterhouse-Friderichsen syndrome), or infection (eg, tuberculosis); congenital absence of the adrenal cortex; or congenital hyperplasia of the cortex associated with glucocorticoid insufficiency and androgen excess. It may occur as a consequence of inadequate secretion of corticotropin (ACTH) due to anterior pituitary or hypothalamic disease. Any acute illness, surgery, trauma, or exposure to excessive heat may precipitate an adrenal crisis. A temporary salt-losing disorder (possibly due to hypoaldosteronism) may occur during infancy.

Adrenogenital syndrome and associated adrenal insufficiency, congenital adrenocortical insufficiency, autoimmune adrenal insufficiency, and neoplasms are the most common causes of chronic adrenocortical insufficiency. Autoimmune Addison's disease may be associated with hypoparathyroidism, lymphocytic thyroiditis, candidiasis, pernicious anemia, ovarian failure, alopecia, and diabetes mellitus. Antiadrenal antibodies and antiparathyroid antibodies may be present.

Clinical Findings

A. Symptoms and Signs:

1. Acute form (adrenal crisis)–Signs and symptoms include nausea and vomiting; diarrhea; dehydration; fever, which may be followed by hypothermia; circulatory collapse; and confusion or coma.

2. Chronic form (Addison's disease)–Signs and symptoms include vomiting (which becomes forceful and sometimes projectile), diarrhea, weakness, fatigue, weight loss or failure to gain weight, increased appetite for salt, dehydration, opisthotonos (rare), increased pigmentation (both generalized and over pressure points and scars and on mucous membranes), hypotension, and small heart size.

B. Laboratory Findings:

1. Adrenal insufficiency–Findings suggestive of adrenal insufficiency include the following:

a. Serum sodium, chloride, and carbon dioxide levels are decreased.

b. Serum potassium* and blood urea nitrogen levels are increased.

c. Urinary sodium levels are increased despite low serum sodium levels.

d. Eosinophilia and moderate neutropenia occur.†

e. Fasting blood glucose levels are generally normal but may be low in crisis.

f. There is inability to excrete a water load.

2. Adrenal cortex function–Results of confirmatory tests to measure the functional capacity of the adrenal cortex include the following:

a. Blood cortisol and urinary 17-hydroxycorticosteroid levels and ketogenic steroid excretion levels are decreased. ACTH levels are increased in primary adrenal insufficiency.

b. Urinary 17-ketosteroid levels are decreased (see Appendix) except in cases due to congenital hyperplasia or tumor of the cortex. Determination of urinary 17-ketosteroids is of no value in younger children, who may normally excrete less than 1 mg/d.

c. Circulating eosinophil counts are elevated. If the blood eosinophil count is under 50/μL, the diagnosis of primary adrenocortical insufficiency is doubtful.

d. Corticotropin and metyrapone test results are outlined on pp 825–826 of the Appendix.

e. In the prolonged corticotropin (ACTH) test, blood levels of cortisol and 17-hydroxycorticoids or 17-ketogenic steroids on the day before and on the day of ACTH infusion are compared. A rise of 150% or more in 17-hydroxycorticoids excludes primary adrenal insufficiency. Acute allergic disorders will not affect this test.

Treatment

A. Acute Form (Adrenal Crisis):

1. Treat infections with large doses of the appropriate antibiotics or other antimicrobial agents.

2. Treat hypovolemia with adequate fluid and electrolyte therapy. Avoid overtreatment. Infusion of a solution of human albumin may be necessary in severe cases (see Chapter 5).

3. In Waterhouse-Friderichsen syndrome with fulminant infections, adrenal steroids and isoproterenol should be used in the presence of adrenal insufficiency but not for fulminant infections alone.

4. For replacement therapy, use the following:

a. Hydrocortisone sodium succinate (Solu-Cortef), 2 mg/kg diluted in 2–10 mL of water intravenously, is given over 2–5 minutes.

*Hyperkalemia may persist for 2 or 3 months in infants with adrenogenital syndrome despite treatment with cortisone, desoxycorticosterone acetate, and supplemental salt.

†Failure to depress the number of eosinophils significantly the first day after operation or in the presence of a severe infection is also suggestive of insufficiency.

Follow this with an infusion of normal saline and 5–10% glucose, 100 mL/kg/24 h intravenously. Cortisone acetate, 1 mg/kg intramuscularly, may be used after initial replacement therapy; the onset of action of this preparation given intramuscularly is delayed, and its effect may continue for several days.

b. Hydrocortisone sodium succinate, 1.5 mg/kg (12.5 mg/m^2), is given intravenously every 4–6 hours until stabilization is achieved and oral therapy tolerated.

c. Desoxycorticosterone acetate, 1–2 mg/d intramuscularly, is given as part of initial therapy. This is repeated every 12–24 hours depending on the state of hydration, electrolyte states, and blood pressure.

d. Ten percent glucose in normal saline, 20 mL/kg intravenously in the first 2 hours, may be of value, particularly in infants with adrenal crisis who have congenital adrenal hyperplasia. Avoid overtreatment.

5. Fruit juices, ginger ale, milk, and soft foods should be started as soon as possible.

B. Chronic Form (Addison's Disease): There may be variable response to different glucocorticoids in some patients. (See Table 22–6

Table 22–6. Corticosteroids.

Generic and Chemical Name	Potency per Milligram Compared to Hydrocortisone* Glucocorticoid Effect	Mineralocorticoid Effect
Glucocorticoids		
Hydrocortisone	1	1
Betamethasone†	33	
Cortisone	4/5	1
Dexamethasone	30	Minimal
Fluprednisolone	13	
Methylprednisolone†	5	Minimal
Paramethasone	10–12	
Prednisolone	4	Minimal
Prednisone	4	Minimal
Triamcinolone†	5	Minimal
Mineralocorticoids		
Aldosterone	30	500
Desoxycorticosterone		15
Desoxycorticosterone acetate		15
Desoxycorticosterone pivalate		15
Fludrocortisone		15–20

*To convert hydrocortisone dosage to equivalent dosage in any of the other preparations listed in this table, divide by the potency factors shown.

†There is no indication that these preparations offer any advantage over prednisone and prednisolone.

for conversion of other corticosteroids to hydrocortisone equivalents.) Maintenance therapy following initial stabilization generally requires the use of a corticosteroid together with a liberal intake of salt and supplementary desoxycorticosterone acetate or a fluorinated steroid. Children requiring prolonged adrenocorticosteroid administration should have periodic determinations of height, weight, and blood pressure (taken in the recumbent position) and assay of blood glucose and serum sodium and potassium.

1. Cortisone acetate–Give an aqueous suspension or give orally, 20 mg/m^2. Increase to 2–4 times regular dosage during periods of intercurrent illness or other periods of stress.

2. Hydrocortisone–Dosages are as follows:

a. Physiologic replacement–
(1) Intramuscularly–0.44 mg/kg or 13–20 mg/m^2 once daily.
(2) Orally*–0.66 mg/kg or 20 mg/m^2/d.

b. Therapeutic use–
(1) Intramuscularly–4.4 mg/kg or 130 mg/m^2 once daily.
(2) Orally*–6.6 mg/kg or 200 mg/m^2/d.

c. Therapeutic maintenance–
(1) Intramuscularly–1.3–2.2 mg/kg or 40–65 mg/m^2 once daily.
(2) Orally*–2–3.3 mg/kg or 60–100 mg/m^2/d.

d. Development of infection–If infection occurs while the patient is receiving a large dose of steroid, give about 1½–2 times the physiologic maintenance dose for 3 or 4 days and then resume the larger dose.

e. Long-term maintenance–Except when used for replacement therapy (ie, in the treatment of Addison's disease and the adrenogenital syndrome) and in the treatment of certain malignant states, the total 2-day dose of corticosteroid for long-term maintenance therapy may be administered as a single dose once every 48 hours. This will not diminish the therapeutic efficacy but will diminish the side effects; there may be normal growth and decreased tendency to cushingoid appearance.

3. Fludrocortisone–Give fludrocortisone, 0.05–0.2 mg daily in 2 divided doses.

4. Desoxycorticosterone acetate–This may be used in place of fludrocortisone.

a. Give desoxycorticosterone acetate in oil, 0.5–3 mg/d intramuscularly, and increase or decrease gradually to the amount needed to maintain hydration, normal blood pressure, heart size, and weight. This agent also comes in propylene glycol for sublingual administration.

b. Desoxycorticosterone pivalate may be given following prolonged regulation (25 mg/mL of this long-acting macrocrystalline sus-

*In 4 doses 6 hours apart (preferred) or 3 doses every 8 hours, providing approximately 50% of the total dose in the early morning.

pension given intramuscularly every 3–4 weeks corresponds to about 1 mg of desoxycorticosterone acetate in oil given intramuscularly daily). In patients with congenital adrenal hyperplasia, hypertension (without hypernatremia) may occur following the administration of mineralocorticoids and may persist for months following their discontinuation.

c. Pellets of desoxycorticosterone acetate may be implanted.

5. Sodium chloride–Give 1–3 g/d (as enteric-coated salt pills if they can be taken). Reduce the dose if edema appears.

6. Increased dosages–Additional desoxycorticosterone acetate, sodium chloride, or cortisone may be necessary with acute illness, surgery, trauma, exposure to sudden change in temperature, or other stress reactions after optimal glucocorticoid stabilization has been achieved.

C. Other Recommendations:

1. If corticosteroids have been administered for more than 1 month, terminate their use gradually. Abrupt withdrawal may cause a severe "rebound" of the disease or produce symptoms of adrenal insufficiency.

2. Give corticosteroids to any child undergoing surgery, severe infection, or other significant stress who has received prolonged therapy with corticosteroids in the past.

3. If a child receiving maintenance doses of steroids develops chickenpox, the dosage of the steroid should be increased to pharmacologic levels (eg, 3 times maintenance). Steroid withdrawal in these circumstances may have a fatal outcome.

4. Use of topical corticosteroids for the treatment of inflammatory skin conditions may result in absorption of significantly large amounts of corticosteroid through both normal and inflamed skin.

D. Corticosteroids in Patients Requiring Surgery: In patients with current or previous adrenocortical insufficiency who undergo surgery, corticosteroids are given as follows:

1. Preoperatively–Give cortisone acetate intramuscularly in a single dose (100% of maintenance) 24 hours before surgery and in a single dose (200% of maintenance) 1 hour before surgery.

2. During operation–Give hydrocortisone sodium succinate (Solu-Cortef), 1–2 mg/kg by intravenous infusion over a 6- to 12-hour period.

3. Postoperatively–Give cortisone acetate intramuscularly, 100–200% of maintenance daily, for 1–2 days. Begin oral preparation as soon as possible, and give full maintenance doses daily. If the maintenance dose is unknown, give 1.25 mg/kg intramuscularly as follows: 100% of total at 8:00 AM and 50% of dose at 2:00 PM and at 10:00 PM. If significant stress occurs postoperatively, give 3–5 times the maintenance dose.

ADRENOCORTICAL HYPERFUNCTION

CUSHING'S SYNDROME

The principal findings in Cushing's syndrome in children result from excessive secretion of glucocorticoid and androgenic hormones, leading to varying degrees of abnormal carbohydrate, protein, and fat metabolism and virilization. There may also be lesser degrees of overproduction of mineralocorticoids.

Cushing's syndrome is more common in females; in children under 12 years of age, noniatrogenic disease is usually due to adrenal tumor or to an ectopic ACTH-producing tumor. Hemihypertrophy may be present. Cushing's syndrome is a common result of therapy with corticotropin or one of the corticosteroids. Rarely, it may be associated with an apparently primary adrenocortical hyperplasia or hyperplasia secondary to basophilic adenoma of the pituitary gland. Spontaneous remission has been reported.

Clinical Findings

A. Symptoms and Signs:

1. Due to excessive secretion of the carbohydrate-regulating hormones–"Buffalo type" adiposity, most marked on the face, neck, and trunk, may occur; a fat pad in the interscapular area is characteristic. Other findings include easy fatigability and muscle weakness, striae, plethoric facies, easy bruisability, osteoporosis, hypertension, growth failure, diabetes (usually latent), psychologic disturbances, and pain in the back.

2. Due to excessive secretion of androgens–Findings include hirsutism, acne, varying degrees of clitoral or penile enlargement, advanced skeletal maturation, and deepening of the voice. Menstrual irregularities occur in older girls.

3. Due to excessive production of mineralocorticoids–Sodium retention with hypertension (rarely edema) occurs.

B. Laboratory Findings:

1. Serum chloride and potassium levels may be low.

2. Serum sodium, pH, and carbon dioxide content may be elevated.

3. Plasma cortisol levels are increased, and plasma and urinary diurnal variation may not occur.

4. Excretions of urinary 17-ketosteroids, 17-hydroxycorticosteroids, 17-ketogenic steroids, and free cortisol are generally increased; the test for free cortisol is the assay of choice. Increased secretion of ACTH occurs in patients with adrenal hyperplasia and with ACTH-secreting nonendocrine tumors but not with other adrenal tumors. Sup-

pression of blood cortisol and 17-hydroxycorticosteroids by high doses of dexamethasone occurs with adrenal hyperplasia but not with adrenal tumors.

5. Eosinophil counts are below 50/μL.

6. Glycosuria alone or with carbohydrate intolerance and hyperglycemia may be present ("diabetic" type of glucose tolerance curve).

7. Abdominal ultrasonography, CT scan, and radioactive cholesterol uptake studies may be helpful in localizing a tumor.

Treatment

Since almost all cases of primary hyperfunction in childhood are due to tumor, surgical removal, if possible, is indicated. Corticotropin has been recommended for pre- and postoperative use to stimulate the nontumorous adrenal cortex, which is generally atrophied. Corticosteroids should be administered for 1 or 2 days before surgery and continued during and after operation. Supplemental potassium, normal saline solution, and desoxycorticosterone acetate may be necessary. (See p 537.)

Pituitary irradiation or cyproheptadine may be of value to control Cushing's disease resulting from adrenal hyperplasia. If these measures are ineffective, bilateral adrenalectomy and hypophysectomy may be tried. The use of mitotane (Lysodren; *o,p'*-DDD) for the treatment of adrenal hyperplasia and tumors has been suggested.

Prognosis

If the tumor is malignant, the prognosis is poor. If it is benign, cure should result following proper preparation and surgery. Following total bilateral adrenalectomy, pituitary tumors may appear.

ADRENOGENITAL SYNDROME

Adrenogenital syndrome may result from tumor or congenital adrenal hyperplasia.

The congenital form of adrenogenital syndrome is an autosomal recessive disease due to an inborn error of metabolism with a deficiency of an adrenocortical enzyme. Various types are recognized, including the following:

(1) Deficiency of 21-hydroxylase (approximately 90% of cases), resulting in inability to convert 17-hydroxyprogesterone into 11-deoxycortisol. Mild forms result in androgenic changes (virilization) alone, but severe cases are associated with salt loss and electrolyte imbalance.

(2) Deficiency in 11β-hydroxylation and a failure to convert 11-deoxycortisol to cortisol. This is associated with virilization and usually

with hypertension.

(3) A defect in 17-hydroxylase, with the enzyme deficiency in both the adrenals and the gonads. Hypertension, virilization, amenorrhea, and eunuchoidism may be present.

(4) A partial or complete defect in 3β-hydroxysteroid dehydrogenase activity and a failure to convert Δ^5-pregnenolone to progesterone. This is associated with incomplete masculinization, hypospadias, and cryptorchidism in the male. Some degree of masculinization may occur in the female. Severe sodium loss occurs, and the infant mortality rate is high in the complete form.

(5) Cholesterol desmolase deficiency with congenital lipoid adrenal hyperplasia. Clinical features are similar to those of 3β-hydroxysteroid dehydrogenase deficiency (above).

Adrenogenital Syndrome in Females

A. Congenital Bilateral Hyperplasia of the Adrenal Cortex (Pseudohermaphroditism): Abnormalities of the external genitalia include an enlarged clitoris with partial to complete labial fusion and a common urogenital sinus. Growth in height is excessive and "bone age" advanced, and patients may have excessive muscularity and sexual development. Pubic hair appears early; acne may be excessive; and the voice may deepen.

Pseudohermaphroditism in the female may also be produced as a result of the administration of androgens, progestins, diethylstilbestrol, and related hormones to the mother during the first trimester of pregnancy or as a result of virilizing maternal tumors. In these cases, the condition regresses after birth.

B. Postnatal Adrenogenital Syndrome (Virilism): This syndrome may be due to adrenal hyperplasia or tumor or to arrhenoblastoma (extremely rare). Enlargement of the clitoris occurs, but other changes of the genitalia are not found. The family history is negative. If a tumor is present, it may be palpably enlarged. Other findings are similar to those of pseudohermaphroditism.

Adrenogenital Syndrome in Males (Macrogenitosomia Praecox)

In males, precocious sexual development is along isosexual lines. With congenital bilateral hyperplasia of the adrenal cortex, the infant may appear normal at birth; however, during the first few months of life, the penis enlarges, the scrotum darkens, the rugae become more prominent, and acne and pubic and axillary hair appear. The testicles generally remain small, and spermatogenesis does not occur. Other symptoms and signs are similar to those of the congenital form in females. If an adrenal or testicular tumor is the cause, the tumor may be palpable. Rarely, an adrenal tumor in either sex produces feminization, with gynecomastia resulting in males.

Laboratory Findings

A. Urine:

1. 21-Hydroxylase deficiency–17-Ketosteroid, 17-ketogenic steroid, pregnanetriol, and testosterone levels are increased. (**Note:** Urinary pregnanetriol levels are sometimes normal in the neonatal period. During the first 3 weeks of life, normal infants may excrete up to 2.5 mg/d. Aldosterone may be reduced, and excessive sodium loss occurs in salt-losing forms.)

2. 11β-Hydroxylase deficiency–11-Deoxycortisol (and its tetrahydro derivative), 17-hydroxycorticoid, deoxycorticosterone, 17-ketosteroid, and testosterone levels are increased.

3. 17-Hydroxylase deficiency–17-Ketosteroid and 17-hydroxycorticoid levels are decreased; aldosterone, corticosterone, and deoxycorticosterone levels are increased.

4. 3β-Hydroxysteroid dehydrogenase deficiency–Urinary 17-ketosteroid, 17-hydroxycorticoid, and 17-ketogenic steroid levels are decreased.

5. Cholesterol desmolase deficiency–All steroid excretion is markedly decreased.

6. Tumor–Excretion of dehydroepiandrosterone may be greatly elevated.

7. Other findings–Urinary excretion of gonadotropins may be elevated for age.

B. Blood:

1. 21-Hydroxylase deficiency–Levels of circulating cortisol are decreased. Levels of 17-hydroxyprogesterone, androstenedione, and dehydroepiandrosterone are increased. Plasma renin activity may be elevated.

2. 11β-Hydroxylase deficiency–11-Deoxycortisol levels are increased.

3. 17-Hydroxylase deficiency–Serum progesterone levels are increased.

4. 3β-Hydroxysteroid dehydrogenase deficiency–Serum pregnenolone levels are increased.

5. Other findings–Blood excretion of gonadotropins may be elevated for age.

C. Dexamethasone Suppression Test: If the administration of dexamethasone, 2–4 mg/d orally in 4 doses for 7 days, reduces 17-ketosteroid levels to normal, hyperplasia rather than adenoma is the probable diagnosis.

D. Buccal Smear: In female pseudohermaphrodites, the nuclear chromatin pattern is positive.

X-Ray Findings

Genitograms using contrast media may indicate the presence of a urogenital sinus. Displacement of the kidney and calcification in the area of the adrenal may be seen on urograms or plain films of patients with tumors. "Bone age" is typically advanced with 21- and 11β-hydroxylase defects after the first year of life.

Treatment

A. Congenital Hyperplasia of the Adrenal Cortex:

1. Cortisone acetate–Approximately 25–35 mg/m²/d orally will produce adrenal suppression and normal linear growth. Dosages of 10–25 mg/d for infants and 25–100 mg/d for older children initially are usually necessary. The drug should be given orally in divided doses several times a day, two-fifths of the total dose given as the first morning dose and two-fifths as the last dose at night.

2. Mineralocorticoids–For patients with salt-losing forms of adrenogenital syndrome, therapy with desoxycorticosterone or fludrocortisone and sodium chloride is necessary (see pp 536–537).

3. Glucocorticoids–Glucocorticoids should be increased (by 3–4 times) during acute severe stress or infection.

4. Surgical measures–Recession or partial clitoridectomy is occasionally indicated in a girl with an abnormally large or sensitive clitoris but may be delayed for 1 or 2 years until the effect of therapy is determined. Surgical correction of the labial fusion and urogenital sinus may require several operations.

B. Tumor: Because the malignant lesions cannot be distinguished clinically from the benign ones, surgical removal is indicated whenever a tumor has been diagnosed. Preoperative and postoperative treatment are as for Cushing's syndrome due to a tumor (see Cushing's Syndrome, above).

Course & Prognosis

Untreated patients with congenital hyperplasia will show precocious virilization throughout childhood. Because of excessive skeletal maturation, these individuals will be tall as children but short as adults. Adequate corticosteroid treatment permits normal growth and sexual maturation.

Female pseudohermaphrodites mistakenly raised as males for more than 3 years may have serious psychologic disturbances if their sex role is changed after that time.

When the adrenogenital syndrome is caused by a tumor, progression of signs and symptoms will cease after successful surgical removal; pubic hair, pigmentation, and deepening of the voice may regress or persist.

PRIMARY ALDOSTERONISM

Primary hyperaldosteronism may be caused by an adrenal tumor or by adrenal hyperplasia. It is characterized by paresthesias, tetany, weakness, periodic "paralysis," polyuria, low serum potassium levels, hypertension, alkaline urine, proteinuria, metabolic alkalosis, carbohydrate intolerance, suppressed plasma renin activity, and hyposthenuria that does not respond to vasopressin. The urinary aldosterone level is increased, but other steroid levels are variable. Treatment of the tumor is by surgical removal. With hyperplasia, subtotal or total adrenalectomy is recommended if pharmacologic doses of glucocorticoid are ineffective after 2 months.

A form of secondary hyperaldosteronism, possibly due to increased prostaglandins, occurs in which both renin and aldosterone levels are elevated in the absence of hypertension (Bartter's syndrome). There is associated renovascular disease, with hyperplasia of the juxtaglomerular apparatus and renal electrolyte wasting.

DISEASES OF THE ADRENAL MEDULLA

PHEOCHROMOCYTOMA
(Chromaffinoma)

Pheochromocytoma is an uncommon tumor that may be located wherever there is any chromaffin tissue (eg, adrenal medulla, sympathetic ganglia, carotid body). The condition may be familial (eg, multiple endocrine adenomatosis type II), and in children the tumors are often multiple and bilateral.

Clinical Findings

Clinical manifestations of pheochromocytoma are due to excessive secretion of epinephrine or norepinephrine. Attacks of anxiety and headaches should arouse suspicion. Other findings are palpitation, dizziness, weakness, nausea, vomiting, diarrhea, dilated pupils with blurring of vision, abdominal and precordial pain, rapid pulse, hypertension (usually persistent), and discomfort from heat. The symptoms may be sustained, producing all of the above findings plus papilledema, retinopathy, and cardiac enlargement.

Urine and serum catecholamine levels are increased. The 24-hour urine collection shows markedly increased urinary excretion of metanephrines and vanillylmandelic acid. ***Caution:*** Attacks may be provoked by mechanical stimulation of the tumor or by histamine or tyramine. Results of the phentolamine (Regitine) test are positive, but the test is not specific for pheochromocytoma and may not be necessary for diagnosis. Displacement of the kidney may be shown by routine x-ray. The tumor may be defined by ultrasonography of the abdomen or by CT scan.

Treatment

Surgical removal of the tumor is the treatment of choice, but a sudden paroxysm and death during surgery are not uncommon. The oral administration of propranolol and phentolamine preoperatively has been recommended to prevent the extreme fluctuations of blood pressure that sometimes occur during surgery. Medical treatment includes phenoxybenzamine to reduce hypertension and propranolol to lessen tachycardia and ventricular arrhythmias.

Prognosis

Complete relief of symptoms, except those due to long-standing vascular or renal changes, is the rule after recovery. If no treatment is given, severe cardiac, renal, and cerebral damage may result.

• • •

DIABETES MELLITUS*

Diabetes mellitus is a generalized hereditary metabolic disorder that leads to derangement of carbohydrate, protein, and fat metabolism, followed by glycosuria, dehydration, ketoacidosis, coma, and eventually death. The administration of insulin corrects these deficiencies but is not curative.

Diabetes in the newborn may be transient, may not require insulin, and may disappear after weeks or months. In some cases, diabetes has resulted from ingestion of inappropriately diluted powdered formula. Transient hyperglycemia, acetonuria, and glycosuria have been noted in young children who have received phenylephrine or asparaginase and in patients who have had infections or hyperglucagonemia.

Heredity is an important predisposing factor in the onset of diabetes, but the precise mode of inheritance has not been determined; environmental factors may be important.

Clinical Findings

A. Symptoms and Signs:

1. Early manifestations–Early manifestations in patients with

*Revised with the assistance of H. Peter Chase, MD.

chemical and overt disease (1–2 months or less) include thirst and polydipsia, polyuria and nocturia or enuresis, loss of weight or failure to gain, increase in appetite (less common in children than in adults; anorexia is often noted), lassitude and easy fatigability, cramping pains in the limbs or abdomen, dizziness, confusion, hyperventilation, and sudden coma or stupor (due to diabetic acidosis).

2. Chronic complications–Stunting of growth and poor development occur in patients with uncontrolled diabetes of long standing (Mauriac's syndrome). Many children with diabetes develop contractures of finger joints. Serious psychologic difficulties are not infrequent. Characteristic "small vessel" changes occur. Diabetic retinopathy develops in most juvenile diabetics 10–20 years after onset of symptoms. Premature atherosclerosis and coronary vascular disease may also develop, as well as intercapillary glomerulosclerosis (Kimmelstiel-Wilson syndrome), with hypertension, edema, proteinuria, and atherosclerosis.

B. Laboratory Findings: Findings include glycosuria, fasting hyperglycemia, and hyperglycemia 2 hours after a meal. (A fasting blood glucose level of > 120 mg/dL in the absence of obesity or drugs is generally indicative of diabetes mellitus; however, a normal fasting blood glucose level does not rule out diabetes.) Other findings include abnormal results in glucose tolerance tests, ketonuria, hyperlipidemia, hemoconcentration, and lactic acidemia. Hemoglobin A_{1c} levels may be elevated in new, long-standing, or poorly controlled patients or in patients with partial remission. Insulin concentration is usually low but may be elevated, especially in obese adolescents.

Treatment

A. Insulin: Insulin therapy (Table 22–7) is necessary in almost all cases of childhood diabetes. Initially (7–14 days), the insulin requirements may be high, followed by a period of considerably lower needs, but requirements will soon rise again after that. The initial dose of insulin may be determined primarily by trial and error in relation to urine glucose and occasional blood glucose determinations; in many cases, it will be approximately 0.5 unit/kg initially with a gradual increase to 1

Table 22–7. Summary of bioavailability characteristics of the insulins.

	Insulin Type	Onset	Peak Action	Duration
Short-acting	Regular, Actrapid, Velosulin	15–30 min	1–3 h	5–7 h
	Semilente, Semitard	30–60 min	4–6 h	12–16 h
Intermediate-acting	Lente, Lentard, Monotard	2–4 h	8–10 h	18–24 h
	NPH, Insulatard, Protophane	2–4 h	8–10 h	18–24 h
Long-acting	Ultralente, Ultratard, PZI	4–5 h	8–14 h	25–36 h

unit/kg in later years. Patients with type I diabetes mellitus (insulin-dependent diabetes mellitus, juvenile-onset diabetes) should usually be started on long-acting preparations, preferably equal proportions of semilente and ultralente or 1 part of regular to 3 or 4 parts of neutral protamine Hagedorn or isophane (NPH) insulin as soon as the initial ketoacidosis has cleared. Regular insulin should be available for emergency situations and as a supplemental dose with injections for other critical changes. Older children may achieve better control on a regimen of 2 injections daily, with two-thirds of the total dose given in the morning and one-third given before dinner. Initially, insulin is often given as 1 part of regular insulin to 2 parts of NPH insulin. Injections should be given 20–30 minutes before meals, enabling the regular insulin to act at the time of food intake. In patients who require more insulin than 60 units/d or who develop rashes following injections, use of pork insulin may be more effective than beef insulin.

B. Oral Hypoglycemic Agents: These drugs play a minimal role in the management of insulin-dependent diabetes, although they are occasionally employed in the adolescent with type II diabetes mellitus (non-insulin-dependent diabetes mellitus, maturity-onset diabetes).

C. Diet: The diet should be well balanced and consistent in amount from day to day, allowing approximately 1000 kcal plus an additional 100 kcal per year of age. Give 50–55% as carbohydrate, 25–30% as fat, and 20% as protein. Many believe that the patient may be allowed freedom to eat according to appetite within sensible limits but that foods high in sugar should be limited. Intermittent mild glycosuria (without ketosis) is permitted and is preferred in the infant, in whom hypoglycemia may be particularly harmful. The patient should know about the American Diabetes Association exchange diet, which uses household measurements rather than weights. With the use of long-acting or intermediate-acting insulin, one must give a bedtime feeding to prevent hypoglycemia during the night. A small feeding in the afternoon or before exercise may also be indicated. In general, weight should be kept at normal or slightly subnormal levels. An attempt should be made to maintain normal serum lipoprotein, cholesterol, and triglyceride levels.

D. Outpatient Management: In most children and adolescents, urine should be tested 3 times each day (in the morning, before supper, and at bedtime). Recently, monitoring of blood glucose levels at home has gained in popularity and importance. This can be done with diagnostic paper strips (eg, Chemstrip bG strips), which permit visual estimation of the glucose concentration when compared to a color chart, or by use of a meter (eg, Glucometer, Ames Co.). If the blood glucose concentration is above 250 mg/dL, urine ketone levels should also be checked. Many investigators recommend that blood tests be done on 3 days of each week (in the morning and in either the afternoon or evening or both) and that urine be tested on the other 4 days of each week. Examination every 3 months of the retinas, thyroid, liver, injection sites, fingers (for contractures), and lower extremities (for edema and for reflexes) is recommended. The patient's understanding of the disease should be reviewed. After puberty, hemoglobin A_{1c} (glycosylated hemoglobin) levels should be determined every 3–6 months. Prior to puberty, when the rate of tissue change from high glucose levels is not as great, hemoglobin A_{1c} levels should be determined once or twice yearly.

E. Other Factors Influencing the Regulation of Diabetes:

1. Activity–Strenuous exercise tends to lower the insulin requirement. Exercise in moderation (and without significant day-to-day variations) is beneficial. However, patients should be cautioned against strenuous exercise unless they take extra carbohydrate beforehand or reduce the insulin dosage.

2. Infection–Any infection is serious in a diabetic patient; it completely upsets the equilibrium established by therapy, usually increasing the need for insulin, and is one of the most common precipitating causes of ketosis and acidosis. During severe infections, it is often necessary to add small doses of supplemental regular insulin every 2–4 hours until acetonuria clears. When vomiting is present without ketoacidosis, it is often best to reduce the daily insulin dose by half; regular insulin may be supplemented later if high glucose and ketone levels develop.

3. Surgery–Prior to elective surgery, the patient should be given half the usual dose of long-acting insulin in the morning; following this, 5 or 10% dextrose in water should be administered slowly intravenously before, during, and after surgery to cover the insulin. Blood glucose levels should be monitored during surgery and the early postoperative period. If blood glucose levels exceed 300 mg/dL or if abnormally high levels of ketones appear, regular insulin may be administered intravenously at the rate of 0.05 unit/kg/h. If the patient is unable to return to oral food intake promptly, intravenous glucose and electrolytes are continued and intravenous insulin may be continued as necessary. On the day after surgery, if the patient is able to resume eating, the usual amount of long-acting insulin should be administered. As soon as possible, feedings by mouth should be reinstituted and an early return to the exclusive use of long-acting insulin anticipated.

4. Control of glucose level–Suspect hypoglycemia and post-hypoglycemic hyperglycemia (Somogyi's reflex) may be due to overdosage with insulin or failure to administer insulin as instructed in diabetic children with poor control of glucose levels.

DIABETIC ACIDOSIS
(Diabetic Coma)

Clinical Findings

A. Symptoms and Signs: Diabetic acidosis is characterized by marked thirst and polyuria, followed by nausea and vomiting, abdominal pain, and general malaise. Dehydration and acidosis develop rapidly. Respirations then become long, deep, and labored; headache, irritability, drowsiness, stupor, and finally coma may develop. On physical examination, the patient is irritable, drowsy, or unconscious, and there is marked dehydration. The skin and mucous membranes are usually dry, lips cherry-red, eyeballs soft, blood pressure low, pulse usually rapid and thready, hyperventilation present, temperature low, and a sweetish ("fruity") acetone breath may be detected. The abdomen may show diffuse spasm and tenderness suggestive of an acute abdominal disorder. The signs and symptoms of the precipitating cause (infection, trauma, emotional upset, etc) will usually be found.

A syndrome of hyperosmolar nonketotic diabetic coma in children has been described. It is characterized by the presence of severe hyperglycemia, severe dehydration, and metabolic acidosis and may occur secondary to hypernatremia. The duration of illness is short. There is little or no polydipsia and polyuria, and these children are frequently insulin-resistant. In treatment, sufficient insulin (and isotonic parenteral fluid initially) should be used to normalize glucose metabolism; insulin may not be necessary when the disorder follows hypernatremia.

B. Laboratory Findings: Findings include glycosuria, ketonemia, ketonuria, and hyperglycemia. Serum sodium and chloride levels and the plasma carbon dioxide content are low. Serum potassium and inorganic phosphorus levels may be increased initially, but there is a major total body depletion of these elements, and levels usually decline rapidly with correction of acidosis. Total protein, hemoglobin, and blood urea nitrogen levels may be increased. Leukocytosis and increased hematocrit are often present.

Treatment

A. Objectives: Objectives are the restoration of circulation, correction of fluid and electrolyte deficit, reestablishment of normal carbohydrate metabolism, and eradication of the cause of acidosis and the hyperosmolar state.

B. Emergency Measures:

1. Hospitalize the patient if diabetic acidosis is severe. Most patients can be treated without hospitalization. Keep the patient warm, but avoid excessive warmth. Do not give narcotics or barbiturates.

2. Treat shock, if present, with plasma and other antishock measures (see Chapter 2).

3. Evaluate the degree of dehydration and shock by physical examination and by close inquiry to determine if there is a history of recent weight loss.

4. Obtain urine for estimation of glucose and ketone levels, specific gravity, and evidence of infection.

5. Take blood for measurement of pH and determination of levels of carbon dioxide, sodium chloride, potassium, glucose, inorganic phosphorus, urea nitrogen, and ketone bodies. Measurement of the blood lactic acid level may also be of value, especially in the acidotic nonketotic patient.

6. Insulin is given as follows:

a. Intravenous insulin should not be given until the blood glucose level is known, particularly if subcutaneous injections were given previously. If the glucose level is high (> 250 mg/mL) and the serum acetone level is moderately or greatly increased, an initial loading dose of regular insulin, 0.1–0.2 unit/kg, is given intravenously.

b. A constant intravenous infusion of regular insulin, 0.1–0.2 unit/kg/h, is given by use of a constant infusion pump if that method of delivery is available. Regular insulin, 30 units, is added to 150 mL of 0.9% sodium chloride to give a dilution of 1 unit/5 mL. If 50 mL of this solution is run through the tubing prior to use, the insulin binding sites on the tubing will be saturated. A similar dose of insulin may be given intramuscularly instead of intravenously but will then need to be repeated every hour. With either route of administration, blood glucose and acetone levels should be determined hourly, if possible. Insulin may be given subcutaneously every 2–4 hours in less severely involved patients, except in markedly dehydrated patients who may have varied absorption of the drug.

7. Gastric lavage may be necessary to relieve distention of the stomach and to reduce vomiting.

8. Fluids and electrolytes are given as follows:

a. First correct extracellular dehydration, shock, anoxia, and impaired renal function with normal saline solution or, if acidosis is severe (pH < 7.0), a solution containing the following: sodium, 150 mEq/L; chloride, 100 mEq/L; and bicarbonate, 50 mEq/L. Give 20–40 mL/kg over the first 1 or 2 hours of therapy. If shock is present, the use of plasma or other volume expander is essential.

b. Then give 50% physiologic solution (usually without bicarbonate) at a rate calculated to restore deficits, supply maintenance amounts, and replace intercurrent losses.

c. When urine flow and circulatory efficiency are satisfactory, the blood pH level is above 7.1, and signs of hyperpnea have begun to subside (generally in 1–2 hours), replace intracellular electrolytes (potassium and phosphorus). Although serum potassium and phosphorus concentrations are usually normal or high early in acidosis, they may fall to low levels following correction of acidosis. (Serum phosphorus levels tend to parallel potassium levels; therefore, a mixture of half potassium phosphate and half potassium chloride is recommended.)

d. Replace the remainder of the water deficit, and when the blood glucose level falls below 250 mg/dL, 5% glucose may be added to the intravenous fluids.

C. General Measures:

1. Ascertain the precipitating cause of the acidosis, and initiate appropriate treatment.

2. Use an indwelling catheter if spontaneous voidings are not possible (rarely necessary).

3. Measure urinary glucose and acetone, blood glucose and carbon dioxide, and serum electrolytes at frequent intervals.

4. Continuous or intermittent monitoring of the ECG is helpful to follow the effect of potassium therapy.

5. After 12–18 hours, if there is no vomiting, the remainder of the day's fluid and electrolyte requirements may be given orally in a suitable vehicle (orange juice, ginger ale, or milk). Vomiting generally subsides after ketosis has been corrected.

6. For continued fluid and electrolyte therapy, see Chapter 5.

Prognosis

With prompt and adequate therapy, the prognosis is good. The largest number of serious side effects and sequelae result from the administration of potassium when the serum level is still high, from delayed or inadequate correction of fluid and electrolyte losses, or from overzealous correction of the hyperglycemia, dehydration, or acidosis. Recurrent episodes of acidosis are due to failure to take the proper insulin or diet, to emotional problems, to omitting insulin altogether, or to chronic or repeated infections.

HYPOGLYCEMIA

(See also Neonatal Hypoglycemia, Chapter 9.)

Low blood glucose levels can occur when a patient with diabetes receives excessive insulin, fails to eat, or exercises too strenuously. In children who do not have diabetes, the diagnosis of hypoglycemia *should not be made* unless the blood glucose level is below 40 mg/dL or, in a newborn, below 30 mg/dL. The diagnosis is unfortunately assigned frequently to children with behavioral or other problems who have never had a documented low blood glucose level.

The most common known cause of hypoglycemia in infants during the first year of life is inappropriate insulin secretion. During episodes of hypoglycemia, the insulin level remains above 20 μU/mL even though the blood glucose level is low. When the pancreas is examined histologically, the islet cells may be hypertrophied in some cases; in other cases, there may be excessive numbers of islet cells, which may be arising from pancreatic ductules (nesidioblastosis). A trial of small amounts of sucrose (table sugar) in combination with diazoxide, 10–20 mg/kg, to inhibit insulin release should be attempted. Because leucine may stimulate insulin production, it is also necessary to restrict leucine intake in some infants. If this is unsuccessful, partial pancreatomy may be indicated.

The most frequent known cause of hypoglycemia in children between 1 and 5 years of age is the presence of ketones in the urine. Ketotic hypoglycemia is more common in males and in children who had birth weights below 2500 g, who were small for gestational age, or who have minor neurologic or behavioral disorders. There is often a history of vomiting or of decreased appetite or failure to eat during the previous 24 hours. Ketotic hypoglycemia is characterized by early morning seizures with the concurrent appearance of ketones in the urine. Treatment should consist of preventing excessive fasting and monitoring the urine for ketones whenever the child is ill or appears to be deviating from normal behavior patterns. If ketones are present, foods high in simple sugars should be encouraged. If the child is vomiting, parenteral glucose should be administered.

Islet cell adenoma represents an increasingly more frequent cause of primary-onset hypoglycemia in patients over 4 years of age and probably is the most frequent known cause in patients over 6 years of age. Inappropriate ratios of insulin to glucose are noted, and the tumor can sometimes be detected by means of ultrasonography or arteriography. Treatment is surgical removal.

There are some cases in which a cause for hypoglycemia cannot be found (group IV, idiopathic spontaneous hypoglycemia; Table 22–8). Sometimes a genetic metabolic disorder (group VI; Table 22–8) is suspected on the basis of the family (or other) history or the physical examination (eg, large liver). In other cases, particularly in association with poor growth, a primary endocrine deficiency (group VII; Table 22–8) or nutritional liver disease (group VIII; Table 22–8) may be the suspected cause of hypoglycemia.

Clinical Findings

A. Symptoms and Signs: Findings include weakness, hunger, irritability, faintness, sweating, changes in mood, epigastric pain, vomiting, nervousness, hypothermia, unsteadiness of gait, semiconsciousness, tremors, and convulsions. All of these are relieved by administration of glucose. If left untreated, hypoglycemia may lead to extensive central nervous system damage. Symptomatic hypoglycemia is more commonly associated with mental deterioration, disintegration of the personality, and death, but some infants may have prolonged and severe hypoglycemia and subsequently develop normally. Brain damage appears to result more frequently from second or subsequent episodes of hypoglycemia than from the first. It has been suggested that in some cases the central nervous system dysfunction is primary and may play a role in the production of hypoglycemia.

B. Laboratory Findings: (See Table 22–8.)

1. Blood glucose levels are low during an attack. There is no sharp dividing line below which a level can be regarded as abnormal, but consistent or repeated levels below 40 mg/dL, except during the neonatal period, generally are considered to be significantly lowered.

2. Serum insulin levels may be inappropriately elevated in hyperinsulinemic states when compared with the simultaneous glucose level.

3. No single test of blood glucose regulation reliably confirms the diagnosis of hypoglycemia, and no combination of tests reliably establishes the mechanism of hypoglycemia.

Treatment

Long-term treatment for specific types of hypoglycemia is outlined in Table 22–8. Acute treatment is usually necessary prior to definitive diagnosis and includes:

A. Glucose:

1. Infuse 10–20% dextrose via peripheral vein, at a constant rate, maintaining a blood glucose level that controls central nervous system symptoms (eg, 30 mg/dL in newborns and 40–50 mg/dL in children). If hyperinsulinemia is suspected or is a possibility, avoid bolus ("push") infusions of concentrated dextrose solutions. (Fifty percent dextrose solutions are seldom necessary for use during infancy and childhood.)

2. Instruct the patient's family to give glucose as follows if the patient is unconscious and a physician is not available: Place Insta-Glucose between the child's cheek and gums or under the tongue. If there is no response in 10 minutes, give an initial deep intramuscular injection of glucagon, usually 0.5 mL (0.5 mg). If there is no response, wait 10 more minutes and inject an additional 0.5 mL of glucagon.

3. If a diagnosis of hypoglycemia not due to hyperinsulinism has been established, carbohydrates can be safely administered via any route without risk of hypoglycemic rebound.

4. If a diabetic patient is unconscious and a diagnosis of coma or insulin reaction is impossible or in doubt, give 50% glucose intravenously, up to 1 mL/kg. This will definitely overcome the insulin reaction and will not harm the patient with diabetic acidosis.

B. Drugs:

1. In general, drug therapy should be employed only after a definite diagnosis (Table 22–8) is established.

Table 22–8. Hypoglycemia.

Classification	Clinical and Laboratory Findings	Treatment
I. Antenatal period disorders (1) Fetal malnutrition (placental insufficiency) (2) Sepsis Offspring of diabetic mothers Erythroblastosis fetalis (3) Neonatal cold injury (4) Hypoglycemia, cardiomegaly, and pulmonary edema	Offspring of diabetic mothers and infants with erythroblastosis fetalis may have hyperinsulinemia with rebound hypoglycemia to insulinogenic stimuli; blood ratios of insulin to glucose are elevated. The other conditions listed have in common depleted hepatic glycogen and fat stores and fasting hypoglycemia.	Infusion of 10–20% glucose by peripheral vein. Frequent oral feedings. Avoidance or cautious administration of insulinogenic agents (eg, arginine, 50% dextrose) in hyperinsulinism states.
II. Hyperinsulin states (1) Islet cell hyperplasia (2) Islet cell adenoma or adenocarcinoma (3) Islet cell nesidioblastosis (4) Leucine sensitivity (5) Beckwith-Wiedemann syndrome	As a whole, this group is prone to fasting hypoglycemia and rebound hypoglycemia to insulinogenic stimuli. Diagnosis is dependent on finding of abnormally elevated insulin or proinsulin levels during the fasting state or following insulin provocation with glucose, amino acids (ie, leucine, arginine), glucagon, or tolbutamide (1–5); or finding of clinical characteristics of the EMG triad, ie, exomphalos, macroglossia, and gigantism with abdominal organomegaly (5).	(1) Avoidance of insulinogenic stimuli. (2) Catecholamines or diazoxide (or both). (3) A diet low in simple sugars and, sometimes, low in leucine. (4) Pancreatectomy.
III. Ketotic hypoglycemia	Findings include a history of low birth weight for gestational age; onset between ages 1 and 6 yr; and triad of hypoglycemia, ketosis, and blunted glycemic response to glucagon. Patients may have abnormalities in gluconeogenesis with abnormalities in hepatic handling of alanine during a fast.	Frequent feedings with diet high in carbohydrates and protein. Avoid periods of prolonged fasting.

IV. Idiopathic spontaneous hypoglycemia	Fasting hypoglycemia occurs within the first 2 yr of life in 90% of cases. There is no determinable cause.	Frequent feedings with diet high in carbohydrates.
V. Primary neurologic disorders ("central")	Hypoglycemia is frequently observed in children with neurologic disorders of various types. No definite pattern or consistent metabolic abnormality has been demonstrated, although hyperinsulinemia has not been a feature.	Frequent feedings. Anticonvulsants when indicated.
VI. Metabolic disorders (1) Liver glycogen storage disease (2) Liver glycogen synthetase deficiency (3) Fructose intolerance (4) Maple syrup urine disease (5) Deficiency of liver 1,6-diphosphatase activity	Definitive diagnosis is dependent on enzyme determination. Blunted hyperglycemia response to glucagon (1, 2, and 5), history of hypoglycemia after fructose ingestion (3), and a characteristic odor (4) are helpful for diagnosis.	(1 and 2) Frequent feedings with diet high in carbohydrates. Hyperalimentation. Portacaval diversion in severe type 1 glycogen storage disease may be indicated. (3 and 4) Rigid avoidance of offending substrate.
VII. Endocrine insufficiency syndromes (1) Hypopituitarism (2) Hypopituitarism and hyperinsulinemia (3) Adrenocortical insufficiency (4) Adrenomedullary insufficiency (Broberger-Zetterström syndrome) (5) Congenital hypothyroidism (6) Glucagon deficiency	Definitive diagnosis is dependent on biochemical establishment of hormone deficiency. History of failure to thrive, growth retardation, and features of hypopituitarism (1 and 2), excessive tanning (3), and abnormal weight for gestational age (4) are helpful for diagnosis.	Replacement of deficient hormone or hormones.
VIII. Severe malnutrition states (1) Chronic diarrhea (2) Liver disease	Characteristics include fasting hypoglycemia and depleted glycogen and fat stores.	Nutritional rehabilitation.

2. If the cardiorespiratory status permits, catecholamines (oral ephedrine sulfate; subcutaneous epinephrine in oil [Sus-Phrine]) may be useful and have the unique advantage in the undiagnosed case of avoiding insulin stimulation.

3. Corticosteroids, corticotropin, and glucagon may be helpful in controlling hypoglycemia, but they may stimulate insulin production, and the action of glucagon in neonates is unpredictable (see Appendix for dosage).

4. In severe chronic hyperinsulinism states, an oral preparation of diazoxide is useful. Diazoxide, a nondiuretic benzothiadiazine, may be of value in controlling chronic idiopathic hypoglycemia and certain cases of hyperinsulinism, including leucine-sensitive hypoglycemia. The dosage has varied from 5 to 20 mg/kg/d. Side effects include hypertrichosis, advancement of epiphyseal maturation, hyperuricemia, fluid retention, neutropenia, and depression of immunoglobulin G. Failure of adequate response to therapy with diazoxide should prompt consideration of subtotal pancreatectomy.

5. Sedatives and anticonvulsant therapy may be helpful to reduce convulsions and neuromuscular irritability. (Phenytoin has the added effect of reducing insulin stimulation.)

C. Diet: In leucine-sensitive patients, a low-leucine diet is indicated. In patients with ketotic hypoglycemia, provide a liberal carbohydrate diet and place a moderate restriction on ketogenic foods.

1. Give no concentrated forms of carbohydrate; these should be avoided because they will stimulate the pancreas to elaborate insulin. Rapidly utilized carbohydrates should be replaced by slow-acting ones.

2. Give small frequent feedings (6 or more meals a day). It may be necessary to feed the patient at regular intervals throughout the 24 hours and to give small carbohydrate feedings 30–45 minutes after regular meals.

D. Surgical Measures: Surgical removal of a portion of the pancreas (or of a tumor if present) should be undertaken for any individual who cannot be controlled by the above measures.

Prognosis

Excellent results have been reported in some treated patients with the idiopathic form of the disease and following removal of a tumor. Otherwise, the results depend on the underlying condition.

• • •

GALACTOSEMIA

Galactosemia is an autosomal hereditary (recessive) disease due to congenital absence of the activity of the enzyme galactose-1-phosphate uridyl transferase, which is necessary to convert galactose 1-phosphate to glucose 1-phosphate. There is decreased activity of the enzyme in heterozygous individuals. Galactosemia is characterized by feeding difficulties, hepatomegaly with or without splenomegaly, cataracts, mental retardation (not universal), and jaundice during the neonatal period. Pseudotumor cerebri may occur. Other findings include hypoglycemia (*total* reducing substance in blood may be normal or even elevated), galactosuria, aminoaciduria, proteinuria, and increased levels of galactose 1-phosphate in erythrocytes. A screening test is available to diagnose the condition during the newborn period.

A second form of galactosemia is due to galactokinase deficiency and does not affect the liver, kidneys, or central nervous system. However, cataracts may develop in patients during the first few months of life.

Treatment consists of excluding galactose (especially milk and its derivatives) from the diet. This prevents development of the signs and symptoms of the disease or may result in improvement after they have developed. A more normal diet may be tolerated later in childhood. Administration of progesterone may minimize progression of cataract formation and mental deficiency.

The mother of a known galactosemic child should be on a restricted galactose diet during subsequent pregnancies.

GLYCOGEN STORAGE DISEASE

There are numerous types of glycogen storage diseases. The following is a partial listing:

Type I, Von Gierke's Disease: Type I, the most common glycogen storage disease, is an autosomal recessive disorder that involves the liver and kidneys. It may be associated with debranching enzyme deficiency. It starts at birth or in early infancy and is characterized by anorexia, weight loss, vomiting, convulsions, and coma. Organomegaly of the liver and kidneys, growth retardation, obesity with a "doll-like" appearance, and bleeding tendencies may be noted. Cardiac failure, intermittent cyanosis, muscular weakness, neurologic abnormalities, hepatic cirrhosis, and marked enlargement of the tongue may occur in some cases. Laboratory findings include a deficiency in glucose-6-phosphatase, flat epinephrine and glucagon tolerance curves, elevated blood lactic and pyruvic acid levels, and abnormal glycogen deposition in the liver. Findings may also include acetonuria, hypoglycemia, hyperlipemia, and impaired glucose tolerance with insulinopenia. Treatment includes frequent high-carbohydrate feedings, sometimes including nighttime intragastric tube feedings. Portacaval shunts have been shown to be helpful in some patients. The prognosis is variable.

Type II, Pompe's Disease (Generalized Glycogenosis): Findings include muscle weakness, cardiomegaly, macroglossia, hepatomegaly, normal mental development, and deficiency of the lysosomal enzyme α1,4-glucosidase.

Type III, Cori's Disease: Type III involves the liver, striated muscle, and red blood cells. The clinical features are similar to those of type I but less severe. A defect in debranching enzymes (amylo-1,6-glucosidase or oligo-1,4-glucantransferase) and hepatomegaly may be present.

Type IV, Andersen's Disease (Amylopectinosis): Findings include abnormal levels of glycogen in the liver and reticuloendothelial system, diminished response to glucagon and epinephrine, a defect in the branching enzyme (amylo-1:4, 1:6-transglucosidase), hepatosplenomegaly, cirrhosis, ascites, and normal mental development.

Type V, McArdle's Syndrome: Type V involves the skeletal muscle. There is a defect in muscle phosphorylase.

Type VI, Hers' Disease: Type VI is clinically similar to type I but less severe. There is a deficiency in liver phosphorylase.

Type VII: Other types involve reduced activity of phosphoglucomutase, phosphofructokinase, or phosphohexoisomerase. Findings include weak muscles, partial defect of other glycolytic enzymes, and elevated levels of SGOT, serum aldolase, and phosphocreatine kinase.

PHENYLKETONURIA
(Phenylpyruvic Oligophrenia)

Phenylketonuria is a hereditary (recessive) familial disease usually caused by a deficiency of phenylalanine hydroxylase.

Clinical Findings

Affected children (most often blond and blue-eyed) appear normal at birth but soon develop vomiting, irritability, a peculiar odor, patchy eczematous lesions of the skin, convulsions, schizoid personality, and abnormal findings on EEG. Mentality is retarded. (An occasional patient may have normal intelligence without treatment.) Affected children are hyperactive, with erratic behavior. Perspiration is excessive. Serum and urinary phenylalanine levels are markedly high as determined by ferric chloride test, Phenistix paper strip, or Guthrie bacterial inhibition assay (of particular value in young infants). Some normal infants, particularly those with physiologic jaundice of the newborn, may have transiently elevated (> 6 mg/dL) blood levels of phenylalanine. Orthohydroxyphenylacetic acid is usually present in the urine.

Treatment

A diet low in phenylalanine (58 ± 18 mg/kg) should be instituted to keep plasma phenylalanine levels between 5 and 10 mg/dL; when started in patients during the first weeks of life, this diet prevents severe retardation. It has also been shown that it is possible to breast-feed an infant in combination with giving a milk substitute that is deficient in phenylalanine. The diet should be titrated against the nutritional status of the child and the serum phenylalanine levels to ensure that the diet is restricted enough to prevent manifestations of the disease but liberal enough to prevent hypophenylalaninemia with resultant malnutrition and cerebral damage. It is now generally recommended that weekly serum phenylalanine assays be done during the first year of life. In established cases, proper diet may arrest the condition and produce improvement in personality and in symptoms other than the mental deficiency. It may be discontinued after several years.

The blood phenylalanine levels of phenylketonuric females should be maintained in the normal range during the childbearing years to decrease the risk of abnormalities (eg, growth and mental retardation, microcephaly) in their offspring who may be nonphenylketonuric.

Hyperphenylalaninemia may be a transient phenomenon in some newborns who have normal urinary metabolites and do not require treatment.

23 | Neoplastic Diseases & Reticuloendothelioses*

Cancer in children differs biologically from cancer in adults. (See Fig 23–1.) Neoplastic disease is the second leading cause of death in the pediatric age group in the USA. Solid tumors represent 60% of cases and acute leukemia the remaining 40%.

NEUROFIBROMATOSIS
(Von Recklinghausen's Disease)

Neurofibromatosis is a hereditary autosomal dominant disorder characterized by the gradual development of numerous pedunculated soft tissue tumors. It is frequently associated with small areas of skin pigmentation (café au lait spots) and sometimes with mental deficiency. Lesions are found in the skin and subcutaneous tissues (mollusca fibrosa), bones, peripheral nerves (neurofibromas), and the spinal canal. Neurofibromas are formed in the sheaths of the peripheral nerves and may rarely undergo malignant degeneration to form sarcomas. Glioma of the central nervous system is frequently associated with neurofibromatosis.

Clinical Findings

Skin lesions are of 2 types: (1) areas of smooth-bordered brown discoloration (café au lait spots) and (2) multiple fibromas. Many findings are caused by pressure on adjacent structures. Their location and size determine the severity of symptoms. There may be loss of function of the area supplied by a nerve that is compressed, or there may be sensory and motor changes due to compression on spinal cord roots. Eighth nerve involvement is common.

Treatment

Localized lesions may be excised to relieve pressure. Recurrences are frequent. Tumors that have undergone malignant degeneration may be treated with chemotherapy (doxorubicin and dacarbazine) and may show transient response.

*Revised with the assistance of David G. Tubergen, MD, and Raleigh Bowden, MD.

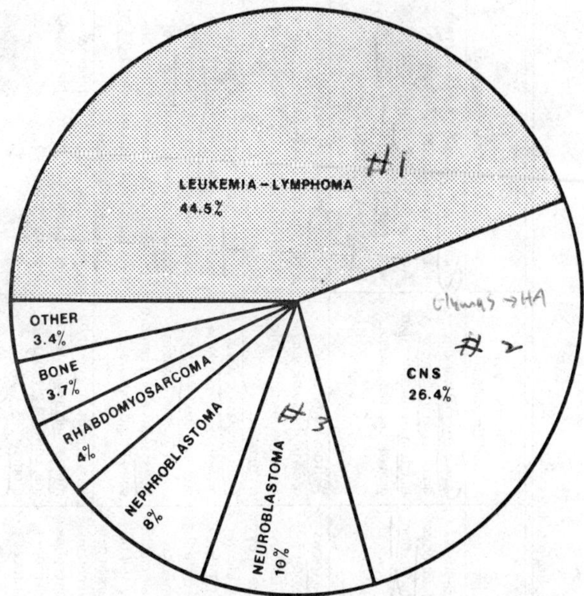

Figure 23–1. Relative frequencies of malignancies in childhood. (Tumor experience at Children's Hospital, Denver, from 1931 to October 1, 1972. Total cases: 867. Courtesy of B Favara, MD.)

Course & Prognosis

The prognosis for life varies, depending on the presence or absence of malignant degeneration and pressure symptoms. Patients with peripheral neurofibromas are generally devoid of serious complications and have a good prognosis. However, in the presence of associated intraspinal or intracranial tumors, the prognosis is poor.

BRAIN TUMORS

(See Table 23–1.)

Over 75% of brain tumors of childhood are gliomas. Almost all of these are characteristically found in the posterior fossa. The most prominent general symptom of central nervous system tumor of childhood is headache. The 2 most prominent physical findings are enlargement of the head and papilledema.

Table 23–1. Brain tumors.

Part Affected	Symptoms and Signs	Radiologic Findings	Tumor Type and Characteristics	Treatment and Prognosis
Brain stem	Cranial nerve palsies (IX–X, VII, VI, V; chiefly sensory root). Pyramidal tract signs (hemiparesis). Cerebellar ataxia. Rarely, signs of increased intracranial pressure or emaciation.	CT scan of posterior fossa shows displacement of cerebral aqueduct and fourth ventricle. Calcifications may be present.	Astrocytoma (varying grades; polar spongioblastoma): usually rapid growth and recurrence.	X-ray therapy to site; remission rate for short periods. Prognosis grave. Average survival 1 yr, particularly when medulla is involved. 25% of patients survive 5 yr.
Cerebellum and fourth ventricle	Evidence of increased intracranial pressure.* Cerebellar signs.† Signs due to pressure on adjacent structures.‡ Personality and behavioral changes. Occasionally, emaciation.	CT scan of posterior fossa shows displacement or obliteration of fourth ventricle and resultant hydrocephalus; mural nodule of cystic astrocytoma is usually identified. Contrast-enhanced CT demonstrates even better the differing densities of tumors common to this region and shows their calcification. Angiography may still be needed to visualize tumors in cerebellopontine angle or cerebellar hemangioblastoma. Air encephalography is also used to demonstrate cerebellopontine or low vermis lesions.	Astrocytoma: slow growth, frequently cystic (depends on histology of tumor).	Surgical removal. Follow by intensive x-ray therapy if removal is incomplete. Prognosis good if removal complete.
			Medulloblastoma: rapid growth; seen mostly in children age 2–6 yr; about 75% of cases in boys; seeds along cerebrospinal fluid pathways.	Surgical decompression of posterior fossa and x-ray therapy to site, cerebrum, and spinal canal. Chemotherapy. Shunt (ventriculopleural, etc) for relief of cerebrospinal fluid obstruction. Prognosis guarded. 50% of patients survive 5 yr.
			Less common: ependymoma, hemangioblastoma, choroid plexus papilloma.	Surgical cure possible with hemangioblastoma and choroid plexus papilloma.

Cerebral hemispheres and lateral ventricles	Evidence of increased intracranial pressure.* Seizures (generalized, psychomotor, focal) in about 40% of cases. Neurologic deficits, including hemiparesis (40% of cases), visual field defects, ataxia, personality changes.	CT scan is highly diagnostic (nearly 100% of cases) and shows edema, ventricular deformation, shift. Increased density with contrast enhancement correlates with vascularity of lesion. Tumors as small as 0.5 cm in diameter may be detected.	Gliomas: primary astrocytomas; glioblastomas in 10% of cases. Meningiomas rare. Leptomeningeal sarcoma.	Surgical biopsy or excision where possible. X-ray treatment. Prognosis varies with tumor type. Chemotherapy gaining in trial and usage.
			Ependymoma and choroid plexus papilloma.	Surgical excision of choroid plexus papilloma. Occasionally, hydrocephalus persists and requires shunt.
Diencephalon	Emaciation; good intake. Often, very active and euphoric. Few neurologic findings (occasionally, vertical nystagmus, tremor, ataxia). Pale; without anemia. Frequently, eosinophilia, decreased T_4 and pituitary reserve.	CT scan shows defect in floor of third ventricle and other midline findings.	Usually astrocytomas; less common, oligodendroglioma, glioma, ependymoma, glioblastoma.	X-ray therapy. Shunt for relief of cerebrospinal fluid obstruction. Prognosis variable; generally poor.
Midbrain and third ventricle	Personality and behavioral changes, often early. Evidence of increased intracranial pressure.* Pyramidal tract signs. Cerebellar signs.† Inability to rotate eyes upward. Sudden loss of consciousness. Rarely, seizures.	CT scan shows displacement or obliteration of third ventricle and resultant hydrocephalus. Pineal is rarely calcified in children.	Astrocytomas, teratomas including pinealoma (macrogenitosomia praecox in boys), ependymoma.	Shunt (ventriculocisternal, etc) for relief of cerebrospinal fluid obstruction. Intensive x-ray therapy. Prognosis poor.
			Choroid plexus papilloma and colloid cyst (rare).	Surgical removal. Prognosis good if removal is complete.

*Evidence of increased intracranial pressure includes headache, vomiting (often without nausea and before breakfast), diplopia, blurred vision, papilledema. Personality changes, including irritability, apathy, disturbances in sleep and eating patterns, are frequent. Sudden enlargement of the head if head circumferences have been plotted is detectable when sutures are still open or after sutures have split. Alterations of consciousness and stiff neck with tonsillar herniation may be seen.

†Cerebellar signs include ataxia, dysmetria, and nystagmus. Truncal ataxia in the absence of lateralizing signs is most common in vermis tumors.

‡Signs due to pressure on adjacent structures may include head tilting, cranial nerve signs, pyramidal tract signs, suboccipital tenderness, and stiff neck.

Table 23–1 (cont'd). Brain tumors.

Part Affected	Symptoms and Signs	Radiologic Findings	Tumor Type and Characteristics	Treatment and Prognosis
Suprasellar region	Visual disorders (visual field defects, optic atrophy). Hypothalamic disorders (including diabetes insipidus, adiposity). Pituitary disorders (growth arrest, hypothyroidism, delayed sexual maturation). Evidence of increased intracranial pressure.*	Skull films show suprasellar calcification (about 90% of cases), deformity of sella turcica (frequent), and enlarged optic foramens in optic gliomas. CT scan shows deformity and obliteration of suprasellar cistern; shows hydrocephalus if foramens of Monro blocked. Optic nerves are thickened in optic glioma and may show calcification. CT scan may miss cystic craniopharyngioma, isodense with brain. Use air encephalography if craniopharyngioma is suspected clinically (not shown by CT scan).	Optic glioma: high incidence of café au lait spots; feet and hands may be large in infants and young children if the diencephalon is involved.	X-ray if optic chiasm is involved. Surgical removal if only one optic nerve is involved. Conservative approach advised. Prognosis fair to good.
			Craniopharyngioma: often dormant for years.	Complete excision of craniopharyngioma, with hormone replacement, now often feasible; or drainage of cyst and irradiation. Prognosis good if removal is complete. Repeated surgery often necessary if complete removal cannot be achieved.

*Evidence of increased intracranial pressure includes headache, vomiting (often without nausea and before breakfast), diplopia, blurred vision, papilledema. Personality changes, including irritability, apathy, disturbances in sleep and eating patterns, are frequent. Sudden enlargement of the head if head circumferences have been plotted is detectable when sutures are still open or after sutures have split. Alterations of consciousness and stiff neck with tonsillar herniation may be seen.

†Cerebellar signs include ataxia, dysmetria, and nystagmus. Truncal ataxia in the absence of lateralizing signs is most common in vermis tumors.

‡Signs due to pressure on adjacent structures may include head tilting, cranial nerve signs, pyramidal tract signs, suboccipital tenderness, and stiff neck.

In the newborn, the various forms of hydrocephalus are the most common causes of abnormal enlargement, but tumors may cause enlargement. If abnormal skull enlargement occurs in children between 2 months and 1 year of age, subdural hematoma is more likely responsible. The most common cause of abnormal increase in the size of the head after 1 year of age is tumor.

Diagnostic Points

An elevated white blood cell count and a rapid sedimentation rate, even in the absence of fever, suggest a diagnosis of pyogenic brain abscess rather than neoplasm.

Papilledema occurs in internal hydrocephalus due to brain tumor but not in idiopathic internal hydrocephalus.

The "cracked pot" percussion note elicited in internal hydrocephalus (Macewen's sign) has previously been considered diagnostic of this condition, but it is also present in subdural hematoma and in some normal children with open sutures.

Differential Diagnosis of Intracranial Lesions

The entire symptom complex of an intracranial space-consuming lesion, including vomiting, increase in intracranial pressure, and papilledema, can be caused by lesions that are not neoplastic. The principal ones are granulomatous abscess (including tuberculoma), pyogenic abscess, hemorrhage (subdural hematoma), central nervous system infections, and venous sinus thrombosis.

TUMORS OF THE SOFT TISSUE

The most common malignant soft tissue tumor seen in children is rhabdomyosarcoma. The child usually presents with a firm mass on an extremity, in the head and neck region, or in the pelvic area. Patients should be evaluated by use of skeletal survey; intravenous urograms; chest x-ray with oblique views; bone marrow aspiration and biopsy; and liver function tests, including creatine phosphokinase, lactate dehydrogenase, blood urea nitrogen, and uric acid. Treatment consists of en bloc surgical resection when possible, followed by high-energy radiation therapy of 4000–6000 rads over a period of 5–8 weeks. Chemotherapy with vincristine, dactinomycin, and cyclophosphamide, with the addition of doxorubicin in advanced stages, is used for 1–2 years.

Fibrosarcomas and liposarcomas are rare lesions and should be surgically excised when possible. Electron beam therapy (4000–6000 rads) has also been used.

Benign tumors are slow-growing and nontender. Most commonly seen are the fibromas and lipomas. These may be excised if they are symptomatic.

TUMORS OF BONE

The most frequent age group seen with a malignant bone tumor is the preadolescent, adolescent, and young adult group. Osteosarcoma, Ewing's sarcoma, chondrosarcoma, fibrosarcoma, and synovial sarcoma may all present with a painful mass, limitation of motion, and x-ray changes in the bones involved. Metastatic disease contraindicates radical surgery and should be sought prior to planning therapy. Survival rates with surgery alone have been poor; 5–15% 5-year survivals are reported. These tumors tend to spread to lungs, soft tissues, and other bones. Patients with Ewing's tumor have had an increase in survival rate in recent years with radiation therapy, 5000 rads to the entire bone, along with vincristine, cyclophosphamide, and doxorubicin chemotherapy. Amputation is usually not done, but the entire bone may be removed if the tumor involves a bone such as the clavicle or a rib.

Survival rates for patients with osteosarcoma did not change with surgical amputation alone, but significant improvement has resulted from the combination of aggressive surgery, irradiation, and multiple-drug chemotherapy. The most effective chemotherapeutic agents are high-dose methotrexate with leucovorin rescue and doxorubicin.

Many fibrous, cartilaginous, and osseous benign tumors are seen. Some have classic x-ray findings; others should be excised to rule out the possibility of a malignant tumor.

Osteoid osteoma is a relatively common benign tumor of bone in adolescents and young adults. It is characterized by pain, limp (if the lower extremity is involved), atrophy of muscle, normal laboratory findings, and prompt and dramatic relief of pain in response to aspirin.

OTHER TUMORS

WILMS' TUMOR
(Nephroblastoma)

The most common abdominal masses encountered in early childhood are hydronephrosis, neuroblastoma, and Wilms' tumor. Wilms' tumor is believed to be embryonal in origin, develops within parenchyma, and enlarges with distortion and invasion of adjacent renal tissue. This tumor may be associated with congenital anomalies such as hemihypertrophy, aniridia, ambiguous genitalia, hypospadias, undescended testes, duplications of ureters or kidneys, horseshoe kidney, multiple nevi, and Beckwith's syndrome.

Clinical Findings

A. Symptoms and Signs: Symptoms include abdominal mass, malaise, flank pain, fever, and pallor. A solid or (rarely) cystic, nontender, firm mass is present in the flank. It rarely crosses the midline but may be bilateral in 2% of patients. Hematuria is rare as compared to renal tumors in the adult. Hypertension is unusual.

B. Laboratory Findings: Results of urinalysis are usually normal, but hematuria or pyuria may be found if trauma or infection has occurred within the tumor mass. Blood urea nitrogen levels are usually normal; uric acid and erythropoietin levels may be increased.

C. X-Ray Findings: A soft tissue mass may be seen on a plain film of the abdomen, and calcification may occur in a marginal concentric fashion. Hepatomegaly may be present if the liver has extensive metastases. Intravenous urography may show distortion and displacement of the renal pelvis and calices in any direction; hydronephrosis may also be present. Chest x-ray may reveal metastases; oblique views are often helpful.

Treatment

Surgical excision of the mass after clinical staging is the treatment of choice. A transabdominal approach is essential to allow adequate mobilization, prevent excess manipulation of the tumor, and allow examination of abdominal viscera, nodes, and the opposite kidney. Conservative surgery is appropriate when bilateral disease occurs with nephroblastoma.

Radiation therapy to the tumor bed should be given postoperatively with megavoltage equipment in dosages of 2000–3500 rads depending upon the age of the patient and the stage of the tumor. Radiation therapy is not needed for tumors confined entirely within the kidney. If the tumor is ruptured, the entire abdomen should be treated, with the remaining kidney properly shielded.

Adjunctive chemotherapy with dactinomycin and vincristine (adding doxorubicin in advanced stages) has increased survival rates.

Prognosis

The 2-year survival rate is better in children under 2 years of age with localized disease. Survival rates are improving where radiation and chemotherapy are used concurrently, and the overall 5-year survival rate is now about 80%.

NEUROBLASTOMA

Neuroblastoma is a tumor arising from cells in the sympathetic ganglia and adrenal medulla. It is the third most frequent pediatric neoplasm. The tumors may spontaneously regress in 5–10% of cases. The prognosis is much better in a child under 1 year of age. Presentation in the abdominal area carries a poor prognosis. This tumor may be seen in the newborn period; the highest incidence is at 2 years of age.

Clinical Findings

A. Symptoms and Signs: General symptoms include failure to thrive, anorexia, black eyes, fever of unknown origin, diarrhea, hypertension, pallor, irritability, and masses.

1. Cervical tumors–Tumors commonly present with a mass in the neck and may be associated with Horner's syndrome.

2. Thoracic tumors–Tumors may present with respiratory symptoms such as cough, croup, dysphagia, and fatigue.

3. Abdominal tumors–Tumors may cause abdominal swelling from adrenal or paraspinal tumor. They may be very large and cross the midline or may be deep and difficult to palpate. Other findings include abdominal pain, change in bowel habits, delay in walking, paraplegia, or shock if a large tumor is ruptured.

B. Laboratory Findings: Anemia or pancytopenia may be secondary to marrow involvement with tumor and thus present a myelophthisic picture, or it may be due to dietary factors. Bone marrow may reveal classic rosettes or sheets of anaplastic neuroblasts. The patient should be placed on a restricted catecholamine diet and a 24-hour urine collected for catecholamine levels. Urinary cystathionine should also be measured. Blood urea nitrogen and uric acid as well as liver function should be evaluated as baseline studies.

C. X-Ray Findings: Multiple destructive lesions of bone with a "moth-eaten" appearance may be seen in all bones. Pathologic fracture may also occur.

1. Thoracic tumors–Chest x-ray shows soft tissue areas with clear borders and scattered calcifications close to the spine and in the upper chest. There may be erosion and separation of posterior ribs.

2. Abdominal tumors–Abdominal x-ray reveals a soft tissue mass in the region of the adrenal gland or along the spine. Many tumors show calcification. Intravenous urograms reveal downward and lateral displacement of the kidney.

Treatment

The most important variable in therapy is age. For children under 1 year, a conservative approach with surgery, irradiation, and chemotherapy is best. For older children with localized disease, the whole tumor or as much as possible should be removed, sometimes after shrinkage with chemotherapy or irradiation. Combination chemotherapy is effective in control of disseminated neuroblastoma and should be given aggressively if skeletal metastases are present. The most effective drugs are cyclophosphamide, vincristine, and doxorubicin. So far, chemotherapy has not significantly increased the survival rate. Immunotherapeutic measures and agents that enhance maturation of the tumor are being explored.

Course & Prognosis

Localized tumor that is surgically removed carries a good prognosis. Unfortunately, in children over age 2 years, two-thirds present with metastatic disease, and the prognosis is grave.

ADRENOCORTICAL TUMORS

Tumors of the adrenal cortex are characterized by the excessive production of hormones that, in turn, cause marked physiologic and anatomic changes. Metastases may be local or pulmonary and usually occur relatively early in the disease.

GANGLIONEUROMA

Ganglioneuroma is a functional neurogenic tumor that may cause chronic severe diarrhea owing to an increase in circulating norepinephrine and epinephrine. Renal acidosis and the celiac syndrome may also occur. Urinary levels of vanillylmandelic acid and vanilphenylethylamine are elevated.

PHEOCHROMOCYTOMA
(Chromaffinoma)

(See Chapter 22.)

LEUKEMIAS IN CHILDHOOD

Most leukemias (97.5%) in childhood are acute. The most common types are lymphoblastic, undifferentiated, myelomonocytic, and myeloblastic. Forms with normal or reduced white blood counts (aleukemic or hypoplastic) occur in about one-third of patients. The highest incidence of leukemia occurs in patients between 2 and 5 years of age. There is an increased risk of leukemia in patients with chromosomal abnormalities or immune deficiency states.

Clinical Findings

A. Symptoms and Signs: Initial signs and symptoms may include anemia, fever, weakness, bleeding, and bone or joint pain or swelling. Purpura is common. Lymphadenopathy and hepatosplenomegaly may be prominent, particularly in patients with high white blood counts. Central nervous system infiltration may cause manifestations simulating meningitis and may be associated with findings of pleocytosis, increased protein levels, and lowered glucose levels in cerebrospinal fluid. Septicemia may occur during the course of the disease.

B. Laboratory Findings:

1. Blood–Red blood counts and hemoglobin levels are usually low. Normochromic normocytic anemia is generally seen, and normoblasts are occasionally seen. The white blood count may be elevated, normal, or reduced. In some cases, large numbers of abnormal cells are seen; in others, especially with leukopenia, the leukocytes appear entirely normal. Thrombocytopenia is very frequent.

2. Bone marrow–In almost all cases, 50–98% of nucleated cells are blast forms with marked reduction in the normal erythroid, myeloid, and platelet precursors.

3. Chromosomes–A variety of chromosome abnormalities have been reported in all forms of leukemia.

4. Serum–Levels of uric acid and lactate dehydrogenase are usually elevated.

5. Cerebrospinal fluid–Pleocytosis (consisting of blast forms), elevated levels of protein, and decreased levels of glucose may be seen.

Treatment of Acute Leukemias

Present-day treatment of leukemia is complex, multimodal, and multidisciplinary and should, if possible, be carried out in centers specializing in the care of children with neoplastic diseases.

A. Specific Measures:

1. Acute lymphoblastic or undifferentiated leukemia–Most patients (85–95%) achieve complete remission following treatment with vincristine, prednisone, asparaginase, and intrathecal methotrexate.

2. Central nervous system leukemia–Because of the significant incidence of central nervous system leukemia (50%), some patients should be treated prophylactically with intrathecal methotrexate or central nervous system irradiation (or both), despite the risk of complicating encephalopathy.

3. Maintenance–Continuation or maintenance therapy lasts 2–3 years, with oral mercaptopurine and methotrexate as mainstays of treatment. Other drugs may be used on a periodic basis.

4. Relapse–If the disease recurs, another remission may be induced with selected combinations of the above drugs or other antineoplastic agents.

B. General Measures: Give transfusions of packed red blood cells and platelets as needed. Treat infections with antibiotics. Regulate diet and activity as needed or tolerated by the patient. Hyperuricemia due to the degradation of nucleic acid purines may occur, especially following the initiation of antileukemic therapy. Allopurinol (Zyloprim), 100–150 mg/m² orally twice daily, is effective in reducing the hyperuricemia. Urinary alkalinization (with intravenous fluids) and mannitol diuresis may also be of value. Pain due to leukemic infiltration of bone may be relieved by local x-ray radiation.

Course & Prognosis

Aggressive combination chemotherapy and supportive therapy with blood products and antibiotics have contributed to improved survival. As many as 90% of children with acute lymphocytic leukemia will achieve remission within 1 month of starting therapy, and long-term "cure" rates are between 50 and 60%. Children with nonlymphocytic leukemia have a somewhat poorer prognosis. Conventional chemotherapy and bone marrow transplants, when possible, may contribute to the increasing survival seen in this group of children.

HODGKIN'S DISEASE

Hodgkin's disease occurs twice as frequently in men as in women, with its peak incidence in the third decade. It has been reported in children as young as 3 years of age. The cause is not known. The clinical staging and histologic classification are shown in Tables 23–2 and 23–3.

Clinical Findings

A. Symptoms and Signs: Variable degrees of anorexia, weight loss, fatigue, weakness, fever, malaise, pruritus, night sweats, and pain on ingestion of alcohol are noted. The most common site of nodal involvement is the cervical region. Involved nodes are usually firm and nontender and may produce pressure symptoms depending upon their location, which may be anywhere. Hepatosplenomegaly and extranodal disease in any organ may be present.

B. Laboratory Findings: Hematologic findings may be normal or may show anemia, leukocytosis, leukopenia, thrombocytosis, thrombocytopenia, eosinophilia, or elevated sedimentation rate. Kidney and liver function tests or scans may reflect abnormalities if these organs are involved with disease. Immunologic defects as a reflection of abnormalities of the cell-mediated immune responses may be seen in delayed hypersensitivity to PPD, candidal extract, and streptokinase skin test antigens. Hemolytic anemia and abnormal levels of immunoglobulins may also occur. The diagnosis of Hodgkin's disease is confirmed by biopsy of the involved node followed by bone marrow biopsy, clinical

Table 23–2. Histologic classification of Hodgkin's disease.*

Designation	Distinctive Features	Relative Frequency
Lymphocyte depletion	Reed-Sternberg and malignant mononuclear cells usually, though not always, numerous; marked paucity of lymphocytes; diffuse fibrosis and necrosis may be present.	5–15%
Lymphocyte predominance	Abundant stroma of mature lymphocytes, histiocytes, or both; no necrosis; Reed-Sternberg cells may be sparse.	10–15%
Mixed cellularity	Usually numerous Reed-Sternberg and atypical mononuclear cells with a pleomorphic admixture of plasma cells, eosinophils, lymphocytes, and fibroblasts; foci of necrosis commonly seen.	20–40%
Nodular sclerosis	Nodules of lymphoid tissue partially or completely separated by bands of doubly refractile collagen of variable width; atypical Reed-Sternberg cells in clear spaces ("lacunae") in the lymphoid nodules.	20–50%

*Reproduced, with permission, from Kempe CH, Silver HK, O'Brien D (editors): *Current Pediatric Diagnosis & Treatment,* 7th ed. Lange, 1982.

Table 23–3. Staging classification for Hodgkin's disease.*
(Ann Arbor classification.)

Designation†	Distinctive Features
Stage I	Involvement of a single lymph node region (I) or a single extralymphatic organ or site (I_E).
Stage II	Involvement of 2 or more lymph node regions on the same side of the diaphragm (II) or localized involvement of an extralymphatic organ or site (II_E).
Stage III	Involvement of lymph node regions on both sides of the diaphragm (III) or localized involvement of an extralymphatic organ or site (III_E) or spleen (III_{SE}).
Stage IV	Diffuse or disseminated involvement of one or more extralymphatic organs with or without associated lymph node involvement. The organs involved should be identified by a symbol.

*Reproduced, with permission, from Kempe CH, Silver HK, O'Brien D (editors): *Current Pediatric Diagnosis & Treatment,* 7th ed. Lange, 1982.

†Stages are also classified as IA, IB, IIA, IIB, etc, on the basis of symptoms and signs: A = asymptomatic; B = fever, sweats, weight loss > 10% of body weight.

staging, and laparotomy with multiple abdominal node biopsies, liver biopsy, and splenectomy.

C. X-Ray Findings: Chest x-rays may show parenchymal or mediastinal nodal disease. Skeletal surveys may show bone involvement. The intravenous urogram may show diversion of the ureter or bladder; a lateral view is often helpful to show anterior displacement. Lymphangiography may reveal a "foamy" enlarged node, which implies tumor filling the node.

Treatment

After proper staging, the patient should receive extended field megavoltage irradiation or involved field irradiation plus chemotherapy if the disease is stage I or IIA. Irradiation and multiple-drug chemotherapy should be given for stage IIB or higher. To minimize side effects, irradiation should be performed by a therapist skilled in the treatment of the growing child. Chemotherapeutic agents commonly employed in combination are vincristine, mechlorethamine or cyclophosphamide, procarbazine, and prednisone. Other effective agents include lomustine (CCNU), vinblastine, bleomycin, and doxorubicin (Table 23–4).

Prognosis

In adequately treated patients, 5-year survival rates have improved greatly. In stages I and II, rates range from 85 to 90%. In stages III and IV, rates range from 50 to 70%.

NON-HODGKIN'S LYMPHOMA

Classification of this diverse group of lymphomas is based on the architecture of the node, on whether the disease is nodular or diffuse, on the cytologic differentiation of lymphocytes and histiocytes, and on the surface membrane markers (T cell, B cell, null cell) of lymphocytes. This group includes the former "lymphosarcomas"—reticulum cell sarcomas or tumors with giant follicular cell patterns.

Burkitt's tumor (African lymphoma) is a special type of childhood lymphoma found principally in Africa. This tumor is responsible for half of all cancer deaths in children in Uganda and Central Africa. A viral cause has been assumed, and Epstein-Barr virus is under scrutiny. The tumor is characterized by (1) predilection for the facial bones and mandible *or* (2) primary involvement of abdominal nodes and viscera and (3) massive proliferation of primitive lymphoreticular cells and phagocytosis on histologic examination. When Burkitt's tumor is seen in patients in the USA, it generally presents as an abdominal tumor.

Table 23–4. Antineoplastic agents.*

Agent	Indications	Toxicity
Asparaginase (Elspar)	Acute lymphoblastic leukemia.	Nausea, vomiting, fever, hypersensitivity, pancreatitis, hyperglycemia.
Bleomycin (Blenoxane)	Hodgkin's disease, non-Hodgkin's lymphoma, testicular tumors.	Nausea, vomiting, stomatitis, fever, chills, pulmonary fibrosis, hyperpigmentation, alopecia.
Carmustine (BCNU)	Malignant gliomas, medulloblastoma, advanced Hodgkin's disease and other sarcomas, neuroblastoma, malignant melanoma.	Nausea, vomiting, hepatotoxicity, chemical dermatitis. Bone marrow depression (3- to 4-wk delay).
Cyclophosphamide (Cytoxan)	Leukemia, Hodgkin's disease, neuroblastoma, sarcomas, retinoblastoma, hepatoma, rhabdomyosarcoma, Ewing's sarcoma.	Nausea, vomiting, anorexia, alopecia, bone marrow depression, hemorrhagic cystitis.
Cytarabine (cytosine arabinoside; Cytosar)	Acute myeloblastic and acute lymphocytic leukemia.	Nausea, vomiting, anorexia, bone marrow depression, hepatotoxicity.
Dactinomycin (Cosmegen)	Wilms' tumor, sarcomas, rhabdomyosarcoma.	Nausea, vomiting, anorexia, bone marrow depression, alopecia. Chemical dermatitis if leakage at intravenous site. Tanning of skin if used with radiation therapy.
Daunorubicin (daunomycin)	Acute myelogenous, monomyelogenous, and monoblastic leukemias.	Same as for doxorubicin (below).
Doxorubicin (Adriamycin)	Acute lymphoblastic and myelocytic leukemia, lymphoma, Hodgkin's disease, Wilms' tumor, neuroblastoma, ovarian or thyroid carcinoma, Ewing's sarcoma, osteogenic sarcoma, rhabdomyosarcoma, other soft tissue sarcomas.	Alopecia, stomatitis, esophagitis, nausea, vomiting. Severe chemical cellulitis and necrosis if extravasated. Bone marrow depression, myocardial damage if dose exceeds 550 mg/m². Monitor ECG.
Fluorouracil (Adrucil)	Hepatoma, gastrointestinal carcinoma.	Nausea, vomiting, oral ulceration, bone marrow depression, gastroenteritis, alopecia, anorexia.

*Since the dosage of these agents varies widely depending on number of drugs used simultaneously, type of tumor being treated, bone marrow reserve, and previous toxicities and therapies (eg, irradiation), the dosages are not given in this handbook. It is best to use a protocol from a major pediatric oncology center or to consult a specialist at such a center to determine safe and effective doses for these agents.

Table 23–4 (cont'd). Antineoplastic agents.*

Agent	Indications	Toxicity
Lomustine (CCNU; CeeNu)	Brain tumors, Hodgkin's disease.	Nausea, vomiting, alopecia, stomatitis, hepatotoxicity. Bone marrow depression (4- to 6-wk delay).
Mechlorethamine (nitrogen mustard)	Hodgkin's disease, non-Hodgkin's lymphoma.	Nausea, vomiting, bone marrow depression, strong vesicating effect on skin and veins.
Mercaptopurine (Purinethol)	Acute myeloblastic and acute lymphocytic leukemia.	Nausea, vomiting, rare oral ulcerations, bone marrow depression.
Methotrexate	Acute lymphocytic leukemia, central nervous system leukemia, lymphoma, choriocarcinoma, brain tumors, Hodgkin's disease.	Oral ulcers, gastrointestinal irritation, bone marrow depression, hepatotoxicity. Do not use in presence of impaired renal function.
Prednisone	Acute myeloblastic and lymphocytic leukemia, lymphoma, Hodgkin's disease, bone pain from metastatic disease, central nervous system tumors.	Increased appetite, sodium retention, hypertension, osteoporosis, provocation of latent diabetes or tuberculosis.
Procarbazine (Matulane)	Hodgkin's disease, lymphoma.	Nausea, vomiting, anorexia. Bone marrow depression (3-wk delay). Do not give with narcotics or sedatives; has "disulfiram effect." Monitor liver and renal function.
Vincristine (Oncovin)	Acute lymphocytic and myeloblastic leukemia, lymphoma, Hodgkin's disease, rhabdomyosarcoma, Wilms' tumor, neuroblastoma, Ewing's sarcoma, retinoblastoma, hepatoma, sarcomas, osteogenic sarcoma, brain tumors.	Alopecia, constipation, abdominal cramps, jaw pain, paresthesia, myalgia, muscle weakness, neurotoxicity, decrease in deep tendon reflexes, chemical dermatitis. Do not use in presence of severe liver impairment.

*Since the dosage of these agents varies widely depending on number of drugs used simultaneously, type of tumor being treated, bone marrow reserve, and previous toxicities and therapies (eg, irradiation), the dosages are not given in this handbook. It is best to use a protocol from a major pediatric oncology center or to consult a specialist at such a center to determine safe and effective doses for these agents.

Clinical Findings

A. Symptoms and Signs: The primary site of involvement differs from that of Hodgkin's disease in its mode of presentation. The gastrointestinal tract in the region of the terminal ileum, cecum, appendix, ascending colon, and mesenteric nodes is the most common site. Boys are more commonly affected than are girls (ratio of 9:1). Acute abdominal pain, intussusception, gastrointestinal tract perforation, and hemorrhage may occur. Involvement of the tonsillar region, cervical nodes, and nasopharynx may be diagnosed by the presence of a mass or compression symptoms. The mediastinum and retroperitoneal nodes may be involved as well as any superficial nodal chain. The incidence of marrow involvement with a leukemialike picture is 20–50% of cases; this is most frequently seen when the mediastinum is the primary site of involvement. Central nervous system involvement is also more common with primary mediastinal lymphoma.

B. Laboratory Findings: These patients should be evaluated as is done for Hodgkin's disease patients, with the exception of routine exploratory laparotomy and splenectomy. Laboratory findings depend on organ, nodal, or marrow involvement. Lumbar puncture with cytocentrifuge examination or brain scan may be helpful in confirming the diagnosis of central nervous system disease.

Treatment

Surgical resection of extranodal disease, when possible, is advocated. If surgical resection is not feasible at diagnosis, the tumor size should be decreased first by chemotherapy with or without irradiation. Multiple-drug chemotherapy should be started as soon as possible and continued for 2–3 years. The drugs most commonly employed are vincristine, cyclophosphamide (especially effective in patients with Burkitt's lymphoma), doxorubicin, prednisone, methotrexate, and bleomycin. In patients at high risk for central nervous system involvement, prophylactic therapy should be given as soon as remission is achieved; therapy consists of cranial irradiation, 2400 rads, and concurrent intrathecal methotrexate. Irradiation to the site of the primary lesion is often part of initial therapy, but many oncologists now reserve its use for tumor areas that do not completely regress with drug therapy.

Prognosis

The prognosis in patients with non-Hodgkin's lymphoma is not as good as that in patients with Hodgkin's disease, and many children die with a conversion to a leukemic phase.

TUMORS OF THE OVARY

Tumors of the ovary constitute only 1% of all childhood tumors. The 3 main types are benign teratoma (dermoid), cysts, and malignant tumors. Granulosa cell tumors may be malignant or benign.

Tumors of the ovary are characterized by an enlarging palpable mass in the lower abdomen or pelvis. Severe abdominal pain may occur owing to a twisted pedicle. Sexual precocity, uterine bleeding, and advanced bone age as a result of excessive estrogen production occur only in patients with granulosa cell tumors (which are almost always large enough to palpate).

Treatment is by surgical removal of the tumor. If the tumor is malignant and found to be inoperable at exploration, postoperative irradiation may be used. Combination chemotherapy has been helpful in some patients. Intracavitary chemotherapy is no longer advocated.

TUMORS OF THE TESTICLE

Testicular tumors vary from highly malignant (adenocarcinoma, seminoma, or malignant teratoma) to relatively benign (Leydig cell tumor or benign teratoma). Paratesticular rhabdomyosarcoma may also present as a scrotal mass in the male child. Tumors are characterized by painless, solid swelling of the testicle, which does not transilluminate and appears to have a purplish discoloration. Although evidence of endocrine activity usually is absent, pseudoprecocious puberty occasionally occurs. Pregnancy tests yield positive results in embryonal carcinoma and choriocarcinoma. α-Fetoprotein levels may be elevated in embryonal carcinomas and some teratomas and may be followed for activity of disease.

Orchiectomy with high ligation of the cord is indicated in all testicular tumors. Retroperitoneal node dissection is indicated for staging and adequate resection. Radiation therapy to involved nodes and chemotherapy are also useful.

The prognosis is best in seminomas but has substantially improved in the other forms with the use of vinblastine, cisplatin, and bleomycin. Metastases may occur to the lungs, mediastinum, and regional and abdominal lymph nodes.

CARCINOMA OF THE THYROID

Carcinoma of the thyroid may occur spontaneously or following irradiation of the neck or upper chest. Any thyroid nodule should be suspected of being a tumor. If it occurs in an adolescent with goiter, therapy with thyroid preparations is indicated. If the nodule does not respond to therapy, surgical removal is indicated. Thyroid carcinoma occurring at other ages or in adolescents without an accompanying goiter nodule should be treated by subtotal thyroidectomy. Lesions found in the cervical lymph nodes should be treated by radical radiation therapy. Palliative treatment with radioiodine is indicated for distant metastases that take up radioiodine or can be induced to do so by thyroidectomy plus the use of thyrotropin or one of the thiourea derivatives. However, only about 10% of metastatic cancers of the thyroid will take up radioiodine in quantities sufficient to warrant treatment with this agent.

The prognosis for patients with completely removed thyroid tumors is excellent. The prognosis for patients in whom metastases have occurred is questionable. The prognosis for patients with widespread tumor, regardless of method of treatment, is poor.

RETICULOENDOTHELIOSES (Histiocytosis X)

The diseases to be discussed under this heading comprise a heterogeneous group of proliferative disorders of the reticuloendothelial system. The disorders are of unknown cause. Eosinophilic granuloma of bone, Hand-Schüller-Christian disease, and Letterer-Siwe disease constitute a complex of diseases of unknown cause, of histiocytic proliferation, and of unpredictable prognosis. Lichtenstein has grouped them under the term histiocytosis X. Although foam cells containing cholesterol are found in these disorders, it is currently believed that the storage cells are not the result of a primary disturbance of lipid metabolism but are secondary to increased intracellular cholesterol synthesis or to ingestion of cholesterol from necrotic tissue.

Certain patients present primarily with signs and symptoms of lytic lesions limited to the bones—especially the skull, ribs, clavicles, and vertebrae. These lesions are well demarcated and occasionally painful. Biopsy reveals eosinophilic granuloma, which may be the only lesion the patient will develop, although further bone and even visceral lesions may occur.

Another group of patients often present with otitis media, seborrheic skin rash, and evidence of bone lesions, usually in the mastoid or skull area. They frequently also have visceral involvement, which may be indicated by lymphadenopathy and hepatosplenomegaly. This chronic disseminated form is usually known as Hand-Schüller-Christian disease and is associated with "foamy histiocytes" on biopsy. The classic triad of Hand-Schüller-Christian disease (bony involvement, exophthalmos, and diabetes insipidus) is rarely seen; however, diabetes insipidus is a common complication.

A third group of patients present early in life primarily with visceral involvement. They often have a petechial or macular skin rash, generalized lymphadenopathy, enlarged liver and spleen, pulmonary involvement, and hematologic abnormalities such as anemia and thrombocytopenia. Bone lesions can occur. This acute visceral form, Letterer-Siwe disease, is often fatal.

In all 3 groups, the tissue abnormalities are proliferation of histiocytes; aggregations of eosinophils, lymphocytes, and plasma cells; and collection of foam cells.

The principal diseases to be differentiated from histiocytosis X are bone tumors (primary or metastatic), lymphomas or leukemias, granulomatous infections, immune deficiency states, and storage diseases. The diagnosis is established by biopsy of bone marrow, lymph node, liver, or mastoid or other bone.

Almost any system or area can become involved during the course of the disease. Rarely, these will include the heart (subendocardial infiltrates), bowel, eyes, mucous membranes such as the vagina or vulva, and dura mater.

Isolated bony lesions, if progressive or symptomatic (or both), are best treated by curettage and local radiotherapy. Multiple bony involvement and visceral involvement often respond well to prednisone, vinblastine, cyclophosphamide, and methotrexate. Whether chemotherapy substantially changes the course of the disease is controversial.

If diabetes insipidus occurs, treatment with vasopressin gives good control.

In patients with idiopathic histiocytosis, the prognosis is often unpredictable. Many patients with considerable bony and visceral involvement have shown apparent complete recovery. In general, however, the younger the patient and the more extensive the visceral involvement, the worse the prognosis.

• • •

INFECTIONS IN THE IMMUNODEFICIENT PATIENT

Immunodeficiency may be congenital but more often is due to suppression of the immune system by diseases or drugs. Deficiencies of polymorphonuclear (PMN) cells, T lymphocytes, or B lymphocytes tend to predispose the host to infection with different agents. For example, PMN deficiency predisposes to infection with gram-negative or gram-positive bacteria; B lymphocyte deficiency, infection with extracellular bacteria such as pneumococci and staphylococci; and T lymphocyte deficiency, infection with intracellular bacteria (mycobacteria, *Listeria,* etc), fungi (*Candida, Aspergillus,* etc), protozoa (*Pneumocystis,* etc), and viruses (herpes simplex, etc).

Many opportunistic organisms (ie, organisms that rarely produce invasive infections in an uncompromised host) do not produce disease except in the immunodeficient host. Such hosts are often infected with a number of pathogens simultaneously.

Infections caused by common organisms may present uncommon clinical manifestations. Determination of the specific infecting agents is essential for effective treatment.

Immunodeficient Hosts

Immunodeficient patients fall into several groups:

(1) Children with congenital immune defects of cellular or humoral immunity or a combination of both (eg, Wiskott-Aldrich syndrome).

(2) Patients with malignancy, particularly lymphoreticular malignancy.

(3) Patients receiving immunosuppressive therapy. These include patients with neoplastic disease and those bearing transplants who are receiving corticosteroids or other immunosuppressive drugs.

(4) Patients who have very few PMNs ($< 1000/\mu L$) or those whose PMNs do not function normally with respect to phagocytosis or the intracellular killing of phagocytosed microorganisms (eg, chronic granulomatous disease).

(5) A larger group of patients who are not classically immunodeficient but whose host defenses are seriously compromised by debilitating illness, surgical or other invasive procedures (eg, intravenous drug abuse or intravenous hyperalimentation), burns, massive antimicrobial therapy, or acquired immune deficiency syndrome (AIDS).

Infectious Agents

A. Bacteria: Any bacterium pathogenic for humans can infect the immunosuppressed host. Furthermore, noninvasive and nonpathogenic organisms (opportunists) may also cause disease in such cases. Examples include gram-negative bacteria, particularly *Pseudomonas, Serratia,* and *Aeromonas.* Many of these come from the hospital environment and are resistant to antimicrobial drugs.

B. Fungi: *Candida, Aspergillus, Cryptococcus, Nocardia,* and *Mucor* can all cause disease in the immunosuppressed host. Candidiasis is by far the most common and is often found in patients receiving intensive antimicrobial therapy.

C. Viruses: Cytomegalovirus is the most common, but varicella-zoster and herpes simplex viruses are also important. Vaccinia virus may cause serious problems if inadvertently inoculated.

D. Protozoa: *Pneumocystis carinii* is an important cause of pneumonia in many immunodeficient patients. It is particularly important to make this diagnosis early, because reasonably effective therapy is available. *Toxoplasma gondii* is also important in this group of patients.

Approach to Diagnosis

A systematic approach is necessary, including the following steps:

(1) Review carefully the patient's current immune status, previous antimicrobial therapy, and *all* previous culture reports.

(2) Obtain pertinent cultures for bacteria, fungi, and viruses.

(3) Consider which of the serologic tests for fungal, viral, and protozoal diseases are pertinent.

(4) Consider special diagnostic procedures, eg, lung biopsy or lung puncture or endobronchial brush biopsy to demonstrate *Pneumocystis*.

(5) Consider whether the infection (eg, candidiasis) is superficial or systemic. Therapeutic considerations are quite different in each case.

Approach to Treatment

Caution: It is essential to avoid aggravating the patient's underlying condition and to avoid gross alterations of the host's normal microbial flora.

Provide general therapeutic measures to improve host defenses, correct electrolyte imbalance, offer adequate caloric intake, etc. Improve the patient's immune status whenever possible. This includes a temporary decrease in the immunosuppressive drug dosage in transplant patients and modification of chemotherapy in cancer patients.

Granulocyte transfusions may be able to tide the patient over a period of PMN deficiency. Injection of immune globulin at regular intervals may compensate for certain B cell deficiencies.

Antimicrobial drug therapy should be specific for the infecting agent and should be lethal for it. Combinations of chemotherapeutic agents may be necessary, since multiple infectious agents may be involved in some cases.

Note: Many of the drugs used for treatment of patients with these infections are seldom used in general practice, and some are quite toxic (eg, amphotericin B). Great care should be exercised in using these agents, especially if they are used in combination.

24 | Infectious Diseases: Viral & Rickettsial

VIRAL DISEASES

ROSEOLA INFANTUM
(Exanthema Subitum)

Roseola infantum, an acute febrile disease of infants and young children, is characterized by a high sustained or spiking fever of 1–5 days' duration followed by a faint rash. The incubation period is estimated to be 7–17 days.

Clinical Findings

A. Symptoms and Signs: The onset is sudden, with fever as high as 41.1 °C (106 °F). Fever persists for 1–5 days (average, 3 days), falls by crisis, and then is usually subnormal for a few hours just before the rash appears. Rash appears when the temperature returns to normal. It is faintly erythematous, macular, and diffusely disseminated, starting on and principally confined to the trunk. Individual macules resemble those of rubella. Physical findings may be entirely normal except for the rash, although many children have mild pharyngitis, enlargement of the postoccipital nodes, and irritability.

B. Laboratory Findings: Findings include progressive leukopenia to 3000–5000 white cells, with a relative lymphocytosis as high as 90%.

Complications

Convulsions are the principal complication (may be the first sign of illness) and are related to the rapidly rising temperature. A parainfectious type of encephalopathy has been reported (see Chapter 21).

Treatment

A. Specific Measures: None available.

B. General Measures: Restrict activity until the rash appears. Give aspirin for temperatures of over 39.4 °C (103 °F). Give tepid water sponge baths or alcohol rubs for high fever uncontrolled by aspirin.

C. Treatment of Complications: Barbiturate sedatives may prevent convulsions resulting from hyperpyrexia, especially in children with convulsive tendencies (see Table 21–4).

Prognosis

The prognosis is excellent.

MEASLES
(Rubeola)

Measles is a highly communicable disease with the highest incidence between the ages of 2 and 14 years. It is easily spread from person to person by droplets and by contact with articles freshly soiled by nose and throat secretions of an infected individual during a prodromal period of 3–5 days. The incubation period is 8–14 days, with a majority of cases occurring 10 days after exposure.

Clinical Findings

A. Symptoms and Signs:

1. Prodrome–The prodromal period is 3–5 days. Fever is usually the first sign and persists throughout the prodrome. It ranges from 38.3 to 40 °C (101 to 104 °F), tends to be higher just before the appearance of the skin rash, and may be lower after eruption of the rash. Sore throat, nasal discharge, and dry, "barking" cough are common during the prodrome. Nonpurulent conjunctivitis appears toward the end of the prodrome and is accompanied by photophobia. Lymphadenopathy of the posterior cervical lymph nodes may occur.

2. Koplik's spots–Fine white spots on a faint erythematous base appear first on the buccal mucosa opposite the molar teeth and later may spread over the entire inside of the mouth by about the third or fourth day of the prodrome. They usually disappear as the exanthem becomes well established.

3. Rash–Rash appears on about the fifth day of disease. The pink, blotchy, irregular, macular erythema rapidly darkens and characteristically coalesces into larger red patches of varying size and shape. The eruption fades on pressure. The rash first appears on the face and behind the ears; it then spreads to the chest and abdomen and, finally, to the extremities. It lasts 4–7 days and may be accompanied by mild itching. A fine branny desquamation, especially of the face and trunk, may follow, lasting 2 or 3 days; light brown pigmentation may then appear.

B. Laboratory Findings: Leukopenia is present during the prodrome and early stages of the rash. There is usually a sharp rise in the white cell count with the onset of any bacterial complication. In the absence of complications, the white cell count slowly rises to normal as the rash fades.

Complications

A. Bacterial Infection: Most common in the respiratory tract, bacterial infection is manifested by recurrence of fever and leukocytosis.

1. Otitis media–This appears toward the end of the prodrome or during the course of the rash (see Chapter 14).

2. Tracheobronchitis–Besides the specific inflammation due to rubeola, there may be secondary bacterial involvement. This is usually accompanied by more productive cough.

3. Bronchopneumonia–While rubeola virus itself often causes a specific pneumonitis, involvement of the lower bronchial tree by secondary bacterial invasion with resultant bronchopneumonia is a relatively common complication.

B. Encephalitis: Encephalitis (see Chapter 21) occurs in about 1 of 3000 cases (no relation to severity of measles). The first sign may be increasing lethargy or convulsions. Lumbar puncture shows 0–200 cells, mostly lymphocytes. Subacute sclerosing panencephalitis (SSPE) is a late degenerative central nervous system complication.

C. Hemorrhagic Measles: This rare form with a high mortality rate is characterized by generalized bleeding and purpura.

D. Tuberculosis: Active pulmonary tuberculosis may be aggravated by measles.

Treatment

A. Specific Measures: None available.

B. General Measures: Measures include isolation for 1 week from onset of rash, bed rest until the patient is afebrile, aspirin for temperatures over 39.4 °C (103 °F), saline sponges for the eyes (darkness is not necessary but may make the child more comfortable), and warm moist air (steam) for cough. Sedative cough mixtures may be necessary.

C. Treatment of Complications: Bacterial complications are usually due to group A streptococci. Prophylaxis of bacterial infection may be instituted in children with preexisting pulmonary conditions or other debilitating diseases. For treatment of patients with encephalitis, see Chapter 21.

Prophylaxis

Measles vaccine should be given routinely as outlined in Chapter 7. Passive immunization with immune globulin may prevent the disease or result in a mild, modified rubeola syndrome with reduced incidence of bacterial complications (see Chapter 7). Give vaccine 8 weeks later.

Prognosis

In uncomplicated cases or those with bacterial complications, the prognosis is excellent. In patients with encephalitis, the prognosis is guarded; the incidence of permanent sequelae is high.

RUBELLA
(German Measles)

Rubella is a mild febrile virus infection that frequently occurs in epidemics but is not as contagious as rubeola or chickenpox (Table 24–1). Transmission is probably by the droplet route. The incubation period is 12–21 days (average, 16 days).

Clinical Findings

A. Symptoms and Signs:

1. Prodrome–The prodrome, if present, lasts only a few days and is characterized by slight malaise, occasional tender postero-occipital lymph nodes, and no catarrhal symptoms. In younger children, the prodrome may not be noted by parents. Rash may be the first sign of disease and consists of faint, fine, discrete, erythematous macules appearing first on the face and spreading rapidly over the trunk and extremities. Macules are only slightly raised; eventually they blend. The rash may suggest measles on the first day and scarlet fever on the second. It generally disappears by the third day. The temperature rarely exceeds 38.3 °C (101 °F) and usually lasts less than 2 days.

2. Rubella without rash–Rubella sine eruptione occurs as a febrile lymphadenopathy that may persist for a week or more. During epidemics, this syndrome may represent over 40% of cases with infection.

3. Congenital rubella–This is a syndrome involving infants born to mothers affected with rubella in the first trimester of pregnancy. The majority of infants show growth retardation, hepatosplenomegaly, and purpura, in addition to congenital defects of the heart, eye, and ear. Marked thrombocytopenia is a common finding. X-ray of the long bones shows an irregularity of trabecular pattern, with longitudinal areas of radiolucency in the metaphysis. Rubella virus is easily isolated from such patients, and they must be considered to have a highly contagious disease that can spread to other patients and to hospital personnel. A late-onset congenital rubella syndrome, with minimal signs at birth and an acute onset of severe clinical disease after 3–6 months, has been reported.

B. Laboratory Findings: Transient leukopenia is generally noted.

Complications

If rubella occurs during the first month of pregnancy, there is a 50% chance of fetal abnormality (cataracts, congenital heart disease, deafness, mental deficiency, microcephaly). By the third month of pregnancy, the risk of abnormalities decreases to less than 10%.

Encephalitis and thrombocytopenic purpura are rare. Polyarthritis occurs in 25% of cases in persons over 16 years of age.

Table 24–1. Diagnostic features of some acute exanthems.

Disease	Prodromal Signs and Symptoms	Nature of Eruption	Other Diagnostic Features	Laboratory Findings
Chickenpox (varicella)	0–1 d of fever, anorexia, headache.	Rapid evolution of macules to papules, vesicles, crusts; vesicles extremely fragile; all stages simultaneously present in successive outcroppings; lesions superficial; distribution centripetal.	Lesions on scalp and mucous membranes.	Specialized complement fixation and virus neutralization in tissue culture. Fluorescent antibody test of smear of lesions.
Drug eruption	Occasionally fever.	Maculopapular rash resembling rubella, rarely papulovesicular.		Eosinophilia.
Eczema herpeticum	No prodrome.	Vesiculopustular lesions in area of eczema.		Herpes simplex virus isolated in tissue culture; complement fixation. Fluorescent antibody test of smear of lesions.
Enterovirus infection	1–2 d of fever, malaise.	Maculopapular rash resembling rubella, rarely papulovesicular or petechial.	Aseptic meningitis.	Virus isolation from stool or cerebrospinal fluid; complement fixation titer rise.
Erythema infectiosum	No prodrome. Usually in epidemics.	Red, flushed cheeks; circumoral pallor, maculopapules on extremities.	"Slapped face" appearance.	White blood count normal.
Exanthema subitum	3–4 d of high fever.	As fever falls by crisis, pink maculopapules appear on chest and trunk; fade in 1–3 d.		White blood count low.
Infectious mononucleosis	Fever, adenopathy, sore throat.	Maculopapular rash resembling rubella, rarely papulovesicular; distribution scattered, asymmetrical.	Splenomegaly, tonsillar exudate.	Atypical lymphs in blood smears; heterophil agglutination. Slide agglutination test.
Meningococcemia	Hours of fever, vomiting.	Maculopapules, petechiae, purpura.	Meningeal signs, toxicity, shock.	White blood count high. Cultures of blood and cerebrospinal fluid.

Rocky Mountain spotted fever	3–4 d of fever, chills, severe headache.	Maculopapules, petechiae; distribution centrifugal.	History of tick bite.	Agglutination (OX19, OX2), complement fixation.
Rubella (German measles)	Little or no prodrome.	Maculopapular, pink; begins on head and neck, spreads downward, fades in 3 d. No desquamation.	Lymphadenopathy, postauricular or occipital.	White blood count normal or low. Serologic tests for immunity and definitive diagnosis (hemagglutination inhibition, complement fixation).
Rubeola (measles)	3–4 d of fever, coryza, conjunctivitis, cough.	Maculopapular, brick-red; begins on head and neck; spreads downward. In 5–6 d, rash is brownish, desquamating.	Koplik's spots on buccal mucosa.	White blood count low. Virus isolation in cell culture. Antibody tests by hemagglutination inhibition and complement fixation or neutralization.
Scarlet fever	½–2 d of malaise, sore throat, fever, vomiting.	Generalized, punctate, red; prominent on neck, in axilla, groin, skin folds; circumoral pallor; fine desquamation involves hands and feet.	Strawberry tongue, exudative tonsilitis.	Group A hemolytic streptococci cultures from throat; antistreptolysin O titer rise.
Smallpox (variola)	3 d of fever, severe headache, malaise, chills.	Slow evolution of macules to papules, vesicles, pustules, crusts; all lesions in any area in same stage; lesions deep-seated; distribution centrifugal.		Virus isolation. Serologic tests for immunity. Fluorescent antibody test of smear of lesions.
Typhus fever	3–4 d of fever, chills, severe headache.	Maculopapules, petechiae; distribution centripetal.	Endemic area, lice.	Agglutination (OX19), complement fixation.

Treatment

A. Specific Measures: None available.

B. General Measures: Isolation is usually not necessary, but susceptible women must not be exposed during the first trimester of pregnancy. Symptomatic measures are rarely necessary.

C. Treatment of Complications: For treatment of encephalitis and purpura, see Chapters 21 and 17, respectively.

Prophylaxis

A live attenuated rubella virus vaccine should be given to children between age 1 year and puberty. Particular emphasis should be directed to girls before the onset of menses and the possibility of pregnancy (see Chapter 7). A history of "German measles" should not be considered a contraindication to the use of this preparation.

Immune globulin given to pregnant women after exposure is not recommended. Determination of rubella antibody in the serum of exposed women may establish a state of immunity; in the absence of such antibody, therapeutic abortion should be considered. Pregnant women should avoid exposure to clinical rubella regardless of their presumed immunity.

Prognosis

The prognosis in patients with acquired infection is excellent. In patients with congenital disease, the prognosis is universally poor. A progressive, degenerative panencephalitis has been reported. Late manifestations of brain damage such as behavior problems, increasing mental retardation, and minimal brain dysfunction (see Chapter 21) may occur.

ERYTHEMA INFECTIOSUM
(Fifth Disease)

Erythema infectiosum is a mild, usually afebrile contagious disease of presumed viral etiology, usually occurring in family or institutional epidemics. The incubation period is estimated to be 7–14 days.

Clinical Findings

A. Symptoms and Signs: There is usually no prodrome. The first symptom is the rash, which has a characteristic appearance and course. It appears first on the cheeks and ears as very red coalescent macules that are warm and slightly raised. Circumoral pallor is marked, leading to the "slapped cheek" appearance. This eruption fades within 4 days. Following the eruption on the face by 1 day, a maculopapular erythematous rash appears on the extensor surfaces of the extremities and spreads, over

2–3 days, to the flexor surfaces and trunk. Macules develop a pale central area, producing a reticular appearance. Palms and soles are rarely involved. Rash lasts 3–7 days and may recur after 7–10 days, with irritation of the skin. Pruritus, headache, and arthralgia are occasional additional symptoms.

B. Laboratory Findings: The white blood cell count is normal.

Treatment & Prognosis

No treatment is indicated. There are no complications, and the prognosis is excellent.

VARICELLA (Chickenpox) & HERPES ZOSTER (Shingles)

Varicella is an acute, extremely communicable disease caused by the varicella-zoster virus. It is spread from person to person by droplets from a respiratory source or by direct contact with freshly contaminated articles. Varicella is communicable from 24 hours before until 6 days after appearance of the rash. The incubation period is 12–21 days (average, 15 days).

With rare exceptions, immunity to varicella after attack is probably lifelong, although the individual with a history of varicella may later develop herpes zoster.

Clinical Findings

A. Symptoms and Signs:

1. Prodrome–The prodrome is usually not apparent; there may be slight malaise and fever for 24 hours.

2. Rash–Usually, the first sign is rash. Lesions tend to appear in crops (2–4 crops in 2–6 days), and all stages and sizes may be present at the same time and in the same vicinity. Lesions occur first on the scalp and mucous surfaces and then on the body. They are numerous over the chest, back, and shoulders; less numerous on the extremities; and seldom seen on the palms and soles. Successive stages (usually over a period of 1–4 days) are as follows:

a. Macular–Blotches are small and red.

b. Papular–Raised skin eruptions occur.

c. Vesicular–Lesions are very fragile, generally not umbilicated, and appear as drops of water on a slightly red base; the top may be readily scratched off.

d. Pustular–Lesions have crust formation. This stage may be reached within a few hours after the appearance of the macule. Scabs fall away by the 9th–13th days.

3. Pruritus–Pruritus is minimal at first but may become severe in the pustular stage.

4. Fever–Fever may occur when most vesicles reach the pustular stage, but constitutional reactions are usually minimal; the rash is often noted by chance.

5. Herpes zoster–Herpes zoster (shingles) occurs in individuals who have had varicella and is rarely seen in very young children. There may be pain in the area of the rash before the vesicles erupt. Lesions resemble those of varicella but are confined to the dermatomal distribution of a specific sensory nerve. The most common site is the chest, but lesions may also follow the distribution of the trigeminal nerve root. The vesicles have usually dried and are healing by the fourth or fifth day.

B. Laboratory Findings: Leukopenia occurs early. The white blood count may rise with extensive secondary infection of vesicles.

Complications

There may be secondary infection of vesicles. Encephalitis is rare. Severe disease, with high mortality rates, occurs in individuals receiving immunosuppressive therapy and in patients with any one of the leukemias.

Treatment

A. Specific Measures: None available.

B. General Measures: Pruritus may be relieved by local application of calamine lotion, mild local anesthetic ointments, or systemic antihistamines. Cut nails short, and have the patient wear gloves if necessary to prevent excoriation. Mouth and perineal lesions may be treated by use of rinses, gargles, and saline soaks. Sponge baths with antiseptic detergent (eg, pHisoHex) relieve itching and reduce the incidence of secondary bacterial infection.

C. Treatment of Complications: Treat secondary infection of the skin with local broad-spectrum antibiotics (see Chapter 6). If secondary infection is suspected, give antibiotics systemically (penicillin for group A streptococcal infection). For general measures of treatment in patients with encephalitis, see Chapter 21.

Prophylaxis

Zoster immune globulin (ZIG) may modify the progressive disease or prevent it in immunodeficient individuals exposed to the virus (see Chapter 7). A live attenuated virus vaccine is under investigation at present but is not commercially available. Intravenous vidarabine has been reported to interrupt the progress of varicella and herpes zoster in immunosuppressed individuals.

Prognosis

In uncomplicated disease, the prognosis is excellent. Scarring from secondary infection of eruptions is not uncommon. In encephalitis, the prognosis is poor, with a high incidence of sequelae in surviving patients. Death has been reported in cases of varicella occurring in children receiving long-term therapy with cortisone. In patients with herpes zoster, pain along the nerve root may persist for several months.

SMALLPOX
(Variola Major)

Smallpox was an acute disease with a sudden onset of high fever lasting up to 5 days, followed by the appearance of a rash that rapidly spread centrifugally. It has now been eradicated throughout the world, although the possibility of local outbreaks resulting from laboratory accidents must still be considered.

Vaccination against smallpox may still be practiced (see Chapter 7), which means that occasional cases of vaccinia may be seen.

EPIDEMIC PAROTITIS
(Mumps)

Mumps is an acute virus disease that may involve many organ systems but commonly affects the salivary glands, chiefly the parotid gland (about 60% of cases), and frequently the central nervous system. It is uncommon before 3 and after 40 years of age. It is probably not as contagious as measles and chickenpox. Mumps is spread directly from person to person and by direct contact with contaminated articles. It is communicable from 2 days before the appearance of symptoms to the disappearance of salivary gland swelling. Disease without salivary gland involvement is also communicable. The incubation period is usually 12–24 days (average, 16–18 days).

Clinical Findings

A. Symptoms and Signs:

1. Gland involvement–Parotid gland involvement is common. (Submaxillary and sublingual glands may be involved also or in the absence of parotid gland involvement.) A prodrome of 1 or 2 days may precede the parotid swelling and is characterized by fever, malaise, and pain in or behind the ear on chewing or swallowing. Involvement of the salivary glands, with tender swelling and brawny edema, contrasts with the more sharply defined enlargement of a lymph node. Pain is referred to the ear and is aggravated by chewing, swallowing, or opening the mouth. Aggravation by sour substances (eg, lemon) is not a reliable symptom. Tenderness persists for 1–3 days, and swelling is present for 7–10 days. Skin over the gland is normal. Openings of ducts of the involved gland and especially the papilla of Stensen's duct (opposite the upper second molar) may be puffy and red. Fever may be absent or as high as 40 °C (104 °F). Malaise, anorexia, and headache may be present.

2. "Inapparent" mumps infection–This infection has a short course, with fever lasting 1–5 days.

3. Central nervous system involvement–Mumps encephalitis may precede, accompany, or follow inflammation of the salivary glands but may occur without such involvement. Asymptomatic central nervous system inflammation with pleocytosis may be found in over half of cases of mumps. The onset of meningeal irritation is usually sudden. Headache, vomiting, stiff neck and back, and lethargy are characteristic. Fever recurs or increases, up to 41.1 °C (106 °F). Symptoms seldom last more than 5 days. Central nervous system involvement by mumps virus must be suspected in every case of nonbacterial "meningitis." Transient paresis may suggest poliomyelitis.

4. Other organ involvement–Mastitis and thyroiditis may occur. Other organs may be involved, including the following:

a. Testicles and ovaries–Involvement is usually during or after adolescence, but orchitis can occur in childhood. This may occur in the absence of distinctive salivary gland involvement.

b. Pancreas–There is a sudden onset of pain in the mid or upper abdomen, with vomiting, prostration, and usually fever.

c. Kidney–Nephritis is rare and mild, with complete recovery in most cases.

d. Ear–Deafness occasionally occurs and may be permanent.

B. Laboratory Findings: The white blood cell count usually shows leukopenia and relative lymphocytosis. Serologic tests will confirm the diagnosis. Skin testing is unreliable as an indication of immunity in exposed persons. For cerebrospinal fluid findings, see Appendix, Table 4.

Complications

With central nervous system involvement, paresis of the facial nerve has been reported. A fatal outcome with central nervous system involvement is extremely rare. Testicular involvement (usually unilateral) may produce atrophy, but sterility is rare.

Treatment

A. Specific Measures: None available.

B. General Measures: Measures include bed rest during the febrile period, isolation of the patient until the salivary swelling is gone, local warm or cold applications to areas of salivary gland swelling, aspirin or codeine analgesics when pain is severe, mouth wash with fat-free broth or slightly saline solution, and avoidance of highly flavored and acid foods and drinks.

C. Treatment of Complications:

1. Central nervous system involvement–Treatment is symptomatic for mild encephalitis. Lumbar puncture may be useful in reducing headache.

2. Orchitis–Cortisone may be very effective in some cases. Suspension of the scrotum in a sling or suspensory and use of analgesics (codeine or morphine) may be indicated. Infiltration around the spermatic cord at the external inguinal ring with 10–20 mL of 1% procaine solution may produce dramatic relief.

3. Pancreatitis and oophoritis–Treatment is symptomatic only.

Prophylaxis

A live attenuated mumps virus vaccine is highly effective (see Chapter 7). It is especially recommended for children approaching adolescence who have no history of mumps. Mumps hyperimmune globulin is not recommended.

Prognosis

The prognosis is excellent even with extensive organ system involvement. Sterility very rarely results from orchitis in the postadolescent male.

COXSACKIEVIRUS INFECTION

Coxsackieviruses have been shown to be the cause of several general types of clinical disease (Table 24–2), usually occurring in epidemic form during the summer months. There are many immunologic types, which are classified as group A and group B. Coxsackieviruses (a

Table 24–2. Enteroviral enanthems and exanthems.*

Infection	Source	
	Coxsackieviruses	Echoviruses
Enanthem		
Herpangina	A2, 4, 5, 6, 8, 10; B4	17
Nodular pharyngitis	A10	
Stomatitis	A3, 5	
Exanthem		
Petechial	A9; B3	4, 9, 11
Rubelliform	A; B	All types
Urticarial	A9, 16; B5	11
Vesicular	A4, 5, 9, 16; B1, 4	

*After Horstman.

subgroup of the enteroviruses) are found in the stool for up to 8 weeks after onset of symptoms and are transmitted by the fecal-oral route.

Clinical Findings

A. Herpangina: In herpangina due to group A virus infection, the onset of fever (up to 40 °C [104 °F]) is abrupt and lasts 1–4 days. Older children may complain of moderately severe sore throat. There may be vomiting and abdominal pain. The pharynx shows characteristic hyperemia of the anterior pillars of the fauces, with discrete vesicular eruptions. The gingival or buccal mucous membranes are not involved, as they are in herpes simplex infection.

B. Hand-Foot-Mouth Syndrome: In this syndrome caused by group A virus, there is papulovesicular eruption in the areas of the hand, foot, and mouth.

C. "Summer Grippe": An acute, brief febrile illness lasts 1–4 days without other signs or symptoms. This may represent the most common form of infection with these viruses. Diagnosis depends upon knowledge of a community or family epidemic with more characteristic syndromes present in other individuals.

D. Pleurodynia: Pleurodynia (epidemic myalgia, Bornholm disease) due to group B virus infection is more common in older children and adults. Onset is abrupt, with fever, dyspnea, and often headache. Acute pain occurs most commonly around the lower ribs and is intensified by respiratory movement. The thoracic type may simulate pneumonia or pleuritis. Abdominal pain occurs in about 50% of cases and may simulate appendicitis, cholecystitis, or hepatitis. After fever subsides, pain may recur up to 2 weeks after onset. Pleurodynia may be accompanied by central nervous system symptoms (see below).

E. Aseptic Meningitis: Onset is usually abrupt, with fever, headache, nausea, and vomiting. Abdominal or chest pain may be an early symptom. Stiffness of the neck or back may follow after 24 hours. Spinal fluid may show an increase in cells, usually monocytes, but rarely exceeding 100/mL. Aseptic meningitis must be differentiated from poliomyelitis and bacterial meningitis. Asymmetric flaccid paralysis has been reported in rare cases.

F. Myocarditis and Pericarditis: These infections (see Chapter 13) may be caused by group B virus. Except in the neonatal period, the prognosis is generally good, although sudden death has been reported.

G. Generalized Infection: Myocarditis, encephalitis, hepatitis, and pneumonia due to group B virus infection have been reported as epidemic in newborn nurseries. The mortality rate is high.

Treatment

A. Specific Measures: None available.

B. General Measures: Measures include bed rest during the febrile period and aspirin or codeine when pain is severe. Warm applications to the back and chest may bring relief.

Prophylaxis

Since transmission is by the fecal-oral route, careful disposal of stools is required to minimize spread of infection in the family and hospital.

Prognosis

The prognosis is excellent. The disease is usually self-limited, and recovery is complete. In small infants, myocarditis due to these viruses often has a fatal outcome. Transient paresis has been reported.

ECHOVIRUS INFECTION

Many types of echoviruses have been found on tissue culture of human stools. Several types have clearly been shown to cause human disease of different clinical categories. Transmission from human to human is by the enteric-oral route. Like poliomyelitis virus and coxsackievirus epidemics, infections are most common during the summer months.

Clinical Findings

A. Aseptic Meningitis Syndrome: This syndrome usually is due to echovirus type 6 but is common with type 4 and has been rarely found with types 9 and 16. Onset is sudden, with fever to 39.4 °C (103 °F), vomiting, headache, and stiff neck. There may be a morbilliform rash resembling that of rubella and lasting 1–6 days. The rash is found mostly on the face and trunk. All symptoms usually subside within 1 week. Paralytic disease, consisting of paresis in the extremities, has been described involving types 2, 4, 6, 9, and 16. The weakness is usually temporary and does not persist beyond 1 month in most cases.

B. Exanthematous Disease: Echovirus types 4, 9, and 16 (Boston exanthem) have been found to be the cause of a febrile disease characterized by sudden onset of fever to 39.4 °C (103 °F), sore throat, and nausea. A discrete macular, morbilliform rash soon appears, with distribution mostly over the face and trunk. This rash lasts 1–10 days. The disease may be differentiated from rubeola by absence of catarrhal respiratory symptoms and Koplik's spots; it is differentiated from rubella by persistence beyond the third day.

C. Diarrheal Disease of Infants: Type 18 echovirus has been associated with epidemic diarrheal disease in infants under 1 year of age. There is a sudden onset of diarrhea unaccompanied by fever. Stools show no pus and rarely blood.

D. Respiratory Tract Infection: Echovirus types 8 and 20 have been shown to cause outbreaks of acute upper respiratory tract disease.

Treatment

No specific measures are available. General measures include bed rest during the febrile period and, in the case of the diarrheal disease, infants' dietary measures as for other enteric infections (see Chapter 16).

Prognosis

The prognosis is excellent. Asymmetric paresis with complete recovery has been reported but is rare.

VIRAL HEPATITIS

Viral hepatitis is an acute contagious disease often occurring in epidemics, always involving inflammation of the liver, and often accompanied by jaundice. At least 2 viruses are presently recognized, with distinct morphologic and antigenic characteristics (Table 24–3). In addition to hepatitis A and hepatitis B, one or more additional types (non-A, non-B) are suggested on an epidemiologic basis.

Table 24–3. Hepatitis A and hepatitis B.

Characteristic	Hepatitis A	Hepatitis B
Antibodies	Anti-HAV	Anti-HBs Anti-HBc Anti-HBe
Antigens	Whole virus particle	HBsAg (surface) HBcAg (core) HBeAg DNA polymerase
Chronic, persisting and recurrent disease	0	+
Heat resistance	56 °C for 1 h	60 °C for 4 h
Heterologous immunity	0	0
Homologous immunity	+	?
Incubation period	15–50 d, average 28–30 d	45–160 d, average 60–90 d
Standard immune globulin (IG) protection	+	?
Susceptibility	General. Low in infants and preschool children.	General. Transmission across placenta and during labor.
Virus in blood	+	+
Virus in feces	+	+
Virus in saliva	+	+
Virus size	27 nm	42 nm

Clinical Findings

A. Symptoms and Signs: Fever, malaise, chills, anorexia, vomiting, and headache may occur. Upper abdominal pain and hepatomegaly are common. Jaundice appears in 2–5 days, when fever is subsiding, and may last several weeks. Infection without jaundice is probably most common in childhood and may be detectable only by laboratory tests of liver function. Fulminant infection, with rapid onset of liver involvement, acute yellow atrophy, and death, is rare. Type B hepatitis is characterized by a slow onset with low-grade fever and mild symptoms often ignored until the appearance of jaundice. A morbilliform rash and arthralgia may precede the appearance of jaundice.

B. Laboratory Findings: The sedimentation rate is increased. Liver function studies show evidence of hepatocellular disease. The sulfobromophthalein test result is the first to become abnormal and the last to become normal. Occasionally, false-positive results in the Wassermann or Kahn test are reported. The SGOT level is increased early, usually to above 200 units. Numerous laboratory tests are available for the detection of hepatitis B surface antigen and antibody in patients' sera. Antigens and antibodies are listed in Table 24–3.

Complications

There may be hemorrhagic manifestations due to low prothrombin levels. Acute hepatic failure and acute yellow atrophy are usually fatal with widespread hemorrhage.

Differential Diagnosis

Type A and type B hepatitis (Table 24–3) must be differentiated from hepatitis caused by other infections (eg, infectious mononucleosis, leptospirosis, amebiasis, Q fever, cytomegalovirus disease) and from hepatitis caused by toxins, drugs, collagen diseases, obstructive disorders, and neoplastic disease.

Treatment

A. Specific Measures: None available.

B. General Measures:

1. Physical activity–Reduce physical activity and stress bed rest in children with moderate to severe symptoms. In these children, sedatives may be necessary. Give phenobarbital, but avoid sedatives and hypnotics that are detoxified by the liver (eg, pentobarbital). In children without moderate to severe symptoms, physical activity as tolerated will probably not interfere with a smooth convalescence.

2. Diet–Institute a balanced and palatable diet with adequate protein-sparing carbohydrates. If the patient is unable to retain oral feedings, give 5% glucose and 5% protein hydrolysate solutions by intravenous infusion. A mixture of protein hydrolysate and skimmed milk may be given by plastic nasogastric tube. When the patient is able to take food by mouth, give restricted oral feedings. Finally, give a full diet high in carbohydrates and proteins.

3. Vitamins–Supplementary vitamins, particularly B complex, may be indicated.

4. Corticosteroids–In severely ill patients with anorexia, nausea, and vomiting, give corticosteroids for 5 days, and then rapidly reduce the dosage.

C. Treatment of Complications:

1. Hemorrhagic manifestations–Give transfusions of fresh whole blood (see p 18). If possible, increase the donor prothrombin level by administration of vitamin K to the donor prior to drawing blood. Irradiated plasma has limited value and should not be used in view of the danger of superimposed hepatitis B.

2. Acute hepatic failure and acute yellow atrophy–Although the prognosis is extremely poor, liver function can improve and recovery can take place in some cases. Protein intake should be sharply restricted. Protein breakdown by bacteria in the bowel should be inhibited by enema as well as by administration of neomycin. Corticosteroids should be administered in full dosage. Intravenous glucose should be stressed. Exchange transfusions may be most useful.

Prophylaxis

Immune globulin will protect individuals exposed to hepatitis A if it is given soon after exposure (up to 6 weeks). Give 0.02 mL/kg intramuscularly and repeat at 2-month intervals if exposure continues. Epidemics of hepatitis in children in day-care centers may be controlled by administration of immune globulin to staff and children when the first case is diagnosed. When several cases occur within a few days, household contacts of the staff and children should also be given immune globulin.

Hepatitis B immune globulin will reduce the incidence of hepatitis B in exposed individuals. The dose is 0.06 mL/kg intramuscularly within 7 days after exposure, repeated in a second dose 30 days later. Individuals receiving multiple transfusions may benefit from hepatitis B immune globulin.

Inactivated hepatitis B vaccine (Heptavax-B) is now available and is given in 3 intramuscular doses of 0.5 mL each in children 3 months to 10 years of age, 1 mL each in older children and adults, or 2 mL each in dialysis patients and immunocompromised patients. The second dose is given 1 month after the first, and a third dose is given 6 months after the first dose. This may be useful in high-risk patients such as health care staff, dialysis patients, and those receiving multiple transfusions.

Prognosis

Viral hepatitis is usually a self-limited disease. In the absence of acute hepatic failure, the prognosis is good. Chronic progressive or recurrent liver disease is common with hepatitis B and may lead to cirrhosis.

HERPES SIMPLEX INFECTIONS

(See also Table 9–1.)

Herpes simplex virus type 1 (HSV-1) typically produces a subclinical or clinical primary infection, followed by latent persistence of the virus in a sensory ganglion. Subsequently, recurrences are triggered in the dermatome supplied by the respective sensory fibers when fever, trauma, stress, etc, occur. Once infected, people carry the virus throughout their lives and, during active recurrent episodes, are able to transmit the virus. HSV-1 occurs principally around the mouth and produces lesions on the face and upper part of the body; it is transmitted commonly by saliva or respiratory droplets. Herpes simplex virus type 2 (HSV-2) occurs principally on genital areas and lower parts of the body and is often a sexually transmitted disease. It also causes neonatal herpes infection. During and after a primary infection, there is a rise in antibody titer, which subsequently remains elevated. A typical lesion is a vesicle that lasts for several days and then crusts in 7–10 days. Diagnosis rests on clinical impression, finding of multinucleated giant cells at the base of the lesion, or isolation of the virus in cell culture.

Clinical Findings

A. Symptoms and Signs:

1. HSV-1 infection–HSV-1 produces the following entities, among others:

a. Acute herpetic gingivostomatitis–This is a typical primary infection of young children, with extensive vesicles and ulcers on the gums, palate, and buccal mucous membranes; pain; bleeding; and fever. It is self-limited and heals in 1–2 weeks. Primary oral infection is often subclinical.

b. Recurrent "cold sores"–These are most common at mucocutaneous junctions of the lips or nose. They recur at the same site in a given person, with the virus latent in the trigeminal ganglion between recurrences. Individual vesicles develop 36–60 hours after a "trigger" (eg, sunburn), persist for 2–4 days, and then rupture, leaving an ulcer that crusts and heals without scarring.

c. Eczema herpeticum–There is widespread vesication (usually primary infection) in a child with atopic lesions or eczema. Unless the child is immunodeficient, these widespread lesions usually heal.

d. Keratoconjunctivitis–This may be a primary or recurrent infection, usually with HSV-1. Recurrent lesions often take the form of dendritic lesions or ulcers of the corneal epithelium. Sometimes the corneal stroma may be involved, leading to opacity and impairment of vision or to blindness. Virus is easily isolated from the cornea.

e. Encephalitis–This may be a primary infection with HSV-1 or occur years later. It begins with headache, fever, impairment of the sensorium, seizures, or signs pointing to a lesion of the temporal lobe (aphasia, behavioral disorders, psychomotor convulsions). This is a necrotizing encephalitis that is often fatal. Brain biopsy permits virus isolation, but cerebrospinal fluid findings are often negative. HSV-1 may be responsible for 2–5% of cases of viral aseptic meningitis with an almost universally favorable outcome. (For HSV-2 encephalitis in newborns, see below.)

f. Whitlow–This is a paronychia caused by primary or secondary infection of a finger with HSV-1 (eg, thumb-sucking in a child with gingivostomatitis; finger infection of a nurse suctioning a patient) or HSV-2 (finger contact with a genital lesion).

2. HSV-2 infection–HSV-2 produces the following entities, among others:

a. Neonatal herpes–This is a primary HSV-2 infection transmitted from lesions on the mother's genitalia to the child during birth. The spectrum is very wide, ranging from subclinical or minimal skin lesions to widespread involvement of surfaces and many organs including the brain, with fatal outcome. It is postulated that in order to prevent neonatal infection, cesarean section should be done in any woman who has lesions of genital herpes near the time of delivery. (See Table 9–1.)

b. Genital herpes–Primary HSV-2 infection produces vesicles and ulceration on the genitalia, with much surrounding inflammation. Recurrent lesions occur at the same site (penis, vulva, cervix), liberating virus and serving as a source of infection for sexual contact. Recurrent lesions may have minimal inflammation and symptoms but cause much emotional stress. Genital herpes and HSV-2 antibodies occur at a later age than do HSV-1 antibodies. (The role of genital herpes in neonatal infection is described above.)

B. Laboratory Findings: Scrapings from ulcerations or the base of vesicles show multinucleated giant cells in Giemsa-stained smears. Swabs or aspirates from early lesions (first to fourth days) inoculated into cell cultures permit growth of the virus in 1–3 days. Such isolates are readily obtained from mucous membrane, skin, or corneal lesions or by brain biopsy. The isolates can be identified by serologic tests (neutralization, immunofluorescence, etc) and typed by laboratory means. Antibody determinations establish that the person has been infected with herpes simplex virus in the past. Only during primary infections can one detect a rise in antibody titer in paired serum specimens.

Treatment

Several drugs can inhibit herpes simplex virus replication.

Idoxuridine and trifluridine ophthalmic preparations, applied topically for herpetic keratitis, and local debridement will greatly accelerate corneal healing but will not affect the rate of recurrence.

Vidarabine can be applied topically for corneal herpetic infections; it can also be given systemically, since it is relatively nontoxic. Vidarabine, 15 mg/kg/d intravenously, has been used for treatment of newborns with disseminated herpes simplex virus and for treatment of immunosuppressed patients and can limit the progression of lesions. In patients with herpetic encephalitis diagnosed early (before onset of coma), vidarabine can significantly reduce mortality; however, neurologic findings are close to normal in only 40% of survivors.

Acyclovir, 15 mg/kg/d intravenously, can delay the onset or limit the progression of mucocutaneous herpes simplex lesions in immunocompromised patients (eg, after organ transplants). Acyclovir given intravenously can also reduce pain and accelerate healing of primary herpes simplex genital infections, but it does not affect the establishment of latency or the frequency of recurrence. Given by mouth, acyclovir may have similar effects.

Topical application of 5% acyclovir ointment can limit the progression of mucocutaneous herpes simplex lesions in immunosuppressed individuals but not in patients with normal immunity. It can also shorten the healing time in primary genital herpetic lesions but not in recurrent lesions. Acyclovir-resistant herpes simplex viruses have been isolated.

Prophylaxis

In view of the wide distribution of HSV-1 among all human populations, preventive measures are difficult. Contact of susceptible individuals and surfaces with open lesions should be avoided. HSV-2 behaves as an agent of sexually transmitted disease; precautions suitable for the latter are applicable. Cesarean section may prevent some neonatal infections in women with active lesions near the time of delivery.

Prognosis

In most cases, the prognosis is excellent. In patients with severe generalized eruptions, the prognosis depends upon control of secondary bacterial infection. In patients with central nervous system involvement and in newborns with systemic disease, the prognosis is very poor.

CAT-SCRATCH FEVER
(Benign Lymphoreticulosis)

Cat-scratch fever is an acute illness of unknown cause, characterized by low-grade fever, malaise, an erythematous papular or pustular cutaneous lesion at the site of contact, and regional adenopathy occurring about 2–4 weeks later. The lymph nodes are usually not painful, but they may become warm, fixed to surrounding tissue, and suppurative; the enlargement may persist for 1 week to several months. A history of cat scratch, cat bite, or contact with healthy cats a few days before onset is characteristic.

An encephalopathy associated with cat-scratch fever has been reported, and a conjunctivitis associated with inoculation on the face has also been described.

Heat-inactivated purulent material from enlarged and fluctuant lymph nodes has served as a skin test antigen under research conditions and produces a tuberculinlike reaction in convalescent cases. No specific therapy is known. Surgical removal or needle evacuation of the affected node will usually be followed by marked improvement.

Complete recovery usually occurs within a few months.

DENGUE

Dengue is an acute febrile disease with sudden onset, short duration, and excellent prognosis, occurring potentially wherever the vectors and infected individuals exist (mostly in the tropics and subtropics). Dengue is characterized by the triad of morbilliform rash, bradycardia, and leukopenia. Transmission of the virus is through the bite of a mosquito, and prophylaxis consists of mosquito control.

Clinical Findings

A. Symptoms and Signs: The incubation period is 5–9 days after the bite of the mosquito. Onset is very sudden, with a rise in temperature to 38.9–40.6 °C (102–105 °F), severe headache, and joint pains. The initial rash is an irregular blotchy congestion on the face. On the third or fourth day, the temperature falls to normal, with profuse diaphoresis. After 1–3 days, fever recurs, accompanied by a faint morbilliform rash that spreads from the hands and feet to the trunk and by a definite bradycardia (around 50/min). This stage lasts 4–6 days. Convalescence is marked by depression and anorexia.

B. Laboratory Findings: Leukopenia occurs by the second day of fever.

Treatment

Control temperatures above 39.4 °C (103 °F) to prevent possible convulsions due to hyperpyrexia. Increase fluid intake to allow for deficiency caused by profuse diaphoresis.

YELLOW FEVER

Yellow fever is an acute febrile disease that is of varying severity but usually causes hepatic necrosis and renal damage. It is endemic in Brazil, Colombia, Venezuela, and parts of Africa. The virus is transmitted through the bite of the *Aedes aegypti* mosquito. Blood of an infected individual is infectious from 2 days prior to fever until 4 days after onset. The mosquito may transmit the disease 10–20 days after biting an infected person. The incubation period is 3–6 days after the mosquito bite.

Clinical Findings

A. Symptoms and Signs: There is a short prodrome with mild malaise, followed by a rise in temperature, headache, and joint pains. The temperature rises to about 40 °C (104 °F) by the second day and persists for about 4 days. The pulse rate falls as the temperature rises. The second phase follows after 1–3 days, with increasing fever at onset and jaundice by the fifth day of disease. Nausea and vomiting are prominent. Icterus is not intense. Bleeding tendency may be prominent, with gastrointestinal hemorrhage. Hypoglycemia is common at this stage. The disease ends by crisis in the second week. In mild cases with only slight fever and headache, clinical diagnosis is almost impossible.

B. Laboratory Findings: Initial polymorphonuclear leukocytosis is followed in 6 days by leukopenia, urinary casts and increasing proteinuria, and hypoglycemia.

Complications

Hemorrhage, usually from the gastrointestinal tract, may be extensive and fatal. Severe renal damage with anuria may occur.

Treatment

A. Specific Measures: None available.

B. General Measures: Measures include strict bed rest and ample fluid intake, with stress on glucose to combat the hypoglycemia. The parenteral route should be used without hesitation.

C. Treatment of Complications: Give transfusions to compensate for gastrointestinal bleeding (see p 18).

Prophylaxis

Prophylactic measures include control of the insect vector, control of individuals entering from endemic areas, and active immunization (see Chapter 7).

Prognosis

The prognosis is guarded until 7 days after onset, when severity of liver involvement will be apparent. Hemorrhagic tendency at this stage may be the cause of death. Clinical improvement after 10 days is an excellent sign. One attack produces lifelong immunity.

INFECTIOUS MONONUCLEOSIS

Infectious mononucleosis is an infectious but not very contagious disease caused by the Epstein-Barr (EB) virus of Burkitt's lymphoma syndrome in West Africa. It may occur at any age up to 30 years but is rare in infancy and most common in the later years of childhood and early adult years.

Clinical Findings

A. Symptoms and Signs: There is usually a gradual onset of malaise and fever to 38.9 °C (102 °F). A sore throat becomes apparent and sometimes becomes severe, with swelling of the neck and a membrane on tonsils and pharynx. There is generalized lymphadenopathy, especially of the cervical nodes. The spleen is characteristically enlarged, usually after the first week of symptoms. A morbilliform, scarlatiniform, or petechial rash may appear. A benign type of "hepatitis" frequently occurs, owing to swelling of the reticuloendothelial tissues in the liver, with resultant obstruction. Hepatocellular involvement does not occur.

B. Laboratory Findings: A leukocytosis develops very early, with a predominant lymphocytosis. The stained smear of the blood shows increasing numbers of large immature vacuolated lymphocytes. A rising titer of heterophil agglutinins usually appears in the serum by the second week. A titer against sheep red blood cells of 1:112 is significant, and a titer of 1:160 is diagnostic. The heterophil agglutinin is usually apparent when the peripheral white blood cell count is most abnormal. Serum sickness from the injection of horse serum will stimulate a similar antibody, which can be differentiated by absorption tests. A simple slide agglutination test is commercially available; it demonstrates the same antibody and can be used for diagnostic purposes.

Complications

A secondary infection in the throat with group A streptococci is the most common complication. Myocarditis and encephalitis have been reported. Rupture of the spleen may occur from trauma to the abdomen and represents a surgical emergency.

Differential Diagnosis

Toxoplasmosis (see Chapter 26) and cytomegalovirus disease (see below) may cause a very similar clinical picture. The throat is usually not as sore. Laboratory findings are similar, but a heterophil antibody does not appear.

Treatment

A. Specific Measures: None available.

B. General Measures: Bed rest should be continued until the patient has been afebrile for 4 days. In severe cases, give methylprednisolone (Medrol), 1 mg/kg immediately and the same dosage daily for 5 days. Pharyngitis complicated by group A streptococci should be treated with penicillin (see Chapter 6). Patients with symptoms of liver involvement require no treatment or special diets.

Prognosis

The disease usually runs its course in 10–20 days. The prognosis is excellent in most cases. Rupture of the spleen is a serious complication requiring surgical intervention.

CYTOMEGALOVIRUS DISEASE

Cytomegalovirus disease, once thought to be a rare type of congenital infection that was usually fatal, is now recognized as the cause of several types of disease of which the congenital variety is perhaps the least common.

Cytomegalovirus is isolated easily from the urine of the acutely ill patient as well as from the body tissues. The virus can also be isolated from the urine for many months after the acute illness or after birth in the case of the congenital disease. Characteristic large inclusion bodies are present in the epithelial cells found in the urinary sediment.

Clinical Findings

A. Congenital Disease: There is rapid onset of jaundice shortly after birth, with hepatosplenomegaly, purpura, hematuria, and signs of encephalitis. Laboratory findings include thrombocytopenia, erythroblastosis, bilirubinemia, and marked lymphocytosis. Downey type abnormal lymphocytes are present in large numbers. Sequelae include intracranial calcifications, microcephalus, mental retardation, convulsive states, and optic atrophy. The prognosis is poor.

B. Acute Acquired Disease: This resembles the syndrome of infectious mononucleosis (see above). There is a sudden onset of fever, malaise, joint pains, and myalgia. Pharyngitis is minimal, and respiratory symptoms are absent. Lymphadenopathy is generalized. The liver shows enlargement and often slight tenderness. Laboratory findings include the hematologic picture of mononucleosis as well as bilirubinemia. Heterophil antibody does not appear.

C. Generalized Systemic Disease: This occurs in immunosuppressed individuals, especially following organ transplant procedures. The syndrome includes pneumonitis, hepatitis, and leukopenia, often with a lymphocytosis. The condition is occasionally fatal. Transplant patients without serologic evidence of previous infection from the acquired disease represent a higher risk of serious if not fatal systemic disease.

Treatment

No specific treatment measures are available. General measures should include analgesic and antipyretic procedures and control of convulsions (see Table 21–4). Corticosteroids have been reported to produce amelioration of symptoms and are especially indicated in the congenital disease where the prognosis is so poor.

Prognosis

Ninety percent of survivors of the congenital disease are neurologically impaired, with microcephaly and mental retardation the most common defects. Neuromuscular disorders, hearing loss, and optic atrophy are also common.

INFLUENZA

Influenza is an acute systemic viral disease that usually occurs in epidemics and is caused by a distinct class of viruses divided into 3 main serotypes (A, B, and C) based on the ribonucleoproteins. Further classification of each type is based on the surface proteins, hemagglutinin and neuraminidase. The clinical disease is characteristic of all serotypes; in epidemics, the symptoms are very consistent. In the absence of an established epidemic, the diagnosis should be considered with great care to rule out other specific diseases in which the prodrome has similar clinical findings.

Clinical Findings

The onset is abrupt, with sudden fever to 39.4–40 °C (103–104 °F), extreme malaise, myalgia, headache, and a dry, nonproductive cough. Small infants may exhibit only fever, cough, and marked irritability. Physical findings are minimal and usually include only a red pharynx. In small children, the neck and back may appear to be stiff (myalgia).

Complications

Primary complications due specifically to the influenza virus are rare but may include an extensive hemorrhage type of pneumonia with rapid downhill course, myocarditis, and toxic encephalopathy. Secondary complications due to bacterial agents include bronchial pneumonia and otitis media. The bacterial agent most often responsible is *Staphylococcus aureus*. Bacterial complications should be considered if the temperature remains elevated longer than 4 days and if the white blood cell count is greater than 12,000/μL.

Treatment

No specific measures are available. General measures include analgesic and antipyretic measures, use of mist and steam, as in croup (see Chapter 15), and bed rest for at least 1 week. If bacteriologic laboratory diagnosis is not available, treat with penicillin and chloramphenicol (see Chapter 6 for dosage). In the rare event of encephalopathy, treat as for toxic encephalopathy. Amantadine hydrochloride (Symmetrel) has been reported to show promising results when given during the first 24 hours of symptoms in the same dosage used for prophylaxis (see below).

Prophylaxis

Influenza vaccine has been demonstrated to have varying efficacy in the past, but improved techniques offer continuing promise for more reliable active immunization in the future. It is recommended for any child with chronic respiratory tract or cardiovascular disease.

Amantadine hydrochloride (Symmetrel) has been shown to prevent infection with influenza type A_2 when given after exposure, especially in previously immunized individuals. It appears to exert its effect by preventing penetration of the virus into the host cell. For children under 9 years of age, give 4.5–9 mg/kg/d (2–4 mg/lb/d) in 2 or 3 equal doses. For children 9 years of age and over, give 100 mg twice a day. Continue this drug for at least 10 days following a known exposure. It can be used for a maximum of 30 days in a persistent epidemic with recurrent exposure.

ACUTE INFECTIOUS LYMPHOCYTOSIS

Acute infectious lymphocytosis is a rare benign disease, probably of viral origin, with symptoms lasting 1–3 days and a distinct lymphocytosis lasting 3–7 weeks. Few symptoms are found, but the onset may be marked by fever and irritability. Abdominal pain or symptoms of upper respiratory tract infection may also occur. The condition must be differentiated from lymphatic leukemia and mononucleosis. The white blood cell count is diagnostic, with totals to 40,000/μL and occasionally to over 100,000/μL, predominantly adult lymphocytes. Lymph node or splenic enlargement is absent. The heterophil agglutination test results are negative. The prognosis is excellent; long-term follow-up shows no evidence of leukemia or other blood disease.

MUCOCUTANEOUS LYMPH NODE SYNDROME (MLNS)

Mucocutaneous lymph node syndrome was first described in Japan in 1960 and is now reported with increasing frequency in the USA and Europe. The cause is not known, and a variety of viruses and toxic or allergic causes have been postulated. The association of the syndrome with clinical varicella, herpes simplex, and Epstein-Barr infections has suggested that this disease might be the result of an abnormal immunologic response.

The onset is abrupt, with fever as high as 40 °C (104 °F) and a diffuse rash over the body. The lips are very red, and the tongue has a bright "strawberry" appearance. The conjunctiva and the palms and soles are red and swollen. The lymph nodes in the neck are usually enlarged. The fever usually subsides in 1–3 weeks, and there is a characteristic peeling of the skin, beginning around the fingertips and toenails. Associated symptoms or findings may include carditis, diarrhea, arthralgia, proteinuria, and pyuria.

Complications include coronary arteritis, with abnormal electrocardiographic findings in over half of the patients investigated. Serial coronary angiograms show that most cases have healed spontaneously. Sudden death, however, may occur during convalescence or months later.

Treatment is entirely symptomatic, with sponging and aspirin for the fever.

The prognosis is guarded. Fatalities have been reported, but the fatality rate is unestablished.

COLORADO TICK FEVER

Colorado tick fever is an acute viral disease, relatively common in the western USA, that is transmitted by a wood tick. It is characterized by a sudden onset of fever lasting 2–3 days, followed by an afebrile period (24–48 hours) and then a second febrile period of 2 or 3 days. Rarely, central nervous system involvement or maculopapular rash may be present. Leukopenia is invariably present.

There is no treatment. The prognosis is excellent.

VIRAL INFECTIONS OF THE CENTRAL NERVOUS SYSTEM*

POLIOMYELITIS

Poliomyelitis is an acute viral infection of the spinal cord and brain stem. In its severe form, it leads to neuron destruction and irreversible muscular paralysis and, in 10% of the paralytic forms, to death. In countries where the trivalent oral attenuated virus vaccine is widely used, this disease is very rare.

Clinical Findings

There is no common cause other than poliomyelitis for asymmetric, scattered flaccid paralysis accompanied by signs of meningeal irritation and fever.

A. Nonparalytic Poliomyelitis: This is the most common form of the disease. There is no clinical or laboratory evidence of invasion of the central nervous system. Diagnosis can rarely be established except by inference in epidemics.

B. Paralytic Poliomyelitis (Spinal Type): Paralysis may occur without obvious antecedent illness, especially in infants. It usually begins and progresses during the febrile stage of the illness. Tremor upon sustained effort may be the first clue to diagnosis and may be present before weakness occurs. Muscle tightness and pain on stretching may cause malfunction and simulate paralysis. For cerebrospinal fluid findings, see Appendix. The cell count may be normal in 10–15% of cases.

C. Bulbar Polioencephalitis: This is paralytic poliomyelitis that includes involvement of the cranial nerves and brain stem. Significant lower spinal involvement may be absent. Any cranial nerve may be affected, but swallowing difficulties predominate. This form of poliomyelitis is more likely to occur in patients whose tonsils have been removed. Polioencephalitis is the term applied when there is impairment of cerebral function. It follows a fulminant course.

Respiratory Difficulty in Poliomyelitis

Respiratory difficulty may occur with paralysis of intercostal muscles, manifested by anxiety, increased respiratory rate, and reluctance to vocalize. The upper arm and shoulder muscles are often involved. Paralyses of the diaphragm, which are easily overlooked, are usually associated with intercostal paralysis. Weakness of the intercostal muscles and diaphragm is demonstrated by diminished chest expansion and decreased vital capacity. Damage to the medullary respiratory center

*See also Coxsackievirus Infection (p 593) and Echovirus Infection (p 595).

may also occur, sometimes with severe symptoms of irregular, shallow, spasmodic breathing. Obstruction of the pharynx or trachea, due to aspiration of saliva secondary to pharyngeal or palatal paralysis (or both), may occur.

Treatment

A. Specific Measures: None available.

B. General Measures: Many patients with mild forms of poliomyelitis can be cared for in the home. The need for isolation in special hospitals is questionable, since the virus is universally distributed in epidemic conditions. Special facilities and trained professional personnel are required for the more severely involved patient.

Bed rest is indicated, with careful observation for further paralysis during the first week of disease. Hot packs, hot soaks, bedboards, footboards, and splints may be used. Physiotherapy is the most important single factor in recovery. During the acute stage, passive motion is begun to the point of pain only. All extremities must be exercised to prevent joint immobilization. Active motion is begun when pain subsides. Uncoordinated or unnatural function must be avoided as long as possible. Resistance type exercises should be postponed until all tightness has subsided. Braces and surgery are indicated only after physiotherapy has been attempted.

C. Treatment of Respiratory Difficulties: Intercostal or diaphragm paralysis requires artificial ventilation before cyanosis appears. A tank respirator, operated by experienced personnel, may be used. The chest respirator (cuirass) is about 60% as efficient as the tank. It is useful in rehabilitation and simplifies the problem of nursing care. Tracheostomy may be required in patients with paralysis of muscles of swallowing, weakness of muscles of respiration, or bulbar poliomyelitis.

Prophylaxis

The paralytic consequences of infection with poliomyelitis virus can be avoided by prophylactic use of oral vaccine.

Prognosis

The prognosis as to paralysis is guarded until pain subsides. In the bulbar form, prognosis is good if complications are overcome. Patients with polioencephalitis usually have a poor prognosis for survival. If the respiratory center is severely involved, the prognosis is poor.

VIRAL ENCEPHALITIDES

The most important types of viral encephalitides are those carried by an insect vector, usually a mosquito. The arthropod-borne encephalitides include a large number of diseases caused by antigenically distinct viruses: western equine encephalomyelitis virus, eastern equine encephalitis virus, St. Louis encephalitis virus, Australian X disease virus, Venezuelan virus, Japanese B encephalitis virus, and West Nile fever virus. Encephalitis in children is discussed in Chapter 21.

LYMPHOCYTIC CHORIOMENINGITIS

Lymphocytic choriomeningitis is an acute viral infection involving principally the meninges. It is transmitted by direct contact with house mice in certain geographic areas; it occurs rarely west of the Mississippi.

The clinical picture is dominated by signs of meningeal irritation. Malaise and fever are usually not great. Encephalitic symptoms are rare. The course is short and benign.

Cerebrospinal fluid (see Appendix) shows high cell count, predominantly lymphocytes, as in mumps meningoencephalitis. Differentiation from mumps is made on serologic and epidemiologic grounds.

No specific treatment is available. The prognosis is excellent.

RABIES

Rabies, an acute viral encephalitis, is transmitted by saliva of an afflicted animal and gains entry into the body by means of a bite or abrasion. Skunks, foxes, bats, and other wild animals are widely infected in the USA; dogs, cats, and other domestic animals may become infected and are the main reservoir of rabies in some developing countries. Persons in contact with infected animals are at risk. The virus appears in saliva 5–7 days before the development of symptoms. Virtually all symptomatic animals and humans die from the disease, but the incubation period may range from a few days to several months.

The most common problem confronting the physician is the management of a patient bitten by an animal. If the patient develops symptoms (pain and tingling at the site of the bite, restlessness, muscle spasms, convulsions, and coma), it is usually too late for effective measures.

The first step is the evaluation of the patient's exposure to determine if it is "significant." Factors include information regarding the biting animal, whether the attack was provoked or unprovoked, local and individual circumstances, and advice from public health authorities. The bite wound must always be cleansed with soap and water, flushed out, and debrided if necessary. If the exposure is deemed "significant," rabies-killed virus vaccine (human diploid cell [HDC] vaccine; see Chapter 7) is injected on days 0, 3, 7, 14, and 28. If indicated, rabies immune globulin is injected both around the bite wound and intramuscularly. The recommendations of the Rabies Investigation Unit, Centers for Disease Control,* as well as the manufacturer's directions for use of the vaccine and immune globulin, should be followed.

Only if HDC vaccine is not available should duck embryo vaccine be used. It must be given in a series of 23 injections, and its efficacy is probably low. Rabies immune globulin must be given concurrently.

Preexposure prophylaxis with 3 injections of HDC vaccine is recommended for individuals at high risk of exposure (eg, persons residing in a country of high endemicity).

RICKETTSIAL DISEASES

The rickettsiae are very small intracellular organisms that stain irregularly gram-negative. They are divided immunologically into distinct groups and subgroups. While most groups stimulate the production in humans of agglutinins against strains of *Proteus vulgaris,* the determination of complement-fixing antibodies is a more accurate and acceptable serologic testing method.

EPIDEMIC TYPHUS

Epidemic typhus is an acute febrile disease characterized by a generalized rash and caused by *Rickettsia prowazekii,* which is transmitted in louse feces from person to person by inoculation through abraded skin. The incubation period is 5–15 days.

The onset is sudden, with nausea, vomiting, headache, nosebleeds, and cough. Fever rises, although the disease may be very mild in children. A rash appears on the fourth to the sixth day, first on the trunk near the axillae and then spreading to the extremities. The rash appears first as a pale macule, which becomes darker red or hemorrhagic, lasting for about 7 days.

The white blood cell count is normal or reduced during the first week. Agglutinins against *Proteus* OX19 show a rise in titer during the second week.

Complications include myocarditis appearing in the second week, bronchopneumonia from secondary bacterial infection, and renal insufficiency.

*For information in the USA regarding rabies, contact the Centers for Disease Control; telephone (404) 329-3696 or (404) 329-3670 during the day or (404) 329-2888 during nights, weekends, and holidays. Most local health departments can also provide information.

Specific treatment with tetracyclines (see Chapter 6) is highly effective. With bronchopneumonia as a complication, use appropriate antibiotic therapy.

Typhus vaccine is very effective. A booster dosage should be given every 6 months to persons residing in endemic areas. Delousing of exposed persons and clothing in endemic areas will prevent spread of disease.

The prognosis is excellent in vaccinated individuals and those who are treated early in the course of disease.

ENDEMIC TYPHUS

Endemic typhus is an acute febrile disease clinically indistinguishable from mild epidemic typhus and caused by *Rickettsia typhi*. Transmission is through the bite of the rat flea.

Clinically, the disease is a mild one with no complications and excellent prognosis. Treatment is the same as for epidemic typhus. Vaccines are not available; prophylaxis consists of rat control.

ROCKY MOUNTAIN SPOTTED FEVER (Kenya Typhus, South African Tick Fever, Tobia Fever, Pinta Fever, São Paulo Typhus)

Rocky Mountain spotted fever is an acute febrile disease caused by *Rickettsia rickettsii*. Transmission is through a tick bite. In the eastern USA, the dog tick, *Dermacentor variabilis*, is the most common vector; in the western USA, it is the wood tick, *Dermacentor andersoni*.

Clinical Findings

A. Symptoms and Signs: The incubation period is 3–14 days (average, 7 days). Onset is sudden with a febrile course, as in typhus, lasting for 3–7 weeks in untreated cases. In children, Rocky Mountain spotted fever is more severe than typhus. The rash appears on the third or fourth day, first on the extremities and then spreading to the trunk. The lesion is a small, bright red macule that becomes hemorrhagic or even necrotic. Tick or evidence of the bite is present.

B. Laboratory Findings: Findings include white blood cell counts of 12,000–14,000/μL and a rising complement fixation titer by the second week.

Complications

In severe cases, there may be a shocklike state due to markedly disturbed fluid and electrolyte balance.

Treatment

Tetracyclines should be given, and symptoms should be treated. In severe cases with shock and dehydration, liberal but careful use of parenteral fluid therapy, including plasma, is extremely important (see Chapter 2).

Prophylaxis

Vaccine (see Chapter 7) is very effective in children. In tick-infested areas, the body should be examined frequently for ticks.

Prognosis

The prognosis is excellent with early therapy. In severe cases, the outcome will depend upon the success of fluid and electrolyte therapy, in addition to the specific antibiotic in use.

Q FEVER

Q fever is an acute febrile disease caused by *Coxiella burnetii*. Animal reservoirs (eg, sheep, goats, cattle) excrete large numbers of organisms in feces and urine and through the placenta; the dust-borne organisms are transmitted to humans. Infected cattle excrete organisms in milk, and infection is carried to humans in unpasteurized milk.

Clinical Findings

A. Symptoms and Signs: Most cases of Q fever resemble mild attacks of influenza. There may be fever for 2–6 days, with slight respiratory symptoms. In severe cases, the onset is sudden, with high fever, characteristically spiking to 39.4–40 °C (103–104 °F), and chills. Fever in children lasts for 3–7 days. A faint, generalized, morbilliform rash appears rarely. Clinical or x-ray evidence of pneumonitis may be present.

B. Laboratory Findings: The white blood cell count is usually within normal range. The complement fixation titer rises during the second week.

Treatment

Give tetracyclines (see Chapter 6) and symptomatic care.

Prophylaxis

Measures for prophylaxis include vaccine, dust control, detection of animal vector sources, and pasteurization of milk.

Prognosis

The prognosis is excellent with specific antibiotic therapy. Severe cases are very rare in children.

Infectious Diseases: Bacterial & Spirochetal | 25

BACTERIAL DISEASES

STREPTOCOCCAL DISEASES
(Streptococcosis)

A variety of disease states directly or indirectly ascribed to streptococci are very important in the pediatric age groups. These are spread from person to person by droplets but may occasionally be transmitted by contact with soiled articles.

Etiology

Streptococci are gram-positive and characteristically appear in chains. They may be classified as follows:

A. β-Hemolytic Streptococci: These exhibit beta hemolysis on blood agar culture and are divided into a number of groups, of which A, B, and D are the principal pathogens. Group A infections most commonly occur in children and adults, and group B may cause severe disease in infants.

B. Non-β-Hemolytic Streptococci: These commonly exhibit alpha hemolysis or no change on blood agar culture. Viridans streptococci are included in this category.

C. Peptostreptococci: These produce variable hemolysis, are found in the intestinal tract, and are sometimes pathogenic.

Clinical Findings

A. Symptoms and Signs: Streptococci produce a great variety of clinical diseases. Certain entities show a definite concentration in certain age groups.

1. Infection in neonates–Neonatal infections are principally caused by group B streptococci, especially type 3. There are 2 clinical syndromes, early onset and late onset. In the early onset syndrome (at less than 5 days of age), infection is acquired from the maternal vagina. Symptoms in the neonate include apnea, shock, and meningitis. There is a very high mortality rate. In the late onset syndrome (between 2 weeks and 4 months), meningitis, cellulitis, impetigo, and osteomyelitis are common manifestations.

2. Infection in young children–In the early childhood type (group A) infection, the onset is insidious, with mild constitutional symptoms, mucopurulent nasal discharge, and many suppurative complications (otitis media, lymphadenitis). Exudative tonsillitis is uncommon, and sore throat is apparently absent. Rheumatic fever, nephritis, and scarlet fever rarely occur in association with this form of the disease.

3. Infection in older children–In the middle childhood type (group A) infection, the onset is usually sudden, with temperature over 39 °C (102.2 °F). The throat is moderately sore and beefy red, with edema of anterior pillars and palatal petechiae. Exudative tonsillitis, with a white-yellow membrane, is relatively frequent. Anterior cervical lymph nodes are large and tender. Scarlet fever, which occurs in association with this form of disease, consists of streptococcal pharyngitis plus a rash due to susceptibility to erythrogenic toxin. The rash appears 12–48 hours after the onset of fever; it begins in the areas of warmth and pressure, spreads rapidly to involve the entire body below the chin line, and reaches its maximum in 1 or 2 days. It is characterized by a diffuse erythema of the skin, with prominence of the bases of the hair follicles. It fades on pressure and does not involve the circumoral region. Transverse lines that do not fade on pressure are found at the elbow (Pastia's sign). The exanthem usually is followed by desquamation beginning in the second week; peeling of the fingertips has greatest diagnostic significance. The tongue may be coated but then desquamates and becomes beefy red.

4. Infection in adults–The adult type (group A) infection usually occurs in patients over 10 years of age but may occur in much younger children who have had repeated streptococcal infections. The course is similar to the pharyngitis described above; exudative tonsillitis is common.

5. Skin infection–In streptococcal disease of the skin (see Impetigo, Chapter 12), streptococci may enter the skin and subcutaneous tissues through abrasions or wounds and may produce progressive erysipelas with fever, chills, rapidly progressive edema, and erythema. Wound infection with streptococci may result in "surgical scarlet fever" when the organism produces the erythrogenic toxin in a patient without antitoxin.

B. Laboratory Findings: The white blood cell count is usually elevated (12,000–15,000/μL) in patients with uncomplicated upper respiratory tract infection; it may go to 20,000/μL or higher in patients with suppurative complications. Antistreptolysin titers will rise above 150 units in the course of a streptococcal infection of any sort. If the titer later drops, the test may be used as a measure of recent uncomplicated streptococcal infection. The results of throat culture are positive for streptococci. The more predominant this organism is in populations of organisms in culture, the more likely that it is playing a causative role.

Complications

A wide variety of clinical conditions may result from the presence of streptococci in the upper respiratory tract of the patient or from contact with the carrier. There is no relationship to age.

A. Pyoderma: Impetigo may occur. There may be secondary infection of eczema, with multiple papulovesicular lesions resembling Kaposi's varicelliform eruption. Furuncles and cellulitis due to streptococcal infection appear less commonly than those due to staphylococcal infection.

B. Otitis Media: This is commonly caused by streptococci as a complication of upper respiratory tract infection.

C. Adenitis: Streptococci are the most common cause of adenitis (which is usually cervical) in children.

D. Septicemia: Septicemia occurs especially in the debilitated or the very young.

E. "Metastatic Foci": These include meningitis, pyogenic arthritis, and osteomyelitis.

F. Vaginitis: Vaginitis may be due to streptococci.

G. Nonsuppurative Complications: These include rheumatic fever (see Chapter 29) and acute glomerulonephritis (see Chapter 18).

Treatment

A. Specific Measures:

1. Penicillin is the drug of choice.

a. For group A infections (the most common type), including pharyngitis, otitis, impetigo, and adenitis, give a single intramuscular dose of 1.2 million units of one of the following (listed in order of preference): combined procaine and benzathine penicillin; procaine penicillin; or benzathine penicillin. For group B infection in infants, give penicillin G, 150–250 thousand units/kg/d intravenously for at least 10 days. Combined treatment with ampicillin and gentamicin has been recommended. For more severe infection with sepsis, pneumonia, meningitis, or osteomyelitis, use penicillin G, 250–400 thousand units/kg/d intravenously.

b. Oral penicillin may be adequate if there is compliance in giving and taking the prescribed dosage. Give 250 mg every 6 hours between meals for at least 10 days.

2. In cases of penicillin sensitivity, patients may be treated with oral erythromycin, clindamycin, or cephalexin. In severe infections, cephalothin and cefazolin may be used intravenously or intramuscularly (see Chapter 6).

B. General Measures: Irrigation of the throat with warm saline solution may provide some relief in older children. Bed rest is recommended until the patient is afebrile.

C. Treatment of Carriers of Streptococci: Opinion differs on how to manage the carrier state. Some recommend full therapeutic doses of penicillin; others feel that the strain of organism carried does not produce clinical disease and may increase immunity to future infection. Recurrent tonsillitis in a carrier may not respond to antibiotic therapy. Tonsillectomy may be necessary.

Prophylaxis

No immunizing agent against hemolytic streptococci is at present available. In certain cases, antibiotic prophylaxis may be indicated (eg, rheumatic fever; see Chapter 29). The complications and sequelae of streptococcal disease are less likely to occur if the patient is treated promptly and adequately with antibiotics.

Prenatal identification and antibiotic treatment of mothers carrying group B streptococci may be effective in preventing infection of the infant. A vaccine for pregnant carriers is being investigated.

Prognosis

The prognosis for patients with early childhood and adult types of infection is excellent with penicillin treatment. Uncomplicated cases of middle childhood type infection subside in 4–5 days with or without specific treatment.

PNEUMOCOCCAL DISEASES

Streptococcus pneumoniae produces a number of disease entities principally in the respiratory tract. The organism is gram-positive, occurs in pairs, and is divided into more than 83 types on the basis of specific capsular polysaccharides. Types 6, 14, 19, and 23 are more likely to cause disease in children than in adults. The disease is spread from person to person by respiratory droplets.

Clinical Findings

A. Symptoms and Signs:

1. Upper respiratory tract infection–This occurs commonly as a consequence of primary viral infections, with pharyngitis, sinusitis, otitis, or tracheobronchitis increasing at the end of the first week of the viral illness. Pneumococcal disease is associated with a rise in fever and leukocytosis. A profuse, thick, purulent, greenish nasal discharge is characteristic.

2. Bacteremia–*S pneumoniae* is a frequent cause of bacteremia, with fever and leukocytosis in children over 1 month of age. A presumptive diagnosis should be made when a characteristic gingival cystic swelling is found on the posterior buccal surface of the alveolar ridge, and specific therapy should be started after a blood culture is obtained.

3. Pneumonia–Pneumonia is usually peribronchial in the child under 6 years of age. Typical lobar pneumonia occurs more commonly in older children.

4. Meningitis–Meningitis occurs usually as a result of pneumococcal bacteremia accompanying upper or lower respiratory disease.

5. Peritonitis–Peritonitis may occur, especially in patients with chronic glomerulonephritis and nephrosis.

6. Vaginitis–Vaginitis may occur in preadolescent girls.

B. Laboratory Findings: Leukocytosis is the rule in pneumococcal infection. Nasopharyngeal cultures usually yield positive results. Blood cultures should always be done when pneumonia, meningitis, or peritonitis is suspected.

Complications

Localized pneumococcal infection may result from bacteremia accompanying the above manifestations, with abscess in the vitreous, purulent arthritis, pericarditis, and empyema following pneumonia. Sinusitis may be a subtle and almost silent residual complication in older children.

Treatment

A. Specific Measures: Penicillin is the drug of choice, given as in streptococcal infection. In cases of penicillin sensitivity, patients may be treated with oral erythromycin, clindamycin, or cephalexin. In severe infection, cephalothin and cefazolin may be given intravenously or intramuscularly (see Chapter 6).

B. General Measures: Maintenance of a warm, humid environment is important.

Prophylaxis

A polyvalent pneumococcal vaccine is now available. It contains antigens from the 14 different types of *S pneumoniae* that are responsible for 80% of cases. A protective antibody response develops 2 weeks after inoculation and has been shown to persist for 2 years. The vaccine is indicated for immunization of high-risk patients such as those who are immunosuppressed, those with splenic dysfunction due to sickle cell disease or other causes, children with chronic respiratory tract disease such as cystic fibrosis, and children with diabetes mellitus. Administration to individuals under 2 years of age is not recommended, because the antibody response is poor.

Detection of pneumococcal bacteremia in children under 10 years of age with high fever and leukocytosis will permit early antibiotic treatment and prevention of the more serious forms of pneumococcal disease.

STAPHYLOCOCCAL DISEASES

The staphylococci are gram-positive organisms and are divided into several types. Coagulase-producing strains are the most common pathogens. Recently, most strains of this organism produce penicillinase and are thus resistant to penicillin treatment.

Staphylococci are common in the environment and are normally found in the throat and on the skin. In newborn infants, the umbilical stump is colonized, and a carrier state may produce endemic disease in the newborn nursery.

Clinical Findings

A. Symptoms and Signs:

1. Superficial infection–Pyoderma is the most common type of infection with this organism. Furuncles, folliculitis, carbuncles, and impetigo are discussed in Chapter 12.

2. Deep infection–Osteomyelitis can occur following bloodstream spread from a local inoculation or a superficial infection. Pneumonia, usually peribronchial, is common during early infancy. Septicemia, with focal abscesses in the chest, abdomen, and brain, may be present. Enterocolitis in the small infant is often the result of modified intestinal flora through use of broad-spectrum antibiotics.

3. Toxic disease–Food poisoning (see Table 16–4) may be due to production of enterotoxin in contaminated foods, usually gravies or custards. The onset is abrupt, with vomiting, prostration, and diarrhea within 4 hours of ingestion. Ritter's disease (scalded skin syndrome, toxic epidermal necrolysis; see Table 9–1) is an exfoliative skin disease in the newborn and is caused by an exotoxin. Toxic shock syndrome, also caused by an exotoxin, may result from staphylococcal infection in surgical wounds, in the vagina during menstruation and with the use of tampons, and in fulminant staphylococcal sepsis. The onset is sudden, with fever, vomiting, diarrhea, and hypotension, followed by a generalized scarlatiniform rash that desquamates (see p 616).

B. Laboratory Findings: Leukocytosis occurs in patients with deep infection. Culture of the blood yields positive results in most cases of deep infection. A smear of pus from the local infection or a rectal smear in enterocolitis easily demonstrates the organism.

Treatment

A. Specific Measures: Whenever possible, antibiotic sensitivity of the infecting organism should be determined before treatment is undertaken. In the absence of other information, it should be assumed that the infecting strain is resistant to penicillin, especially in infection presumed to be acquired in a health facility or hospital.

1. Pneumonia, osteomyelitis, and meningitis–Give methicillin, 200–300 mg/kg/d intravenously in 6 doses; or give cephalothin, 100–200 mg/kg/d intravenously in 6 doses. (Oxacillin, nafcillin, cloxacillin, or vancomycin may also be used, depending on the determination of antibiotic sensitivity.) In patients with osteomyelitis, continue intravenous therapy for at least 1 week, followed by oral therapy for another 3 weeks; surgical drainage is often necessary.

2. Enterocolitis–Give neomycin orally.

B. General Measures: When there is evidence of localized infection with abscess formation, surgical drainage must be accomplished.

1. Osteomyelitis–If pus is demonstrated by aspiration from the metaphysis or if there is little response to antibiotic treatment, surgical drainage is indicated, with removal of necrotic soft tissue.

2. Pneumonia–Combined antibiotic and surgical treatment by thoracotomy and drainage is usually necessary.

3. Brain abscess–Brain abscess requires surgical drainage.

Prophylaxis

For prophylaxis of recurrent furunculosis, see Chapter 12. Prevent food poisoning by adequate refrigeration and sanitation. Control of heavy contamination, especially from draining lesions, is important in preventing spread and dissemination or contamination of food or fomites. Asepsis, cleanliness, and antiseptic measures can control excessive spread. Hand washing by attendants and other personnel is an important control measure.

Prognosis

In the usual case of local infection with adequate local treatment, the prognosis is excellent. In deep infections with sepsis, pneumonia, brain abscess, or other localization, the prognosis is guarded. Patients with osteomyelitis have an excellent prognosis if they are promptly treated by specific and general measures.

PERTUSSIS
(Whooping Cough)

Bordetella pertussis is a gram-negative bacillus. Transmission is by droplets during the catarrhal and paroxysmal stages of whooping cough. Pertussis is communicable from 1 week before to 3 weeks after onset of paroxysms. The incubation period is 7–10 days. A pertussislike syndrome may be caused by *Bordetella parapertussis, Haemophilus haemolyticus,* or several respiratory tract viruses.

Clinical Findings

A. Symptoms and Signs: Insidious onset of symptoms of a mild catarrhal upper respiratory tract infection occurs, with rhinitis, sneezing, lacrimation, slight fever, and irritating cough. Within 2 weeks, the cough becomes paroxysmal; repeated series of many coughs during one expiration are followed by a sudden deep inspiration with a characteristic crowing sound or "whoop." Eating often precipitates paroxysms, which may also cause vomiting. Tenacious mucus may be coughed and vomited. The paroxysmal stage lasts 2–6 weeks, but a habit pattern of coughing may continue for many weeks.

B. Laboratory Findings: The white blood cell count may be very high, with predominant lymphocytosis. Cultures are best obtained by nasopharyngeal swab. The nasopharyngeal culture on Bordet-Gengou medium yields positive results. Results are generally positive during the catarrhal stage and the first week or 2 of the paroxysmal stage. The fluorescent antibody test may give a rapid diagnosis. The sedimentation rate may be low.

Differential Diagnosis

Pertussis must be differentiated from aspiration of a foreign body, pneumonia, influenza, and acute bronchitis. Lymphocytosis may suggest acute leukemia. Adenovirus, respiratory syncytial virus, *B parapertussis,* and *H haemolyticus* may cause clinical pictures indistinguishable from that caused by *B pertussis.*

Complications

Pneumonia accounts for 90% of the deaths due to pertussis. Atelectasis, emphysema, and bronchiectasis are other pulmonary complications. With convulsions, which are probably due to cerebral anoxia during paroxysms, permanent brain damage may occur. When hemorrhage occurs, it is usually into the conjunctiva or from the nose during paroxysms.

Treatment

A. Specific Measures: Erythromycin will quickly eradicate organisms and reduce the possibility of secondary infection. It will not influence the course of the clinical disease. Pertussis immune globulin is no longer recommended.

B. General Measures:

1. Respiration–Because of anoxic periods during paroxysms, infants under 18 months require constant attendance and sometimes such measures as insertion of airway, artificial respiration, and suction of oropharynx. In severely ill children and all infants under the age of 18 months, use an oxygen tent with high humidity.

2. Parenteral fluids–Severe paroxysms may prevent adequate oral intake of fluids and necessitate parenteral therapy.

3. Sedatives–Phenobarbital for younger children and early in the disease is often of value. Codeine may be used for older children in the latter phases of the illness.

4. Feedings–Frequent small feedings are less likely to cause vomiting than the usual 3-meals-a-day schedule. Thick feedings are often retained better than more fluid ones. If vomiting occurs during or immediately after a feeding, the child should be fed again. Paroxysms are less likely to occur at this time.

5. Other measures–An abdominal binder may help to shorten paroxysms. General hygienic measures are of importance because of the extended course of the disease.

C. Treatment of Complications: Treat pulmonary complications on the basis of identification of the specific organisms involved (see Chapter 6). The liberal use of oxygen in severe cases will reduce the severity of cerebral anoxia and hence the incidence of convulsions and brain damage. If convulsions occur despite the use of oxygen, give parenteral sodium phenobarbital (see Table 21–4).

Prophylaxis

For active immunization in early infancy, see Table 7–1. In exposed susceptible children under 5 years of age, give a 5-day course of tetracyclines or erythromycin.

Prognosis

Untreated severe disease in infants under 1 year of age has a poor prognosis. Adequate treatment in this age group gives a good prognosis. The prognosis is good in patients over 1 year of age with uncomplicated infection.

EXOTOXIC DISEASES (DIPHTHERIA, TETANUS, GAS GANGRENE)

The dominant pathologic process in this group of diseases is due to a product of bacterial metabolism (exotoxin) rather than to the actual invasion of the host by the organism. The successful treatment of these diseases depends primarily upon neutralization of the effects of such toxins rather than upon elimination of the organisms.

DIPHTHERIA

Diphtheria is an acute febrile infection, usually of the throat, and is most common in the winter months in temperate zones. Infants born of immune mothers are relatively immune for about 6 months. With active immunization in early childhood, the disease is becoming more common in adolescents and adults.

Diphtheria is caused by a gram-positive, pleomorphic rod, *Corynebacterium diphtheriae*, which shows barred forms on staining with methylene blue. It grows best on Löffler's medium. The organism produces a powerful necrotizing toxin; unless the toxin is neutralized by circulating antitoxin, it is fixed on tissues. The disease is transmitted by droplets from the respiratory tract of a carrier or patient. The organism resists drying; contaminated articles may therefore serve as transmitting agents. The incubation period is 1–7 days (average, 3 days).

Clinical Findings

A. Symptoms and Signs:

1. Pharyngeal–Findings include mild sore throat, moderate fever to 38.5–39 °C (101.2–102.2 °F), rapid pulse, severe prostration, and exudate. A membrane forms in the throat and spreads from the tonsils to the anterior pillars and uvula. It is typically dirty gray or gray-green when fully developed but may be white early in the course. The edges of the membrane are slightly elevated, and bleeding results if it is scraped off. (This procedure is contraindicated, as it will hasten absorption of toxin.) Rule out infectious mononucleosis (see Chapter 24), usually by laboratory tests.

2. Nasal–Nasal discharge is a potent source of spread of infection to others, and serosanguineous nasal discharge may excoriate the patient's upper lip. The membrane is visible on turbinates, and constitutional manifestations are slight.

3. Laryngeal–Findings of laryngeal involvement are the most serious and include hoarseness or aphonia, croupy cough, fever up to 39.5–40 °C (103–104 °F), marked prostration, cyanosis, difficulty in breathing, and eventually respiratory obstruction. Brawny edema of the neck may occur, and membrane formation may be visible in the pharynx.

4. Cutaneous, vaginal, and wound–Findings include ulcerative lesions with membrane formation. The lesions are persistent and often anesthetic.

B. Laboratory Findings: The white blood cell count is normal, or there may be a slight leukocytosis. A smear of exudate stained with methylene blue shows rods with midpolar bars. Cultures on Löffler's medium yield positive results.

Complications

A. Myocarditis: Myocarditis is a direct result of the effect of the toxin. Clinical diagnosis is discussed in Chapter 13. The ECG shows T wave changes and partial or complete atrioventricular block.

B. Neuritis: Neuritis is usually a late development. Both sensory and motor paralyses develop rapidly once neuritis becomes apparent. Complete recovery is usual.

1. Pharyngeal and palatal muscles–These are the earliest muscles to become involved. Manifestations include nasal voice, dysphagia, and nasal regurgitation of fluids.

2. Extrinsic eye muscles–Diplopia and strabismus are manifestations.

3. Skeletal muscles–Involvement of the legs and arms may end in quadriplegia.

C. Bronchopneumonia: Bronchopneumonia may occur.

D. Proteinuria: Proteinuria usually clears as the temperature returns to normal, but nephritis may occur.

Treatment

A. Specific Measures: The following measures are for treatment of all types of diphtheria.

1. Antitoxin–Antitoxin in sufficient dosage must be given promptly. The longer the time between onset of disease and administration of antitoxin, the higher the mortality. Give antitoxin if disease is considered possible from clinical manifestations; do not wait for reports of cultures. The dosage is 10,000–100,000 units for patients of any age, depending on the site, severity, and duration of the disease. Always test for horse serum sensitivity before administration (see Administration of Animal Sera, Chapter 7). Antitoxin may be given intramuscularly, but the intravenous route is used in patients with laryngeal diphtheria, extensive nasopharyngeal involvement, extensive cervical adenitis, or hemorrhage and in all patients treated after the third day of illness.

2. Antibiotics–Erythromycin (best) or procaine penicillin G should be used in treatment and to shorten the carrier state. The administration of these antibiotics before specimens for culture are collected may prevent diagnosis of diphtheria by inhibiting growth of the organisms.

3. Toxoid–Diphtheria may not confer immunity. Therefore, if results of the Schick test are positive, give toxoid inoculations in convalescence (see Chapter 7).

B. General Measures: Give fluids parenterally if they cannot be taken by mouth. Strict bed rest is indicated for at least 4 weeks, followed by a gradual return to normal activity. During this period, the child should be fed, bathed, and handled with utmost caution. Voluntary activity should be cut down to an absolute minimum. Examine the patient frequently for the appearance of possible complications.

Special measures for the treatment of patients with the laryngeal form of diphtheria include avoidance of sedation, aspiration of the larynx as necessary, tracheostomy for respiratory obstruction, use of an atmosphere with high humidity, and expectorant drugs.

C. Treatment of Complications:

1. Myocarditis–Give oxygen by tent and administer 20% glucose solution, 200–500 mL intravenously daily. Digitalis and quinidine are of questionable value in arrhythmias. It may be necessary to treat the patient for shock (see Chapter 2).

2. Neuritis–Dysphagia may necessitate the use of an indwelling polyethylene nasogastric tube. Intercostal paralysis may necessitate the use of a mechanical respirator.

3. Cutaneous and wound diphtheria–The use of antitoxin is required as for pharyngeal infection.

Prophylaxis

Prophylactic measures include active immunization in early childhood (see Table 7–1) and discovery and treatment of carriers.

Prognosis

The prognosis is always guarded, varying with the day of disease on which antitoxin treatment is given. After 6 days without treatment, mortality is almost 50%. Myocarditis within the first 10 days is an ominous sign.

TETANUS

Tetanus is an acute disease characterized by painful muscular contractions. Individuals of all ages are susceptible, including the newborn. The causative organism of tetanus, *Clostridium tetani,* is an anaerobic, spore-forming, gram-positive organism that produces a very powerful neurotoxin. Bacilli and spores are widely distributed in soil and dust and are present in the feces of animals and humans. Inoculation of a wound with dirt or dust is most likely to occur with puncture wounds. In many cases, the original wound may have been very minor or overlooked entirely. In the newborn, transmission may occur by contamination of the umbilical cord, which, as it becomes necrotic, permits growth of the organism. The exotoxin acts upon the motor nerve end-plates and anterior horn cells of the spinal cord and brain stem.

Clinical Findings

A. Symptoms and Signs: The incubation period varies from 5 days to 5 weeks, depending upon the size of the inoculum and the rapidity of its growth. The onset may be with spasm and cramplike pain in the muscles of the back and abdomen or about the site of inoculation, together with restlessness, irritability, difficulty in swallowing, and sometimes convulsions. A gradual increase in muscular tension occurs in the following 48 hours, with stiff neck, positive Kernig sign, tightness of masseters, anxious expression of the face, and stiffness of the arms and legs. Facial expression is modified by inability to open the mouth (trismus). Swallowing is difficult. Recurrent tetanic spasms occur and last 5–10 seconds; they are characterized by agonizing pain, stiffening of the body, retraction of the head, opisthotonus, clenching of the jaws, and clenching of the hands. Fever is usually low-grade but may rarely be as high as 40 °C (104 °F). Auditory or tactile stimuli may initiate convulsions.

B. Laboratory Findings: The white blood cell count is 8000–12,000/μL. Cerebrospinal fluid shows a slight increase in pressure, with a normal cell count. Anaerobic culture of excised necrotic tissue may yield positive results.

Treatment

A. Specific Measures:

1. For use of antitoxin, see Table 25–1 and Chapter 7. Tetanus immune globulin (human) is preferred in doses of 500–5000 units intramuscularly. If human globulin is not available, give tetanus antitoxin (horse), 50,000 units intravenously, after testing for horse serum sensitivity. The value of antitoxin treatment is questionable in mild cases and when treatment is delayed for several days after appearance of symptoms. The toxin produced by the organism is rapidly fixed upon the tissues and cannot be neutralized by antitoxin.

2. Surgical exploration of the wound, with excision of necrotic tissue and cleaning and drainage, is indicated to eliminate a local source

Table 25–1. Guide to tetanus prophylaxis in wound management.*

History of Tetanus Immunization	Clean, Minor Wounds		All Other Wounds	
	Td†	TIG‡	Td†	TIG‡
Uncertain, or < 2 doses	Yes	No	Yes	Yes
≥ 3 doses; last dose within 10 yr	No	No	Yes§	No

*Modified and reproduced, with permission, from Immunization Practices Advisory Committee, Centers for Disease Control: Diphtheria, tetanus, and pertussis: Guidelines for vaccine prophylaxis and other preventive measures. *Ann Intern Med* 1981; **95**:723.

†Td = tetanus toxoid and diphtheria toxoid, adult form. Use only this preparation (Td-adult) in children over 6 yr of age.

‡TIG = tetanus immune globulin.

§Unless last Td dose was within the past year.

of infection. There is no conclusive evidence that local therapy with antitoxin is indicated.

3. Give intramuscular penicillin for at least 7 days.

B. General Measures:

1. Keep the patient in a quiet, dark room. Minimize handling.

2. Give sedation as follows:

a. Diazepam is an effective muscle relaxant and sedative. Newborns and children up to 5 years of age should receive 0.5–2 mg/kg/d intravenously in 6 doses. Older children may require 10–20 mg/kg/d intravenously in 6 doses.

b. An alternative to diazepam is meprobamate. The parenteral dosage is as follows: in children up to 5 years of age, 50–100 mg every 3 hours; ages 5–12 years, 200–300 mg every 3 hours; and over 12 years, 400 mg every 3 hours.

c. Barbiturates in doses sufficient to overcome spasms can be given if the above are not available.

3. Gentle aspiration of secretions in the nasopharynx should be done as required.

4. Oxygen should be available.

5. Intravenous fluids are given as required.

6. Tracheostomy is a lifesaving measure for removal of secretions in the tracheobronchial tree, prolonged spasm of respiratory muscles, laryngeal obstruction, or coma.

Prophylaxis

Active immunization (see Table 7–1) and an occasional recall as rarely as every 10 years will prevent tetanus in children and adults.

Adequate debridement of wounds is one of the most important preventive measures. In doubtful cases, give a combination of procaine penicillin G, 300,000 units intramuscularly, and benzathine penicillin G, 600,000 units intramuscularly.

Prognosis

The mortality rate in infants is 70%; in other age groups, mortality rates range from 10 to 60%

GAS GANGRENE

Gas gangrene is caused by infection with any of the anaerobic clostridia, which produce powerful necrotizing toxins. It is characterized by a sudden onset of fever to 40 °C (104 °F), tachycardia, and toxemia developing after a contaminated wound (usually deep puncture wounds). The wound is tender, painful, and swollen, with a watery or purulent discharge, and has a musty, sickeningly sweet odor. Gas bubbles are palpable (crepitus). Gas gangrene is less common in children than in adults.

Treatment consists of thorough debridement of all potentially infected wounds, with multiple incisions to aerate the infected part, plus penicillin G, 300,000 units/kg/d in 8 doses given every 3 hours intravenously. Polyvalent gas gangrene antitoxin and hyperbaric oxygen therapy are of unproved value. Hemolysis may be profound and may require aggressive transfusion therapy.

Unless specific measures are started early, the prognosis is poor.

• • •

BOTULISM

Three clinical syndromes due to the neuromuscular paralytic effects of the neurotoxins produced by *Clostridium botulinum* are now recognized:

A. Endogenous Toxin Syndrome: Infant botulism is the result of colonization of the infant's intestinal tract with *C botulinum,* probably from food sources other than milk. Contaminated honey has been implicated in several cases. Toxin is produced in the infant bowel and absorbed to produce symptoms.

B. Exogenous Toxin Syndrome: Poisoning from contaminated food, with growth of the organism and production of toxin, may occur especially if the food is improperly processed or canned.

C. Wound Infection: Botulism may result from wound infection.

Clinical Findings

A. Symptoms and Signs:

1. Endogenous toxin syndrome–Onset of infant botulism is between 1 and 2 months of age. Manifestations include apathy, weakness, constipation, floppiness, and (occasionally) sudden apnea.

2. Exogenous toxin syndrome–Sudden onset of food poisoning occurs 12–36 hours after ingestion of contaminated food. Double vision, nystagmus, dry mouth, and dysphagia may occur. There may be progressive motor paralysis with no sensory impairment or meningeal signs.

3. Wound infection–Onset is 12–24 hours after injury. Symptoms are similar to those found in patients with exogenous toxin syndrome.

B. Laboratory Findings: All possible food sources should be sampled for culture when botulism is suspected. Exogenous toxin can be demonstrated in the wound, vomitus, and serum. In infant disease, endogenous toxin is found in the intestinal tract only. The organism can sometimes be cultured from the feces in the infant. Other laboratory findings are usually normal. Cerebrospinal fluid findings are normal. Electromyography shows responses characteristic of neuromuscular block.

Treatment

A. Specific Measures: Although the value of antitoxin is questioned, a polyvalent preparation should be given in the exogenous diseases. See Table 7–2 regarding dosage and administration of the preparation. Endogenous disease in the infant does not require antitoxin.

B. General Measures: Respiratory paralysis requires mechanical aids. Tracheostomy may be necessary to remove pooled secretions. Tube feeding may be necessary with prolonged paralysis. In infant disease, the possibility of sudden death due to respiratory arrest dictates constant and careful observation. The use of aminoglycoside antibiotics (gentamicin) may exacerbate symptoms.

Prognosis

The mortality rate in exogenous disease is over 50% in the USA. In endogenous disease, all infants recover after an illness that may last several weeks.

SALMONELLOSIS

Salmonellosis designates the group of disease states caused by organisms of the genus *Salmonella,* gram-negative bacilli. Salmonellosis is spread from the feces of the infected person or fecal carrier to the mouths of other individuals. Epidemics have been traced to contaminated water, ice, milk, and various improperly prepared foods. Flies, ducks, turkeys, pet turtles, and egg preparations have been sources of infection. Chocolate products contaminated with the organism have been implicated in some epidemics.

Etiology

There are more than 1500 serotypes of salmonellae pathogenic for humans and divided into groups, replacing the old terminology in which only 2 types (paratyphoid A and paratyphoid B) were described. Grouping is as follows: group A, *Salmonella paratyphi A* (uncommon); group B, *Salmonella typhimurium* (common) and *Salmonella schottmülleri* (formerly *Salmonella paratyphi B;* uncommon); group C, a large number of sporadically encountered species; and group D, *Salmonella typhi* (the cause of typhoid fever). Other species of *Salmonella* are rarely encountered in human disease.

Clinical Findings

A. Symptoms and Signs: *Salmonella* infections are of 4 types:

1. Enteric fever–This type includes typhoid fever. After an incubation period of 8–16 days, fever to 40 °C (104 °F) appears and is accompanied by anorexia, vomiting, abdominal distention, and extreme malaise. In many cases, these are the only symptoms. However, after about 5 days, a rash may appear, usually on the abdomen and consisting of red macules that blanch easily ("rose spots"). At this point, the patient is usually very ill, sometimes with coma or convulsions. Physical findings include splenomegaly and a relative bradycardia. Diarrhea is rarely prominent but may develop in the third week of the untreated case.

2. Septicemia–Septicemia is particularly common in children. The onset is sudden, often with convulsions and spiking fever to 39.5–40.5 °C (103–105 °F). Septicemia may accompany localized infectious processes (see below).

3. Gastroenteritis–Acute gastroenteritis and enterocolitis are probably the most common forms of salmonellosis and are probably much more common than statistics indicate. After an incubation period of 1–3 days, there is a sudden onset of vomiting, diarrhea, and fever to 40 °C (104 °F). Abdominal cramps and prostration are common. Stools usually contain pus and blood (see Table 16–3).

4. Localized infection–Salmonellae may cause localized infections in practically any part of the body. These include osteomyelitis, meningitis, pyelitis, appendicitis, peritonitis, bronchitis, and pneumonia. Children with sickle cell anemia are particularly susceptible to *Salmonella* osteomyelitis.

B. Laboratory Findings:

1. Enteric fever–Leukopenia occurs at the onset of typhoid fever. Results of blood, stool, urine, or bone marrow cultures are positive. The serologic test for antibodies (Widal test) is best done with H and O antigens. The classic Widal test includes both antigens and does not differentiate antibodies from active immunization (H). A single specimen any time during illness with a titer above 1:100 against O antigen is indicative of acute enteric fever.

2. Septicemia–Blood cultures yield positive results during the febrile phase.

3. Gastroenteritis–Findings include moderate leukocytosis and white blood cells in the rectal smear. Culture of stools often yields positive results. Multiple negative results on culture do not rule out this etiology.

4. Localized infection–Leukocytosis occurs. Serologic tests and cultures of specimens from involved areas are positive.

Complications

In the third week of typhoid fever, hemorrhage or perforation of the intestines may occur (rare in childhood). With septicemia, there may be a localized infectious process such as meningitis, osteomyelitis, pleural infection, or abscess in any organ. Gastroenteritis may be accompanied by dehydration and acidosis, as in any severe diarrhea.

Treatment

A. Specific Measures: For patients with enteric fever, septicemia, and meningitis, give ampicillin or chloramphenicol. Both drugs should be given intravenously 4 times a day for 10 days, if possible, followed by oral ampicillin to a total of 4 weeks. The dosage is 100 mg/kg/d for chloramphenicol and 250 mg/kg/d for ampicillin. For patients with gastroenteritis, dietary therapy is the most important factor. Antibiotics and antispasmodics seem to be of no value. A prolonged carrier state is often found despite antibiotic therapy.

B. General Measures: Provide a high-calorie, low-residue diet, parenteral fluids as needed, and proper skin care. Hydrocortisone, 100 mg intravenously every 8 hours, may be given in cases of severe toxicity. Transfusions for hemorrhage or surgery for perforations may be required. Strict isolation of patients and careful disposal of excreta will protect other patients.

Prophylaxis

Prophylactic measures include discovery and supervision of cases and carriers, sanitary disposal of excreta, protection and purification of food and water supplies, and supervision of food handlers. Active immunization is discussed in Chapter 7.

Prognosis

In enteric fever, the prognosis is usually good with antibiotics. In septicemia, the prognosis is guarded; local *Salmonella* infections are particularly difficult to treat. In gastroenteritis, the prognosis is usually good with adequate measures to control diarrhea. The carrier state is common in young children. Treatment of the carrier is unsuccessful and not necessary. Family hygiene in such cases should be reviewed and improved by instruction.

SHIGELLOSIS
(Bacillary Dysentery)

Bacillary dysentery is spread from human feces of the infected person or fecal carrier to the mouths of other individuals. Epidemics have been traced to contaminated water, ice, milk, and various foods. Flies frequently carry the organisms.

There are more than 40 serotypes of shigellae. *Shigella sonnei* is the most common in the USA. *Shigella dysenteriae,* type 1, is common in Central and South America. The incubation period is 1–6 days (usually less than 4 days).

Clinical Findings

A. Symptoms and Signs: In severe and fulminant cases, the onset is sudden, with prostration, fever to 39.5 °C (103 °F), vomiting, profuse bloody diarrhea, colic, and tenesmus. The patient may be in shock very early in the course of the illness. Meningismus, deep drowsiness, coma, or convulsions may occur. Generalized abdominal tenderness is usually present, and rigidity may be present at times. Patients with the mild form of the disease may show only slight fever and a mild, watery diarrhea.

B. Laboratory Findings: An increase in the white blood cell count (10,000–16,000/μL) and number of polymorphonuclear leukocytes occurs in most patients. Pus and blood may be seen in the smear of stool. Cultures of the stool usually yield positive results. Several cultures should be obtained in suspected cases before antibiotics are administered.

Complications

A chronic, recurrent form of shigellosis may occur.

Treatment

A. Specific Measures: Ampicillin (see Chapter 6) is the antibiotic of choice if the strain is ampicillin-sensitive. For ampicillin-resistant strains, give trimethoprim-sulfamethoxazole (co-trimoxazole; Bactrim, Septra), 8 mg/kg/d of trimethoprim and 40 mg/kg/d of sulfamethoxazole, every 12 hours for 5 days. For older children and adults, tetracycline may be used (see Chapter 6). Since most cases are mild and self-limited, antibiotics should be reserved for unresponsive severe cases.

B. General Measures: Parenteral hydration and correction of electrolyte disturbances are essential in all moderately or severely ill patients. Dietary measures (see Chapter 16) are most important. Antispasmodics such as paregoric, tincture of belladonna, or diphenoxylate with atropine (Lomotil) may control diarrhea but prolong *Shigella* excretion.

Prophylaxis

Control of cases and carriers is most important. No active immunizing agent is available.

Prognosis

When treatment is begun early in the disease, the prognosis is good. In infancy and old age, the mortality rate is highest if therapy is delayed. Relapse or reinfection occurs in 10% of cases.

CHOLERA

The causative agent of cholera is *Vibrio cholerae (Vibrio comma)*, a gram-negative, curved organism with a terminal flagellum that is actively motile in suspension. Transmission, as in other enteric infections, is by contaminated food or water.

Clinical Findings

A. Symptoms and Signs: During the incubation stage (1–3 days), mild diarrhea may be present. During the diarrheal stage, there is severe cramping and profuse diarrhea, the stools becoming almost clear fluid and albuminous ("rice water"). Vomiting is severe. In the collapse stage, diarrhea ceases and shock appears within 2–12 hours after onset of diarrhea. During the recovery stage, the stools become more normal within the course of a week.

B. Laboratory Findings: There is marked hemoconcentration, with rising specific gravity of plasma, metabolic acidosis, and often elevation of nonprotein nitrogen levels. The stools rarely show pus cells, but the vibrios can be easily cultured.

Treatment

A. Specific Measures: Use of trimethoprim-sulfamethoxazole (co-trimoxazole; Bactrim, Septra) as in shigellosis (see above) or use of tetracycline in older children (see Chapter 6) may shorten the duration of disease.

B. General Measures: Give oral glucose/electrolyte solution as in other diarrheal conditions (see p 347). The absorption of glucose and sodium occurs despite massive secretion by the intestine in patients with cholera. Children strong enough to drink will voluntarily ingest an appropriate volume of the glucose/electrolyte solution to produce rehydration and maintenance. The solution need not be sterile and can be administered by nonprofessionals. Intravenous therapy with massive infusions of physiologic saline solution should be given when shock or coma prevents oral therapy. Potassium and bicarbonate supplements may be necessary.

Prophylaxis

Prophylactic measures include active immunization, boiling all water and potentially contaminated foods, and screening in endemic areas. Use of tetracycline in full dosage (see Chapter 6) for 5 days may prevent infection in close contacts of cholera patients.

Prognosis

In untreated cases, the mortality rate is 25–50%. With early and adequate treatment, the prognosis is good.

GONORRHEA

Neisseria gonorrhoeae is a gram-negative, coffee bean-shaped diplococcus usually found both intracellularly and extracellularly in purulent exudate. The neonatal infection may be acquired during delivery by direct contact with infected material in the mother's vagina. In childhood, infection may be acquired by contact with infected vaginal or urethral discharge or from infected bedpans, toilet seats, and towels.

Clinical Findings

A. Symptoms and Signs: For gonococcal conjunctivitis of the newborn, see Chapter 19. Urethritis with purulent discharge may occur in males, and gonorrheal vulvovaginitis may occur in females. While the vaginal mucosa in adults is resistent to gonococcal infection, both the vagina and the vulva are readily infected before puberty, most commonly from birth to 5 years of age. The infection is spread by contact with contaminated articles or infected children or adults and is manifested by itching and burning of the vulva and vagina. The mucous membranes of the vulva and vagina are red and edematous, and there is a profuse yellow purulent discharge. Vulvovaginitis due to gonococci must be differentiated from nonspecific vulvovaginitis due to improper hygiene. Acute salpingitis (pelvic inflammatory disease) may develop suddenly after several weeks or months of inapparent infection. Nongonococcal salpingitis may have an identical clinical picture. Perihepatitis in conjunction with salpingitis is characterized by right upper abdominal tenderness and occasionally abnormal results in liver function tests.

B. Laboratory Findings: A smear of purulent exudate may show intracellular organisms. Cultures on Thayer-Martin medium should be carried out for any suspected case. In cases of pelvic pain, ultrasonography may clearly demonstrate the presence of a tubo-ovarian cyst.

Complications

Complications of conjunctivitis include corneal ulceration and opacity. Vaginitis may spread to regional organs or (through the bloodstream) to joints. Septicemia with purulent arthritis and distinctive skin lesions can occur. The skin lesions have an erythematous base, with central hemorrhage. They later become necrotic and vesicular. Arthritis involves ankles, knees, and wrists and is migratory. Tenosynovitis is also common.

Treatment

A. Specific Measures:

1. Conjunctivitis, vaginitis, and urethritis–In children under 8 years of age, give procaine penicillin G, 2.4 million units in a single dose at several intramuscular sites if necessary. Give probenecid, 25 mg/kg, 1 hour before penicillin. In patients over 8 years of age (including young adults), give procaine penicillin G, 4.8 million units as a single dose preceded by probenecid as above. If there is sensitivity to penicillin, give one of the tetracyclines every 6 hours for 4 days.

2. Salpingitis, arthritis, and sepsis–Give penicillin G, 20 million units/d intravenously for at least 5 days or until symptoms subside. Therapy may be continued with ampicillin (see Chapter 6) orally for a total of 10 days. If there is sensitivity to penicillin, give one of the tetracyclines every 6 hours for 10 days. In patients with arthritis that persists or recurs, intra-articular injection of penicillin G, repeated 3 times every 2 days, may be useful.

B. General Measures: Give additional supportive treatment for complications, if indicated.

Prophylaxis

For prophylaxis of conjunctivitis, see Chapter 19. To prevent recurrence of vaginitis or infection of other children, examine contacts and perform bacteriologic cultures. Pregnant women with vaginitis should be examined and cultures performed prior to delivery. Examination and treatment of sexual partners must also be carried out. Asymptomatic vaginal or urethral infection is common.

Prognosis

The prognosis is excellent with penicillin treatment. Untreated conjunctivitis may result in corneal scarring. Salpingitis as a result of spread from the vagina may be asymptomatic and chronic and lead to sterility.

TULAREMIA

The causative agent of tularemia is *Francisella tularensis,* a gram-negative rod. The infection is transmitted through direct contact with the blood of an infected rabbit, ground squirrel, or (more rarely) any one of many species of wild mammals; through bites of infected ticks; or through ingestion of improperly cooked meat from wild mammals, usually rabbits. The incubation period is 1–7 days (average, 3 days).

Clinical Findings

A. Symptoms and Signs: Onset is sudden, with fever to 40–40.5 °C (104–105 °F), vomiting, chills in older children, and convulsions in the rarely infected infant. Cutaneous eruptions of various types occur in about 10% of children. The clinical picture depends upon portal of entry.

1. Ulceroglandular type– The lesion on the extremity where the bacteria enter the skin is at first papular but rapidly breaks down and becomes a punched-out ulcer. It is accompanied by enlargement and tenderness of regional lymph nodes and sometimes by nodules along the course of the lymphatics. Without therapy, suppuration of the lymph nodes frequently occurs. In some cases, there is lymphadenopathy, but no primary lesion can be detected.

2. Pharyngotonsillar type–Ulceration and formation of a membrane on the pharynx and tonsils are accompanied by enlargement of the cervical lymph nodes.

3. Oculoglandular type–Infection is acquired when material is rubbed into the eye. Findings include acute conjunctivitis with edema; photophobia; itching and pain in the eye; swelling of the upper lid, which may show scattered small yellow nodules; and enlargement of lymph glands of the neck, axilla, and scalp.

4. Cryptogenic type–The point of entry of the organisms cannot be recognized, and the symptoms are entirely systemic.

B. Laboratory Findings: The white blood cell count may be normal, or there may be a slight leukocytosis. The agglutination test shows a positive rising titer, beginning around 7 days from onset. The test strains may cross-react with brucellar strains.

Differential Diagnosis

Tularemia must be differentiated from rickettsial and meningococcal infections, cat-scratch disease, infectious mononucleosis, and various pneumonias and fungal diseases. Epidemiologic considerations and rising agglutination titers are the chief differential points.

Treatment

A. Specific Measures: Give streptomycin, 30–40 mg/kg/d intramuscularly for 3 days, followed by 15–20 mg/kg/d intramuscularly for 4 days. Tetracyclines or, in older children, chloramphenicol may be given concurrently.

B. General Measures: Treatment is symptomatic and supportive.

Prophylaxis

Prophylactic measures include proper handling and cooking of meat from wild mammals, wearing rubber gloves in handling potentially infected animals, using extreme care in handling laboratory materials from the case, and avoiding the early surgical incision of suppurating lesions.

Prognosis

The mortality rate in patients with untreated ulceroglandular tularemia is 5%, and that of patients with the pneumonic type is 30%. Early chemotherapy eliminates fatalities. Skin tests and agglutination tests suggest that subclinical infection is common in endemic areas.

PLAGUE

Plague is a disease primarily of rats and other small rodents. It is transmitted to humans by a variety of fleas. The organism is present in ground squirrels and other rodents in the USA. The pneumonic form of the disease may be transmitted from person to person by the inhalation of infected droplets.

The causative agent is *Yersinia pestis,* a gram-negative, bipolar-staining, pleomorphic bacillus.

Clinical Findings

A. Symptoms and Signs: The incubation period is 2–10 days, and there are 3 clinical syndromes of the disease:

1. Bubonic plague–Onset is sudden, with chills, fever to 40 °C (104 °F), vomiting, and lethargy. There is tender, firm enlargement of the inguinal, axillary, and cervical lymph nodes (buboes) by the third day. Meningismus, convulsions, and delirium may occur.

2. Pneumonic plague–Findings are as above but with the absence of buboes and onset of cough on the first day. Blood-tinged, mucoid or thin, bright red sputum may be brought up. Clinical signs of pneumonia may be absent at first.

3. Fulminant (septicemic) plague–Onset is as above but with overwhelming bloodstream invasion before enlargement of nodes or pneumonia.

B. Laboratory Findings: Leukocytosis appears early, with counts as high as 50,000/μL (mostly polymorphonuclear leukocytes). Early blood cultures show positive results. Organisms are isolated on smears of lymph node contents and sputum and can sometimes be isolated from cerebrospinal fluid.

C. X-Ray Findings: Pulmonary infiltration in a person suspected of having plague implies a grave prognosis and requires strict isolation and prompt treatment.

Differential Diagnosis

The lymphadenitis of plague is most commonly mistaken for the lymphadenitis accompanying staphylococcal or streptococcal infections of an extremity, venereal diseases (eg, lymphogranuloma venereum and syphilis), and tularemia. The systemic manifestations resemble those of enteric or rickettsial fevers, malaria, or influenza. The pneumonia resembles other severe gram-negative or staphylococcal pneumonias or psittacosis.

Treatment

A. Specific Measures: Streptomycin, 50 mg/kg/d in 4 intramuscular doses, is the drug of choice and should be given for 10 days. A tetracycline (for older children) or chloramphenicol may be used as an alternative, but these drugs are less reliable for treatment (see Chapter 6).

B. General Measures: Treatment is symptomatic, with strict isolation of patients with pneumonic plague and disinfection of all discharges.

Prophylaxis

Periodic surveys of rodents and their ectoparasites in endemic areas will provide guidelines for extensive rodent and flea control measures. Total eradication of plague from wild rodents in an endemic area is rarely possible. Active immunization in endemic areas may be indicated (see Chapter 7). Antibiotic prophylaxis with tetracycline or sulfisoxazole may provide temporary protection for those exposed to plague infection, especially by the respiratory route. Upon recovery from plague, the patient will be immune.

Prognosis

If treatment can be started early enough in the disease, the prognosis is excellent. Delay in treatment may result in death from the fulminant form of disease. Without treatment, the prognosis is poor.

BRUCELLOSIS
(Undulant Fever, Malta Fever)

Brucellosis is caused by one of the 3 strains of gram-negative brucellae *(Brucella abortus, Brucella melitensis,* and *Brucella suis).* Although these varieties are most commonly found in cattle, goats, and hogs, respectively, they have also been isolated in other species of animals. The incubation period is 5–20 days.

Transmission is by direct contact with diseased animals, their tissues, or unpasteurized milk or cheese from diseased cows and goats.

Clinical Findings

A. Symptoms and Signs: In the acute disease, the onset is gradual and insidious, with fever and loss of weight. Fever at first may be low-grade and present in the evening only, but in the course of days or weeks it may reach 40 °C (104 °F) and present a wavelike character over a period of 2–4 days. The chronic disease is manifested by low-grade fever, sweats, malaise, arthralgia, depression, splenomegaly, and leukopenia.

B. Laboratory Findings: The white blood cell count is usually normal to low, with a relative or absolute lymphocytosis. The organism can be recovered from the blood, bone marrow, urine, and local abscesses, usually with difficulty and requiring long incubation in a special medium. An agglutination titer greater than 1:100 or a rising titer will support the diagnosis. A prozone phenomenon in which the agglutination occurs in high dilutions but not in low ones is common. Skin tests are of no value and should not be carried out. Serologic tests may give a cross-reaction with tularemia.

Differential Diagnosis

Brucellosis must be differentiated from many other acute febrile diseases, especially influenza, tularemia, acute fever, and salmonellosis. In its chronic form, it resembles tuberculosis, malaria, Hodgkin's disease, infectious mononucleosis, and chronic urinary tract infection. The chronic form may also be diagnosed and treated as a psychologic disturbance.

Treatment

A. Specific Measures: Tetracyclines are the drugs of choice. Continue treatment for 2–3 weeks. For dosages, see Chapter 6. In severe illness, add streptomycin, 20 mg/kg/d intramuscularly in 4 doses for 5 days.

B. General Measures: Bed rest during the acute stage and high intake of vitamins (B complex and C) are indicated.

Prophylaxis

Milk and milk products should be pasteurized.

Prognosis

In patients with the acute form of infection, the prognosis is good with adequate treatment. In patients with the chronic form, response to treatment may be poor, although the disease is not fatal.

NOCARDIOSIS

Nocardia asteroides was formerly classified as a fungus but is in fact a gram-positive filamentous aerobic bacterium causing chronic pulmonary and systemic disease or local infection of the skin. The lungs are the most common site of initial infection, with systemic spread common in the course of a chronic febrile illness, especially in immunologically deficient children. Local skin infection or mycetoma (Madura foot) occurs by inoculation through an abrasion. Systemic disease includes multiple abscesses in the lungs, liver, and lymph nodes. If the cause of immunologic deficiency is not apparent, as in lymphoma, Hodgkin's disease, leukemia, or immunosuppressive treatment, it should be carefully sought.

Treatment is with triple sulfonamides or sulfisoxazole in full dosage for 6 weeks to 3 months. Streptomycin or tetracycline, given as for brucellosis (see above), may be added if response to sulfonamides is not satisfactory. Surgical drainage and excision of abscesses and necrotic tissues are also necessary in some cases.

Prognosis for control of infection is good.

MYCOPLASMA PNEUMONIAE INFECTIONS

Mycoplasmas are free-living organisms. The common clinical disease caused by mycoplasmas is pneumonia, which is most frequent in persons 5–18 years of age and especially in young adults.

Clinical Findings

A. Symptoms and Signs: There is gradual onset of moderate fever, with malaise and sore throat. Onset of nonproductive cough is after 3–5 days. The cough becomes persistent and sometimes paroxysmal, resembling pertussis. Other findings include abdominal pain, vomiting, nausea, and dry rales occasionally accompanied by friction rub.

B. Laboratory Findings: The white blood cell count is normal early in the disease but later may show leukocytosis, especially with complications such as otitis media abscess. Autohemagglutinins for type O human erythrocytes (cold agglutinins) appear usually after the first 10 days of disease. Complement fixation, indirect hemagglutination, and metabolic inhibition antibody tests are all useful when available. The organism may be grown on special media and will indicate either present or recent infection.

C. X-Ray Findings: The x-ray findings are those of pneumonitis, with a linear infiltrate developing around the hilum and gradually spreading in a wedge-shaped manner. Pleural effusion may be apparent.

Complications

Otitis media is common in younger individuals. Central nervous system disease, hemolytic anemia, exanthems, and arthritis have all been reported. Lung abscess may develop after 2–4 weeks of disease.

Treatment

Erythromycin in young children or tetracycline in those over 10 years of age is the drug of choice (see Chapter 6).

Prophylaxis

An inactivated vaccine is under investigation at present and shows some promise.

Prognosis

With adequate treatment, the prognosis is excellent.

intracell. bacteria

CHLAMYDIAL INFECTIONS

The 2 species of the genus *Chlamydia* are obligate intracellular bacteria and are classified as *Chlamydia trachomatis* and *Chlamydia psittaci*. These agents cause several disease entities.

Clinical Findings

A. Symptoms and Signs:

1. Inclusion conjunctivitis and trachoma–Neonatal inclusion conjunctivitis (inclusion blennorrhea) and trachoma are caused by *C trachomatis*. The neonatal infection is acquired during passage through the cervix and causes a purulent conjunctivitis after 7–10 days (see under Conjunctivitis, Chapter 19).

2. Pneumonitis–Neonatal pneumonitis is characterized by onset during early infancy, with progressive tachypnea, staccato cough, cyanosis, and vomiting.

3. Lymphogranuloma venereum–Infection is caused by *C trachomatis*, and there is inguinal and pelvic lymph node involvement after sexual contact with penile, vaginal, or rectal surfaces. The inguinal nodes in the male and the perirectal nodes in the female become infected, enlarge, and suppurate. This is apparent as buboes in the male and proctitis in the female or in the homosexual male.

4. Urethritis and cervicitis–Infection is caused by *C trachomatis*. It is clinically similar to disease produced by gonococci and may be mistaken for penicillin-resistant gonococcal infection.

5. Psittacosis–Psittacosis (ornithosis) is caused by *C psittaci* and is acquired by contact with parrots, parakeets, pigeons, chickens, ducks, and other wild birds. There is a sudden onset of fever, chills, and nonproductive cough, with clinical signs of pneumonia or bronchiolitis (see Chapter 15).

B. Laboratory Findings: The white blood cell count is usually normal. Chlamydiae can be cultured, with difficulty, on special media. Characteristic inclusion bodies are found on Giemsa-stained smears of discharge in neonatal conjunctivitis and trachoma. Complement fixation tests are diagnostic in lymphogranuloma venereum and psittacosis. Results of an intradermal skin test (Frei test) will become positive in lymphogranuloma venereum and psittacosis.

C. X-Ray Findings: Findings are identical to those seen with mycoplasmal pneumonia (see above).

Complications

Neonatal inclusion conjunctivitis and trachoma may produce corneal scarring and vision problems if untreated. Untreated lymphogranuloma venereum in boys may produce extensive scarring around draining inguinal nodes; in girls, perirectal scarring may cause rectal stricture. Untreated urethritis in boys may cause chronic discharge and dysuria persisting for many weeks. Untreated cervicitis in girls may spread to cause salpingitis with resultant scarring and sterility.

Treatment

A. Specific Measures:

1. Inclusion conjunctivitis–In neonatal infection, a 10% suspension of sulfacetamide, instilled in the eyes 4 times daily for 7 days, is usually effective. Combined therapy with oral erythromycin continued for 10 days (see Chapter 6) has also been recommended.

2. Trachoma–Give oral tetracyclines in addition to local treatment (as above). Therapy may have to be continued for as long as 30 days.

3. Lymphogranuloma venereum–Give tetracyclines orally (see Chapter 6).

4. Urethritis and cervicitis–Oral tetracyclines may reduce symptoms but may not eradicate the organisms.

5. Psittacosis–Give tetracyclines orally (see Chapter 6).

B. General Measures: Give additional supportive treatment for complications, if indicated.

Prognosis

With early diagnosis and treatment, complications are minimal and the prognosis excellent.

BACTERIAL INFECTIONS OF THE CENTRAL NERVOUS SYSTEM

GENERAL CONSIDERATIONS IN MENINGITIS

The most important step in diagnosis of infection of the central nervous system is to suspect that it may be present.

Symptoms & Signs of Meningitis

A. "Meningeal" Signs: Signs include stiffness of the neck (inability to touch the chin to the chest), stiffness of the back (inability to sit up normally), a positive Kernig sign (inability to extend the knee when the leg is flexed anteriorly at the hip), and a positive Brudzinski sign (when the head is bent forward, flexure movements of the lower extremity are produced).

B. Increased Intracranial Pressure: Findings include bulging fontanelles in small infants, irritability, headache (may be intermittent), projectile vomiting (or vomiting may be absent), diplopia, "choking" of the optic disks, "cracked pot" percussion note over the skull (sometimes in normal children also), slowing of the pulse, and irregular respirations.

C. Change in Sensorium: Changes range from mild lethargy to coma.

D. Convulsions: Convulsions usually are generalized and are more common in infants.

E. Fever: Onset of high- or low-grade fever may be sudden or insidious, or there may be a marked change in pattern during a minor illness.

F. Shock: Shock may appear in the course of many types of infection of the central nervous system.

G. Other: In the child under 2 years of age, irritability, persistent crying, poor feeding, diarrhea, or vomiting may be the *only* symptom. Fever may be absent or low-grade, and meningeal signs as above may not be found.

Examination of Cerebrospinal Fluid (See Appendix.)

When infection of the central nervous system is suspected, lumbar puncture and examination of the cerebrospinal fluid must be performed to establish the diagnosis. The gross examination, cell count, and microscopic examination of a concentrated sediment for bacteria may all be performed immediately after this procedure. Counterimmunoelectrophoresis is a rapid and specific diagnostic procedure that may be used to identify a capsular antigen of meningococci or *Haemophilus influenzae* in cerebrospinal fluid. This test may be applied also to joint fluid and serum. The determination of glucose content should be done *at once;* the degree of depression of the glucose level will determine the urgency of treatment. A poor prognosis is related to the degree of depression.

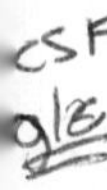

Culture of Cerebrospinal Fluid & Blood

Cerebrospinal fluid must be cultured both aerobically and anaerobically. The organism causing the central nervous system infection may grow in a blood culture and not in cultures of the cerebrospinal fluid.

Differential Diagnosis

Bacterial meningitis must be differentiated from other types of central nervous system infection and disease (eg, granulomatous meningitis due to tuberculosis, coccidioidomycosis, cryptococcosis, histoplasmosis, and syphilis) and from aseptic meningitis and viral encephalitis (see Tables 21–1, 21–2, and 21–3).

Leptospiral infection with meningeal involvement shows lymphocytic cellular response (see Leptospirosis, below).

Partially treated bacterial meningitis may present with the same course and same laboratory findings as aseptic meningitis following inadequate antimicrobial therapy.

The "neighborhood reaction" (ie, a response to a purulent infectious process in close proximity to the central nervous system) introduces elements of the inflammatory process—white cells or protein—into the cerebrospinal fluid. Such an infection might be brain abscess, osteomyelitis of the skull or vertebrae, epidural abscess, or mastoiditis.

Meningismus or noninfectious meningeal irritation may occur in such infections as pneumonia, shigellosis, salmonellosis, otitis media, and meningeal invasion by neoplastic cells. In the latter instance, there may be not only increased numbers of cells in the spinal fluid but also a lowered glucose level.

Complications of Meningitis

Central nervous system infection may produce hydrocephalus, especially in infants (uncommon since the advent of specific therapy; see Chapter 21); subdural accumulation of fluid, especially in a patient under 2 years of age (see Chapter 21); deafness (see Chapter 14); paralysis of various muscles, mental retardation, or focal epilepsy (see Chapter 21); or psychologic residua. Persistent fever may be due to brain abscess, lateral sinus thrombosis, mastoiditis, drug reaction, or continued sepsis.

General Plan of Treatment

A. Emergency Measures: Treat shock (see Chapter 2). For treatment of possible endotoxic shock, see below. Avoid overhydration and aggravation of brain edema.

B. Specific Measures:

1. Infection with known organism–Treat according to recommended programs given below.

2. Suspected infection with undetermined bacterial organism–Obtain all diagnostic material possible before instituting antimicrobial therapy. Urgency depends upon the presumed duration of disease, the presence and depth of coma, and the age of the patient, with infancy as an absolute indication for urgency. An additional factor of urgency is the degree of depression of the cerebrospinal fluid glucose level. Meningitis of unknown cause in premature infants and infants under 1 month of age should be treated with ampicillin plus erythromycin. Infants over 1 month of age should be given ampicillin plus chloramphenicol, since half of these cases are due to *Haemophilus influenzae,* against which chloramphenicol is effective. Chloramphenicol blood levels should be monitored. If tuberculosis is a strong possibility, add streptomycin as set forth below.

3. Increased intracranial pressure–Increased pressure may cause death before antimicrobial treatment takes effect. Treat as for encephalitis (see Chapter 21).

HAEMOPHILUS INFLUENZAE MENINGITIS

Haemophilus influenzae meningitis is the most common type of bacterial meningitis in children. It usually occurs in children under 2 years of age and is rarely seen in those over 10 years of age.

Clinical Findings

A. Symptoms and Signs: Onset may be insidious or quite abrupt following an upper respiratory tract infection (usually mild). Coma occurs within a few hours. Any of the findings listed above may be present. Young infants may have persistent unexplained fever, irritability, difficulties with feeding, or a high-pitched cry and no clear evidence of meningitis.

B. Laboratory Findings: Nose and throat cultures usually yield positive results. Smears of spun sediment from cerebrospinal fluid usually show gram-negative, pleomorphic, encapsulated coccobacilli in pairs or chains. A positive quellung reaction occurs with specific antiserum. Blood cultures frequently yield positive results. Severity of infection may be determined by glucose test (see above) on cerebrospinal fluid; the lower the cerebrospinal fluid glucose level, the more severe the infection. Counterimmunoelectrophoresis and latex agglutination tests may provide rapid identification of the specific capsular antigen in the cerebrospinal fluid.

Complications

Subdural effusion, a collection of fluid (often sterile) in the subdural space, may occur especially if initial therapy has been delayed or inadequate. Symptoms include recurrence of fever, vomiting, and lethargy; there may be enlargement of the head in infants. In younger children with open fontanelles, a subdural tap (see Chapter 32) will establish the diagnosis. In older children, bur holes are required. Recent reports suggest that postmeningitis effusions are more likely to occur when large amounts of cerebrospinal fluid (> 5 mL) are removed at the time of the "diagnostic" spinal puncture.

Treatment

A. Specific Measures:

1. Treat children and infants over 1 month of age with ampicillin plus chloramphenicol. Give an initial dose of ampicillin, 100 mg/kg (rapidly infused) intravenously, followed by 300 mg/kg/d given intravenously in 6 divided doses. The dosage of chloramphenicol is 100 mg/kg/d intravenously in divided doses every 12 hours. Continue for 10 days. Chloramphenicol blood levels should be monitored.

2. Do not give chloramphenicol to premature infants or infants under 1 month of age. Give ampicillin plus erythromycin (see Chapter 6).

3. Since strains of *H influenzae* resistant to ampicillin have been reported with increasing frequency from widely separated locations in the USA, the infecting organisms should be tested immediately for sensitivity to antibiotics and in particular ampicillin. An alternative treatment regimen is streptomycin and sulfonamides given simultaneously for 5 days and followed by chloramphenicol by mouth for an additional 10–14 days. Chloramphenicol may also be given in addition to the first 2 drugs during the first 5 days and continued when the latter drugs are stopped. (For dosages, see Chapter 6.)

B. General Measures: Give symptomatic therapy, as indicated.

C. Treatment of Complications: In patients with otitis media, perform myringotomy. Subdural empyema (see Chapter 21) is treated by repeated aspiration.

Prognosis

The fatality rate in patients with *H influenzae* meningitis is 5%. With early and adequate therapy, the prognosis is good.

MENINGOCOCCAL MENINGITIS

Clinical Findings

A. Symptoms and Signs: Any of the findings described under General Considerations in Meningitis (above) may be present. Most cases have a sudden onset, high temperature, and petechial or purpuric rash. Herpes labialis is commonly associated. Meningococcemia with petechiae and morbilliform rash without central nervous system involvement may occur.

B. Laboratory Findings: Cerebrospinal fluid abnormalities are usually characteristic of acute purulent bacterial meningitis (see Appendix, Table 4). Organisms usually can be seen in smears of cerebrospinal fluid and may be demonstrated within polymorphonuclear leukocytes in blood smears obtained by puncturing the center of the petechiae. Leukocytosis is present. Blood cultures usually yield positive results.

Complications

Any of the complications listed under General Considerations in Meningitis (above) may develop. In addition, arthritis, conjunctivitis, pneumonia, osteomyelitis, pericarditis, and toxic myocarditis may be present. Diffuse thromboembolic lesions with disseminated intravascular clotting may involve many organs. The course may be fulminant, with Waterhouse-Friderichsen syndrome, in which case the bloodstream may be so infected with organisms that they can be seen in a blood smear. Hemorrhagic phenomena are a prominent feature of this form of the disease, with rapidly spreading purpura and hemorrhage into body cavities and organs. Hemorrhage of the adrenal glands creates a shocklike state. The chronic, recurrent form is uncommon.

Treatment

A. Specific Measures: Combination therapy with penicillin G in the maximum parenteral dosage (see Chapter 6) should be instituted. If penicillin allergy is present, give chloramphenicol. Continue antimicrobial therapy for 10 days.

B. General Measures: Give symptomatic therapy as indicated.

C. Treatment of Complications:

1. Arthritis–Perform paracentesis for relief of pain.

2. Conjunctivitis–See Chapter 19.

3. Toxic myocarditis–There are no specific measures of treatment.

4. Endotoxic shock–Shock may occur with any gram-negative organism, including meningococci. The clinical picture is that of shock plus hemorrhagic phenomena, including purpura. Treat disseminated intravascular clotting as follows:

a. Treat for primary shock (see Chapter 2). Use dextran-70 as a plasma expander; this substance will inhibit platelet aggregation and adherence to injured surfaces.

b. Give hydrocortisone intravenously, 50 mg/kg in a single dose, followed by 100 mg/kg given over the next 24 hours.

c. Give heparin sodium intravenously in repeated doses of 100 units/kg every 4 hours. An increase in platelet count will indicate the success of this agent; the dosage should be reduced or discontinued, depending on repeated counts.

d. Give isoproterenol (1 mg of isoproterenol in 250 mL of isotonic solution) at a rate of 1 mL/min. Dopamine may be used as an alternative to decrease peripheral vascular resistance and central venous pressure.

5. Cerebral edema–Give mannitol (see p 487).

6. Other complications–Cardiac failure due to increased central venous pressure and possibly myocarditis should be treated (see Chapter 13).

Prophylaxis

For close contacts in the family and exposed attendants, rifampin (Rifadin, Rimactane) should be given twice daily for 2 days, 600 mg for adults or 10–20 mg/kg for children. Minocycline has been shown to be highly effective in clearing asymptomatic carriers, but vestibular side effects have been reported. Give minocycline twice daily for 3 days, 200 mg for adults or 4 mg/kg for children.

An effective polysaccharide vaccine for meningococci groups A and C has been approved. (Preparations are available containing the Y and W serotypes in addition.) Immunity requires at least 5 days for development after inoculation. If the infecting organism can be shown or is suspected to be a member of these serogroups, prophylaxis should include inoculation with the appropriate vaccine to prevent long-term development of disease in a carrier temporarily protected by chemoprophylaxis.

Prognosis

Except for patients with the fulminating type of infection, the prognosis is good. The prognosis for patients in endotoxic shock is poor but improves markedly if the patient can survive the first 24 hours.

PNEUMOCOCCAL, STREPTOCOCCAL, & STAPHYLOCOCCAL MENINGITIS

Clinical Findings

Clinical findings are similar in all 3 types. Differential diagnosis is made on the basis of laboratory examination.

A. Symptoms and Signs: A history of upper respiratory tract infection, sinusitis, pneumonia, otitis, or other infection or a history of skull fracture or meningocele may be obtained. Any of the findings described under General Considerations in Meningitis (above) may be found. Onset is less acute than with meningococcal meningitis. Petechial rash is rare.

B. Laboratory Findings: Cerebrospinal fluid abnormalities are characteristic of acute purulent bacterial meningitis (see Appendix, Table 4). Smears usually show large numbers of gram-positive cocci in pairs (pneumococci), chains (streptococci), or clumps (staphylococci).

Complications

Any of the complications listed under General Considerations in Meningitis (above) may develop, particularly if therapy is inadequate or started late. Infection of the middle ear and sinusitis are common. There may also be arthritis or localization in the pleural, pericardial, or peritoneal cavity.

Treatment

A. Specific Measures: Use penicillin G in a large dosage. Give 300,000 units/kg/d intravenously in 8 divided doses for 10 days or until cerebrospinal fluid glucose levels are normal. An intrathecal dose of penicillin is occasionally used at onset in young children or small infants; for dosage, see Chapter 6. In staphylococcal infection, use methicillin, oxacillin, or nafcillin.

B. General Measures: Give symptomatic therapy, as indicated.

C. Treatment of Complications: Give large doses of drugs. In some instances, surgical drainage of abscess or empyema is indicated. In patients with pneumococcal or streptococcal meningitis, mastoidectomy should be considered even in the absence of localizing signs.

Prognosis

With early, adequate therapy, complete recovery occurs. Otherwise, the prognosis for life or residua depends on the severity and duration.

MENINGITIS DUE TO GRAM-NEGATIVE BACTERIA

Meningitis may be caused by *Escherichia coli, Pseudomonas aeruginosa, Enterobacter aerogenes, Proteus morgani,* and *Klebsiella pneumoniae*. Any of the findings listed under General Considerations in Meningitis (above) may be present. A history of local infection (infected navel, diaper area pyoderma), meningomyelocele (in infants), or urinary tract infection (in older children) can be obtained. Laboratory confirmation is very important. Smears of cerebrospinal fluid show numerous gram-negative rods. Growth on culture is usually rapid. Results of the "*Limulus* test" for endotoxin are frequently positive. Sensitivity to various antibiotics should be determined.

Treatment of choice is ampicillin, 300 mg/kg/d intravenously in 6 divided doses, combined with gentamicin, 6 mg/kg/d intramuscularly in 3 divided doses. Kanamycin or amikacin (see Chapter 6) may be substituted for gentamicin, depending on the results of sensitivity tests and clinical experience with these agents. For treatment of endotoxic shock, see p 648.

The prognosis depends upon the type and severity of infection.

MENINGITIS DUE TO *LISTERIA MONOCYTOGENES*

Listeria monocytogenes produces a clinical picture resembling those of the other purulent meningitides (see General Considerations in Meningitis, above). Sepsis and meningitis due to this organism occur in the neonatal period with onset as early as a few hours after birth and as late as 3 weeks of age. Only bacteriologic studies can identify the organism, which is gram-positive, rod-shaped, and non-spore-forming. The organism may be misidentified as a "diphtheroid" and concluded to be a contaminant.

Treatment of choice is ampicillin combined with gentamicin, given as for meningitis due to gram-negative bacteria. Intravenous erythromycin may be used if the patient is allergic to ampicillin. Treatment should be continued for at least 10 days.

TUBERCULOUS MENINGITIS

Clinical Findings

A. Symptoms and Signs: A history of exposure to an adult with pulmonary tuberculosis is common. Any of the findings listed under General Considerations in Meningitis (above) may be present. Onset is often gradual, with irritability, change in personality, and drowsiness. Symptoms referable to the central nervous system may be minimal or may suggest encephalitis. As the disease advances, the irritative symptoms subside, and stupor becomes more pronounced. A positive tuberculin skin test result (see Chapter 7) in a child under 10 years of age with central nervous system disease is very suggestive of tuberculous meningitis. An associated tuberculous pneumonitis is often present.

B. Laboratory Findings: Lumbar puncture should be performed in any child with known tuberculosis who shows a change in temperature pattern or any central nervous system symptoms. The cerebrospinal fluid is frequently yellowish, with increased pressure and 100–500 cells/μL. The glucose content is usually very low. The fluid may later form a web and pellicle in which organisms may be demonstrated by smear or culture. Chest x-ray may reveal a tuberculous focus or miliary disease.

Differential Diagnosis

Tuberculous meningitis may resemble any other type of meningitis, but the gradual onset and evidence of tuberculosis in other parts of the body will clarify the diagnosis. Other forms of granulomatous meningitis must be considered.

Complications

After recovery, there may be residual brain damage resulting in motor paralysis, convulsive states, mental impairment, and abnormal behavior. The incidence of complications increases with delay in instituting therapy.

Treatment

A. Specific Measures: Give the following drugs in combination (for 18 months unless otherwise noted). Oral drugs can be eventually adjusted to a single daily dose.

1. Isoniazid (INH), 8 mg/kg orally for 1 day and then 20 mg/kg/d orally (maximum, 300 mg/d) for 1 year.
2. Ethambutol (Myambutol), 25 mg/kg/d orally for 1 month and then 15 mg/kg/d. Check vision monthly.
3. Rifampin, 15 mg/kg/d orally (maximum, 600 mg/d).
4. Streptomycin sulfate, 200 mg/kg/wk intramuscularly in daily doses for 3 months, or kanamycin, 15 mg/kg/d intramuscularly.

5. Dexamethasone (Decadron), 2–5 mg intravenously, depending on age and weight, repeated at 4-hour intervals for 14 days.

If treatment has been delayed or if the patient is severely ill, more intensive therapy may be necessary. Among the recommended methods are intrathecal streptomycin, 2 mg/kg/d; intrathecal isoniazid, 20–40 mg/d; fibrinolytic enzymes (streptokinase); ventricular drainage for relief of intracranial pressure; and intrathecal tuberculin (PPD). The exact value of these procedures has not been determined.

B. General Measures: Maintenance of nutrition is important because of the protracted course. Gavage feedings may be necessary. Blood transfusion and electrolyte management are indicated. Give pyridoxine, 10–25 mg/d, and thiamine, 10 mg/d. Occupational and play therapy is indicated according to the physical and psychologic tolerance of the patient.

Prognosis

Without treatment, mortality is 100%. With early, adequate treatment, recovery is to be expected. Long-term follow-up is necessary to determine recurrences; treat as the initial disease.

BRAIN ABSCESS

Brain abscess is usually caused by one of the common pyogenic bacteria: streptococci, pneumococci, staphylococci, *Escherichia coli*, or *Bacteroides* species. The source of infection is usually a septic focus elsewhere in the body (eg, otitis media, pneumonia, osteomyelitis, subacute infective endocarditis, furuncles). After skull fracture, organisms may enter through the sinuses or middle ear.

Clinical Findings

A. Symptoms and Signs: Findings may be few and diagnosis difficult. Onset is gradual, with fever, vomiting, lethargy, and coma. Increased intracranial pressure is usually present, manifested by bulging fontanelles (infants) or papilledema (older children). Neurologic signs related to special areas of the brain may be present, and a focal type of convulsion may occur (see under Convulsive Disorders, Chapter 21). A history of infection elsewhere in the body should be sought.

B. Laboratory Findings: Leukocytosis and cerebrospinal fluid changes may occur (see Appendix, Table 4).

C. X-Ray Findings: Cranial sutures may be widened. Brain scan, CT scan, and arteriography may give specific diagnosis and location.

Treatment

A. Specific Measures: If the organism is known, treat the patient with the specific antibiotic of choice (see Chapter 6). If the causative organism is not known, treat the patient with large doses of penicillin, as for streptococcal meningitis (see above), until specific etiologic diagnosis can be made. Surgical drainage will usually be necessary.

B. General Measures: Give anticonvulsants (see Table 21–4).

Prognosis

When the organism is known and is susceptible to antibiotics and treatment is early, the prognosis is good. Otherwise, the prognosis is at best guarded. Extensive brain damage may occur, with resultant mental retardation.

SPIROCHETAL DISEASES

SYPHILIS

Congenital syphilis is transmitted from mother to infant by direct inoculation into the blood through the placenta during the latter half of pregnancy. If infection of the mother has occurred recently, the infant is almost always affected. The longer the interval between infection of the mother and conception, the greater the likelihood that the infant will be free of the disease.

Syphilis may be acquired in childhood through an abrasion or laceration, by contact with infected nipples, through kissing, or by sexual contact.

Clinical Findings

A. Symptoms and Signs: Childhood syphilis may occur in early or late congenital forms or may be transmitted in the same way as the adult disease.

1. Early congenital syphilis—Signs appear before the sixth week. The more severe the infection, the earlier the onset. Rhinitis or "snuffles," a profuse, persistent, mucopurulent nasal discharge, is usually the first symptom. The discharge may be blood-tinged. Skin rash follows onset of rhinitis and appears as a maculopapular or morbilliform eruption, heaviest over the back, buttocks, and backs of thighs. Bullous lesions on the hands and feet are suggestive. Other findings include bleeding ulcerations and fissures of mucous membranes of the mouth, anus, and contiguous areas; anemia, with erythroblasts often present in large numbers; osteochondritis or periostitis (or both), with pseudoparalysis, pathologic fractures, and a characteristic x-ray appearance of increased density, widening of the epiphyseal line, and scattered areas of decreased density; hepatomegaly and splenomegaly (jaundice may be prominent); and chorioretinitis, with eventual optic atrophy.

2. Late congenital syphilis–Symptoms do not usually occur until after the third month. There may be maldevelopment of bones of the nose (saddle nose) and legs (saber shins). Neurosyphilis may occur, with clinical evidence of meningitis, paresis, or tabes, or with a slowly developing hydrocephalus. Deciduous teeth are normal. Permanent dentition may show Hutchinson's teeth, in which upper central incisors have a characteristic V-shaped notch in a peg-shaped tooth. The first permanent molars may have multiple cusps ("mulberry molar"). Other findings include rhagades, or scars around the mouth and nose; interstitial keratitis, usually occurring in children between 6 and 12 years of age; and early conjunctivitis, which gradually infiltrates deeply into the cornea and produces opacity.

3. Acquired syphilis–Symptoms in children are similar to and as variable as those in adults.

B. Laboratory Findings: A routine serologic test on cord blood obtained at birth will detect passively acquired antibodies from treated or untreated syphilis in the mother as well as actively acquired antibodies from the infection in the infant. If the mother has been adequately treated during pregnancy and the infant shows no evidence of disease, repeated serologic testing should be performed for 2 or 3 months. This will verify the absence of congenital disease by demonstrating a declining antibody titer. If there is any doubt about whether treatment of the mother has been adequate, treatment of the infant should be instituted without delay.

Scrapings from mucous lesions and nasal discharge may show *Treponema pallidum*.

C. X-Ray Findings: Findings are characteristic. All of the long bones may be affected. Changes are apparent early in the disease. The epiphyseal line shows increased density, with decreased density proximal to it. In severe cases, destructive lesions occur near the ends of long bones. Periostitis appears as a widening of the shaft of the long bones, with eventual calcification and distortion of the normal curvature.

Treatment

A. Specific Measures:

1. Early congenital syphilis–Give aqueous penicillin G, 50 thousand units/kg/d intravenously in 2 divided doses, or procaine penicillin G, 100 thousand units/kg/d intramuscularly in one dose, for 10 days.

2. Late congenital syphilis, including neurosyphilis–Give procaine penicillin G, 50 thousand units/kg/d intramuscularly for 14 days.

3. Acquired syphilis–Give benzathine penicillin G, 2.4 million units in intramuscular injections of 1.2 million units each.

4. Penicillin sensitivity–In individuals sensitive to penicillin, give tetracycline or erythromycin for 14 days.

B. Complications of Specific Therapy: Jarisch-Herxheimer reaction, with fever due to the sudden destruction of spirochetes by drugs, occurs within the first 24 hours and subsides within the next 24 hours. Treatment should not be discontinued unless aggravation of laryngitis, if present, obstructs the airway.

C. Follow-Up Treatment: Serologic tests should be done at intervals of 3 months for at least 1 year. Disease in the mother should also be evaluated and treated.

Prophylaxis

If syphilis is diagnosed early in pregnancy, treatment may be completed before delivery. The chances of preventing the disease in the newborn are excellent even if the mother is not treated until the seventh or eighth month of pregnancy.

Prognosis

Rapid treatment of infants with early congenital syphilis will usually result in a cure and normal growth and development. In children with late congenital syphilis, the prognosis for cure of the spirochetal infection is good, but pathologic changes in the bones, nervous system, and eyes will remain throughout life.

LEPTOSPIROSIS

Leptospirosis is an acute febrile disease caused by *Leptospira* species or serovariants of *Leptospira interrogans*. The most common species (or serovariants) implicated are *Leptospira canicola*, *Leptospira icterohaemorrhagiae*, and *Leptospira pomona*. The infection is transmitted through the ingestion of food or water contaminated with the urine of the reservoir animals (dogs, rats, cattle, and swine). Ingestion may occur while bathing in contaminated water. Rat bites are also a source. The incubation period is 6–12 days.

Clinical Findings

A. Symptoms and Signs: Onset is abrupt, with fever to 39.5–40.5 °C (103–105 °F). Pharyngitis, cervical lymphadenopathy, and conjunctivitis accompany this first phase of the disease, which lasts 3–5 days and is followed by subsidence of fever and symptoms. The second phase of the disease appears after 2 or 3 days, with recurrence of fever and the onset of joint pains, vomiting, headache, and often a rash, which is morbilliform and sometimes purpuric. Meningitis and (more rarely) uveitis may develop at this phase of the disease.

B. Laboratory Findings: The white blood cell count usually is markedly elevated (as high as 50,000/μL), sometimes with immature forms. Cerebrospinal fluid may show 100–200 cells/μL. Leptospirae may be seen on Wright's stain of blood, urine, or cerebrospinal fluid during the first 10 days of symptoms. Serum bilirubin levels may be elevated, and the SGOT level may be abnormal. A rapid agglutination test is available, and antibody is detectable after the first 7 days of disease.

Complications

Renal involvement, with hematuria, proteinuria, and oliguria, occurs in about 50% of cases. Jaundice, with an enlarged and tender liver, is also common. Symptomatic meningitis with any of its findings may become apparent in the second phase of the disease.

Treatment

A. Specific Measures: Give procaine penicillin G, 50,000 units/kg/d intramuscularly in 4 divided doses for 10 days. If started within the first 4 days of illness, this treatment may minimize symptoms during the second phase of the disease. In patients with penicillin sensitivity, give tetracyclines for 10 days. In patients with severe renal and hepatic involvement, vigorous treatment will be necessary (see under Acute Renal Failure, Chapter 18).

B. Complications of Specific Therapy: Jarisch-Herxheimer reaction may occur, as in the treatment of syphilis (see above).

Prognosis

In the absence of renal or hepatic involvement, recovery is complete after 10–15 days. With severe kidney and liver involvement, the mortality rate may be as high as 30%.

RELAPSING FEVER

Relapsing fever is endemic in many parts of the world, especially in mountainous areas. The causative organism is *Borrelia recurrentis*, and the reservoir is rodents or other human beings with relapsing fever. Transmission to humans occurs by lice or ticks and occasionally by contact with the blood of infected rodents.

After an incubation period of 2–14 days, the onset of disease is abrupt, with fever, chills, tachycardia, nausea, vomiting, arthralgia, and cough. A morbilliform rash appears usually within the first 2 days and maximally over the trunk and extremities. Petechiae may also occur. Without treatment, the fever falls by crisis in 3–10 days. Relapse then characteristically occurs at intervals of 1–2 weeks and may involve as many as 10 such episodes in the absence of treatment.

Diagnosis depends upon the clinical course and the observation of spirochetes in the peripheral blood by darkfield examination or by use of Wright's stain.

Treatment with penicillin, tetracyclines, or chloramphenicol is successful. As with syphilis and leptosporosis, the Jarisch-Herxheimer reaction may occur in the first 24 hours of treatment.

Prognosis is good except in patients with debilitated states.

RAT-BITE FEVER

There are 2 forms of rat-bite fever, both rare in children. One is caused by a gram-negative spiral organism, *Spirillum minor*, and the other is caused by a gram-negative bacterium, *Streptobacillus moniliformis*. Transmission is through the bite of a rat, which may be a household pet or wild rat. In addition, the bites of squirrels, mice, cats, and weasels have resulted in this disease. The onset is about 3 days after the bite, with fever, morbilliform rash, and joint pain. *S minor* can sometimes be found in darkfield examination of blood. *S moniliformis* may grow in enriched media. Treatment is with procaine penicillin in full dosage for 7 days (see Chapter 6). The prognosis is excellent.

26 | Infectious Diseases: Protozoal & Metazoal

PROTOZOAL DISEASES

MALARIA

Malaria is an acute or chronic febrile disease caused by one of 4 types of plasmodia: *Plasmodium vivax, Plasmodium malariae, Plasmodium falciparum,* and *Plasmodium ovale*. Transmission occurs through the bite of the female *Anopheles* mosquito, in which the sexual cycle of the parasite occurs. The asexual cycle occurs in humans.

Clinical Findings

In children, malaria does not always present the classic clinical picture seen in adults.

A. Symptoms and Signs: Sudden onset of paroxysms of fever to 39.5–40.5 °C (103–105 °F) is accompanied by convulsions in the very young. Chill is sometimes present, lasts at least 2–4 hours, and is followed by sweating. In young children, paroxysms may be continuous or very irregularly recurrent. In older children, recurrence of paroxysms varies with type of infection: 48 hours for *P vivax, P falciparum,* and *P ovale* infections and 72 hours for *P malariae* infection. Diarrhea and vomiting are frequent, and splenomegaly is usually present.

B. Laboratory Findings: There is rapid onset of anemia, and serum bilirubin levels are increased. Thin and thick blood smears and bone marrow smears show parasites.

Complications

"Blackwater fever" is rare in childhood. It is usually associated with *P falciparum* infection and is characterized by hemoglobinuria and a shocklike state.

Treatment

A. Specific Measures:

1. Chloroquine–

a. Chloroquine phosphate (Aralen)–Given once daily orally for 4 days, this is the drug of choice for *P vivax* and *P falciparum* infections, which it completely eradicates. Give 10 mg/kg as the initial dose, followed by 5 mg/kg once daily for 3 days. Toxic symptoms include nausea, vomiting, and diarrhea.

b. Chloroquine hydrochloride–If oral therapy is not possible, give chloroquine hydrochloride, 2 mg/kg intramuscularly or intravenously immediately, and continue the same dosage once daily for 2 days.

2. Quinine, pyrimethamine, and sulfadiazine–In chloroquine-resistant *P falciparum* infection, fever will persist for more than 48 hours. Stop chloroquine; start quinine and pyrimethamine (Daraprim).

a. Quinine sulfate–Give 25 mg/kg/d in 3 doses for 5 days.

b. Quinine dihydrochloride*–Dilute in 100 mL or more of physiologic saline. Give 8 mg/kg intravenously up to 3 doses every 8 hours. Give slowly. Use only for patients unable to take oral medication. Follow with oral medication. ***Caution:*** Quinine dihydrochloride is a very dangerous drug.

c. Pyrimethamine–Dosages, according to patient's weight and age, are as follows: under 10 kg, 6.25 mg/d; 10–20 kg, 12.5 mg/d; 4–10 years of age, 25 mg/d; and over 10 years of age, 50 mg/d.

d. Sulfadiazine–Give 100 mg/kg/d in 4 divided doses for 5 days.

3. Primaquine phosphate– Use with chloroquine to prevent relapses in patients with *P vivax* infections. Give orally once daily for 14 days. Dosages, according to patient's weight, are as follows: up to 10 kg, 2 mg/d; 11–20 kg, 4 mg/d; 21–40 kg, 6 mg/d; 41–55 kg, 10 mg/d; over 55 kg, 20 mg/d. ***Caution:*** Primaquine is a toxic drug; its use must be monitored, with careful laboratory follow-up. Never use this drug for treatment of black patients. If anemia, leukopenia, or methemoglobinemia appears, immediately discontinue use of the drug. Never use the drug with quinacrine hydrochloride or within 5 days of quinacrine therapy.

B. General Measures: Fluid therapy is most important. Urge oral intake and, if not satisfactory, give parenteral fluids. Control high fever. Treat anemia with iron.

Prophylaxis

Measures include control of mosquito vectors and use of suppressive therapy. Most of the drugs used to treat the disease may be used prophylactically in endemic areas. Chloroquine phosphate, 5 mg/kg/wk, may be given; it is preferable to start therapy in patients 2 weeks before they enter an endemic area. To prevent infection with *P vivax* or *P ovale*, give primaquine in the same dosage as for treatment (above) for 2 weeks after the patient leaves the endemic area. For prophylaxis of

*Quinine dihydrochloride (parenteral) is available in the USA from the Centers for Disease Control. Telephone (404) 329–3670 during the day or (404) 329–2888 during nights, weekends, and holidays.

chloroquine-resistant malaria, which is widespread in Southeast Asia and South America, give pyrimethamine (Daraprim), 0.5 mg/kg/wk. Chloroquine phosphate, 10 mg/kg, is indicated for use in patients before they receive a transfusion of whole blood in an endemic area or from a donor recently arrived from an endemic area.

Prognosis

In the majority of cases, the prognosis is excellent with proper therapy. In small infants and in the presence of malnutrition or chronic debilitating disease, the prognosis is more guarded.

AMEBIASIS

Amebiasis is an acute and chronic enteric infection with *Entamoeba histolytica*. Transmission from an infected person or a carrier is through the cysts, which are excreted in feces. The cyst may survive as long as 1 month in water. The disease is acquired by oral route through contamination of food or drinking water.

Clinical Findings

A. Symptoms and Signs: Acute amebic dysentery is characterized by a sudden onset of diarrhea, which is not usually explosive or accompanied by tenesmus and which lasts about 1 week. The frequency of stools varies with the age of the child, being higher in infants and occurring only 2 or 3 times daily in older children. This diarrheal phase is followed by an asymptomatic phase and, usually, a recurrence. Fever is usually not significant. Hepatomegaly may be present. Atypical amebiasis, common in children, presents with mild recurrent diarrhea, irritability, anorexia, and slight abdominal pain (most often in the right upper quadrant).

B. Laboratory Findings: In the acute stage of infection, stool examination may show trophozoites. Cysts are excreted in cycles, and repeated stool examinations may be necessary. Biopsy of rectal mucosa sometimes provides a definitive diagnosis.

Complications

Amebic abscess is rare in early childhood but should always be considered. Early symptoms include relief of hunger by extremely small amounts of food and hiccupping as a result of diaphragmatic irritation. Liver scanning with radioisotopes and CT scans may provide useful diagnostic findings.

Treatment

A. Specific Measures: Combined treatment with one of the tetracyclines and chloroquine is the most commonly used regimen. There are, however, wide variations in recommendations, and a variety of other drugs are reported to be effective.

1. Metronidazole (Flagyl)–Give 40–50 mg/kg/d in 3 doses for 5–10 days. *Caution:* Metronidazole has been reported to be associated with cancer in experimental animals; nevertheless, it is the only drug effective against infection in the bowel lumen, the bowel wall, and the liver.

2. Tetracycline–Give 3 times daily for 10 days with or followed by chloroquine, emetine, or diloxanide furoate (see below).

3. Chloroquine phosphate (Aralen)–Give for 10 days. Dosages, according to patient's age, are as follows: up to 5 years, a correspondingly smaller dosage than for older children and adults; 5–10 years, half the adult dosage; and over 10 years, the full adult dosage. Adult dosage is 1 g, followed by 0.5 g after 6–8 hours, and then 0.5 g on the next 2 days (2.5 g total in 3 days).

4. Emetine hydrochloride–This drug, given 1 mg/kg subcutaneously or intramuscularly, is of value (with chloroquine) in treatment of patients with acute dysentery. Like chloroquine, it has less effect on the intestinal phase and should therefore be used with tetracycline as above. The patient should be in the hospital during administration of emetine. Pulse and blood pressure should be followed carefully. Upon increase in pulse rate or fall in blood pressure, discontinue the drug. An ECG should be taken at the start of therapy and after 4 days of treatment. Changes in QRS complex, ST segment, and conduction time are indications for cessation of treatment.

5. Diloxanide furoate*–Give 20–25 mg/kg/d in 3 oral doses for 10 days. This drug is highly effective for treatment of patients with amebiasis. It is used in combination with tetracycline and chloroquine as above.

B. General Measures: Institute dietary measures for diarrhea (see Chapter 16) and take precautions as to disposal of stools and care of diapers.

C. Treatment of Complications: Patients with amebic hepatitis should be treated with erythromycin or chloroquine. Regulate diet as for other types of acute hepatitis.

Prognosis & Prophylaxis

The prognosis is excellent with adequate treatment and follow-up. Proper disposal of excreta and precautions in regard to drinking water are preventive measures.

*Diloxanide furoate is available in the USA from the Centers for Disease Control. Telephone (404) 329–3670 during the day or (404) 329–2888 during nights, weekends, and holidays.

GIARDIASIS

Giardiasis is caused by a flagellate, *Giardia lamblia*.

Clinical Findings

The organism may infest the human bowel without producing symptoms, or (especially in children) it may cause a chronic watery diarrhea or steatorrhea, abdominal cramping, and malaise. The diagnosis is usually based upon identification of cysts and trophozoites in the stool. Duodenal aspiration may be necessary to demonstrate the cysts if stools are repeatedly negative.

Treatment

A. Specific Measures: Any one of the following treatment procedures is usually highly effective for immediate relief of symptoms.

1. Furazolidone (Furoxone)–This is the drug of choice for use in children under 5 years of age. Give 6–8 mg/kg/d in 4 divided doses for 10 days. The drug is available in tablet or liquid form.

2. Quinacrine (Atabrine)–Give 8 mg/kg/d in 3 divided doses for 5 days.

3. Metronidazole (Flagyl)–Give 15 mg/kg/d in 3 divided doses for 10 days (see warning under Amebiasis, above).

B. General Measures: Recurrence in 3 to 4 weeks is not unusual and should be an indication for repeat therapy.

TRICHOMONIASIS

Trichomoniasis is caused by *Trichomonas vaginalis*, a flagellate protozoon. Infection is usually spread by sexual intercourse with an asymptomatic male carrier.

Clinical Findings

The symptoms are vaginitis with intense itching and a frothy discharge that is usually yellow-green with a characteristic "mousy" odor. *Candida albicans* may occur in a mixed infection with more intense inflammatory reaction in the vaginal mucosa and more painful burning symptoms. Trichomoniasis, alone or combined with candidiasis, is very rare in patients before the menarche.

Treatment

Treatment with metronidazole (Flagyl), 250 mg 3 times each day for 10 days, is most effective (see warning under Amebiasis, above). The male sexual partner should be treated concomitantly with the same course. Mixed infection with *Candida* should be treated with nystatin

(Mycostatin) vaginal suppositories, 100,000 units each, once daily for 2 weeks.

Prognosis

The prognosis for patients with vaginal trichomoniasis is excellent unless there is reinfection.

TOXOPLASMOSIS

Toxoplasma gondii, an obligate intracellular parasite, is found worldwide in humans and in many species of animals and birds. The parasite is a coccidian of cats, the definitive host. Human infection occurs by ingestion of oocysts, by ingestion of cysts in raw or undercooked meat, by transplacental transmission, or, rarely, by direct inoculation of trophozoites, as in blood transfusion. The incidence of congenital toxoplasmosis in the USA is about one per 1,000 live births.

Clinical Findings

A. Symptoms and Signs:

1. Congenital toxoplasmosis–Congenital transmission occurs only as a result of acute infection *during* pregnancy and may occur in any trimester. Infection has been detected in up to 1% of women during pregnancy; about 45% of women who acquire the *primary* infection during pregnancy and who are *not* treated will give birth to congenitally infected infants. Signs of congenital toxoplasmosis are present at birth in 10% of infected infants. The others develop symptoms in the first months of life: microcephaly, seizures, mental retardation, hepatosplenomegaly, pneumonitis, rash, fever, chorioretinitis, and cerebral calcification. Chorioretinitis is usually a late sequela of congenital infection, with symptoms being first noted in the second or third decade of life.

2. Toxoplasmosis in the immunocompromised host–Toxoplasmosis may present as a disseminated disease, particularly in patients given immunosuppressive drugs or patients with lymphoreticular, hematologic, or other malignancies. Encephalitis is the most common manifestation; pneumonitis and myocarditis may also occur.

3. Acquired toxoplasmosis–

a. There may be febrile lymphadenopathy resembling infectious mononucleosis but with a more prolonged course (sometimes 2–6 months) and with intermittent exacerbations.

b. There may be febrile disease without symptoms or signs of specific organ system involvement. Transient morbilliform rash may appear. A prolonged and recurrent course is not uncommon.

c. Chorioretinitis, with acute onset in children or young adults, may be recurrent and prolonged (almost pathognomonic of toxoplasmosis).

B. Laboratory Findings: The white blood cell count and differential may resemble infectious mononucleosis (see Chapter 24) or be entirely normal. The heterophil antibody titer is rarely elevated. The Sabin-Feldman dye test results become positive after initial infection and are positive in the mother of the child with congenital infection. Complement fixation, indirect hemagglutination, immunofluorescent antibody (IFA), and IgM-IFA tests are available in special laboratories and research institutes. A rise in titer with any test or a very high single test titer will confirm a clinical diagnosis. In congenital infection, IgM antibody will be present and is diagnostic. Toxoplasmosis can be diagnosed occasionally by histologic examination of tissue or by isolation of the parasite in bone marrow aspirates, cerebrospinal fluid sediment, sputum, blood, and other tissue and body fluids. Only isolation from body fluids confirms acute infection; isolation from tissues could represent chronic infection.

C. X-Ray Findings: Skull x-rays show intracranial calcifications in recovered congenital infection.

Treatment

Treatment is indicated in immunocompromised patients, in pregnant women with acute infection, in congenitally infected infants with or without symptoms, and in patients with acquired disease whose symptoms persist for over 2 weeks or who have active chorioretinitis.

A. Specific Measures:

1. Pyrimethamine, folinic acid, and sulfadiazine or trisulfapyrimidines–Treatment is with a combination of pyrimethamine (Daraprim), folinic acid (calcium leucovorin), and either sulfadiazine or trisulfapyrimidines (Terfonyl). In patients with significant organ involvement, dosages are as follows: pyrimethamine, 15 mg/m^2 or 1 mg/kg (up to 50 mg) twice daily for the first 2 days and 15 mg/m^2 or 1 mg/kg (up to 25 mg) every other day thereafter; folinic acid, 5–10 mg for the first 2 days and every other day thereafter; and sulfadiazine or trisulfapyrimidines, 75 mg/kg (up to 4 g) for the first day and 100 mg/kg (up to 6 g) in 2 or 3 divided doses every day thereafter. The duration of therapy is determined by the severity of illness; it is a minimum of 6 months in congenitally infected infants.

2. Spiramycin–This drug is available in Europe and is given in a dosage of 6 mg/kg/d in 4 divided doses for 14 days.

3. Trimethoprim-sulfamethoxazole and clindamycin–These drugs are under study.

4. Prednisone–For patients with chorioretinitis, give prednisone, 1 mg/kg/d for 10 days, and reduce the dosage to stop the drug in 3 more days.

B. General Measures: Toxicity of pyrimethamine includes thrombocytopenia, agranulocytosis, and leukopenia. Pyrimethamine should not be used in the first trimester of pregnancy because it has been shown to be teratogenic in animals. Spiramycin is a safe drug for use in pregnancy.

Prophylaxis in the Pregnant Woman

Since approximately 90% of women infected during pregnancy are asymptomatic, diagnosis in the pregnant woman can only be made by serologic (screening) methods. Pregnant women may have their serum examined for *Toxoplasma* antibody, and an IgM test can be done (if facilities are available) when conventional tests are positive at any titer. If the IgM test result is negative and the conventional test yields results of less than 1:1000, no further evaluation is necessary. Those with negative titers by conventional tests should take measures to prevent infection: Avoid contact with or wear gloves when handling materials that are potentially contaminated (eg, cat litter boxes) or when gardening. Avoid eating raw or undercooked meat. Wash hands thoroughly after handling raw meat. Wash fruits and vegetables before consumption.

Prognosis

Nearly all children with congenital toxoplasmosis who are asymptomatic or have only mild abnormalities in the first year of life will subsequently develop untoward sequelae such as ophthalmologic and neurologic handicaps.

VISCERAL LEISHMANIASIS
(Kala-Azar)

Visceral leishmaniasis is an infection with a protozoon, transmitted from human to human and animal to human by the *Phlebotomus* sandfly found in North Africa, India, and the Mediterranean region. The organism multiplies in the reticuloendothelial system and in the bone marrow.

Clinical Findings

A. Symptoms and Signs: The onset is abrupt, with high fever, vomiting, and diarrhea. Lymphadenopathy and splenic enlargement are early findings. These symptoms usually persist to a fatal outcome.

B. Laboratory Findings: The organism *Leishmania donovani* will be found in smears of the bone marrow or lymph node aspirates. Agglutination tests are available in the USA from the Centers for Disease Control, Atlanta, GA 30333.

Treatment

A. Specific Measures:

1. Sodium antimony gluconate*–Give 10 mg/kg/d in 6 intravenous doses for 5–8 days. This may cause vomiting and diarrhea.

2. Pentamidine isethionate*–Give 3 mg/kg/d intramuscularly for 10 days. This drug may be given in combination with sodium antimony gluconate, or it may be given alone for treatment of patients with antimony-resistant infections.

B. General Measures: Complicating bacterial infection should be treated with appropriate antibiotics. Nutritional problems and anemia are common and must be treated vigorously.

PNEUMOCYSTIS PNEUMONIA

Pneumocystis is an interstitial pneumonitis occurring in infants or children with low resistance syndromes (eg, when receiving corticosteroids, prolonged antibiotic therapy, or cytotoxic drugs for neoplasms). The causative organism, *Pneumocystis carinii,* has not been classified definitely, although it is most commonly believed to be either a fungus related to the yeasts or a sporozoon. Multiple cases in newborn nurseries have been reported.

Clinical Findings

X-rays show an interstitial pneumonitis, but physical signs are rare. The diagnosis may be established by lung puncture biopsy or open lung biopsy.

Treatment

A. Specific Measures: Trimethoprim-sulfamethoxazole is the treatment of choice. Give trimethoprim, 20 mg/kg/d, and sulfamethoxazole, 100 mg/kg/d, in 4 divided doses for 14 days.

Addition of pentamidine isethionate (Lomidine)* to the treatment regimen has also been recommended; give 4 mg/kg/d intramuscularly for 14 days.

B. General Measures: Oxygen, sedatives, and digitalization are important supportive measures. Transfusions and immune serum globulin increase the patient's resistance to *Pneumocystis*. The cause of lowered resistance should be eliminated if known and possible.

*Sodium antimony gluconate and pentamidine isethionate are available in the USA from the Centers for Disease Control. Telephone (404) 329–3670 during the day or (404) 329–2888 during nights, weekends, and holidays.

Prophylaxis

Use of trimethoprim, 5 mg/kg/d, combined with sulfamethoxazole, 25 mg/kg/d, in 2 divided doses, may prevent infection in patients at risk.

METAZOAL DISEASES

I. NEMATODES

ENTEROBIASIS
(Pinworms)

Asymptomatic infestation with *Enterobius vermicularis* is a common disease. Symptoms occasionally do occur and may require treatment.

The adult worms reside in the cecum and colon. The fertile eggs, laid outside the anus, are distributed from person to person by dust; by transfer to the mouth from contaminated articles, food, drink, or hands; and by direct contact with infected individuals. About 20% of children in the USA harbor the worm.

Clinical Findings

A. Symptoms and Signs: Several members of the family are usually infected. Pruritus ani is the most common symptom and is usually most intense at night, when the worms are laying their eggs. There may be involvement of the vagina, with itching and discharge or dysuria. Massive infestation may cause abdominal pain or even appendicitis, as well as variable, vague nervous symptoms.

B. Laboratory Findings: Demonstration of eggs should be attempted. The customary technique is to press a small piece of pressure-sensitive cellulose tape (Scotch tape) around the anus in the early morning, preferably before bowel movement, and to examine the tape under the microscope on a glass slide. Eggs appear as elongated ovals with the embryonic worm inside. Eosinophilia may be present.

Treatment

A. Specific Measures: Use one of the following methods:

1. Pyrantel pamoate–This drug is highly effective and is given in a single dose of 11 mg/kg to a maximum of 1 g.

2. Mebendazole–Also highly effective, this drug is given in a single dose of 100 mg irrespective of weight or age. ***Caution:*** No information is available on toxicity in infants.

3. Pyrvinium pamoate (Povan)–Give a single dose of 5 mg/kg to a maximum of 250 mg; repeat the dose in 2 weeks. Nausea, vomiting, and cramping may occur.

4. Piperazine–Piperazine citrate or phosphate is available in syrup form (Antepar), 100 mg/mL. Give daily for 7 days, withdraw for 7 days, and then give again for 7 days. Dosages, according to patient's age, are as follows: 1–5 years, 2.5 mL 3 times daily; 5–10 years, 5 mg 3 times daily; and over 10 years, 7.5 mL 3 times daily.

B. General Measures: Patients should be instructed to wash their hands carefully before each meal and after each bowel movement, keep their fingernails short and well scrubbed, launder and boil all bed linen twice weekly, avoid shaking the bed linen when removing it from the bed, scrub toilet seats daily, and avoid scratching the involved area and putting their hands in their mouth and nose.

Prognosis & Prophylaxis

The prognosis is excellent, and complications are extremely rare. Most infestations are not recognized or treated. A high carrier rate makes control measures difficult.

ASCARIASIS
(Roundworms)

Infestation with *Ascaris lumbricoides,* a large roundworm, may produce no symptoms. The eggs are excreted in feces, and the highly infective larvae are developed in the soil. Human-to-human transmission occurs in childhood by ingestion of larvae from soil-contaminated fingers, toys, etc.

Clinical Findings

A. Symptoms and Signs: Passage of the adult worm is usually the only sign of infestation. Colicky, recurrent abdominal pain may occur owing to adult worms in the intestine, and respiratory symptoms may occur owing to passage of the larval stage through the lungs in the course of the normal life cycle. Bile duct obstruction with the adult worm may occur.

B. Laboratory Findings: Eggs found in feces are round and have a prominent outer membrane with a wavelike contour.

Treatment

A. Specific Measures: Treat as for enterobiasis (see above).

B. General Measures: Intestinal decompression with a Levin tube may be helpful in cases of massive infestation with partial intestinal obstruction and during the first 24 hours of drug therapy.

Prognosis

The prognosis is excellent for eradication by the first course of drug therapy.

ANCYLOSTOMIASIS
(Hookworms)

Hookworm disease, widespread in the tropics and subtropics, is caused by *Ancylostoma duodenale* or *Necator americanus*. Eggs are passed in the feces and develop in the soil to form larvae. Larvae pass through the intact skin of bare feet in contact with contaminated soil. Coexisting deficiency diseases and malnutrition may contribute to some of the symptoms.

Clinical Findings

A. Symptoms and Signs: Passage of larvae through the skin of the feet may produce itching and papular eruption. An early sign is soft and sometimes tarry feces (melena). Apathy, pallor, anorexia, and failure to grow are noted, and the abdomen may be protuberant.

B. Laboratory Findings: Examination of stool reveals eggs in great quantity. They are oval and thin-walled, with cells or embryos inside. Early, leukocytosis with eosinophilia is present. Later, hypochromic microcytic anemia appears.

Treatment

A. Specific Measures: Treatment should be undertaken only after general supportive measures have been carried out.

1. Mebendazole (Vermox)–Treat as for ascariasis (see above).

2. Bephenium hydroxynaphthoate (Alcopar)–This drug is highly effective against *Ancylostoma* and may be used with tetrachlorethylene in *Necator* infection. Give a 5-g dose twice in a single day. For children weighing less than 22 kg, give a 2.5-g dose twice. The drug is best given mixed with some flavored liquid, fruit juice, or milk.

3. Tetrachlorethylene–Do not give tetrachlorethylene for treatment of hookworm in the presence of *Ascaris* infection; in mixed infections, treat ascariasis first. No purgation should be given before or after treatment. Withhold all food. Give 0.2 mL per year of age as a single dose, in capsule form or as liquid with syrup, followed by bed rest for 24 hours.

B. General Measures: Give iron for hypochromic anemia, with transfusions if the degree of anemia is severe. Institute or maintain a good diet with supplementary vitamins.

Prognosis & Prophylaxis

The prognosis is excellent for cure, and anemia responds to therapy with eradication of disease. Reinfection can occur. Shoes should be worn in endemic areas.

TRICHINOSIS

Trichinosis is a very common infestation, most often unrecognized, with *Trichinella spiralis* acquired through ingestion of inadequately cooked, infested hog meat. Larvae migrate from bowel to bloodstream to muscle, where they encyst to form a fibrotic nodule.

Clinical Findings

A. Symptoms and Signs: Acute manifestations may be quite mild or may be fatal. Gastrointestinal symptoms appear early, followed in a few days by nausea, vomiting, cramps, diarrhea, flatulence, chills and fever, weakness, rash, edema (especially of the face and about the eyes), conjunctivitis and photophobia, splinter hemorrhages, pain and tenderness in the muscles, and central or peripheral nerve involvement with severe headache. Most patients with chronic trichinosis have no symptoms. Weakness may be present, as well as other symptoms referable to multiple organ involvement.

B. Laboratory Findings: Eosinophilia is present in patients with the acute or chronic form. In the acute form, the *Trichinella* skin test gives a delayed reaction (12–24 hours) early in the disease (third to seventh days). In the chronic form, the *Trichinella* skin test gives an immediate reaction (5 minutes) late in the disease (17th day on). Muscle biopsy may demonstrate organisms. Complement fixation and precipitin tests are of value after the fourth week of infection.

Treatment

A. Specific Measures:

1. Thiabendazole (Mintezol)–Use of 25 mg/kg/d in 2 doses for 5 days will eradicate larvae from the bloodstream.

2. Mebendazole (Vermox)–Mebendazole is effective against larvae in the bloodstream and encysted in the muscle and possibly is effective against the adult worm.

3. Corticotropin or corticosteroids–Corticotropin or one of the corticosteroids (cortisone, hydrocortisone, prednisone) will provide effective relief for acute symptoms of trichinosis (see Chapter 22). A reduction of the eosinophil count, disappearance of fever and splinter hemorrhages, if present, and a general improvement in the clinical state of the patient are guides that should be employed to determine the efficacy of treatment. Patients with the acute form should be treated with relatively large doses of either drug for the first 24–48 hours. In patients with the subacute form, therapy may have to be continued for several days or weeks on a reduced dosage to prevent recurrence of symptoms.

B. General Measures: Hospitalization and optimal nursing care may be necessary in severe cases.

Prognosis & Prophylaxis

The prognosis is excellent for subsidence of symptoms. All pork should be thoroughly cooked and stored at subfreezing temperatures to kill the larvae.

II. CESTODES

TAENIASIS
(Tapeworms)

Taeniasis (Table 26–1) is caused by infestation with *Taenia saginata* (beef tapeworm) and *Taenia solium* (pork tapeworm). Transmission is by ingestion of larvae in inadequately cooked beef or pork. Larvae develop into adult tapeworms in about 3 months.

Clinical Findings

A. Symptoms and Signs: There is usually a history of consumption of raw or incompletely cooked beef or pork. Acute manifestations include diarrhea and fever. Chronic manifestations include vague gastrointestinal and central nervous system symptoms.

B. Laboratory Findings: Leukocytosis and eosinophilia may be present during the acute phase. In patients with chronic taeniasis, findings include mild to severe anemia and gravid proglottids in the feces or on the underclothing.

Treatment

A. Specific Measures:

1. Niclosamide (Niclocide, Yomesan)–Niclosamide is the drug of choice. Give 1 g for children 2–8 years of age, 1.5 g for children over 8 years, and 2 g for older children and for adults. The drug is given orally on an empty stomach on the morning after a light nonresidue supper. Posttreatment purgation is required only in the case of *T solium* infection. The toxicity of niclosamide is slight in therapeutic doses.

2. Paromomycin–Paromomycin is an alternative drug that also works, but niclosamide is definitely preferred. The dosage of paromomycin is 11 mg/kg every 15 minutes for a total of 4 doses.

Table 26–1. Tapeworm diseases.*

Agent	Definitive Host (Mature Worms in)	Intermediate Host (Larval Stages in)	Humans Infected by Eating	Directly Communicable Human to Human	Eggs in Human Feces	Diseases in Humans		
						Stage of Parasite Causing	Pathology	Specific Treatment (Drugs Listed in Order of Preference)
Diphyllobothrium latum	Humans.	Water, copepods, fish.	Fish containing larval worms.	No.	Yes.	Adult.	Vitamin B_{12} deficiency, intestinal irritation, anemia.	Niclosamide, paromomycin.
Dipylidium caninum	Dogs, cats, humans.	Fleas.	Fleas containing larval worms.	No.	Yes.	Adult.	Intestinal irritation.	Niclosamide, paromomycin.
Echinococcus granulosus	Dogs, wolves.	Domestic and wild herbivores, humans.	Worm eggs from canine feces.	No.	No.	Larva (hydatid).	Circumscribed unilocular hydatid disease.	Surgical removal.
Echinococcus multilocularis	Foxes, dogs.	Field rodents, humans.	Worm eggs from canine feces.	No.	No.	Larva (hydatid).	Invasive multilocular hydatid disease.	Surgical removal.
Hymenolepis diminuta	Rodents, humans.	Arthropods.	Arthropods containing larval worms.	No.	Yes.	Adult.	Intestinal irritation.	Niclosamide, paromomycin.
Hymenolepis nana	Humans, rodents.	Humans, rodents.	Worm eggs from human feces.	Yes.	Yes.	Adult.	Intestinal irritation.	Niclosamide, paromomycin.
Taenia saginata	Humans.	Cattle.	Beef containing larval worms.	No.	Yes.	Adult.	Intestinal irritation.	Niclosamide, paromomycin.
Taenia solium	Humans.	Hogs.	Pork containing larval worms.	Yes.	Yes.	Adult.	Intestinal irritation.	Paromomycin.
		Humans.	Worm eggs from human feces.	No.	No.	Larva (cysticercus).	Cysticercosis.	Surgical removal.

*Adapted from *Report of the Committee on Infectious Diseases,* 17th ed. American Academy of Pediatrics, 1974.

B. General Measures: Sometimes several courses of treatment may be necessary.

Prognosis

The prognosis is excellent with successful eradication of all worms.

VISCERAL LARVA MIGRANS
(Toxocariasis, Larval Granulomatosis)

Visceral larva migrans usually occurs in young children as a result of ingestion of embryonated *Toxocara* eggs, which are present in soil contaminated with excrement of infected cats and dogs. In most cases, infection is characterized by hepatomegaly; chronic, persistent leukocytosis; eosinophilia; hyperglobulinemia; and eosinophilic granulomatous lesions of the liver. The disease is self-limited.

For treatment in severe symptomatic cases, give thiabendazole (Mintezol), 25 mg/kg/d in 2 doses for 5–10 days. In patients with a history of ingestion of material contaminated with dog or cat feces, give diethylcarbamazine, 5–10 mg/kg/d in 3 doses for 15–20 days to eradicate larvae from the bloodstream.

CUTANEOUS LARVA MIGRANS

Cutaneous larva migrans is caused by infection with the dog or cat hookworm, *Ancylostoma braziliense*. This disease is principally found in the southern USA. The larvae invade superficial lymphatics, producing winding tunnels visible on the skin. Papules may also develop in the vicinity of the tunnels. Pruritus is severe. It may be necessary to use ethyl chloride spray or a cream preparation of thiabendazole.

FILARIASIS

Filariasis is caused by infection with filarial worms *(Wuchereria bancrofti* and *Brugia malayi)* that are transmitted by mosquitoes. The worms mature in the lymphatics and produce large numbers of microfilariae (motile larvae), which appear in the peripheral blood; in the case of *W bancrofti*, the appearance is at night. Microfilariae of *Dirofilaria immitis*, the heartworm of dogs, may (rarely) infect humans and cause fibrous nodules in the lung. *D immitis* is found in the southern and western USA where mosquito vectors are present.

Clinical Findings

A. Symptoms and Signs: Asymptomatic infection is probably the most common form of disease, with lymphadenopathy of the inguinal nodes as the only finding. Sensitivity to antigens from living and dead filariae develops, and lymphangitis, fever, chills, vomiting, and weakness may occur and last for a few days to several weeks. Obstruction of lymphatic vessels over a long period of time will result in swelling of the extremities and in elephantiasis.

B. Laboratory Findings: Eosinophilia is common in the early stages of infection. A search for microfilariae in blood specimens (especially specimens taken at night) may yield diagnostic results. Antibody determinations can be carried out in special laboratories, and a skin test using *Dirofilaria* antigen may be helpful.

Treatment

A. Specific Measures: Diethylcarbamazine is the drug of choice. Give 6 mg/kg/d in 3 doses for 14–21 days. Since this drug does not affect the adult worm, relapses are common. Retreatment is often necessary for a period of 2–3 years.

B. General Measures: Patients with secondary bacterial infection of the lymphatics should be treated with appropriate antibiotics.

Prognosis

The asymptomatic disease, especially in young children, is without sequelae. Patients with chronic disease and elephantiasis may require surgical treatment.

SCHISTOSOMIASIS
(Bilharziasis)

Schistosomiasis is an infection caused by one of several species of blood flukes (eg, *Schistosoma japonicum, Schistosoma mansoni, Schistosoma haematobium*) whose infective swimming larvae (cercariae) are found in fresh water. Infection is transmitted to humans by contact with cercariae, which invade through the skin and spread to the liver or bladder, where they mature and reproduce.

Clinical Findings

A. Symptoms and Signs: An itchy, maculopapular rash may be seen at the sites of cercarial entry. Spread of the larvae to the liver and other organs may occur over a period of several weeks and will be accompanied by fever, prostration, and (occasionally) bloody diarrhea.

B. Laboratory Findings: In *S mansoni* infection, the ova are demonstrable in the stool and occasionally in the urine. *S haematobium* eggs are frequently found in the urine.

Treatment

A. Specific Measures:

1. Niridazole*–For *S japonicum* infection, give niridazole, 25 mg/kg/d in 3 doses for 7 days. Urine will turn brown during treatment.

2. Oxamniquine–For *S mansoni* infection, give oxamniquine, 20 mg/kg in 2 doses 3 hours apart. For children weighing over 30 kg, a single dose of 15 mg/kg should be given. Drowsiness may occur for a few hours after oral administration of this drug.

3. Metrifonate*–For *S haematobium* infection, give metrifonate in a single oral dose of 7.5 mg/kg, repeated 3 times at intervals of 2–4 weeks.

B. General Measures: Surgery may be necessary to correct fibrotic changes in the liver, urinary tract, and intestines.

Prognosis

For patients with mild infection, the prognosis is good with early and adequate treatment. For patients with complications in the urinary tract and liver, the prognosis is poor.

*Niridazole and metrifonate are available from the Centers for Disease Control. Telephone (404) 329–3670 during the day or (404) 329–2888 during nights, weekends, and holidays.

27 | Infectious Diseases: Mycotic

Several systemic mycoses, including coccidioidomycosis, histoplasmosis, cryptococcosis, and paracoccidioidomycosis, share a number of characteristics. Infection of humans occurs through inhalation of free-living infectious spores of the fungus, which are present in the dust in endemic areas. Primary pulmonary infections are usually mild or asymptomatic, and most infections have a tendency to heal, mainly through cellular immune mechanisms. Results of specific skin tests become positive after primary infection and remain positive during life. In a few specifically predisposed persons, the disease progresses after primary infection, becomes disseminated and involves many organs, and may be fatal. Similar dissemination may occur years after primary infection if the person is immunosuppressed by disease (eg, lymphoma) or drugs.

COCCIDIOIDOMYCOSIS

Coccidioidomycosis is caused by inhalation of arthrospores of *Coccidioides immitis*, a fungus that grows in the soil of certain arid regions of the southwestern USA, Mexico, and Central and South America. Two-thirds of infections are subclinical and diagnosed only by positive skin test results.

Clinical Findings

A. Symptoms and Signs:

1. Primary infection–About 10–30 days after exposure, there may be symptoms of respiratory tract infection, with fever, headache, muscular aches and pains, nasopharyngitis, and bronchitis with cough. One to 2 weeks later, there may be arthralgia, erythema nodosum, or erythema multiforme. All of these tend to subside spontaneously, but a thin-walled pulmonary cavity develops in about 5% of pulmonary lesions. These may take months to close.

2. Disseminated disease–Dissemination occurs in 0.1% of white and 1% of nonwhite persons after primary infection. Racial susceptibility is high in Filipinos, Mexicans, and blacks, and dissemination usually begins within 1–2 years after infection or following immunosuppression by disease or drugs. Pneumonia, empyema, involvement of bones and soft tissues (with abscesses and sinus tracts), and meningitis (with a high mortality rate) may occur as a result of dissemination.

B. Laboratory Findings: In primary infection, the sedimentation rate is elevated, there may be mild leukocytosis, and chest x-rays may show parenchymal densities and enlarged hilar nodes. Precipitating antibodies develop within a few weeks and then decline as the patient recovers. At the same time, results of the coccidioidin skin test (1:100 dilution) become positive and remain so for many years in the well person. Antibody titers in the complement fixation (CF) test rise and fall more slowly. However, if dissemination occurs, the antibody titer in the CF test characteristically rises and remains high, while the coccidioidin skin test results are often negative. Culture of sputum, drainage fluid, or biopsy specimens requires extreme caution. Laboratory-grown *Coccidioides* are *extremely* infectious.

Treatment

A. Primary Infection: Primary coccidioidomycosis is usually a self-limited illness. As the person recovers, substantial cellular immunity develops; results of the delayed-type skin test with coccidioidin are positive.

B. Disseminated Disease: In dissemination, cellular immunity is defective. Unrestrained multiplication of the fungus takes place, producing lesions in many organs. The only established drug of benefit is amphotericin B, 0.5–1 mg/kg/d intravenously. This is given in an intravenous drip of 5% glucose in water over 4–6 hours. To reduce the serious toxic effects (nausea, vomiting, fever), the patient is premedicated with aspirin, diphenhydramine, chlorpromazine, and a corticosteroid. Total daily drug doses are often kept at 35–40 mg, and treatment is continued for 3–4 months, with totals of up to 2 g of amphotericin B or more. Nephrotoxicity, hypokalemia, and other toxic effects are common. If meningitis is present, amphotericin B, 0.05–0.1 mg, must be given intrathecally or cisternally 3 times weekly, or by Ommaya reservoir. This is continued until results of serologic studies of spinal fluid are negative. Miconazole, 2–3 g/d intravenously, has been of benefit in patients with disseminated disease. Surgical excision of focal lesions and drainage of abscesses may be helpful.

Prognosis

The prognosis is excellent in patients with primary infection, fair for prolonged survival in patients with disseminated disease who are intensively treated and show active cell-mediated reactions, and poor for cure of patients with meningitis.

HISTOPLASMOSIS

Histoplasmosis is caused by inhalation of spores of *Histoplasma capsulatum* in dust. The organism grows profusely in bird feces, bat guano, and farm silos, and inhalation of dust from these sources causes massive infection. In the USA, most infections originate in the Midwest and South.

Clinical Findings

A. Symptoms and Signs:

1. Primary infection–Primary histoplasmosis is commonly asymptomatic or presents as a nonspecific influenzalike illness. Massive primary infection may produce pneumonitis with fever, cough, chest pain, and prostration. There may be enlargement of the lymph nodes, spleen, and liver. In most cases, all primary lesions heal.

2. Disseminated disease–Disseminated histoplasmosis develops in a small percentage of heavily exposed or immunodeficient persons, most commonly white males over 40 years of age. Fever, anemia, diffuse lymphadenopathy, splenomegaly, pneumonitis, and severe prostration occur. Tumorlike granulomas in the skin may ulcerate, and there may be multiple bone lesions. The course is progressive and often fatal.

B. Laboratory Findings: Leukopenia is common and anemia marked in progressive disease. The erythrocyte sedimentation rate is commonly elevated during activity. Intracellular budding of yeast cells may be seen in biopsies of bone marrow, lymph nodes, or skin and (rarely) in sputum. The fungus can be cultured from such specimens. During primary infection, results of the histoplasmin skin test become positive and remain so for many years. Skin test results may be negative in disseminated disease. Repeated application of the histoplasmin skin test in nonreactors stimulates antibody development. Antibodies to histoplasmin can be demonstrated by immunodiffusion or complement fixation. A rising titer is associated with progressive disease.

C. X-Ray Findings: Chest x-rays may show scattered patches of consolidation. After healing of primary lesions, calcification may be visible on x-rays of lung.

Treatment

Most mild primary infections heal spontaneously. In widespread histoplasmosis, treatment with amphotericin B (as for coccidioidomycosis; see above) has sometimes arrested the progress. Surgical excision or drainage can be a valuable adjunct to treatment.

NORTH AMERICAN BLASTOMYCOSIS

The soil fungus *Blastomyces dermatitidis* causes a pulmonary/cutaneous syndrome and a disseminated disease, principally in North and Central America. The disease is rare in children. The cutaneous lesion is a papule that soon ulcerates and may be surrounded by very small abscesses. This is accompanied by pulmonary disease that appears on x-ray as massive densities radiating from mediastinal lymph nodes. The disseminated disease may follow the pulmonary/cutaneous syndrome and presents with cough, fever, spread of the cutaneous lesions, and sometimes central nervous system involvement with brain abscesses and coma.

Treatment with amphotericin B (as for coccidioidomycosis; see above) may be useful. In severe disseminated disease, miconazole, 2–3 g/d intravenously, should be considered. The prognosis is always poor, and the disseminated disease is almost always fatal.

PARACOCCIDIOIDOMYCOSIS
(South American Blastomycosis)

Paracoccidioidomycosis is an infection caused by the soil organism *Paracoccidioides brasiliensis*. It occurs in Central and South America. In children, there are frequently skin and mucous membrane lesions that may disseminate to the lymph nodes, lung, and gut. The organism, seen as a yeast cell with multiple buds, can be cultured from biopsy material or pus.

Treatment with sulfonamides, amphotericin B, or miconazole effectively suppresses lesions, but relapses are common.

CRYPTOCOCCOSIS

Cryptococcus neoformans lives in soil and grows profusely in bird feces. Inhalation of dust results in pulmonary infection, which is usually asymptomatic but sometimes causes an influenzalike illness, with pulmonary consolidation visible on x-ray. The most common clinical presentation is an indolent fungal meningitis in a patient with lymphoma. The spinal fluid shows an increase in pressure, cell count, and protein content and a decrease in glucose content. Budding yeast cells with a large capsule can be seen in India ink preparations of the cerebrospinal fluid, and cryptococcal polysaccharide may be present in high concentration in cerebrospinal fluid. Cryptococcal meningitis is typically characterized by exacerbations and remissions. There may also be bone or skin lesions.

In patients with meningitis, treatment for months with amphotericin B, 0.5–1 mg/kg/d intravenously, or with flucytosine, 100–150 mg/kg/d orally, has induced protracted remissions. The 2 drugs have been used in combination to prevent rapid emergence of resistance to flucytosine. Intrathecal amphotericin B, 0.5–1 mg 3 times weekly, may help to speed the initial response. Miconazole (as for coccidioidomycosis; see above) may also be useful. Surgical removal of local tissue granulomas can be effective. Remissions for many years have occurred, but absolute eradication of the organism is probably rare.

CANDIDIASIS

Candida albicans and other *Candida* species are found in the normal flora of human mucous membranes, especially in the respiratory, gastrointestinal, and female genital tracts. In these locations, *Candida* may proliferate and produce local lesions. Moist, warm, eroded skin in intertriginous areas, the diaper area, or nails is subject to chronic surface infection. Mucous membranes of the mouth (thrush) and vagina (vaginitis) are made more susceptible to overgrowth of *Candida* by use of antimicrobial agents that suppress normal flora or by use of corticosteroids. Rarely, *Candida* invades tissues or the bloodstream, as in hyperalimentation, immunodeficiency, leukemia, or parenteral drug abuse, and may then cause progressive systemic lesions, pneumonia, endocarditis, and involvement of other organs.

Treatment consists of keeping local lesions dry and applying topical nystatin, tolnaftate, candicidin, miconazole, or other antifungals. Combined treatment with flucytosine and amphotericin B (as for cryptococcosis; see above) may control some tissue invasion. Miconazole, 2–3 g/d intravenously, has been reported to be effective. Patients with endocarditis require the resection of the infected valve under drug "cover" and the use of a prosthesis.

The prognosis is good for patients with local lesions but poor for those with systemic dissemination.

SPOROTRICHOSIS

Sporothrix schenckii is a fungus that lives on plant matter. Human infection occurs when infected plants are traumatically introduced into the skin. Series of subcutaneous nodes form along the lymph channels, but there is little systemic illness. Results of cultures from biopsy specimens or drainage of lesions will establish the diagnosis.

The lesions often regress spontaneously or after treatment with oral potassium iodide solution.

ACTINOMYCOSIS

Actinomyces israelii is not a fungus but a branching, anaerobic, filamentous bacterium that is found in the normal flora of human tonsils and oropharynx. After local trauma, organisms may invade tissues to form cervicofacial abscesses and draining sinuses. If organisms are aspirated, lesions may develop in the lung; after gut operations, abdominal lesions may occur. The lesions tend to be hard and painless, draining pus through the sinuses. Fever and anemia are the systemic manifestations of infection. The diagnosis rests on microscopic observation of a mass of filaments ("sulfur granules") in pus or growth of the organism in anaerobic culture.

Administration of penicillin, 10–20 million units daily for 2–4 weeks, tends to be curative, but surgical drainage, excision, or revisions may also be required.

28 | Allergic Diseases*

GENERAL CONSIDERATIONS

Predisposing Factors

The development of allergic symptoms depends upon hereditary factors; the nature of the allergen; the degree, duration, and nature of exposure; and a number of poorly understood nonhereditary factors. All persons are potentially allergic, but the susceptibility to certain types of allergic disorders, such as hay fever and asthma (atopic disorders), varies widely. The allergic reaction involving IgE and IgG4 antibodies is only one of several possible mechanisms that may result in an adverse response. Many nonallergic reactions may be confused with true IgE-mediated disorders.

Atopic disorders involve the following: (1) recognized specific symptom complexes (eg, asthma, pollinosis, perennial allergic rhinitis, atopic eczema); (2) a clear hereditary predisposition; (3) frequent association with increased IgE antibody response to environmental antigens; and (4) abnormal physiologic response of target cells to methacholine, histamine, and prostaglandins.

Active sensitization can be effected by inhalation, ingestion, absorption through mucous membranes, or parenteral injections of foreign substances. Characteristically, the antibody response is delayed. Transient hypersensitivity may be acquired through blood transfusions. Increased permeability of the intestinal wall after severe gastrointestinal tract disturbances may permit the ready entrance of protein into the bloodstream and thereby facilitate the development of sensitivity. Psychologic factors may influence the clinical expression of atopy.

Methods to detect IgE and to define its role in allergic reactions have prompted additional investigations of clinical syndromes that mimic classic allergy but involve nonallergic mechanisms (eg, aspirin intolerance). The symptoms of aspirin intolerance (hives, nasal congestion, asthma, and shock) are indistinguishable from those seen in patients with penicillin or horse serum sensitivity. Nevertheless, reactions to penicillin and horse serum are clearly immunologic in origin, while

*Revised with the assistance of John C. Selner, MD.

the reaction to aspirin is nonimmunologic and probably mediated by phospholipid-related pathways. The effects of naturally occurring toxins in food have not been subjected to intensive clinical investigation. Pharmacologic properties of common foods may have important implications for successful treatment of complex "allergic" problems. Chemicals of low molecular weight, such as toluene diisocyanate (TDI) and trimelletic anhydride (TMA) have been reported to induce asthma, rhinitis, and influenzalike symptoms in patients exposed at very low levels. The response to TMA is clearly antibody-related. The presence of TDI-specific antibody was detected in 15% of cases studied, but the inducing mechanism may be pharmacologic (direct effect of the chemical is on β-adrenergic receptors). Sulfur dioxide in levels found in drinks, foods, and aerosolized bronchodilators induces asthma in about 7% of all asthmatic patients; this may be due to a vagal effect or possibly an enzyme deficiency (sulfate oxidase).

Clinical Findings

A. Atopic Disorders: Most allergic children have a family history of allergic disorders. (However, there is also a relatively high incidence [10–35%] of a family history among nonallergic individuals.) In allergic children, the child's allergens need not be the same as those of other allergic members of the family, nor are the allergic manifestations always the same. In addition, different allergic symptoms and signs may appear at different ages. For example, a patient may have eczema as an infant, hay fever as a child, and asthma as an adult. New sensitivities may appear, while previous sensitivities may remain or be lost. Nonallergic factors (irritants, infections, psychologic conditions) characteristically play significant roles in exacerbating symptoms.

B. "Tension-Fatigue" Syndrome: It has been suggested that sensitivity to certain foods, especially milk and chocolate, may cause a "tension-fatigue" syndrome, with chronic fatigue, leg aches and pains, recurrent headache, abdominal discomfort, and, occasionally, low-grade fever. Variations from normal behavior patterns (attention deficit disorders; see Chapter 10) have been noted in a small group of children with this syndrome, and an IgE-mediated mechanism of action has been postulated. It remains to be determined if allergic or pharmacologic mechanisms are involved in behavior and cognitive disorders ascribed to foods and food additives.

Laboratory Findings

Eosinophilia of peripheral blood, nasal mucous membrane secretions, and bronchial mucus may be present in patients with allergic respiratory symptoms. The role eosinophils play in allergic disease is not fully understood. However, the presence of increased numbers of eosinophils in IgE-mediated reactions is recognized. Elevated serum IgE levels in infants during the first year of life may be an indication of an allergic disorder. Severe atopic dermatitis complicated by infection is often associated with elevated IgE levels and abnormal neutrophil chemotaxis (hyperimmunoglobulinemia E).

Diagnostic Tests

A. Scratch or Intradermal Skin Test: Significant positive skin test results for inhalant antigens correlate well with a predisposition to symptoms on exposure to these antigens. Positive skin test reactions to food correlate with gastrointestinal complaints associated with exposure to specific foods, but a significant correlation between respiratory symptoms and positive reactions to food has not been clearly established. Reactions must be interpreted in the light of clinical findings. As a general rule, an intense reaction (especially on scratch testing) is more likely to reflect clinical sensitivity than is a minimal reaction. However, the intensity of a given reaction is not an absolute indicator of the severity of symptoms elicited by the allergen. A positive reaction to a particular antigen does not necessarily indicate a clinical problem.

B. Radioallergosorbent Test (RAST): The RAST test can be used to detect specific IgE antibody in vitro. The test is not as sensitive as a standard allergy skin test, is expensive, and has technical limitations.

C. "Provocative Test": Allergic patients usually react positively to skin and mucous membrane tests with appropriate allergens. "Provocative tests" (nasal, conjunctival, or bronchial challenge; ingestion of possible food allergens) are helpful but may be dangerous; they should only be performed under close supervision. ***Caution:*** Even though skin reactions to specific antigens may be fairly mild, direct mucous membrane challenge tests may provoke marked reactions.

D. Use of Elemental Diets: Elemental diets (eg, Vivonex, which contains corn residuals) may be used for therapy (see below) or diagnosis. Some investigators have found dietary manipulation helpful in identifying foods involved in allergy syndromes. These strategies are taxing, patient compliance is often uncertain, and results are often difficult to interpret. Nutritional requirements must not be overlooked, and selective reintroduction of suspect foods must be monitored.

General Principles of Prophylaxis & Treatment

Removal of the offending allergens is potentially the most effective method of managing patients with any allergic syndrome. Allergic disorders are rarely "cured" but may be kept under control so as not to produce symptoms. Some hypersensitive persons may be forced to avoid allergens completely, but most allergic patients can tolerate slight or moderate contact with allergens. Relief of symptoms can be expected to be proportionate to the extent of allergen removal and depends on the sensitivity to the allergen.

A. Diet: If members of the family are known to be allergic, breast feeding is especially advisable in offspring. The infant should not be given cow's milk in the period before breast feeding is established. What the mother eats may result in symptoms for the breast-feeding infant. In potentially allergic children, the avoidance in early infancy of milk and milk products, eggs, soy, and wheat-containing foods appears to result in a lower incidence of asthma and allergic rhinitis. The early introduction (before 6–9 months) of other foods known to be of high allergic potential, such as fish, chocolate, nuts, eggs, and oranges, should be avoided. New foods should be added to the diet individually and not in mixtures. When dietary manipulation is deemed necessary, care must be taken to ensure that the diet is nutritionally adequate.

B. Immunizations: Patients with atopic disorders should receive routine childhood immunizations (see Chapter 7). Only patients with demonstrated severe anaphylactic reactions to eggs should be considered for special handling; these patients should not be immunized with egg-grown vaccines. Smallpox vaccination is contraindicated in children with eczema (as in all children).

C. Environmental Control*: The preparation of a dust- and irritant-free room is usually of benefit to the allergic child. Some of the following guidelines refer specifically to the patient's bedroom, but the principles are applicable to the rest of the house as well.

1. Remove the following from the patient's bedroom: rugs (especially if underlying pads contain horse or cattle hair), fabric wall or window coverings, cleaning equipment, overstuffed furniture, and unnecessary furniture and clothes (especially furs). Only the patient's clothes in daily use should be left in the room.
2. Clean the bedroom once a week in the patient's absence.
3. Use a wood or metal bed without cloth or fabric covering. Clean the mattress and box springs and enclose each with dustproof, nonporous encasing. Wash the blankets, bedspreads, and sheets often.
4. Use wood or metal chairs without fabric covers, and dust them frequently.
5. Use plain light curtains of nonallergenic, washable material.
6. Do not allow pets with hair or feathers in the room or house, even if the patient shows no evidence of existing sensitivity.
7. Allow the child to play only with washable toys (not fuzzy) and toys stuffed with synthetic materials.
8. Keep the doors closed to prevent excessive passage of dust into the rooms.
9. Close off forced-air furnace inlets or cover them with several thicknesses of cheesecloth. Room filters specifically designed to avoid

*The house dust mite, a major allergen in house dust, is found in homes at altitudes of less than 1700 feet with average relative humidity greater than 50%.

ozone, used in conjunction with a recirculating air conditioner, may be of considerable value.

10. Sleep with the windows shut during the pollen season if pollen sensitivity is observed.

11. Avoid the use of products that contain irritant chemicals (eg, cosmetics, cleansers, pesticides, fertilizers, herbicides, air fresheners), since these may contribute to respiratory symptoms in allergic and nonallergic patients.

12. Avoid the use of gas stoves and kerosene lamps or stoves. These may emit nitrous oxide and sulfur dioxide, which have been shown to contribute to respiratory symptoms.

D. Hyposensitization (Immunotherapy): Hyposensitization (immunotherapy), aimed at reducing the allergic child's sensitivity to offending allergens, is frequently of value. Allergen is injected subcutaneously at frequent intervals and in increasing amounts until a maintenance dose is reached. A safe initial dose of allergen usually equals the smallest amount that will produce a positive intradermal skin test result. Each subsequent dose is increased by 50% (unless the previous dose produced a severe reaction), up to the highest tolerated dose (maintenance dose). The interval between doses is 3–7 days while dosage is being increased and 1–4 weeks when the maintenance dose is given. During the pollen season, it may be necessary to reduce the dose in pollen-sensitive patients. In these patients, treatment may be given preseasonally or perennially (preferred), but the maximum dose should be reached before the start of the pollen season. (Neutralization therapy and use of sublingual drops have been advocated by some allergists. To date, in controlled studies, there is no evidence that these methods are more effective than placebo.)

E. Drug Therapy: Use of certain drugs, including antihistamines, methyl xanthines, sympathomimetic amines, and corticosteroids, may be beneficial for treatment of specific allergic conditions (see below).

ECZEMA
(Atopic Dermatitis)

Atopic dermatitis more commonly appears in patients during the second or third month of life and is more common in infants fed with cow's milk than in breast-fed infants. Most cases begin to clear spontaneously by the third to fifth year of life. When infantile eczema does not clear, this can become a problem of major importance for the child in relation to personal and social development.

The cause of most cases of infantile eczema is obscure. Foods, inhalants, contact with various irritants, trauma, infection, and abnormalities of immunity all may play a role. In the older child, environmental factors (eg, inhalants, various irritants, trauma) appear to be more important.

Clinical Findings

In many cases, initial lesions are on the cheeks, forehead, and scalp. Flexor surfaces of arms and legs are frequently involved; later, the entire skin surface, with the exception of the palms and soles, may be covered. The lesions are very pruritic, and the child may be very uncomfortable. In older children, lesions may be limited to flexor surfaces. Early findings include an erythematous, papular, and subsequently exudative eruption of the skin, which becomes crusted. Secondary infection may occur. The skin later becomes dry, thickened, and scaly. Adenopathy may be marked in areas draining the infected lesions. Adenopathy is often not present if secondary infection does not occur, even in the presence of marked eczematoid inflammatory reactions.

Differential Diagnosis

A. Hyperimmunoglobulinemia E: This is a rare abnormality of T and B cell immunity and is associated with extremely high levels of IgE, recurrent infections (particularly those due to *Staphylococcus aureus*), and pneumatoceles. It must be differentiated from forms of atopic eczema in which recurrent superficial infection and very high levels of IgE are sometimes noted. Leukocyte chemotaxis is not a feature of either condition.

B. Wiskott-Aldrich Syndrome: This is a familial, X-linked recessive disease. Findings include an eczematoid rash, thrombocytopenia, bloody diarrhea, recurrent infections (especially ear infections), leukopenia with decreased lymphocytes, decreased IgM level, and deficient cellular immunity. Most patients succumb to overwhelming infection at an early age. Those who survive through infancy are apt to develop malignant neoplasms.

C. Phenylketonuria and X-Linked Agammaglobulinemia: Typical eczematoid lesions may occur in these conditions.

D. Seborrhea: Eczema can be confused with seborrhea. Both conditions often exist simultaneously.

Treatment

A. General Measures:

1. Give attention and affection. These children should be handled, fondled, and played with liberally.

2. Prevent scratching. On occasion, restraint may be necessary both day and night. If so, it may be helpful to cut fingernails short, use elbow splints to prevent scratching, and use antipruritic drugs (eg, diphenhydramine, promethazine, trimeprazine, cyproheptadine, hydroxyzine) and sedatives (eg, chloral hydrate) at bedtime.

3. Cover as much of the skin as possible (including part of the face) with nonallergenic, lightweight cloth.

4. Avoid soap. Use soap substitutes (Lowila Cake, Neutrogena, Cetaphil) or mineral oil baths to cleanse and lubricate the skin. Even these may irritate. Avoid excessive bathing. Daily bathing, followed by application of a thin layer of bland cream, may help to hydrate the skin in dry climates.

5. Avoid exposure to skin irritants (including house dust, feathers, wool, epidermals, flannel, silk, and wash-and-wear formalin-treated clothes).

6. Avoid overdressing and overheating.

7. Carefully scrutinize the dietary history for possible offending allergens. Foods can be implicated as a cause or aggravator of existing eczema. Therefore, a trial removal of suspected foods (milk, eggs, wheat) or an elemental diet may be of value. Be certain that the diet is nutritionally adequate during such trials.

8. Treat secondary infection with antibiotics (see Chapter 6). Systemic corticosteroids should be avoided.

9. Herpes simplex infection is being recognized more frequently as a complication of generalized eczema. Protecting the child from such infections is a practical dilemma at this time.

B. Specific Measures: Local therapy is the mainstay of the treatment of eczema.

1. Aluminum acetate (Burow's) solution soaks, applied for 20 minutes as often as every 2 hours in severe cases, may be helpful for treatment of patients with acute inflamed, moist lesions, particularly with severe itching.

2. Topical corticosteroids, applied frequently, are extremely effective in treating patients with subacute and chronic stages of the disease. Avoid the use of fluorinated corticosteroids on the face.

3. Crude coal tar, 1–5% in hydrophilic ointment, may be useful for treatment of patients with chronic dry, thickened, localized areas or lichenified lesions.

4. Iodochlorhydroxyquin cream is used for local infection.

Prognosis

There is a tendency for the condition to clear spontaneously toward the end of the third year of life, with lesions being limited to the flexor surfaces of the elbows and knees. Reassurance to the effect that the patient "will outgrow it" should be offered circumspectly. When the child does not outgrow the affliction, the clinician may be faced with a problem of major psychosexual and social dimensions. Infants with eczema frequently develop asthma or allergic rhinitis.

URTICARIA

Urticaria (hives) is usually transitory, but it may recur over many weeks and months. It may result from exposure to an allergenic or nonallergenic agent. It is most commonly caused by food allergy (especially shellfish, nuts, berries, chocolate, eggs, and milk) or drug allergy (most commonly penicillin). Aspirin has been shown to precipitate urticaria in a high percentage of chronic and acute cases. Insect stings, contact with plants, infections, injected foreign sera, vaccines, physical agents, and ill-defined psychogenic factors may cause urticaria. Some patients with chronic urticaria have been shown to have histologic and immunologic evidence of vasculitis, with immunoglobulin and complement deposition in vessel walls.

Hereditary angioneurotic edema without pruritus is due to a deficiency of C1 esterase inhibitor. It is a rare form of urticaria.

Clinical Findings

A. Urticaria: Lesions may be macular and erythematous, with little edema, or the wheal reaction may be the dominant feature. Wheals are usually multiple but may coalesce to involve large areas of the body. Pruritus usually is marked and may begin prior to the appearance of the skin lesion.

B. Angioneurotic Edema: A "giant hive" appears and may be generalized or localized to the tongue, pharynx, face, or extremities. The lesion is tense and pale and may or may not itch. In extreme cases, laryngeal edema may cause respiratory obstruction and death. Angioneurotic edema represents swelling of deep subcutaneous tissue caused by the same mechanism as typical urticaria.

Treatment

A. General Measures: See General Principles of Prophylaxis and Treatment, p 684.

B. Specific Measures:

1. Urticaria: Epinephrine gives most rapid relief. If necessary, 3 or 4 doses may be given every 20 minutes. (Do not use epinephrine in peanut oil.) Give antihistamines by mouth or injection, or give ephedrine sulfate orally if needed. Hydroxyzine may be of value in treatment of patients with chronic urticaria. Use of cyproheptadine is frequently beneficial in cases of cold urticaria. The corticosteroids may be of value in severe reactions. Saline cathartic and enema may be used if an ingestant caused the urticarial reaction. Cimetidine (an H_2 receptor antagonist) may be beneficial in controlling some urticarial reactions.

2. Angioneurotic edema: The response to epinephrine is poor. Edema can be controlled with stanozolol, 2–3 mg/d given initially and tapered to 1 mg given every other day over many months.

ALLERGIC RHINITIS

Allergic rhinitis may occur in the first year of life but more commonly appears after 1 or 2 years. It may be seasonal and due to pollens (hay fever), or it may be perennial and due to other inhalant allergens such as house dust and animal hair and danders. (See also General Considerations, p 682.)

Clinical Findings

A. Symptoms: Cardinal symptoms of seasonal rhinitis are itchiness of the eyes, nose, palate, or pharynx; nasal congestion; rhinorrhea; and paroxyms of sneezing (especially in the early morning hours). Symptoms may be mistaken for frequent "colds." Nasal stuffiness may be the most prominent symptom of perennial rhinitis. Attacks are recurrent and may be seasonal or perennial or may occur at a certain time of day. There may be a history of recurrent epistaxis or recurrent otitis media. Frequent headaches and lethargy may be noted.

B. Signs: Nasal mucous membranes may show only slight hyperemia (in mild cases) or may be pale, boggy, and swollen. Nasal discharge is typically clear and watery but may become purulent if secondary infection occurs. Erythema of the conjunctiva may occur. Polyps occasionally are found in older children, particularly those with infection of the paranasal sinuses or aspirin sensitivity. Tonsils may be enlarged but not inflamed.

C. X-Ray Findings: Sinus x-rays may show mucosal thickening and even fluid levels, without overt symptoms of sinus disease.

Treatment

A. General Measures: See General Principles of Prophylaxis and Treatment, p 684. Use of air cleaners may be of value. Hyposensitization should be considered when symptoms are severe and when avoidance of allergens is not feasible or effective.

B. Specific Measures: Use antihistamines, with or without decongestants, as symptoms warrant. Application of vasoconstricting agents to the nasal mucous membranes should only be done on a short-term basis. Use of a topical corticosteroid (eg, beclomethasone) may be effective in patients with severe allergic rhinitis unresponsive to other medication. Topical cromolyn sodium solution for treatment of mucous membrane allergy is now available in the USA. Cromolyn eye solution has been demonstrated to be safe and effective in controlled studies but is not yet approved for general use by the FDA.

ASTHMA

Asthma, a diffuse obstructive disease of the airway, is characterized by a high degree of reversibility. The obstruction results from edema of the mucous membranes of the airway, increased secretion of mucus, and smooth muscle spasm. Because the obstruction in asthma is more prominent on expiration, there is a typical expiratory wheeze and prolonged expiratory phase. Inspiratory wheezing is frequently also present. (Overt wheezing does not always occur.) The obstructive process leads to hyperinflation of the lungs. In children, the "barrel chest" deformity that is a result of chronic hyperinflation may be mistakenly diagnosed as emphysema (rarely seen in children with asthma).

Characteristically, the airway of a child with asthma is hyperreactive to a variety of stimuli, both allergenic and nonallergenic. Asthma may be evoked by inhalants (eg, house dust, pollen, mold, feathers, animal danders, cosmetics, smoke, sulfur dioxide in aerosolized bronchodilators and in air pollution, nitrous oxide from gas stoves); ingestants (particularly eggs, wheat, and milk; some foods and beverages, especially those containing sulfur dioxide; some food additives; aspirin); physical factors (cold air, exercise); emotional factors; infections (particularly viral infection); physiologic disturbances involving cAMP, cGMP, and membrane phospholipid-derived mediators (prostaglandins, leukotrienes); and other factors mentioned under General Considerations, p 682.

Clinical Findings

A. Symptoms: The onset may be insidious, characterized by slight cough, sneezing, and nasal congestion; or it may be acute, with dyspnea, cough, and noisy, wheezing respirations. In a severe attack, the patient is anxious, sits up to improve aeration, perspires, and may be markedly cyanotic.

B. Signs: The chest is distended and hyperinflated; expiration is prolonged. Cough may be prominent. Intercostal, supraclavicular, and sternocleidomastoid contraction may be noted. The percussion note is hyperresonant. On auscultation, there is wheezing, with prolonged, sibilant, musical rales, which may only be evident on forced expiration. Wheezing may be absent in children with profound obstruction or with very severe disease in whom air exchange may be so reduced as to diminish the intensity of wheezing. Atelectasis may result from plugging of a bronchus with thick, tenacious mucus; it may be misinterpreted as "pneumonitis" on x-ray.

C. Pulmonary Function Test Findings: During acute attack (and sometimes even when the child is "asymptomatic"), the vital capacity, FEV_1, and peak flows are decreased; residual volume and functional residual capacity are increased; and Pa_{CO_2} is diminished.

Treatment

A. General Measures: See General Principles of Prophylaxis and Treatment, p 684. The patient with a chronic problem should be educated to live with it in the best possible way. Children with chronic or recurrent asthma should be instructed in breathing exercises to ensure maximal ventilation.

B. Specific Measures:

1. Antibiotics–Control of any infections present is very important.

2. Bronchodilators–Children with severe asthma may require continuous bronchodilator therapy with theophylline, alone or in combination with a β-adrenergic agonist or cromolyn sodium (or both) by inhalation. These drugs appear to be effective in inhibiting exercise-induced bronchospasm.

3. Corticosteroids–Corticosteroid therapy may be necessary in refractory cases. Giving the total 48-hour dose once every 2 days in the early morning (6:00–8:00 AM) may be effective treatment for corticosteroid-dependent asthmatic patients and produces less adrenal suppression than does the same dosage in multiple divided doses. Corticosteroids should be used with great caution in both acute and chronic cases; their long-term use may be associated with an increased incidence of status asthmaticus and many other side effects. Corticosteroids administered as aerosols may also be associated with significant adrenal suppression. Beclomethasone is a reasonable alternative to daily use of corticosteroids or alternate daily therapy that exceeds 10 mg of prednisone daily. Two metered whiffs (100 μg) 4 times a day does not produce significant adrenal suppression. Withdraw from therapy with caution.

C. Treatment of Patients With Acute Attack:

1. Epinephrine–Epinephrine, 0.1–0.2 mL of a 1:1000 (0.004 mL/kg) solution given subcutaneously every 20 minutes as required for up to 3 doses, will provide the most effective relief and should be tried first. It may be effective after an initial refractory period. Rebound after initial improvement is fairly common, particularly in patients who have been taking substantial quantities of β-adrenergic agonist drugs for a long period of time.

2. Aerosolized β-adrenergic agents–Agents such as isoproterenol, albuterol, terbutaline, and isoetharine, given by hand or pressurized nebulizer, are effective in relieving acute symptoms. ***Caution:*** The patient must be warned against excessive use of aerosolized catecholamines, since this can increase bronchial obstruction and has been implicated in some asthmatic deaths.

3. Oral β-adrenergic agents–These agents, given at 8-hour intervals, may be effective in controlling asthma.

4. Aminophylline (theophylline)–Aminophylline is absorbed rapidly regardless of route of administration. A dosage of 5–7 mg/kg every 6 hours generally provides therapeutic blood levels (10–20 μg/

mL). If vomiting occurs, obtain blood theophylline determinations and titrate to optimal therapeutic levels. Peak and trough levels are useful in determining optimal therapeutic doses. Dosage guidelines, based on the patient's age, are as follows: 1–9 years, 24 mg/kg/d; 9–12 years, 20 mg/kg/d; 12–16 years, 18 mg/kg/d; and over 16 years, 13 mg/kg/d. On this dosage schedule, 25% of patients achieve toxic levels; for 25% of patients, the levels are subtherapeutic. Regulate the dosage schedule on the basis of blood levels if possible. Rectal theophylline (liquid, not suppositories) is useful in patients with gastrointestinal upset.

5. Cromolyn sodium–Cromolyn sodium, 20 mg in capsules (given by Spinhaler) or in nebulized solution, can be of prophylactic value in patients with asthma when used 4 times a day or as preexercise treatment.

6. Atropine–Atropine in nebulized solution is being tested and may be helpful in reversing bronchospasm.

D. Treatment of Hospitalized Patients: If the response to the above measures is inadequate, the patient should be hospitalized. Treatment in an intensive care unit with an anesthesiologist in attendance and facilities available for assisted ventilation make a favorable outcome more likely.

1. Ventilation–If possible, place the patient in an allergen-free room with humidity that is tolerated best. Humidified oxygen (40%) is indicated for hypoxemia (always present when there is respiratory distress). Isoproterenol by constant intravenous drip or nasotracheal intubation and mechanical ventilation may rarely be necessary. (**Note:** The use of isoproterenol by constant drip should be reevaluated in light of the quantities of sulfite identified in the solution and its recognized potential for causing tachyphylaxis.) The procedures are hazardous and should be performed with extreme caution. Monitoring of Pa_{O_2}, Pa_{CO_2}, and pH from arterial or arterialized blood is mandatory in patients with severe asthma, since clinical signs of the severity of the illness are frequently misleading.

2. Diet–Avoid cold foods and drinks. The patient should be given nothing by mouth initially, then started on fluids as tolerated. Gastric distention and esophageal reflux may aggravate bronchospasm.

3. Fluids and electrolytes–Adequate hydration and electrolyte regulation are of utmost importance to compensate for decreased intake, the increased work of breathing, and greatly increased insensible water loss through the lungs. Parenteral administration may be necessary. Obtain serum electrolyte determinations at intervals.

4. Aminophylline–Give 4 mg/kg intravenously over a 10- to 15-minute period, repeated every 4–6 hours. A continuous drip with monitoring of the theophylline level may be preferred.

5. β-Adrenergic drugs–Give drugs in physiologic saline by inhalation (generally avoiding intermittent positive pressure breathing), followed by postural drainage every 4–6 hours, if well tolerated. ***Caution:*** Avoid overdosage.

6. Corticosteroids–These should be used intravenously in high doses (eg, hydrocortisone sodium succinate, 4 mg/kg every 4 hours), particularly in patients already receiving corticosteroids, in patients who have used corticosteroid therapy for an extended period within the past 4–6 months, and in patients with very severe asthma. Use corticosteroids for as short a time as possible.

7. Sedation–In general, sedation should not be used. If a sedative is required, diazepam can be used in selected patients. The best sedative for the anxious asthmatic patient is the relief of airway obstruction.

8. Chest x-ray–To rule out complications (eg, atelectasis, pneumonia, pneumothorax, pneumomediastinum), obtain a chest x-ray if symptoms persist or there is a sudden change in condition.

Course & Prognosis

The long-term prognosis for patients with childhood asthma is good. The disease lessens in severity in the majority of patients. In some patients, symptoms clear completely. However, pulmonary physiology (methacholine response) remains abnormal in most patients. Because of difficulty in predicting which childhood cases will improve spontaneously, all children with asthma should have the benefit of an allergy investigation designed to determine the cause of the illness. Asthma uncomplicated by infection rarely leads to emphysema.

Hyposensitization therapy may be of value for children with seasonal and perennial allergic bronchial asthma.

INSECT STING ALLERGY

Hymenoptera (bees, wasps, hornets, yellow jackets, and fire ants) is the order of insects most likely to cause serious allergic reactions.

Clinical Findings

Insect sting allergy may be manifested by urticaria, generalized pruritus, laryngeal edema, dysphagia, wheezing, tightness in the chest, dyspnea, nasal congestion, sneezing, abdominal cramps, nausea and vomiting, urinary incontinence, circulatory collapse, and death or a delayed serum sickness type reaction.

Treatment

Venom sensitivity is very specific, and skin testing for specific venom antigens is required. Desensitization procedures with venom antigen are indicated for all patients with systemic—as opposed to local—reactions to Hymenoptera sting. Bees should be avoided. Susceptible individuals should keep as much skin covered as possible; wear white clothes with a hard finish; avoid dark colors; not use scented items; stay away from flowers, flowering trees, and shrubs; avoid walking barefoot in the grass; and not flail at nearby bees.

Emergency treatment includes epinephrine, an antihistamine by injection, and use of a tourniquet when the sting is on an extremity. Highly sensitive individuals should carry kits containing these items. Corticosteroids may be of value after epinephrine and antihistamines have been tried.

SERUM SICKNESS

Serum sickness originally described a symptom complex that occurred following the therapeutic use of horse serum antitoxins. The term is now used to describe a similar clinical picture that may occur following administration of drugs such as penicillin and certain foreign proteins. Serum sickness does not appear to be more common in atopic than in nonatopic individuals, and virtually 100% of the population can develop serum sickness if a sufficient antigenic dose is given repeatedly over a period of time. The symptoms have been shown to be due to biologically active "toxic" antigen-antibody complexes in the circulation. These complexes, acting in conjunction with complement components and polymorphonuclear leukocytes, are responsible for the pathologic lesions.

Clinical Findings

A period of 6–10 days characteristically elapses between exposure to the offending agent and the onset of symptoms. Symptoms may occur sooner if the patient has been previously sensitized. The offending agent frequently produces wheal and flare reactivity on skin testing. Urticarial skin eruption is the most common symptom. Other types of eruptions (erythematous, morbilliform, or scarlatiniform) may occur but are less common. Angioneurotic edema, itching, generalized lymphadenopathy, splenomegaly, fever, and malaise, as well as pain, swelling, and redness of joints, are not infrequent. Neurologic complications (especially peripheral neuritis) and glomerulonephritis may be present in severe cases. Fatal reactions to foreign serum usually occur only in individuals already sensitive to serum or dander from that particular animal species.

Treatment

Give epinephrine for acute symptoms and ephedrine and antihistamines for milder cases or to control symptoms. Corticosteroids are indicated for severe cases. Cold compresses (5% sodium bicarbonate) may give symptomatic relief.

Course & Prognosis

Serum sickness is self-limited, usually lasting 1–7 days. Evidences of damage to the central nervous system may persist for months.

RADIOGRAPHIC CONTRAST MEDIA

Reaction to radiographic contrast media involves activation of the alternative complement pathway. This activation apparently occurs to a greater or lesser degree in all patients exposed. The reaction can almost always be prevented by pretreatment 24 hours before exposure with diphenhydramine, 50 mg, cimetidine, 300 mg, and prednisone, 25 mg, every 8 hours. Medications are continued for 24 hours following exposure. This regimen has been successfully employed in patients—including those undergoing coronary angiography—who previously developed anaphylactic reactions upon exposure to radiographic contrast media.

Collagen Diseases* | 29

Since the "collagen diseases" are not limited pathologically to alterations of collagen but also involve changes in the connective tissue (ie, in the fibrillar and cellular elements as well as the interstitial ground substance), they are often called connective tissue diseases. However, although many diseases involve the connective tissue, 6 disorders with similar characteristics can accurately be called collagen diseases: rheumatic fever, rheumatoid arthritis, polyarteritis (periarteritis) nodosa, systemic lupus erythematosus, scleroderma, and dermatomyositis. The similarities can be summarized as follows: (1) frequently overlapping clinical features, (2) chronicity with relapses, (3) changes in immunologic state, (4) common pathologic features (fibrinoid degeneration, granulomatous reaction with fibrosis, vasculitis with proliferation of plasma cells), and (5) improvement with use of corticosteroids (often only symptomatic).

RHEUMATIC FEVER

Rheumatic fever is the most common cause of symptomatic acquired heart disease in childhood. Even though its incidence has been decreasing, it is still responsible for a significant percentage of deaths due to heart disease in the pediatric age group. It is clear that group A β-hemolytic streptococci are implicated in the etiology of rheumatic fever, but the pathogenetic mechanism remains obscure. There is evidence that the cell wall proteins of group A β-hemolytic streptococci contain antigens that cross-react with the membranes of cardiac muscle cells and with the muscle layers of small arteries. Gamma globulins from rheumatic fever patients and antibodies to these cell wall proteins have been shown to bind to these same myocardial and arterial components. This relation to a specific bacterial component sets rheumatic fever apart from the other collagen diseases.

A β-hemolytic streptococcal infection invariably precedes by 1–3 weeks the initial attack and subsequent relapses of rheumatic fever, although not all of these infections are clinically manifest. Since rheumatic heart disease represents a hypersensitivity reaction, it is reasonable

*Revised with the assistance of J. Roger Hollister, MD.

to assume that several infections with group A β-hemolytic streptococci are necessary to trigger the first episode of rheumatic fever.

Predisposing Factors

A. Family History: Familial predisposition and heredity play important roles in susceptibility to the disease.

B. Age: Rheumatic fever is most common in children 4–15 years of age but may occur, usually in a much milder form, in adults. The median age at onset has apparently decreased over the past decade; initial diagnoses in children under 3 years of age are no longer rare.

C. Race: All racial groups are susceptible.

D. Economic Status: The disease occurs most commonly among children living in crowded areas (probably increasing the number of intimate exposures to β-hemolytic streptococci), especially among economic groups with poor diets.

E. Climate and Geographic Incidence: Rheumatic fever has an eclectic distribution in terms of geography and climate; it is found in abundance in temperate, subtropical, and tropical zones.

F. Season: Peak incidence in the temperate zones is during the winter months.

G. Previous Attacks: Recurrences of rheumatic fever following reinfection with β-hemolytic streptococci are frequent (30–60%) in children who have had a previous acute episode of rheumatic fever, as compared with the relatively small number of cases (0.5–3%) of rheumatic fever occurring as a complication of all cases of streptococcal pharyngitis.

Clinical Findings

The diagnosis is usually certain if the child has either (a) 2 major manifestations or (b) one major and 2 minor manifestations (modified after Jones):

A. Major Manifestations:

1. Signs of active carditis.
2. Polyarthritis. Inflammation of the large joints (ankles, knees, hips, wrists, elbows, and shoulders) is usually in a migratory fashion involving one or 2 joints at a time. Occasionally, involvement is monarticular.
3. Subcutaneous nodules.
4. Erythema marginatum.
5. Chorea (see Chapter 21).

B. Minor Manifestations:

1. Fever and malaise.
2. Arthralgia.
3. Electrocardiographic changes, particularly prolonged P–R intervals (see Table 13–3). Electrocardiographic examination should be

done early in the course of the disease; serial studies may reveal useful information regarding progress. S–T or T wave changes are noted if pericarditis is present. Arrhythmias are usually minor, but occasionally second- or third-degree heart block occurs.

4. Abnormal blood test results. The sedimentation rate is greatly accelerated. The white blood cell count is raised, showing a variable polymorphonuclear leukocytosis. Levels of C-rcactive protein and gamma globulin are elevated. Streptococcal antibody (antistreptolysin [ASO] or streptozyme) titers are elevated. A mild or moderate degree of anemia (normochromic or normocytic) is found.

5. Presence of β-hemolytic streptococci. Organisms are often present and can be isolated from the upper respiratory tract of the child or family contacts.

Associated manifestations include erythema multiforme; abdominal, back, or precordial pain; malaise; dyspnea on exertion; nontraumatic epistaxis; purpura; pneumonitis with or without acute pleural effusion; and a family history of rheumatic fever.

There is no specific laboratory test for rheumatic fever. Combined use of clinical and laboratory findings may aid in diagnosis and subsequent evaluation of the degree of rheumatic activity. Echocardiography is helpful in diagnosis by showing that the posterior mitral valve leaflet thickens and separates from the anterior leaflet.

Treatment

A. Specific Measures:

1. Corticosteroids–Corticosteroids should be administered for management of acute-onset congestive heart failure associated with carditis. They are useful in controlling the exudative phase of acute severe myocarditis in critically ill patients. However, long-term controlled studies show no benefit from corticosteroid therapy in preventing chronic rheumatic heart disease. Thus, corticosteroids are not recommended for patients with carditis who are not in congestive heart failure, since ultimately their use does not modify the incidence or severity of residual cardiac damage.

Once initiated, corticosteroid therapy should be continued for about 6 weeks (although some recommend a much shorter course); thereafter, it should be reduced rapidly. To prevent the typical "rebound phenomenon" accompanying weaning, salicylates should be given in full dosage during the last 2 weeks of therapy.

Since retention of fluid during corticosteroid therapy may aggravate cardiac failure, restriction of dietary salt is recommended. Excessive potassium losses should be replaced if necessary.

2. Salicylates–The salicylates markedly reduce fever, alleviate joint pain, and reduce joint swelling. The rapid response of rheumatic fever to salicylates is usually quite dramatic and is a useful diagnostic test in differentiation from rheumatoid arthritis, which responds much more slowly. Salicylates should be continued as long as necessary for the relief of symptoms. If the withdrawal of salicylates results in a recurrence, they should immediately be reinstituted.

The average dose of aspirin is 90–120 mg/kg/d every 4–6 hours. The highest dosage is recommended for the first 48 hours. Symptomatic improvement, blood levels, and signs of toxicity are useful criteria for modifying dosage. Early symptoms of toxicity include tinnitus, nausea, vomiting, and hyperpnea. Gastrointestinal hemorrhage is rarely seen in patients receiving long-term salicylate therapy, but a small increase in fecal blood loss may contribute to anemia. Guaiac tests should be performed periodically to detect blood in stools.

3. Penicillin–Penicillin in full dosage should be used in all cases for 10 days, followed by daily prophylaxis to prevent recurrences (see below). Serious and inapparent infections may occur during corticosteroid therapy but are uncommon in rheumatic fever treated as described.

B. General Measures:

1. Rest–Resumption of full activity should be gradual and related to the severity of the attack, particularly if a significant degree of carditis is present. Most children with mild to moderate carditis are fully ambulatory 6 weeks after treatment has started. The child's tolerance for exercise will dictate the speed with which activities should be resumed. Strict, prolonged bed rest until biologic signs of rheumatic activity have disappeared is unwarranted and contraindicated.

2. Diet–Maintain good nutrition, with particular emphasis on adequate intake of vitamin C and protein. Overfeeding a child whose activity is reduced frequently leads to obesity and the development of undesirable behavior problems.

3. Emotional factors–Careful planning of a home program will help to prevent behavior disorders during the long therapy period and is particularly important in patients with chorea. Tutoring the child at home, play therapy, and occupational therapy are all of importance in the total care of children with rheumatic fever. Parents and siblings should maintain a cheerful attitude; quiet recreation (eg, radio, record player, or television) should be provided; and too much attention must not be paid to the heart.

Prophylaxis

The main principle of prophylaxis is the prevention of infection with β-hemolytic streptococci.

A. Specific Measures:

1. Penicillin–The unequivocal treatment of choice is benzathine penicillin G, given intramuscularly every 28 days; 1.2 million units is sufficient for school-age children. Oral penicillin G, 200 thousand units twice daily, is considerably less effective and is a poor second choice.

Therapeutic doses of penicillin are recommended before tooth extraction or other surgery if valvular involvement is present.

2. Erythromycin–Use of erythromycin, 125–250 mg/d orally, is of value in children who cannot tolerate penicillin.

3. Sulfonamides–These may be used as more economic prophylactic agents.

B. General Measures: Avoid persons who have upper respiratory tract infections. If possible, live in a warm climate and under relatively uncrowded conditions.

Course & Prognosis

The course varies markedly from patient to patient. It may be fulminating, leading to death early in the course of the acute rheumatic episode, or it may be entirely asymptomatic, the diagnosis being made in retrospect on the basis of pathologic findings. Most attacks last 2–3 months. With adequate penicillin prophylaxis, recurrences are virtually eliminated.

The prognosis for life largely depends on the intensity of the initial cardiac insult and the prevention of repeated rheumatic recurrences. In general, the incidence of cardiac damage is in inverse proportion to the age at onset of the first episode. In the USA and other developed countries in the temperate zone, an actual overall reduction in the incidence of rheumatic fever has recently been observed, presumably because of the early use of antibiotic therapy in children with β-hemolytic streptococcal infections and because of the gradual improvement in social and economic conditions in many areas.

RHEUMATOID ARTHRITIS

Rheumatoid arthritis in childhood is a slowly progressive, generalized collagen disease of unknown cause. It is likely to be related to a normal response of antibody-forming cells to modified autoantigens. Rheumatoid factor is an antibody directed against gamma globulins altered by as yet unknown mechanisms. Classic rheumatoid factor is an IgM immunoglobulin, but antibodies with similar specificities have been found in all 3 major immunoglobulin classes. Rheumatoid arthritis commonly has its onset between 2 and 5 years in both sexes and around adolescence in girls. Although family clustering of arthritis occurs, no definite genetic pattern exists. Other predisposing or triggering factors are not usually found, except rubella or rubella vaccine.

Rheumatoid arthritis should be distinguished from ankylosing spondylitis. Ankylosing spondylitis is 10 times more frequent in males. It is sometimes familial and affects the spine (particularly the sacroiliac joints). Transient and nondeforming peripheral arthritis, usually confined to a few large joints—especially in the lower extremities—occurs in about half of patients; it may occur before back complaints appear. Acute iritis and aortitis are characteristic extra-articular manifestations. Spondylitis has also been associated with psoriasis, inflammatory bowel disease (eg, ulcerative colitis, regional enteritis), and Reiter's syndrome. Autoantibodies are not present, but 90% of affected individuals will carry the HLA-B27 histocompatibility antigen. Treatment with phenylbutazone and indomethacin may be of value.

Clinical Findings

A. Symptoms: The onset may be acute or insidious, and symptoms vary markedly in severity. Prolonged fever, frequently spiking and accompanied by chills, is present in 15% of patients and is associated with a characteristic evanescent morbilliform rash. There may be joint pains and swelling, especially of hands and feet; single joint involvement also occurs for weeks to months at a time. Other symptoms include weight loss, clamminess of skin, and muscle aches and tremors. Patients frequently exhibit marked passivity and depression, with underlying anxiety or great lability.

B. Signs: Joint involvement usually consists of symmetric involvement of various joints, including fingers and toes, knees, ankles, wrists, hips, and mandibular joints. In the very young patient, involvement is often monarticular (usually the knee) or asymmetric. Cervical spondylitis may be present. Joints are slightly swollen and tender and motion limited; increased warmth is often present. Within 1–3 months after onset of involvement of the fingers, the joints become characteristically spindle-shaped with shiny smooth skin over them. Subcutaneous nodules are occasionally present, especially along the ulna, the spine, or occasionally the occiput. A recurrent, fleeting, salmon-pink, discrete maculopapular, nonurticarial rash is frequently present over the extremities, trunk, and face and may precede other signs. Chronic subacute iridocyclitis develops in 30% of patients with monarticular or pauciarticular disease. Pericarditis, lymphadenopathy, and hepatosplenomegaly may occur in patients with the febrile pattern of disease.

C. Laboratory Findings: Findings include polymorphonuclear leukocytosis and accelerated sedimentation rates. Levels of gamma globulin and α_2-globulin are increased in 25% of cases. Moderate anemia is present. HLA-B27 antigen is frequently present in ankylosing spondylitis but is not common in juvenile rheumatoid arthritis. Antistreptolysin levels are low (under 120 Todd units) except in the presence of incidental streptococcal disease. Synovial fluid may show an inflammatory reaction. Synovial biopsy demonstrates chronic inflammation, although it is not specific for rheumatoid arthritis.

D. X-Ray Findings: Findings in the early phase of disease usually include swelling of periarticular soft structures, synovial effusion, and slight widening of the joint spaces. Accelerated epiphyseal maturation, increase in size of ossification centers, and disproportionate longitudinal bone growth may occur. Later findings include obliteration of the joint space, erosions of bone, and generalized osteoporosis of all bones of the involved area.

E. Other Findings: Electrocardiographic findings are usually normal unless cardiac involvement is present. Echocardiography often shows pericarditis.

Treatment

A. Specific Measures:

1. Nonsteroidal anti-inflammatory drugs (NSAIDs)–Aspirin is the most satisfactory anti-inflammatory agent. It should be given in the same dosage as recommended for rheumatic fever (see p 699). The response of rheumatoid arthritis to salicylates occurs within 3–4 days and is usually not as dramatic as in rheumatic fever. In patients who cannot tolerate aspirin, use of tolmetin (Tolectin), 20–30 mg/kg/d, or other NSAIDs should be tried. Flurbiprofen, 4 mg/kg/d, used in England and shortly to be approved in the USA, will be the first liquid preparation available for treatment of very young children.

2. Gold salts and penicillamine–These are being used with increasing frequency in patients who do not respond to salicylates.

3. Cyclophosphamide–Cyclophosphamide (Cytoxan) is being used successfully in adult rheumatoid arthritis but has no established role in the treatment of juvenile rheumatoid arthritis. Its gonadal toxicity must be borne in mind at all times.

4. Corticosteroids–Since corticosteroids do not alter the natural remission rate, the length of the illness, or the ultimate prognosis, they are seldom indicated. However, there is a place for them (eg, prednisone, 2–3 mg/kg/d) in cases of myocarditis, in iritis, and in any case where the disease appears to be life-threatening. To avoid the side effects of long-term daily corticosteroids, a trial of alternate-day therapy should be attempted, although the success rate is lower than in other diseases. Intra-articular corticosteroids have a place in the management of juvenile rheumatoid arthritis when there is a monarticular involvement or when one or 2 joints appear to retard rehabilitation.

5. Other drugs–Phenylbutazone and indomethacin do not have a place in the treatment of rheumatoid arthritis.

B. General Measures:

1. Physical therapy–The patient should exercise even if fever is present. A hospital program for physiotherapy is insufficient; exercise at home daily or twice daily is mandatory. Assisted exercise with no weight-bearing on the joints of the lower extremities should be followed by active exercise and then resisted exercise. Heat and hydrotherapy should be useful adjuncts to a well-planned exercise program.

2. Orthopedic care–The wearing of splints during the night will ensure proper alignment of joints. Cylinder casts are to be avoided.

3. Ophthalmic care–Periodic slit lamp examination is the only means for early diagnosis of iridocyclitis, which may otherwise continue undiagnosed until vision fails.

4. Rest–As fatigue is a frequent symptom, periods of rest should be alternated with periods of activity. However, bed rest should be discouraged, since it can lead to osteoporosis, renal calculi, muscle atrophy, or joint deformities.

5. Psychologic care–In view of the long duration of this disease, the family should understand the necessity of fulfilling the patient's social, educational, and psychologic needs.

6. Diet–There is no special diet. Ferrous sulfate should be given if hypochromic anemia is present.

Course & Prognosis

Rheumatoid arthritis is a chronic disease with waxing and waning of inflammatory activity. The systemic features (fever, rash, pericarditis, etc) remit more often than the joint manifestations. It has been reported that reactivation of the disease is occasionally associated with group A β-hemolytic streptococcal or viral infection.

With good medical management, one can expect that more than 70% of patients will have complete functional recovery and less than 10% will be severely disabled. Deaths are reported in the pediatric age group, but they are rare.

LYME DISEASE
(Lyme Arthritis)

Lyme disease is a form of arthritis that is often chronic. The first case was reported in Connecticut in 1975, and subsequent cases have been observed in at least 15 other states. Lyme disease is known to be due to a spirochete transmitted by a tick (*Ixodes dammini*).

The onset is commonly characterized by influenzalike symptoms (fever, malaise, headache, stiff neck). A target-shaped skin rash (erythema chronicum migrans) develops and may spread at the site of the tick bite to reach a diameter as large as 8 cm. Lesions persist for 1 day to 3 weeks. About 90% of patients experience pain and arthritis, which mainly affects the large joints and may be present for many years (in some patients, since discovery of the disease in 1975). In 7–10% of patients, meningoencephalitis occurs, at times with facial paralysis and altered states of consciousness lasting from a few days to several weeks. No patient has died.

The eruption is arrested by use of either penicillin or tetracycline, but lesions may recur.

POLYARTERITIS NODOSA

Polyarteritis (periarteritis) nodosa is a rare systemic disease characterized by inflammatory damage to blood vessels, with resulting injury to involved organs. Pathologically, there is segmental inflammation of small- and medium-sized arteries, with fibrinoid changes and (more rarely) necrosis in the vessel wall. Mucocutaneous lymph node syndrome bears many pathologic similarities to polyarteritis nodosa.

Clinical Findings

Clinical manifestations vary, depending on the location of the involved arterioles.

A. Symptoms: Symptoms are generally those of a rapidly progressive, wasting disease: fever, lassitude, weight loss, and generalized pains in the extremities or abdomen (or both).

B. Signs: Skin eruptions of the urticarial, purpuric, or macular type occur. Subcutaneous nodules are frequently present along the course of the blood vessels. Findings may also include moderate hypertension, convulsions, hemiplegia, muscular weakness or paralysis, rhinitis, conjunctivitis, pericarditis, congestive heart failure, ischemic gangrene of an extremity, asthma, and pneumonia.

C. Laboratory Findings: These include anemia, with moderate leukocytosis and eosinophilia; accelerated sedimentation rate; proteinuria; intermittent microscopic hematuria and showers of casts; elevated levels of nonprotein nitrogen; sterile blood cultures; and cardiomegaly on x-ray. Muscle, skin, or testicular biopsy may show vasculitis and aid in diagnosis. Hepatitis B surface antigen (HBsAg) has been identified in sera of about half of these patients, but its role in disease expression remains unknown.

Treatment

Treatment with corticosteroids (eg, cortisone, prednisone) usually produces symptomatic improvement and may prolong life, but the response is unpredictable and quite variable. (For dosages and precautions, see Chapter 22.)

Prognosis

Prognosis is poor for patients with renal, cardiac, or central nervous system involvement, although spontaneous and corticosteroid-induced remissions are seen.

SYSTEMIC LUPUS ERYTHEMATOSUS

Systemic lupus erythematosus is a multisystem progressive disease whose protean symptomatology and relentless course present a diagnostic and therapeutic challenge. Pathologically, extensive fibrinoid degeneration and necrosis are found. The disease is 9 times more common in females than in males. A lupuslike syndrome (including positive findings in LE cell preparations and antinuclear antibody tests) may occur during procainamide or anticonvulsant therapy.

Clinical Findings

A. Symptoms: Symptoms include prolonged, irregular fever, with remissions of variable duration; recurrent joint or muscle pains; rash (not restricted to the classic malar type); and mucosal ulcers. Weakness, fatigue, and weight loss frequently occur.

B. Signs: The signs are protean and may be related to any system. There may be an erythematous rash on the face, characteristically over the bridge of the nose and cheeks (butterfly distribution) and especially on areas exposed to sun. Lesions may also be seen on fingers and palms. Oral and nasal lesions are common. Alopecia is characteristic. Renal involvement is seen in two-thirds of cases and central nervous system signs in one-third. Central nervous system involvement is probably the second most common cause of death in children with systemic lupus erythematosus. There may be recurrent appearances of polyarthritis, varieties of carditis, pleural effusion, and pulmonary infiltration. Although generalized lymphadenopathy is relatively rare, hepatosplenomegaly occurs in one-third to one-half of patients.

C. Laboratory Findings: Antinuclear antibodies are present in 100% of active cases; the antinuclear antibody test has replaced the LE cell preparation as the most sensitive diagnostic test. Other findings include anemia (autoimmune hemolytic), leukopenia, and thrombocytopenia; positive Coombs test results; microscopic hematuria, cylindruria, and proteinuria; a sedimentation rate that is markedly accelerated in the presence of a relatively low C-reactive protein response; elevated levels of blood urea and serum globulin; and a biologically false-positive result in nontreponemal serologic tests for syphilis. Determinations of anti-DNA titers and complement levels are useful in assessing disease activity.

Treatment

This disease is now diagnosed more on the basis of a few sensitive, relatively specific laboratory tests than on the severity of thc symptomatology, and a wider spectrum of severity is found.

No treatment should be given to asymptomatic patients. Aspirin should be given to the rare patient with only mild joint pain. Prednisone, given in doses of at least 60 mg/m^2/d, not only suppresses the acute inflammatory manifestations but, in many cases, also modifies or halts progressive glomerular involvement. Antibiotics should be used at the first sign of an infection. Chloroquine may be of value for skin and joint symptoms.

The idea that lupus is the classic autoimmune disorder has led to trials with immunosuppressive agents. Both azathioprine (Imuran) and cyclophosphamide (Cytoxan) are effective in controlling renal and systemic manifestations of the disease in some children who are resistant to corticosteroids alone.

Intravenous pulse therapy with methylprednisolone sodium succinate (Solu-Medrol) and plasmapheresis should be tried in critically ill patients.

It is now known that some drugs (anticonvulsants, hydralazine, methyldopa, and certain long-acting sulfonamides) can produce a lupus-like picture. Patients should not be given these drugs, and, because of their well-known photosensitivity, they should use sunscreens when exposed to the sun.

Course & Prognosis

Renal complications and central nervous system involvement are the most frequent causes of death. With good medical management, the 5-year survival rate increased from 51% at 5 years in 1954 to 71% at 10 years in 1979, and later data are even more encouraging. If at the time of diagnosis the serum creatinine concentration is greater than 3 mg/dL and there is severe proteinuria and severe anemia, survival considerably below the average can be anticipated.

SCLERODERMA

Scleroderma is a collagen disease chiefly involving the skin and characterized by minimal systemic symptoms. Interstitial and perivascular fibrosis may occur in the viscera. In local benign scleroderma (morphea), there is a linear distribution of lesions that first show erythema and edema and subsequently scarring and shrinking. In the progressive generalized form (sclerodactylia), there is more extensive thickening and induration of the skin, followed by contractures.

Trophic ulcers, calcific deposits, and Raynaud's phenomenon are common. Skin involvement is usually greatest, but any organ may be involved. Disturbances in esophageal motility lead to dysphagia, and small bowel involvement leads to malabsorption.

There is no specific therapy. Physiotherapy given early may minimize contractures. Corticosteroids are of little value. Phenoxybenzamine (Dibenzyline) has been used to relieve peripheral vasospasm. Bethanechol has been used for dysphagia.

The prognosis is excellent for patients with local scleroderma but only fair for those with the severe generalized form, in which death may occur within a year. Some deformity may occur with the former and is the rule with the latter. Renal or cardiac involvement implies a poor prognosis.

DERMATOMYOSITIS

Dermatomyositis is a chronic inflammatory disease of unknown cause, involving primarily the muscles, skin, and subcutaneous tissues. It may be an autoimmune disorder. The pathologic process can and sometimes does involve the gastrointestinal tract and the central nervous system. Theoretically, since dermatomyositis in childhood appears to be a vascular process leading to arteritis and phlebitis, any organ could be involved. Muscles show segmental or focal necrosis, inflammation, fibrinoid changes in capillaries of blood vessels, and finally atrophy.

Clinical Findings

The diagnosis is suggested by the presence of muscle weakness and induration accompanied by dermatitis, but a biopsy of the area most intensely involved may be required to establish the diagnosis conclusively.

A. Symptoms: Symptoms include fever; muscle tenderness and pain; malaise and weight loss; weakness or pseudoparalysis, sometimes involving muscles of respiration and deglutition; Raynaud's phenomenon; and arthralgia.

B. Signs: Dermatitis and erythema frequently occur around the eyes (violaceous hue of upper lids) and over the bridge of the nose, accompanied by edema. Skin lesions eventually occur elsewhere as well and include urticaria. Erythematous nodules—areas of dark pigmentation and telangiectasia—are frequently seen over the extensor surfaces of the joints. There may be proximal muscle weakness. Calcinosis eventually occurs along tendons or ligaments and near the joints. Muscles may be firm and atrophic, with contractures.

C. Laboratory Findings: Anemia, increased sedimentation rate, and increased levels of serum globulin may be present. Findings of elevated muscle enzyme levels, myopathy on electromyogram, and inflammation on muscle biopsy will aid in the diagnosis.

Treatment

Corticosteroid therapy is indicated in all patients with acute or active disease. The nonspecific suppressive effect of corticosteroids on systemic and local inflammatory phenomena is best achieved early in the course of the disease. Treatment should be vigorous and be modulated to produce normal muscle enzymes. The immunosuppressive drugs methotrexate and azathioprine may be of value in life-threatening disease and in children whose disease is not adequately controlled with corticosteroid therapy alone.

Physiotherapy is a very important part of the treatment; the principles outlined in the section on rheumatoid arthritis should be followed.

Course & Prognosis

The prognosis in childhood dermatomyositis is favorable in most cases with early treatment. The majority of patients can be returned to functional normality. Calcinosis, contractures, and atrophy produce long-term residua.

30 | Pediatric Emergencies

Most pediatric medical emergencies other than poisonings are associated with coma (Fig 30–1), convulsions (Fig 30–2), dyspnea (Fig 30–3), and cardiac arrests. Others include disorders due to heat or cold, electric shock, and drowning.

Adequate professional help must be promptly mobilized to manage the emergency efficiently. Usually 3 individuals can best perform the many diagnostic and therapeutic steps required.

Emergency Measures

(1) Clear the airway of debris, vomitus, and foreign bodies. Position the patient's head. Intubate or perform cricothyrotomy or tracheostomy if the airway passage is not adequate.

(2) Give oxygen in high concentrations immediately and continue giving oxygen during history-taking, physical examination, and diagnostic procedures.

(3) Establish active ventilation if the patient is not ventilating or is hypoventilating.

(4) Initiate closed chest massage if there is no pulse or if the blood pressure is inadequate.

(5) Establish an intravenous line for administration of drugs and treatment of shock.

Diagnostic Measures

A. History: An essential case history must be obtained before rational treatment is possible. Among other items, the history should include the following:

1. Time and nature of onset.

a. In cases of trauma, the mechanism of injury and time interval since injury was sustained are crucial factors.

b. In cases of suspected poisoning (see Chapter 31), details of exposure are crucial; if possible, obtain and examine the container of the ingested substance, noting the list of contents and manufacturer's name and address.

2. Previous occurrence and method of treatment, if any.
3. History of preexisting disease or recent illness.
4. History of drug therapy, including insulin, penicillin, etc.

Figure 30–1. Management of coma.

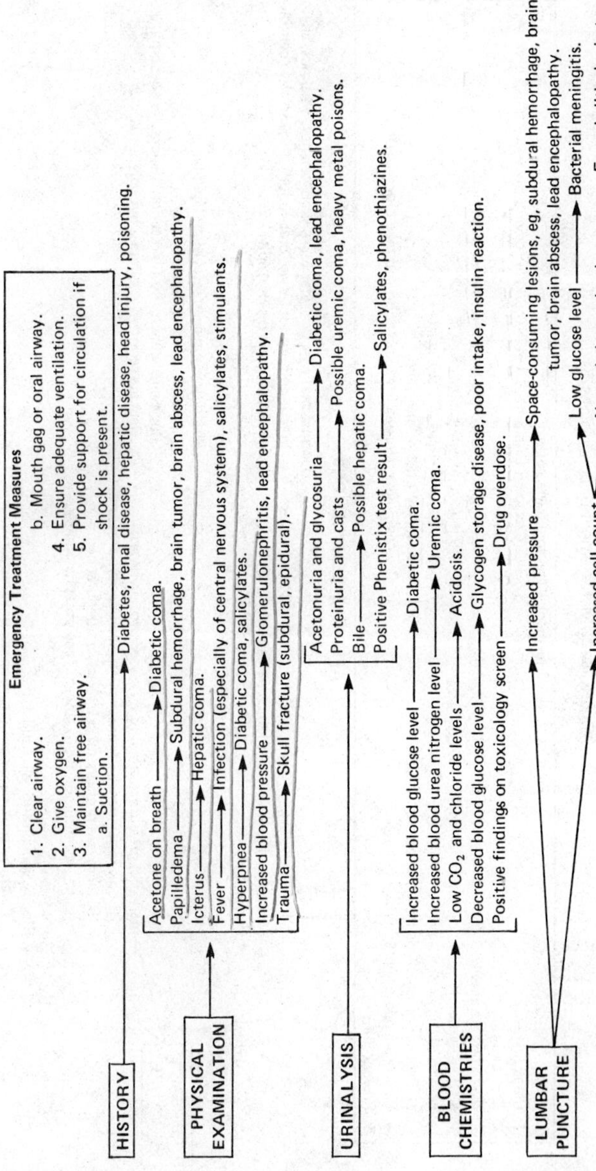

Figure 30–2. Management of convulsions.

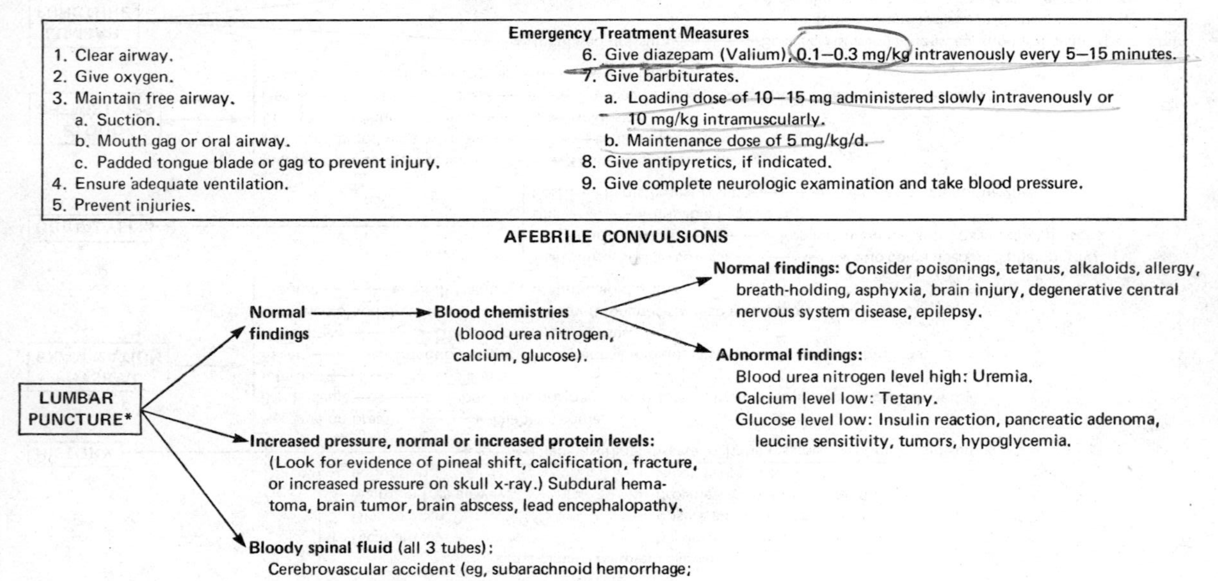

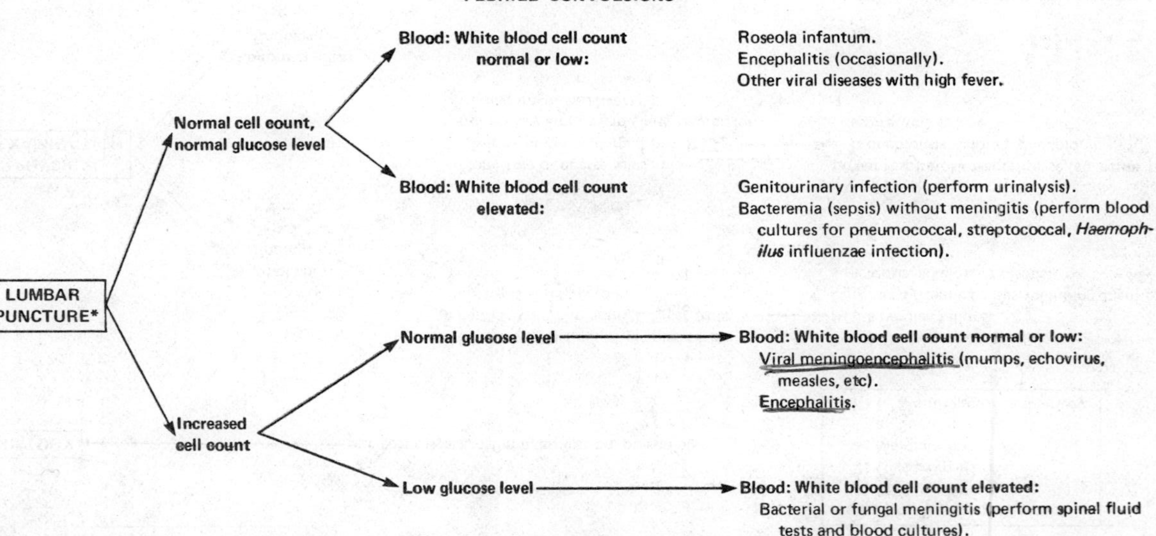

*Caution: Withdraw fluid very slowly or not at all if ophthalmoscopic examination or skull x-ray shows evidence of increased pressure.

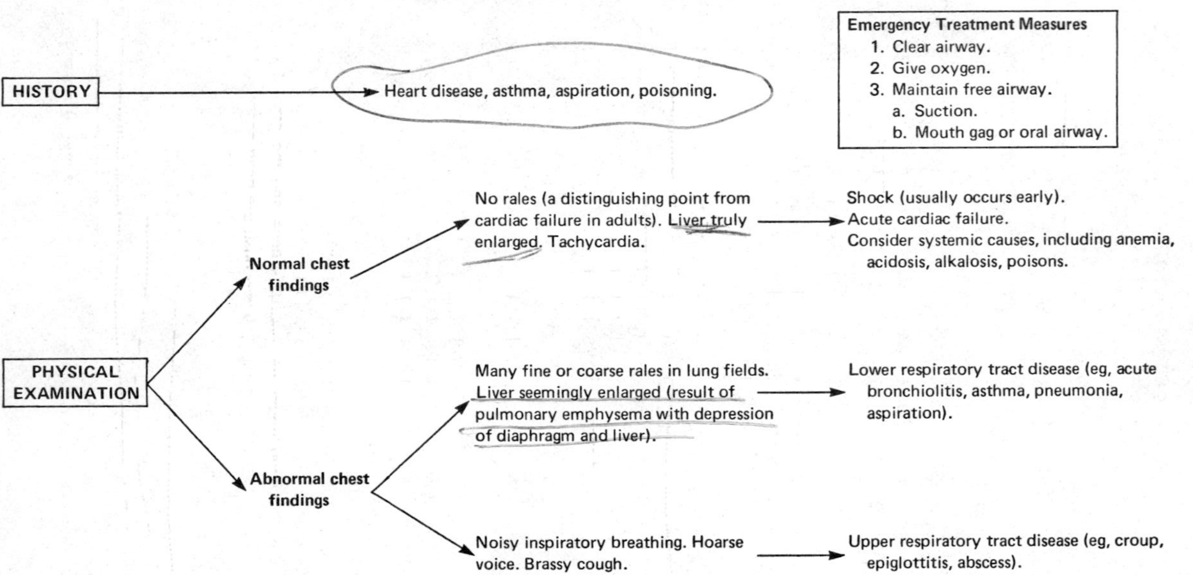

Figure 30–3. Management of dyspnea.

B. Physical Examination:

1. General evaluation of state of consciousness, vital signs (blood pressure, pulse, respiration), hydration status, etc.

2. Careful neurologic examination.

3. Estimation of cardiorespiratory function, including ECG if indicated.

4. Examination of chest for respiratory pattern, retractions, dullness, and rales.

5. Examination of abdomen for size of liver, masses, tenderness, guarding, and rebound tenderness.

6. Examination of skin for evidence of trauma.

7. Complete physical examination after the patient's condition has stabilized.

C. Laboratory Studies:

1. Determination of the hematocrit level. A complete blood count is often of value. A sample of blood for typing and cross-matching should be obtained on admission to the hospital in anticipation of possible future transfusions.

2. Urinalysis for determination of glucose and acetone levels, microscopic examination, and specific gravity. Hematuria due to trauma is associated with many acute medical problems (eg, Henoch-Schönlein purpura). An indwelling catheter may be needed.

3. Blood chemistries, as indicated in Figs 30–1, 30–2, and 30–3.

CARDIAC ARREST*

In children, cardiac arrest is usually secondary to respiratory insufficiency or arrest. Therefore, it is crucial to focus efforts on maintaining the airway and breathing patterns of the patient.

Basic Life Support

(1) Establish patency of the airway. In patients without cervical trauma, this may be achieved by use of the head tilt-neck lift technique. Place one hand under the patient's neck and the other hand on the forehead. Lift the neck gently, and push the head backward by gentle pressure on the forehead.

(2) Evaluate the patient's ventilatory status. If inadequate, begin mouth-to-mouth resuscitation, use a mechanical resuscitator, or deliver oxygen by self-inflating bag (if available).

(3) Rule out infection (including croup and epiglottitis) and foreign bodies as the cause of breathing problems or airway obstruction.

(4) Assess circulation by measuring pulse and, if possible, blood

*Revised with the assistance of Roger M. Barkin, MD.

pressure. If decreased, institute external cardiac compression in conjunction with ventilatory support. In the infant, compression should be done midsternum; in the child, just above the xiphoid process. The rate of compression should be 100/min in the infant and 80/min in the older child. The ratio of compressions to respirations should be 5:1.

Advanced Life Support

Central to the initiation of advanced life support is the coordination of personnel and access to appropriate equipment and drugs. One member of the team must assume leadership.

(1) Give 100% oxygen to all patients.

(2) Perform endotracheal or nasotracheal intubation, if appropriate and safe. The size of the endotracheal tube varies with the patient's age; the following sizes are recommended: under 6 months (newborns), 3 mm; 6 months, 3.5 mm; 18 months, 4 mm; 3 years, 4.5 mm; 5 years, 5 mm; 6 years, 5.5 mm; 8 years, 6 mm; 12 years, 6.5 mm; 17 years, 7 mm; and adults, 8–9 mm.

(3) Establish an intravenous line for administration of drugs.

(4) Correct acidosis. Acidosis has a negative effect on cardiac function and the efficacy of adrenergic drugs. Following cardiac arrest, the reduction of the Pa_{CO_2} may partially reduce acidosis. Correction of the metabolic component requires use of sodium bicarbonate at an initial dose of 1–2 mEq/kg given over 10 minutes, with subsequent infusions reflecting arterial blood gas determinations, if available.

(5) Control bradycardia and hypotension. Sympathomimetic drugs stimulate the β-adrenergic receptors; their effects vary, depending on the relative balance of stimulation achieved. The primary effect of α-adrenergic drugs is vasoconstriction; β_1-adrenergic drugs, tachycardia and increased myocardial contraction; and β_2-adrenergic drugs, vasodilatation and bronchodilatation. The following drugs are commonly utilized:

a. Atropine–This drug has vagolytic action, with increased sinoatrial node discharges and increased atrioventricular node conduction, and is useful in cases of symptomatic severe bradycardia. The dose is 0.01–0.03 mg/kg (maximum, 0.5 mg).

b. Epinephrine–Epinephrine stimulates both α- and β-adrenergic receptors and increases heart rate, force of myocardial contraction, and vascular resistance. It is utilized in cases of ventricular standstill or fine ventricular fibrillation to convert the latter to coarse fibrillation. The dose of epinephrine (1:10,000 solution) is 0.1 mL/kg; it may be repeated every 5–10 minutes.

c. Isoproterenol–This pure β-adrenergic drug increases heart rate and myocardial contraction and produces vasodilatation. The blood pressure is usually maintained by the greater cardiac output. It is particularly useful in cases of bradycardia unresponsive to atropine. Give 1 mg of isoproterenol in 100 mL of 5% dextrose in water (10 μg/mL). Begin with continuous infusion of 0.1 μg/kg/min and increase up to 1.5 μg/kg/min.

d. Dopamine–Dopamine stimulates α- and β-adrenergic receptors as well as specific dopaminergic receptors that maintain renal and mesenteric blood vessel dilatation at low doses (< 10 μg/kg/min). It is particularly helpful in cases of shock and hypotension. Give 200 mg of dopamine in 500 mL of 5% dextrose in water (400 μg/mL). Begin with infusion of 2 μg/kg/min and increase slowly up to 20 μg/kg/min.

(6) Assess myocardial contraction. The use of calcium, which improves myocardial contraction, is particularly important in cases of electromechanical dissociation. Give 10% calcium gluconate solution, 0.1–0.2 mL/kg slowly. The solution should be free of bicarbonate.

(7) Control ventricular arrhythmia, if present (rare in children). Treatment with lidocaine should be initiated when there are more than 5 premature beats per minute and beats are multifocal or come in bursts of 2 or more in rapid succession. An initial dose of 1 mg/kg is infused rapidly; if the patient responds, give continuous infusion of 30 μg/kg/min. If the patient does not respond, give bretylium, 5 mg/kg intravenously. Defibrillation, employing an initial shock of 2 joules (watt-seconds) per kilogram, is indicated in the presence of ventricular fibrillation.

SUDDEN INFANT DEATH SYNDROME (SIDS)*

The incidence of sudden infant death syndrome (SIDS) is approximately 2–3 deaths per 1,000 live births. SIDS accounts for one-third of deaths in infants between 1 week and 1 year of age. The peak incidence is between 1 and 4 months of age. In SIDS, the death is not correlated with a history of illness or disease, and a thorough postmortem examination fails to demonstrate a definitive cause of death. There are probably multiple contributing factors, including respiratory obstruction and central apnea.

When a child is dying of SIDS, it is crucial for the health care provider to help the family members deal with their sense of guilt and grief. Families should be advised of support services in the community that may be useful in adjusting to their loss.

*Revised with the assistance of Roger M. Barkin, MD.

Figure 30–4. Lund and Browder modification of Berkow's scale for estimating extent of burns.

Name________________________ Age__________ Ward__________

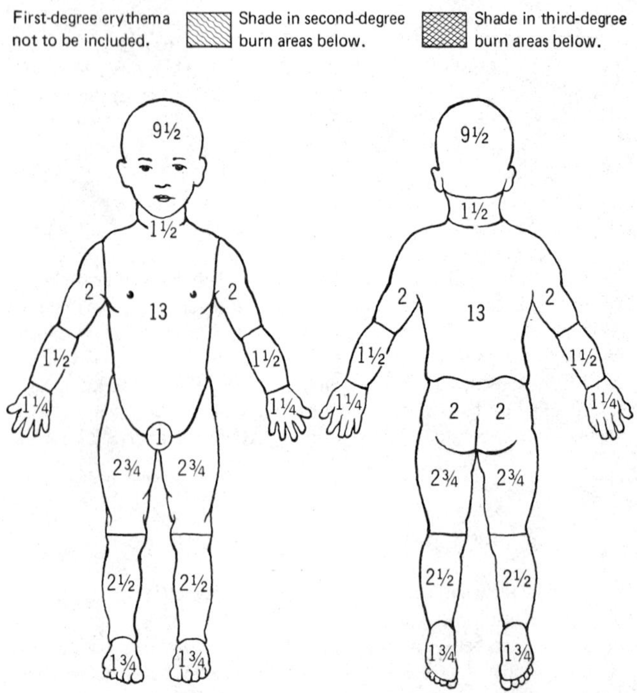

(Above: Infant <1 yr of age)

Area*	Age (yr) 0	1	5	10	15	Adult
Head area	19%	17%	13%	11%	9%	7%
Trunk area	26%	26%	26%	26%	26%	26%
Arm area	7%	7%	7%	7%	7%	7%
Thigh area	5½%	6½%	8½%	8½%	9½%	9½%
Leg area	5%	5%	5%	6%	6%	7%

Total third-degree burns________%

Total second-degree burns________% TOTAL BURNS________%

*The neck, hands, buttocks, genitalia, and feet are not included in this chart.

DISORDERS DUE TO HEAT

BURNS

Burns are tissue injuries due to heat and may be graded as follows:

A. Classification by Depth: In first-degree burns, there is erythema without blistering; in second-degree burns, erythema with blistering; and in third-degree burns, destruction of deeper tissues.

B. Classification by Extent: Minor burns involve less than 10% of the body surface (see Fig 30–4) and are usually first-degree burns. Extensive, major burns involve over 15% of the body surface with second-degree burns or over 10% of the body surface with third-degree burns. A smaller burn with significant involvement of the hands, face, feet, or genitalia qualifies as a major burn because of the difficulty in caring for such injuries.

MINOR (FIRST-DEGREE) BURNS

Local application of ice for 30–60 minutes markedly decreases the development of the burn and may produce relief of pain. Blebs should be protected or, if open, debrided under sterile conditions. Debrided blebs may either be left open or treated with silver sulfadiazine.

EXTENSIVE (SECOND- & THIRD-DEGREE) BURNS

When tissues are burned, plasma is lost into the burned area and from the surface of the burn. This leads to hypoproteinemia, which remains as long as a granulating surface is present. In turn, the granulating surface heals poorly as long as there is hypoproteinemia. The loss of plasma results in a reduced blood volume, hemoconcentration, low cardiac output, decreased blood flow, oliguria, elevated nonprotein nitrogen level, and leukocytosis. Although anemia due to hemolysis may occur in the first 2–4 days, it more commonly becomes apparent about the fifth day. Secondary infection frequently occurs and must be treated promptly. Death may result in an adult when 30% or more of the body surface is involved. In an infant, involvement of 10% may be associated with very severe effects.

The course of a severe burn is usually as follows: (1) neurogenic shock (immediate), (2) burn shock (first 48 hours), (3) toxemia (occurring about the third day), (4) sepsis (also about the third day), and (5) healing and restoration of function.

Treatment

A. Emergency Measures:

1. Promptly hospitalize patients with major or extensive burns.

2. Give meperidine (Demerol) intramuscularly if analgesia is indicated. Morphine is contraindicated since it stimulates antidiuretic hormone and favors fluid retention.

3. Administer oxygen by mask or catheter. Active airway management is rarely indicated.

4. Begin treatment for shock if present. Hypotension is usually delayed in onset. If there is no response to treatment, use of vasopressor agents (see under Cardiac Arrest, above) may be helpful.

5. Promptly cool the affected part (eg, by immersion in cool water or application of ice or cool compresses). This appears to be beneficial.

B. General Measures:

1. Determine levels of hemoglobin or hematocrit and electrolytes.

2. Determine the surface area involved, utilizing Fig 30–4.

3. Determine the urine output. Flow should be maintained at a level of at least 1 mL/kg/h and optimally 2–3 mL/kg/h. Use of a catheter is often indicated.

4. Carefully debride and cleanse all second- and third-degree burns prior to application of topical creams or dressings.

5. Use topical creams or dressings as indicated. Individualization of treatment is essential for each patient. Silver sulfadiazine, 1% cream, is applied topically to most second- and third-degree burns; the frequency of secondary infection is reduced. The approach to dressings is determined by the degree of burns, the areas involved, and the expertise of the health care team. Many prefer to leave burns open, allowing them to air dry. This works particularly well for small burns and in those areas that are difficult to cover (eg, face, genitalia). Some health care teams recommend that large burns be covered with topical creams and dressings or with material such as pig skin.

6. Replace fluid losses. Electrolyte solutions should be given rapidly intravenously, using large-bore catheters. Lactated Ringer's injection (see Table 5–9 for composition) should be initiated at a rate of 4 mL/kg body weight per percentage of body surface area burned. Half of the calculated replacement volume should be given during the first 8 hours after the burn and the remainder over the next 16 hours. Maintenance therapy is given in addition to replacement therapy. The adequacy of fluid therapy is monitored by urinary flow.

7. Give a tetanus toxoid booster if the child is immunized, or give tetanus immune globulin if the child is unimmunized. Dosages, based on the patient's age, are as follows: under 5 years, 75 units; 5–10 years, 125 units; and over 10 years, 250 units. In severe burns, 250 units is usually administered.

8. Maintain the nutritional status in patients with burns. Efforts should be made to maintain normal caloric intake.

9. Use antibiotics only if infection is present. The choice of drugs depends on the demonstration of the etiologic agent by cultures of blood and exudate from the burned area.

HEAT EXHAUSTION

Heat exhaustion is caused by sustained exposure to heat and is characterized by volume depletion and collapse of peripheral circulation, accompanied by salt depletion and dehydration.

Clinical Findings

A. Symptoms and Signs: Findings include weakness, dizziness, and stupor; headache; profuse perspiration; cool, pale skin; oliguria; and tachycardia. There are no muscle cramps.

B. Laboratory Findings: Findings include hemoconcentration and salt depletion. In some instances, serum sodium levels are not strikingly low.

Treatment

A. Emergency Measures: Treat shock when present. Give sodium chloride solution, 0.3%, by mouth (approximately ½ teaspoon of table salt per quart of water); or give physiologic saline solution, 200–1000 mL intravenously. Hypertonic saline solution may be indicated in those instances where there has been a large salt loss with water replacement (see p 90 for calculation of sodium deficit).

B. General Measures: Place the child at rest in a cool, shady place. Elevate the feet and massage the legs.

HEAT STROKE
(Sunstroke)

Heat stroke is caused by prolonged exposure to high temperatures and is characterized by failure of the heat-regulating mechanism. A number of factors increase the risk of experiencing heat stroke; these include drug ingestion (phenothiazines), extremes of age (infancy or old age), and excessive exercise or manual labor.

Clinical Findings

A. Symptoms and Signs: Findings include sudden loss of consciousness; hyperpyrexia; hot, flushed, and dry skin; rapid, irregular, and weak pulse; and cessation of sweating (an index of the failure of the heat-regulating mechanism). There may be premonitory headache, dizziness, nausea, and visual disturbances. Rectal temperatures may be as high as 42.2–43.3 °C (108–110 °F).

B. Laboratory Findings: Hydration and the salt content of the body are normal.

Treatment

A. Emergency Measures: Treatment is aimed at reducing high temperature.

1. Place the child in a cool, shady place and remove all of the child's clothing. Cool the child by fanning after sprinkling with water. Immerse in tepid water or sponge thoroughly to reduce body temperature. ***Caution:*** Discontinue all antipyretic measures when 39 °C (102 °F) is reached.

2. Avoid sedation (unless the child is having convulsions, at which time diazepam may be used). Use of sedation further disturbs the heat-regulating mechanism.

3. Monitor fluid and electrolyte levels. Replace losses if indicated.

B. General Measures: Avoid immediate reexposure to heat. Inability to tolerate high temperatures may remain for a long time.

DISORDERS DUE TO COLD

Keeping the child warm and dry will prevent most disorders due to cold. Children in cold climates should be taught to exercise the extremities (including fingers and toes) to maintain circulation and warmth.

FROSTBITE

Frostbite, an injury of the superficial tissues, is caused by freezing. There are 3 grades of severity: In first-degree frostbite, there is freezing without blistering or peeling; in second-degree, freezing with blistering or peeling; and in third-degree, freezing with necrosis of the skin or deeper tissues (or both).

Mild cases of frostbite are characterized by numbness, prickling, and itching. More severe degrees of frostbite may produce paresthesia and stiffness. As the body part thaws, tenderness and burning pain become severe. The skin is white or yellow, and the involved joints are stiff. Hyperemia, edema, blisters, and necrosis may appear. Localized frostbite may prove difficult to diagnose. The most common areas are on the face under hat straps and buckles.

Treatment

A. Emergency Measures: Treatment is best instituted during the stage of reactive hyperemia, as thawing begins. Rewarming should be done only once. If there is any possibility that the injured part may experience refreezing en route to definitive therapy, rewarming should be delayed.

1. Do *not* rub or massage parts or apply ice, snow, or heat.

2. Protect the injured part from trauma and secondary infection and loosen all constricting garments.

3. Remove the patient to a warm environment.

a. In mild cases, warm the exposed part with natural body heat (eg, place the patient's hands in his or her axillae, next to the abdomen, or in the groin).

b. In severe cases, keep the affected parts uncovered at room temperature (23–27 °C [74–80 °F]). Fairly rapid thawing at temperatures slightly above that of body heat may lessen the extent of necrosis.

4. Elevate the affected part.

5. Give sedation if necessary.

B. General Measures: If indicated, give a tetanus toxoid booster (for immunized child) or tetanus immune globulin (for unimmunized child). Antibiotics should only be initiated when specific infection is present. The use of heparin is controversial, and its effects are not well documented in cases of frostbite.

C. Surgical Measures: The need for amputation should be carefully evaluated; necrosis and gangrene may be very superficial, and the tissue may heal well. Sympathetic and paravertebral block are contraindicated.

DROWNING & ELECTRIC SHOCK

DROWNING

Contrary to some published reports, there is no essential difference between near drowning in salt water or fresh water, and the treatment is the same for both. Differences may arise in the amounts of fresh or sea water absorbed from the stomach. The basic problems are hypoxemia, acidemia, and severe laryngospasm associated with retrograde pulmonary edema.

Treatment

A. Emergency Measures:

1. Clear the upper respiratory tract and pull the tongue forward.

2. Begin artificial respiration (resuscitation) immediately. Do not postpone artificial respiration while waiting for the arrival of a mechanical resuscitator. Resuscitation replaces spontaneous respiration and supplies needed oxygen to the tissues until the paralyzed respiratory center can resume its normal function. Various techniques of artificial respiration have found favor. Mouth-to-mouth insufflation is one of the most efficient methods.

3. Continue artificial respiration for many hours, even in the absence of any signs of life. Only absolute signs of death (ie, rigor mortis and persistent hypothermia) justify discontinuing efforts.

B. General Measures:

1. Administer oxygen during manual artificial respiration if possible. It is necessary only to maintain a free flow of oxygen close to the mouth and nose. Administration of CO_2 is contraindicated.

2. Give external cardiac massage; massaging the legs toward the heart may stimulate circulation.

3. Empty stomach contents to minimize aspiration.

4. Aggressively treat metabolic and respiratory acidosis, which may both develop. Closely monitor blood gas determinations.

5. Treat shock associated with the onset of pulmonary edema. Give plasma or whole blood if indicated. (Mannitol, low-molecular-weight dextran, and diuretics are not indicated.)

6. Give morphine as necessary to control agitation but only if ventilation is being controlled. (Stimulants and corticosteroids are not useful.)

7. Give antibiotics if signs of infection appear. Direct culturing is recommended if near drowning occurs in contaminated water.

8. Treat pulmonary edema with positive pressure (continuous positive airway pressure [CPAP] or volume respiration) and diuretics.

ELECTRIC SHOCK & ELECTRIC BURNS

Direct current is much less dangerous than alternating current. Alternating current of high frequency or high voltage is less dangerous than alternating current of low frequency or low voltage. With alternating currents of 25–300 Hz, low voltages tend to produce ventricular fibrillation; high voltages (> 1000 Hz), respiratory failure; and intermediate voltages (220–1000 Hz), both.

Clinical Findings

A. Symptoms: Electric burns are usually small, round or oval, sharply demarcated, painless gray areas without associated inflammatory reaction. Little happens to them for several weeks; sloughing then occurs slowly and in a fairly wide area. Electric shock may produce loss of consciousness, which may be momentary or prolonged. With recovery, there may be muscular pain, fatigue, headache, and nervous irritability (the so-called postshock psychosis).

B. Signs: The physical signs are often misleading in that the small entry and exit wounds may be associated with major muscle injury (similar to a crush injury), electrolyte imbalance, renal failure, and cardiac arrhythmias. Over a period of days, there may be intravascular thrombosis resulting in necrosis of muscle fibers. In cases of ventricular fibrillation, the patient is unconscious; no heart sounds or pulse can be found; and the respirations continue for a few minutes, becoming exaggerated as asphyxia occurs and then ceasing as death intervenes. In cases of respiratory failure, the patient is unconscious; respirations are absent; the pulse can be felt, although there is a marked fall in blood pressure; and the skin is cold and cyanotic.

Treatment

A. Emergency Measures:

1. Interrupt the current.
2. Give artificial respiration (mouth-to-mouth) and administer oxygen if available.
3. Give external cardiac massage.
4. Treat shock promptly.
5. Treat cardiac arrhythmias.
6. Monitor electrolytes (especially potassium) and renal function.

B. General Measures:

1. Treat simple burns, if indicated, by local therapy to affected areas of skin and mucous membrane.
2. Treat severe burns conservatively. Infection is usually not present early. Granulation tissue should be well established before surgery is attempted. Hemorrhage may occur late and may be severe. Debridement may be necessary and should be left to the surgeon.

SURGICAL EMERGENCIES

DOG BITE

Perhaps the greatest service the physician can render to the patient who has been bitten by a dog is to ensure that the patient has not been exposed to rabies. This may be done by ascertaining the local epidemiologic pattern of rabies and (if there is a risk) having the dog impounded by the local health department so that it may be observed for the development of clinical signs of rabies. The dog must never be destroyed, except in self-defense or to prevent its escape. The examination of the dog's brain by a department of health or university medical center may allow a histologic and immunologic diagnosis of rabies to be made or ruled out.

Treatment

A. Emergency Measures: Evaluate and treat the patient as outlined on p 611.

B. General Measures:

1. Cleanse the wound thoroughly with soap and water, using a syringe to force water into the wound.
2. Debride the wound to remove dead tissue and dirt.
3. Give tetanus toxoid booster if the patient has been immunized previously. Give tetanus immune globulin if immunization has not taken place.
4. Give antibiotics if wounds are on the face or hand or if wounds are extensive. Penicillin or a cephalosporin is preferred.
5. Avoid suturing dog bites; the potential for infection is tremendous if sutures are used. If suturing is done for cosmetic reasons, give antibiotics in large doses.

HUMAN BITE

Minimal abrasions of the skin resulting from bites among children require only local care and generally heal promptly. However, penetrating bites cause some of the most severe of all infections because of the wide variety of pathogenic organisms in the human mouth. Prompt and vigorous treatment is necessary to prevent prolonged infections.

Treatment

A. Emergency Measures: Give antibiotics if wounds are on the face or hand if wounds are extensive. Ampicillin, a cephalosporin, or a combination of both may be given.

B. General Measures:

1. Cleanse the wound thoroughly with soap and water, using a syringe to force water into the wound.
2. Debride the wound as indicated.

ACUTE HEAD INJURIES

Head injuries may be classified as open or closed. Both types are often seen in the same patient and may require consideration jointly. Attention should always be given to the possibility of injury elsewhere, particularly to the cervical spine.

OPEN WOUNDS OF THE HEAD

Treatment

The measures described here represent definitive treatment for extensive wounds and may lead directly to a neurosurgical procedure. Measures should be instituted as the child's general condition permits.

A. Emergency Measures:

1. Apply a compression bandage to control bleeding.

2. Shave the scalp widely about the wound.

3. Cleanse the wound with soap and water and irrigate it thoroughly.

4. Infiltrate margins of the wound with procaine or lidocaine.

5. Debride the wound thoroughly.

6. Gently explore the outer table of the skull for fracture. If no fracture is found, close the wound snugly in one or 2 layers with interrupted sutures of nonabsorbable material.

B. General Measures:

1. Give a tetanus toxoid booster if the patient has been immunized previously. Give 500 units of tetanus immune globulin if a history of immunization cannot be obtained.

2. Give broad-spectrum antibiotics in massive doses (see Chapter 6) only if the wound is dirty.

C. Surgical Measures: Treatment of associated extensive brain injury requires prompt neurosurgical consultation as well as special equipment. Leakage of cerebrospinal fluid from the nose or ears poses a special problem of incipient bacterial meningitis. Prompt use of massive antibiotic prophylaxis is justified to prevent this serious complication. The child should be kept in a sitting position. Leakage usually improves spontaneously within 10 days.

CLOSED WOUNDS OF THE HEAD

The chief dangers of closed head injuries are from immediate destruction of brain tissue (contusions, lacerations); mass effect, compression (subdural, epidural), and progressive secondary damage due to anoxia; and cerebral compression due to intracranial hemorrhage or edema.

Anoxia is one of the most frequent causes of death from head injuries. It is induced by (1) respiratory tract obstruction or involvement, which leads to hypoxia or (2) a decrease in the capacity of the contused brain to utilize oxygen.

The single best indicator of progressive intracranial bleeding is a change in the level of consciousness. The appearance of focal signs such as seizures or weakness is an important diagnostic aid.

Treatment

A. Emergency Measures:

1. Maintain an adequate airway to minimize hypoxia due to mechanical respiratory obstruction. Elevate the head (if possible) to maximize venous drainage of the head. Do *not* elevate the head if secretions are a problem. Surgical management of the airway is indicated if there is major facial trauma and endotracheal or nasotracheal intubation is contraindicated.

2. Give oxygen. Hypoxia of the brain may exist in the absence of noticeable peripheral cyanosis. The most satisfactory route for oxygen administration is by nasal catheter, but this may be difficult in a small child.

3. Treat shock if present. Shock does not occur with closed head trauma unless there is major scalp injury and bleeding or unless the sutures are open, in which case extensive intracranial bleeding may occur. If shock is present, look for other injuries.

4. Treat hyperthermia promptly and energetically. Hyperthermia indicates a disturbed temperature-regulating mechanism. It increases the metabolic and oxygen requirements of tissues that already suffer from lack of oxygen, and it may result in peripheral vascular collapse and may further increase brain hypoxia. Remove the child's blankets, and sponge the child with tepid water or use a cooling blanket. If hyperthermia persists, controlled hypothermia should be employed. Aspirin, given rectally in doses of 65 mg per year of age, may be of some value. Salicylate levels should be monitored carefully to keep them below 25 mg/dL. If hydration and urine output are not normal, chronic salicylism is a danger. Chlorpromazine may be a useful adjunct.

B. General Measures:

1. Perform x-rays of the skull in cases of major head trauma and in patients with neurologic deficits, loss of consciousness for more than 5 minutes, accompanying seizures, or a worrisome or inconsistent history.

2. Perform CT scans in all cases of severe injury and in patients with neurologic deficits, especially those with progressive, altered, or deteriorating neurologic status.

3. Correct fluid imbalance by parenteral administration of fluids

that are designed to provide maintenance sodium requirements and to replace losses through vomiting or via lungs, kidneys, or skin. Do not flood the patient with excessive amounts of fluid. Maintenance fluids should be two-thirds to three-fourths of normal levels to assist in decreasing cerebral edema.

4. Institute gastric feeding of a high-protein diet by nasal catheter in cases of prolonged coma. Tracheostomized patients can more readily be maintained in this fashion, because the danger of aspiration of vomitus is decreased. Small gastric tubes are less likely to contribute to the formation of tracheoesophageal fistula in the presence of a tracheostomy. Intravenous hyperalimentation may also be utilized.

5. Avoid the use of sedatives. If sedation is required in a restless, apprehensive patient, the patient's condition should be monitored by CT scan.

6. Avoid the use of morphine and codeine. They may depress respiration and may cause edema of the larynx, and the attendant alteration of pupil size is undesirable for diagnostic reasons.

C. Follow-Up Measures: Clinical response in the first few hours will generally indicate whether urgent surgical intervention is necessary.

1. Take pulse and respiration every 15 minutes, temperature every 30 minutes, and blood pressure every hour.
2. Test the level of consciousness by ability to rouse.
3. Install an indwelling urinary catheter if indicated (usually necessary).
4. Continue oxygen inhalation. A free airway should be maintained and the patient suctioned when necessary.
5. Use restraints if necessary (not usually indicated).
6. Look for signs of worsening of the child's condition. Patients with signs of progressive stupor, convulsions, focal paralysis, and disturbance of vital signs (such as alterations of pulse, respiration, and blood pressure) require neurosurgical intervention as a lifesaving measure.
7. Do not institute hypothermia therapy. This is contraindicated, since the oxygen requirements at 34 °C (93 °F) are much greater than at the isothermic temperature of 37 °C (98.6 °F). True hypothermia of 28–30 °C (82–84 °F) is of questionable value in this situation.
8. Always consider the possibility of an inflicted head injury, including injury resulting from violent shaking of a small child.

31 | Poisons & Toxins*

Poisons of all types are the third most common cause of accidental deaths in the home; 350–500 children die each year from poisoning. Nonfatal poisonings are 100–200 times as frequent as fatal poisonings. Medicines account for about 50% of all cases of poisoning; cleaning and polishing products, 17%; pesticides, 10%; and petroleum products, 10%.

Accidents involving household poisons, especially in children under age 5 years, are attributable to 4 main factors: improper storage, failure to return a poison to its proper place, failure to read the label properly, and failure to recognize the substance as poisonous. It is clearly the responsibility of the parents to create a safe environment for the child.

The child who survives ingestion of poison may be permanently disabled, eg, with stricture of the esophagus after ingestion of lye, permanent liver and kidney damage after ingestion of poisons such as chlorinated hydrocarbons, and bone marrow depression after benzene poisoning.

GENERAL MANAGEMENT OF POISONINGS

Prophylaxis

Instructions in poison prevention and poison-proofing of homes should be given to the parents prior to or during the child's 6-month checkup. As a child grows developmentally, further areas of discussion should be raised with the parents, eg, when the child begins climbing, the danger of storing medicine in the medicine cabinet should be discussed; after the child is walking, storage in other areas of the house should be discussed. Parents should be asked about the poison-proof status of each of the following areas: under the sink (drain cleaners, etc); kitchen pantries (cleaning supplies, etc); bathroom cabinets (medicines, antiseptics, etc); basements and utility rooms (paints, thinners, etc); garages (antifreeze, automotive supplies, etc); and storage sheds (garden sprays, etc).

*Revised with the assistance of Barry H. Rumack, MD.

Following the discussion of these areas, general concepts should be discussed, such as provision of locked storage; safe disposal of old medicines and products; labeling of containers, especially when a substance is not in its original container; impropriety of the child's tasting or eating things without parental consent; and how and when to use syrup of ipecac—always following a call to the doctor or poison control center. The physician should give the parent (or prescribe) a 1-oz bottle of syrup of ipecac.

The peak age of accidental poisoning is age 2 years. If a child ingests a poison, there is a 56% chance of repeat poisoning in the family within 1 year and a 25% chance of repeat poisoning in the same child. If adequate prevention has been discussed, child battering or neglect should be considered when a second ingestion occurs.

Diagnosis

A child does not usually sit down and "eat" a poison. Rather, the child "textures" and "tastes" the poison, using the mouth as a sensitive organ. That is why most children, even with pills in their mouths, have ingested very little and have no symptoms in 95% of cases.

In the absence of a definite history of ingestion or of contact with the poison, the diagnosis of poisoning presents many difficulties. Most symptoms of poisoning are not diagnostic and may occur also in a number of diseases of childhood. Frequent clues to the presence of an unsuspected poisoning are included in the following:

A. History: The child is frequently found near the source of the poison shortly after having eaten it. Containers suspected of containing the poisonous substance should be brought to the hospital or office with the patient, since poisonous ingredients are almost always listed on the labels and specific antidotes are frequently given. If the ingredients are not listed on the label or the label has been obliterated, call the nearest poison control center or call the manufacturer or the manufacturer's local representative. The initial history correlates with the actual agent ingested less than half of the time. It is best to compare the clinical condition of the patient with the probable signs and symptoms of poisoning with a suspected ingestant and determine if they correspond. A computer-updated system such as Poisindex will provide the most up-to-date information.

B. Symptoms and Signs: These include gastrointestinal disturbances (eg, anorexia, abdominal pain, nausea, vomiting, diarrhea) and circulatory or respiratory symptoms (eg, cyanosis, shock, collapse, sudden loss of consciousness, convulsions). Alopecia is present in a few cases of chronic thallium, arsenic, and selenium poisoning. (See Table 31–1.)

C. Laboratory Findings: Evidence may be obtained from the appearance, smell, or chemical analysis of blood, urine, vomitus, gastric

Table 31–1. Symptoms and signs of acute poisoning by various substances.*

Symptoms and Signs	Substance or Other Cause
Albuminuria	Arsenic, mercury, phosphorus.
Alopecia	Thallium, arsenic, selenium, radiation sickness.
Blood changes	
Anemia	Lead, naphthalene, chlorates, favism, solanine and other plant poisons, snake venom.
Cherry-red blood	Cyanide. (The lips in carbon monoxide poisoning are usually dusky and not cherry-red.)
Hematuria or hemoglobinuria	Heavy metals, naphthalene, nitrates, chlorates, favism, solanine and other plant poisons.
Hemorrhage	Warfarin, thallium.
Methemoglobinemia	Nitrates, nitrites, aniline dyes, methylene blue, chlorates, pyridium.
Breath odors	
Bitter almonds odor	Cyanide.
Garlicky odor	Arsenic, phosphorus, organic phosphates, selenium.
Burns of skin and mucous membranes	Lye, hypochlorite, phenol, sodium bisulfate, etc.
Cardiovascular collapse	Arsenic, boric acid, iron, phosphorus, food poisoning, nitrates.
Cyanosis	Barbiturates, opiates, nitrites, aniline dyes, chlorates.
Eye manifestations	
Lacrimation	Organic phosphates, nicotine, mushrooms.
Ptosis	Botulism, thallium.
Pupillary constriction	Opiates, parathion and other organic phosphates, mushrooms and some other plant poisons.
Pupillary dilatation	Atropine, nicotine, antihistamines, phenylephrine, mushrooms, thallium, oleander.
Strabismus	Botulism, thallium.
Visual disturbances	Atropine, parathion and other organic phosphates, botulism.
Fever	Atropine, salicylates, food poisoning, antihistamines, tranquilizers, camphor.
Flushing	Atropine, antihistamines, tranquilizers.
Gastrointestinal tract symptoms	
Abdominal cramps	Corrosive substances, food poisoning, lead, arsenic, black widow spider bite, boric acid, carbon tetrachloride, organic phosphates, phosphorus, nicotine, castor beans, fluorides, thallium.
Diarrhea	Food poisoning, iron, organic phosphates, arsenic, naphthalene, castor beans, mercury, boric acid, thallium, nicotine, nitrates, solanine and other plant poisons, mushrooms.
Dry mouth	Atropine, antihistamines, ephedrine, furosemide.
Hematemesis	Corrosive substances, warfarin, aminophylline, fluorides.
Stomatitis	Corrosive substances, thallium.
Vomiting	Aminophylline, food poisoning, organic phosphates, nicotine, digitalis, arsenic, boric acid, lead, mercury, iron, phosphorus, thallium, DDT, dieldrin, nitrates, castor beans, mushrooms, oleander, naphthalene.

*Adapted from Arena JM: The clinical diagnosis of poisoning. *Pediatr Clin North Am* 1970;17:477.

Table 31–1 (cont'd). Symptoms and signs of acute poisoning by various substances.*

Symptoms and Signs	Substance or Other Cause
Headache	Carbon monoxide, organic phosphates, atropine, lead, dieldrin, carbon tetrachloride.
Heart abnormalities	
Bradycardia	Digitalis, mushrooms, organic phosphates.
Tachycardia	Atropine, tricyclic antidepressants.
Other irregularities of rhythm	Nitrates, oleander.
Jaundice	Phosphorus, chlordane, favism, mushrooms, acetaminophen.
Muscle involvement	
Cramps	Lead, black widow spider bite.
Spasm or dystonia	Phenothiazines.
Nervous system involvement	
Ataxia	Lead, organic phosphates, antihistamines, thallium.
Coma	Barbiturates, carbon monoxide, cyanide, opiates, ethyl alcohol, salicylates, hydrocarbons, parathion and other organic phosphates, lead, mercury, boric acid, antihistamines, digitalis, mushrooms.
Convulsions	Aminophylline, amphetamine and other stimulants, atropine, camphor, boric acid, lead, mercury, parathion and other organic phosphates, nicotine, phenothiazines, antihistamines, arsenic, DDT, dieldrin, kerosene, fluorides, nitrates, barbiturates, digitalis, salicylates, solanine and other plant poisons, thallium.
Delirium	Aminophylline, antihistamines, atropine, salicylates, lead, barbiturates, boric acid.
Depression	Barbiturates, kerosene, tranquilizers, arsenic, lead, boric acid, DDT, naphthalene.
Mental confusion	Alcohol, barbiturates, atropine, nicotine, antihistamines, carbon tetrachloride, mercury, digitalis, mushrooms.
Paresthesias	Lead, thallium, DDT.
Weakness	Organic phosphates, arsenic, lead, nicotine, thallium, nitrates, fluorides, botulism.
Pallor	Lead, naphthalene, chlorates, favism, solanine and other plant poisons, fluorides.
Proteinuria	Arsenic, mercury, phosphorus.
Respiratory tract symptoms	
Aspiration pneumonia	Kerosene.
Cough	Hydrocarbons, mercury vapor.
Respiratory difficulty	Barbiturates, opiates, salicylates, ethyl alcohol, organic phosphates, dieldrin.
Respiratory failure	Cyanide, carbon monoxide, antihistamines, thallium, fluorides.
Respiratory stimulation	Salicylates, amphetamine and other stimulants, atropine, mushrooms.
Salivation and sweating	Parathion and other organic phosphates, muscarine and other mushroom poisoning, nicotine.
Shock	Food poisoning, iron, arsenic, fluorides.
Skin erythema	Boric acid.

*Adapted from Arena JM: The clinical diagnosis of poisoning. *Pediatr Clin North Am* 1970;17:477.

Table 31–2. Emergency treatment for poisoning.

Ingested Poisons
1. Syrup of ipecac in all cases except corrosives, coma, or seizures.
2. Lavage only if semiconscious or in coma, after endotracheal tube is inserted.
3. Activated charcoal.

Inhaled Irritants
1. Oxygen therapy.
2. Mouth-to-mouth resuscitation.
3. Humidity.
4. Observe for pneumonitis and pulmonary edema.

Local Irritants
1. Copious water irrigation.
2. Careful eye examination.
3. No chemical "antidotes."

Available Consultants
1. Poison control centers.
2. State health departments.
3. Medical center consultants.
4. Pharmaceutical houses.
5. US agricultural office.
6. Medical examiner (coroner's office, toxicologist).
7. See references below.

Specific "Antidote" Treatment Available
1. Amphetamines (see p 739).
2. Arsenic (see p 740).
3. Belladonna derivatives (see p 742).
4. Carbon monoxide (see p 742).
5. Cyanide (see p 743).
6. Ferrous sulfate (see p 744).
7. Lead (see p 481).
8. Mercury (see p 748).
9. Narcotics (see p 749).
10. Nitrites and nitrates (see p 750).
11. Phosphates, organic (see p 752).
12. Snake bites (see p 753).
13. Spider bites (see p 755).
14. Tranquilizers (see p 756).
15. Tricyclic antidepressants (see p 756).

References Useful in Clinical Poisonings

Arena JM: *Poisoning: Toxicology–Symptoms–Treatments,* 4th ed. Thomas, 1979.

Dreisbach RH: *Handbook of Poisoning: Prevention, Diagnosis, & Treatment,* 11th ed. Lange, 1983.

Gleason MN, Gosselin RE, Hodge HC: *Clinical Toxicology of Commercial Products (With Supplements),* 4th ed. Williams & Wilkins, 1975.

Goodman AG, Goodman LS, Gilman A (editors): *Goodman and Gilman's The Pharmacological Basis of Therapeutics,* 6th ed. Macmillan, 1980.

The Merck Index of Chemicals and Drugs, 9th ed. Merck & Co, 1977. [Very useful for identification and antidotes.]

The Merck Manual, 13th ed. Merck Sharp & Dohme Research Laboratories, 1977.

Rumack BH (editor): *Poisindex.* Rocky Mountain Poison Center, Denver, CO 80204. [A microfiche information system. Revised quarterly.]

washings obtained by lavage, or fat obtained at biopsy. Characteristic odors of some poisons may be detected on the patient's breath. Ingestion of corrosives is suggested by blood in vomitus and stools. Tests for urinary porphyrins (lead), red cell stippling (lead), cholinesterase (organic phosphates), and salicylate levels are available in the general laboratory. The usc of ferric chloride (Phenistix) may be helpful in urine testing for salicylates and phenothiazines.

D. X-Ray Findings: In cases of chronic lead and bismuth poisoning, x-ray examinations of the bones may be of great help.

EMERGENCY TREATMENT

(See Table 31–2.)

Specific types of poisoning are discussed on the following pages. Emergency care should be supervised by a physician (*not* delegated to office personnel, eg, those taking emergency telephone calls). This is best done in a hospital, where complete facilities and antidotes are available.

The immediate management of acute poisoning in children should include the following:

A. Ingested Poisons: Speed is essential for effective therapy. **Note:** Induced vomiting is much more effective than lavage with a small-bore nasogastric tube. However, a large-bore orogastric tube is more effective for emesis.

1. Emesis (in the home)–Contraindications to emesis include absent gag reflex, coma, convulsions, and ingestion of strong acids or strong bases. Telephone instructions must be given when the poisoning is first reported. Instruct the parent to give the child syrup of ipecac, 15 mL orally, followed by fluids, 10–15 mL/kg orally; ambulate the child; and repeat the procedure in 20 minutes if emesis does not occur. Do *not* administer more than 30 mL of syrup of ipecac. Do *not* use mustard water, salt water, etc; these "emetics" may be dangerous. Whether or not vomiting occurs, take the child to the hospital. If vomiting does occur, recover the regurgitated vomitus in a pan for later analysis and bring it to the hospital, along with the remainder of the uningested poison and the poison's container.

2. Emesis (in the hospital)–Give syrup of ipecac and follow the same procedure outlined above. This produces an average recovery of 30% of the ingested agent.

3. Lavage–Place the patient in a left-sided, head-down position, and lavage with a large-bore (28–36F) orogastric tube. (Use of a small [< 16–18F] nasogastric tube is worthless except for lavage of liquids and dispersed powders and solutions.) Orogastric tubes should be employed with a minimum of 5–10 L of warm saline. With each exchange, 100 mL should be instilled and withdrawn. With the patient in the position described, no residue should be left in the stomach. **Note:** Endotracheal intubation should precede lavage if the patient is comatose or convulsive or has lost the gag reflex.

4. Catharsis–Sodium sulfate or magnesium sulfate, 250 mg/kg, should be administered orally.

5. Activated charcoal–Activated charcoal (*not* universal antidote, which is contraindicated) should be given or instilled at 5–10 times the estimated weight of the ingested material or a minimum of 10–15 g in a water slurry. Cherry syrup may be added just before it is given and will not interfere with adsorptive ability. If syrup of ipecac is also used, wait until emesis has been induced.

B. Surface Poisons: Remove poisons by washing the area with large amounts of water or with soap and water. In cases involving water-insoluble substances such as phenol, alcohol is used after the initial copious washing has mechanically removed some of the substance. ***Caution:*** Do not use chemical antidotes; the heat liberated by the reaction may increase the extent of injury.

C. Inhaled Poisons: Remove the patient from exposure, remove constricting clothing, and give artificial respiration (see p 724) or utilize an Ambu bag or other positive pressure device if necessary.

MANAGEMENT OF SPECIFIC COMMON TYPES OF POISONING IN CHILDREN

ACETAMINOPHEN

In large overdoses, this commonly used analgesic antipyretic may produce hepatotoxicity. Because of differences in metabolism, children under age 12 are unlikely to suffer hepatotoxicity even if blood levels of the drug are in the toxic range. Children over age 12 will develop hepatotoxicity if untreated and if blood levels are in the toxic range. (See nomogram, Fig 31–1.)

Initial symptoms during the first 24 hours are nausea, vomiting, diaphoresis, and a feeling of general malaise. If the patient is not treated, hepatotoxicity is observed in laboratory tests at 36 hours, with peak SGOT, SGPT, and bilirubin levels and peak prothrombin time by 3 days. This hepatotoxic event is transient, and even in children with SGOT levels as high as 20,000 IU/L, discharge from the hospital with no sequelae occurs by the seventh day.

The blood drug level should be determined 4 or more hours after ingestion, when it will have reached its peak. If it is in the toxic range, treatment with the antidote must be initiated.

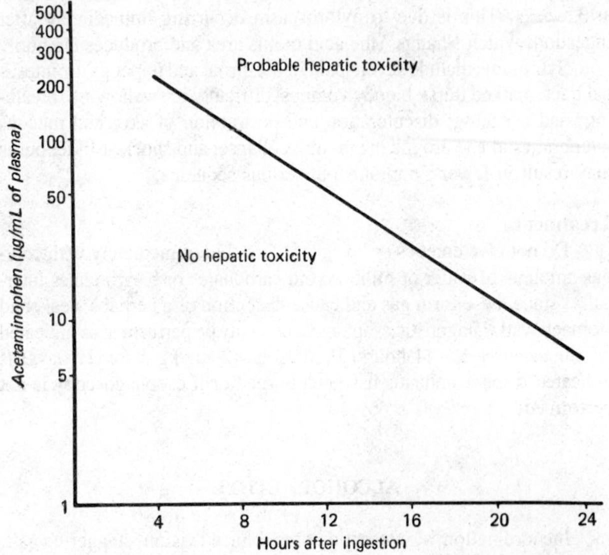

Figure 31–1. Semilogarithmic plot of plasma acetaminophen levels versus time. (Reproduced, with permission, from Rumack BH, Matthew H: Acetaminophen poisoning and toxicity, *Pediatrics* 1975;55:871.)

Treatment

Emesis or lavage should be performed upon arrival at the medical care facility. Activated charcoal should *not* be administered, since it will adsorb the acetylcysteine (Mucomyst, Respaire) antidote. Mucomyst, 140 mg/kg orally, should be administered as a loading dose. It may be diluted in fruit juice or a cola beverage. A drop of peppermint in the final 5% solution will help mask the flavor. Then 70 mg/kg every 4 hours must be administered for 17 additional doses. SGOT, SGPT, and bilirubin levels and prothrombin time should be monitored. Hepatotoxicity should be monitored as for any other transient liver failure.

ACIDS, CORROSIVE

The strong mineral acids exert primarily a local corrosive effect on the skin and mucous membranes. Classically, acids cause oral and gastric (rarely esophageal) burns, the majority of which resolve; however, pyloric constriction with obstruction and vomiting regularly occurs at 3 weeks. This is due to pylorospasm occurring immediately after ingestion, which "hangs" the acid in this area and produces the burn.

Symptoms include severe pain in the throat and upper gastrointestinal tract; marked thirst; bloody vomitus; difficulty in swallowing, breathing, and speaking; discoloration and destruction of skin and mucous membranes in and around the mouth; collapse; and shock. Milder burns may result in fewer symptoms but serious sequelae.

Treatment

Do not give emetics or lavage. Dilute acid immediately with copious amounts of water or milk. Avoid carbonates or bicarbonates internally, since these form gas and cause distention of a perhaps weakened stomach wall. Diagnostic esophagoscopy may be performed as indicated within the first 12–24 hours. Prednisone (2 mg/kg/d for 21 days) is indicated if the esophagus has been burned or if esophagoscopy is not performed.

ALCOHOL, ETHYL

Incoordination, slow reaction time, blurred vision, staggering gait, slurred speech, hypoglycemia, convulsions, and coma are the common results of overdosage. The diagnosis of alcoholic intoxication is commonly overlooked in children.

Treatment

Supportive treatment and aggressive management of any degree of hypoglycemia are usually the only treatment required.

ALCOHOL: FETAL ALCOHOL SYNDROME

Fetal alcohol syndrome is characterized by prenatal and postnatal growth deficiency, developmental delay, microcephaly, ptosis, microphthalmia, and short palpebral fissures. Maxillary hypoplasia, joint anomalies, abnormal palmar creases, cardiac anomalies, hemangiomas, and abnormal external genitalia are frequently found.

Treatment

Supportive care may be required in the newborn nursery. Later management is similar to that recommended for small infants generally.

AMPHETAMINES

Central nervous system stimulation is the most significant result of overdosage. There may be extreme, unmanageable hyperactivity and anxiety as well as flushing, arrhythmias, cardiac pain, hyperpyrexia, hypertension, and eventual circulatory collapse. Abdominal cramps, nausea, and vomiting are frequent.

Treatment

While chlorpromazine has been used in the past, diazepam is safer and more effective. Acid diuresis, while effective, may be dangerous in a child and should be reserved for cases of severe overdose. If there is a question about what has been ingested, do *not* give chlorpromazine, as synergistic hypotension occurs in the presence of congeners such as methylene dioxyamphetamine (MDA), 2,5-dimethoxy-4-methylamphetamine (STP), and dimethyltryptamine (DMT). Hyperpyrexia must not be treated with salicylates.

ANTIHISTAMINES

The effects of poisoning with these agents are variable, but all will show anticholinergic or sympathomimetic effects. Atropinelike toxic effects such as dry mouth, fever, and dilated pupils may predominate. Signs of central nervous system toxicity include ataxia, hallucinations, and convulsions followed by coma and respiratory depression. Especially in older children, depression comparable to that seen with poisoning due to tranquilizers may be prominent.

Prolonged toxic manifestations may be caused by sustained-action tablets.

Treatment

Treatment consists of emesis or lavage, charcoal, and catharsis; the latter are important when prolonged-action tablets have been ingested. Convulsions should be controlled with diazepam (Valium). Stimulants are contraindicated. Avoid salicylates; decrease fever with fluids and sponge baths. Physostigmine, 0.5–2 mg intravenously *slowly,* will reverse coma, hallucinations, arrhythmias, convulsions, and hypertension. Repeat doses should be given to reverse these toxic manifestations only.

ARSENIC

Acute arsenic intoxication is characterized by severe gastrointestinal symptoms and may be accompanied by a metallic taste, hoarseness, dysphagia, renal damage, shock, and fever. Increased capillary permeability, dehydration, protein depletion, garlic odor of breath, and hypotension may be noted. Chronic toxicity is characterized by peripheral neuritis, weight loss, and sometimes involvement of the skin, kidneys, and gastrointestinal tract. Laboratory determination of arsenic levels in vomitus, urine, and tissues is confirmatory.

Treatment

Treatment consists of antishock therapy and specific therapy with penicillamine (Cuprimine), 100 mg/kg/d orally on an empty stomach, to a maximum of 1 g/d for 5 days. Penicillamine is an effective chelating agent when oral medication can be given. Use of dimercaprol (BAL), 2.5 mg/kg intramuscularly immediately and then 2 mg/kg intramuscularly every 4 hours, may be indicated. After 4–8 injections, give BAL twice daily for 5–10 days or until recovery. BAL produces a reaction similar to serum sickness in over 80% of patients.

Arsine gas causes massive hemolysis and must be treated rapidly with exchange transfusion once serum hemoglobin rises or hemolysis is documented.

BARBITURATES

There are 2 categories of barbiturate poisoning: (1) intoxication with short-acting drugs (eg, pentobarbital, secobarbital), which are detoxified in the liver; and (2) intoxication with long-acting drugs (eg, phenobarbital), which are cleared via the kidneys. The general symptoms are similar in both types and consist of drowsiness, ataxia, difficulty in thinking clearly, depression of spinal reflexes, respiratory depression, hypotension, and coma. Coma should be classified by the Reed classification (Table 31–3).

Treatment

Since histories are usually unreliable, treatment decisions based on an estimate of the amount of barbiturate ingested may be risky. Any amount in excess of 10–15 mg/kg may produce more than therapeutic depression. Treatment measures are based on the type of barbiturate ingested (ie, short-acting or long-acting). Following suspected ingestion, close observation should be continued for 4–6 hours.

A. Short-Acting Drugs:

1. Emesis, lavage, charcoal, and cathartics should be administered as under Emergency Treatment (see p 735).

Table 31–3. Clinical classification of coma.*

Symptoms	Class
Asleep; can be aroused and can answer questions.	0
Comatose; does not withdraw from painful stimuli; reflexes intact.	1
Comatose; does not withdraw from painful stimuli; no respiratory or circulatory depression; most reflexes intact.	2
Comatose; no respiratory or circulatory depression; most or all reflexes absent.	3
Comatose; respiratory depression, with cyanosis; circulatory failure or shock (or both); reflexes absent.	4

*After Reed.

2. Analeptic agents (eg, doxapram, nikethamide, caffeine) are contraindicated in all cases.

3. Respiratory assistance should be provided by respirator if necessary. Minute volume of less than 5 mL/kg/min is inadequate.

4. Hypotension is common and should be treated with fluids, plasma, etc. Vasopressors may be utilized if fluids are inadequate.

5. Shock lung with pulmonary edema may occur and may require positive end-expiratory pressure.

6. Forced diuresis is ineffective, since less than 3% is excreted via this route. Fluids should be held to three-fourths of maintenance, since cerebral edema may be a complication, especially following anoxia.

7. Vital signs should be monitored continually until the patient has been free of symptoms for 24 hours and charcoal stools have been passed.

8. Coma lasts approximately 10 hours for each milligram of barbiturate above the therapeutic level of 0.5–2 mg/dL.

B. Long-Acting Drugs:

1–5. As above.

6. Forced alkaline diuresis improves clearance by 3 times. Urine output should be 3–6 mL/kg/h, preferably 6 mL/kg/h. If the urine pH is greater than 7.5, alkalinization may be performed with sodium bicarbonate.

7. Hemodialysis or charcoal perfusion may be useful if the patient is not responsive to the above measures. These procedures are rarely needed, and their use should not be based on blood levels but rather on deteriorating clinical condition.

8. Therapeutic levels of barbiturates are 2–4 mg/dL, but patients with tolerance may have considerably higher levels without toxicity. Correlate levels with clinical status before utilizing them to classify severity of toxicity.

BELLADONNA DERIVATIVES
(Atropine, Scopolamine)

The belladonna alkaloids are parasympathetic depressants with variable central nervous system effects. The patient complains of dryness of mouth, thirst, difficulty in swallowing, and blurring of vision. The physical signs include dilated pupils, flushed skin, tachycardia, fever, delirium, delusions, weakness, and stupor. Symptoms are rapid in onset but may last for long periods, because they delay gastric emptying.

Treatment

Provide emergency emesis as outlined on p 735. Physostigmine, 0.5–2 mg intravenously slowly, dramatically reverses the central and peripheral effects of belladonna alkaloids. Forced diuresis is ineffective with the synthetic alkaloids.

BIRTH CONTROL PILLS

The only toxic effects noted are nausea, vomiting, and vaginal bleeding. These effects are rare. The only treatment is prevention, by keeping all medications out of the reach of children.

BORIC ACID

Toxicity can result from ingestion or absorption of boric acid through inflamed skin. Manifestations include severe gastroenteritis, central nervous system irritation, and fiery red rash (toxic epidermal necrolysis). Shock, convulsions, coma, and death may follow.

Note: There is no justification for keeping boric acid solution or powder where infants and children can be accidentally exposed to it. This drug has no medical value.

Treatment

Gastric lavage or induced emesis (or both) is the immediate therapy. Supportive therapy (for ingestion or absorption) includes maintenance of fluid and electrolyte balance and circulation.

Excretion of ingested or absorbed boric acid can be facilitated with exchange transfusion, hemodialysis, or peritoneal dialysis.

CARBON MONOXIDE

Carbon monoxide combines with hemoglobin to form carboxyhemoglobin, which fails to carry oxygen and results in tissue anoxia. Levels of carboxyhemoglobin can be easily measured, and they correlate well with degree of toxicity. The patient is asymptomatic with levels of 10–20%. Levels of 20–30% cause mild symptoms; 30–40%, moderate symptoms; and 40–50%, severe symptoms. Symptoms are more severe if the patient has exercised or taken alcohol or resides at high altitudes. Symptoms consist of headache, lethargy, depressed sensorium, nausea, vomiting, and occasionally seizures. After prolonged exposure, psychotic behavior may be noted. A bright cherry-red color is typical of blood with high levels of carboxyhemoglobin. Although said to be characteristic of carbon monoxide poisoning, cherry-red lips are rarely seen in living patients. The lips are usually dusky.

Treatment

Therapy consists of exposure to air and administration of oxygen. The half-life of carboxyhemoglobin is 40 minutes in 100% oxygen and 180 minutes in air. Delayed effects are not uncommon and are reflective of anoxia. The levels of SGOT, creatine phosphokinase, and other circulating enzymes will be increased, and variable central nervous system effects will be seen, with residual effects depending upon the degree of anoxia.

CYANIDE

Cyanide specifically inhibits the cytochrome oxidase system, causing cellular anoxia. The onset of symptoms after ingestion or inhalation is rapid. Symptoms include giddiness, hyperpnea, headache, palpitation, and unconsciousness. The breath may smell of bitter almonds. Poisoning may be caused in children by the ingestion of relatively few (5–10) bitter almonds. Death usually occurs in 15 minutes unless treatment is immediate.

Treatment

Initially, inhalation of one ampule of amyl nitrite for 30 seconds of every minute produces 5% methemoglobinemia, which binds cyanide better than hemoglobin. Cyanide antidote packages (Lilly) contain material and directions for therapy; dosage given is for adults, and children should receive proportionately less. Intravenous sodium nitrite (3%) is given first, followed by intravenous sodium thiosulfate (25%). The pediatric dose of sodium nitrite is 10 mg/kg (0.33 mL/kg); it is given at a rate of 2–5 mL/min, which produces approximately 30% methemoglobinemia. The pediatric dose of sodium thiosulfate, 50 mL, then produces a harmless thiocyanate. Oxygen should be administered.

DETERGENTS

Fatalities due to poisoning with anionic and nonionic detergents have not been reported. However, detergents used in the household may contain alkalies. Cationic detergents are common antiseptics (Diaparene, Zephiran, etc), and acute poisoning can cause gastroenteritis, convulsions, burns, and strictures.

Treatment

In cases involving cationic (quaternary ammonium) detergents, dilution with water or, preferably, milk is the primary treatment, followed by esophagoscopy and definitive care if burns are detected.

Anionic and nonionic detergents generally cause emesis but have no toxicity other than gastroenteritis.

FERROUS SULFATE

Accidental ingestion of ferrous sulfate (elemental iron) in amounts as low as 60 mg/kg may cause intoxication. Five phases of intoxication are described: (1) Hemorrhagic gastroenteritis occurs shortly after ingestion (30–120 minutes); shock due to blood loss may be present. (2) A recovery phase occurs and lasts from 2–12 hours after ingestion. (3) Delayed shock may occur 12–24 hours after ingestion and may be due to a vasodepressant action of ferritin or unbound ionic iron. (4) Liver damage occurs at 3–5 days. (5) Delayed gastric obstruction may occur, usually at 3 weeks after ingestion.

The history is the most important diagnostic clue. X-rays of the abdomen may show the radiopaque tablets in the gastrointestinal tract. Laboratory determination of serum iron and total iron-binding capacity allows calculation of free iron, an excess of which is diagnostic.

Treatment

Remove ferrous sulfate by induced vomiting and lavage with a large-bore tube. Sodium bicarbonate as a 5% lavage will precipitate the iron. Phospho-Soda (Fleet) will produce insoluble iron if given orally; 15 mL of a 1:4 dilution should be used, but never use more than one bottle. Supportive measures (blood, plasma, saline, and vasopressors as indicated) are imperative. Exchange transfusion may be useful if the patient does not respond to standard measures. Deferoxamine (Desferal) is useful in cases of severe intoxication. The dose is 15 mg/kg/h as a drip—not a push—during the first 12–24 hours. As long as chelation occurs, the urine shows a reddish "vin rosé" color.

FLEA BITES, FLY BITES; YELLOW JACKET, WASP, BEE, & HORNET STINGS

Insect bites and stings produce a small wheal with a small red dot in the center and cause only itching in most older children and adults. However, in young children and in some hypersensitive children, there may be an allergic response of 2 types: (1) local, with intense swelling and itching and a large wheal; or (2) systemic, in which miliarialike or papular urticaria (small, hard, blanched or pink papules resembling a vesicle but not easily ruptured) may appear over other areas of the skin. A generalized reaction may occur, with fever and intense swelling at the site of the bite or sting, as well as anaphylactic shock with respiratory and circulatory compromise.

Treatment

Treatment is seldom indicated. An excessive local reaction may be treated with anesthetic ointment. For systemic reactions, antihistamines should be given orally or, if necessary, parenterally. Epinephrine, 0.05–0.5 mL subcutaneously, or hydrocortisone intravenously may be lifesaving for anaphylactic reaction to bee sting.

Prophylaxis

Flea or bee antigens may be of value when given to children who are bitten frequently and develop severe reactions. Patients with known severe reactions should carry a kit containing epinephrine when they go on an outing.

FLUORIDES

Fluorides are found in agricultural poisons and insect powders. Clinical reactions produced by fluorides include nausea, vomiting, colicky abdominal pain, diarrhea, cyanosis, excitement, and convulsions. A variable rash may be present, and fever may be significant.

Treatment

Give calcium chloride, calcium gluconate, or milk in large quantities, 10–15 mL/kg orally. Induced vomiting or gastric lavage with a large-bore tube should be employed. Calcium gluconate, 10%, should be injected slowly intravenously as necessary and should be repeated if tetany occurs. Support respiration and treat shock. Give sodium sulfate orally, 15–30 g in 1–2 dL of water, as a cathartic.

GLUE SNIFFING

Toluene was the most common organic solvent used in "glue sniffing," but it has largely been replaced by nontoxic substances. Most frequently, it causes blurred vision, lack of coordination, hallucinations, and renal tubular acidosis.

Treatment

Eliminate exposure to the solvent. Conservative management is indicated. Epinephrine should not be used, since it may have an adverse effect on a sensitized myocardium.

HALLUCINOGENS*

Marihuana has stimulant, depressant, and hallucinogenic properties, but usually the depressant properties predominate. Euphoria, mood swings, and distortion of time and space commonly occur. Performance skills may be affected. Panic states or psychotic reactions are uncommon.

LSD (lysergic acid diethylamide) causes euphoria, mood swings, loss of inhibitions, and depersonalization. Flashbacks (recurrence of initial effects), panic states, and hallucinations occur in some individuals.

DMT (dimethyltryptamine) is a short-acting drug that primarily produces excitation and exhilaration.

STP (2,5-dimethoxy-4-methylamphetamine) is a long-acting hallucinogen that causes euphoria, confusion, and hallucinations.

Mescaline typically produces nausea, vomiting, exhilaration, anxiety, and hallucinations. Mescaline ingestion can sometimes mimic appendicitis.

PCP (phencyclidine) is a veterinary anesthetic that causes a marked paranoid state, hallucinations, and sometimes self-destructive behavior.

Psilocybin causes nausea, vomiting, headaches, and hallucinations.

Histories are often unreliable, and many samples of street drugs supposedly containing one of these agents may contain another. Although most of the commonly abused drugs cannot be readily identified in biologic fluids by standard laboratories, the following can be identified in urine: mescaline, amphetamine, belladonna alkaloids, and tricyclic antidepressants. Others may be identified by laboratories deal-

*Amphetamines, barbiturates, belladonna derivatives, glue sniffing, narcotics, tranquilizers, and tricyclic antidepressants are discussed under individual headings.

ing with forensic cases. Patients ingesting any of these drugs can have hallucinations.

Treatment

Patients ingesting hallucinogens must often be treated without identification of the specific drug used. Most patients are brought to the emergency room because of panic states or uncontrollable hyperactivity. In many cases, the only treatment required is reassurance ("talking the patient down") and placement in a neutral environmental setting. Physical restraints usually do more harm than good. Sometimes diazepam (Valium) is helpful in controlling hyperactivity. Chlorpromazine may cause marked hypotension if STP, MDA, or DMT has been ingested and should not be used unless hard evidence exists that these have *not* been ingested. In planning long-term management of drug abusers, it should be remembered that drug abuse is a symptom, not a disease. Although serious questions have been raised, there is no conclusive evidence that LSD or other hallucinogens cause permanent chromosomal damage or birth defects in humans.

LEAD

(See p 481.)

LYE & BLEACHES

Ingestion of lye and bleaches may result in ulceration and perforation of the gastrointestinal tract and in long-term complications of stricture of the esophagus. Burns in the mouth indicate an absolute need for esophagoscopy, but many cases have been reported in which patients have not sustained oral burns but have developed esophageal burns.

Treatment

Avoid emetics. Dilute with water or, preferably, milk. Then order nothing by mouth and perform esophagoscopy after 12 hours but before 24 hours. Corticosteroids may be helpful and, if used, should be given early and continued for 3 weeks. Antibiotics are not indicated unless an infection is demonstrated. Give supportive therapy with sedation and analgesia as necessary. Intravenous nutrition and fluids may be necessary in early stages. Early tracheostomy may be indicated in cases of severe ingestion. See recommendations under Acids, Corrosive.

MEPROBAMATE
(Equanil, Miltown)

Respiratory depression, coma, cardiac arrhythmia and, occasionally, convulsions associated with hyperexcitability occur. Death results from cardiac or respiratory failure. Severe metabolic acidosis with very rapid onset may occur.

Treatment

Gastric lavage with a large-bore tube should be performed. Recovering patients may relapse and die from delayed absorption of the drug; thus, charcoal and cathartics must be administered (see p 736). Although supportive treatment may be sufficient in mild intoxications, hemodialysis or charcoal perfusion and forced diuresis are indicated in severe cases, especially when they are unresponsive to standard therapy.

MERCURY

Acute symptoms of mercury poisoning include metallic taste, severe gastrointestinal irritation, and shock. Severe acidosis and leukocytosis occur. Delayed symptoms (after 12 hours) include a mercury gum line, lower nephron nephrosis, ulcerative colitis, hepatic damage, and shock. Chronic symptoms are those of gastrointestinal irritability, a blue-black gum line, salivation, stomatitis, nephrosis, and irritability. Acrodynia occurs in children following chronic exposure to small amounts of mercury, including topically applied medication.

Treatment

Treat acute poisoning with dimercaprol (BAL) and penicillamine (Cuprimine) as for arsenic poisoning (see above).

MUSHROOMS

Mushrooms are responsible for rare deaths and somewhat more common nonfatal poisonings. However, a history of mushroom ingestion always arouses concern, which is intensified because some toxins present in mushrooms may not show their effects until many hours after ingestion and because it is often not known exactly what kind of fungus was ingested.

The most common intoxicating American species are delineated. Almost 90% of cases of childhood accidental ingestions involve nontoxic puffballs or nontoxic "little brown mushrooms." The services of a mycologist must be obtained through a botanical garden or poison control center to determine exact identification.

Clinical Findings & Treatment

Clinical findings and treatment vary according to the type of mushroom ingested.

A. Bulb Agarics: These include *Amanita verna* (in the USA) and *Amanita phalloides* (in the USA and Europe). The toxins are cyclopeptides. Vomiting and severe diarrhea occur after a latent period of 6–20 hours, followed by liver and kidney damage. Thioctic acid has been suggested as an antidote, but it is now thought that there is no antidote and that only supportive treatment will help.

B. Fly Agarics: These include *Amanita muscaria* and *Amanita pantherina*. These fungi are variably toxic and may contain muscarine, in which case they will cause parasympathomimetic manifestations. At least as commonly, they contain an atropine isomer, in which case they cause the anticholinergic syndrome (see Belladonna Derivatives, above). Hallucinations may occur with ingestion of either type of mushroom. Atropine sulfate, 50 μg/kg subcutaneously immediately and then as required, should be used *only* if muscarinic signs appear. Discontinue if signs of atropine poisoning appear. If patients have atropinic signs, physostigmine may be used as for antihistamines (see above).

C. False Morels: These are variably toxic, causing hemolysis and gastrointestinal irritation. The toxin can sometimes be removed by cooking or drying. Pyridoxine, 25 mg/kg intravenously, or methylene blue (see Nitrites and Nitrates, below), or both may be used to treat methemoglobinemia.

D. Hallucinogens: Psilocybin, a serotonin congener, is the active principle of the ritual mushroom found in Mexico and has also been implicated in poisoning in a West Coast incident. Hallucinations rarely last more than 3–6 hours. Treatment is usually unnecessary.

NARCOTICS

Intoxication with narcotics (eg, morphine, codeine, and diphenoxylate [in Lomotil]) produces respiratory depression, hypotension, pinpoint pupils, skeletal muscle relaxation, decreased urinary output, and occasionally shock. Additionally, propoxyphene (Darvon) is associated with convulsions in 40–60% of cases of overdosage.

Treatment

Acute overdosage is treated similarly to barbiturate intoxication. Respiratory assistance and maintenance of adequate blood pressure are mandatory. Naloxone (Narcan), 5 μg/kg, is an effective narcotic antagonist that does not cause respiratory depression and has no known toxicity even in overdosage. In refractory cases, naloxone can be given in high doses, eg, 1–4 mg intravenously. Nalorphine should no longer be used because it causes synergistic depression with barbiturates and may cause depression itself if used too frequently. Diazepam (Valium) may be of value to reduce withdrawal symptoms in heroin abusers.

NITRITES & NITRATES

Methemoglobin is produced by the administration of a nitrite compound or a nitrate that is converted to a nitrite in the large bowel. Sodium nitrite, food preservatives, phenacetin, home remedies such as spirits of nitre, and high concentrations of nitrite in water have been reported to cause production of methemoglobin. The onset may be gradual, and symptoms may be deceiving. The color of the child gradually changes to an ashen gray. There are no specific clinical findings other than a weak, lethargic child with some respiratory and cardiac difficulty. Symptoms depend on the amount of available normal hemoglobin to carry oxygen but generally do not occur until approximately 30% of the hemoglobin has been converted to methemoglobin. A drop of patient's blood dried on filter paper will appear brown if levels are 15% or greater.

Treatment

Intravenous methylene blue allows electron transfer to reverse methemoglobinemia. A 1% solution is administered in the amount of 0.1 mL/kg and may be repeated 30 minutes later to reverse symptoms. Persistence of methemoglobinemia at high levels in a symptomatic patient is an indication for exchange transfusion. Laboratory determinations for methemoglobin are available. This is the only known condition in which a colorless solution (spirits of nitre) produces a gray infant with brown blood and a blue medication turns the child pink. The results of treatment are dramatic.

PETROLEUM DISTILLATES
(Charcoal Starter, Kerosene, Paint Thinner, Turpentine, & Related Products)

The petroleum distillates are mixtures of saturated and unsaturated hydrocarbons of the aliphatic and aromatic series. The following products are common causes of poisoning: kerosene, light oils, turpentine and other pine products, gasoline, lighter fluid, insecticides with petroleum distillate bases, benzine, naphtha, and mineral spirits.

It is essential to remember that just a few drops aspirated into the pulmonary tree can cause a severe and fatal pneumonia, a complication to which infants and children are particularly prone. In fatal poisonings, death usually occurs in 2–24 hours.

Pulmonary complications are reported with greater frequency among children who ingest kerosene or mineral seal oil than in those who ingest other petroleum distillate products with higher viscosity. Studies in experimental animals suggest that significant pulmonary complications do not occur secondary to gastrointestinal absorption of kerosene. Kerosene and other products are more likely to cause spontaneous emesis in about 90% of patients in 1 hour.

In general, ingestion of more than 30 mL (1 oz) of a petroleum distillate is associated with a higher incidence of central nervous system complications. Central nervous system involvement is reported most frequently among patients who ingest light oils and kerosene.

Clinical Findings

Ingestion of petroleum distillates causes local irritation with a burning sensation in the mouth, esophagus, and stomach; vomiting; and occasionally diarrhea with blood-tinged stools. With central nervous system involvement, lethargy is found in over 90% of cases, semicoma in 5%, coma in 3%, and convulsions in 1%; other findings include confusion and disorientation. Death may occur (usually owing to respiratory arrest). Pulmonary involvement is usually indicated by cyanosis, rapid breathing, tachycardia, and fever. Basilar rales may rapidly progress to massive pulmonary edema or hemorrhage, infiltration, and secondary infection. In severe poisoning, there may be cardiac dilatation, hepatosplenomegaly, proteinuria, formed elements in the urine, and cardiac arrhythmias associated with congestive heart failure.

Treatment

Although controversial, induced emesis is more effective in life-threatening ingestions and is less dangerous than gastric lavage. Gastric lavage should be performed only if a cuffed endotracheal tube is inserted, because there is no such thing as a "careful gastric lavage" in children. If the amount ingested is small—a difficult thing to estimate in children—a saline cathartic is all that is necessary (see p 736). The American Academy of Pediatrics recommends emesis if more than 1 mL/kg has been ingested.

For central nervous system depression, supportive care is indicated. Do not give epinephrine as a stimulant because it may have adverse effects on the sensitized myocardium.

"Prophylactic" antibiotic therapy is of questionable value and does not speed resolution when pneumonitis exists. Oxygen and mist are helpful. Corticosteroids are probably useless and may be harmful. Hospitalization is only indicated if the child has taken a large amount or is symptomatic. Fever and other symptoms may continue for as long as 10 days without infection, and pneumatoceles may develop 3–5 weeks after pneumonitis.

Withhold digestible fats, oils, and alcohol, which may promote absorption from the bowel or cause aspiration pneumonitis on their own.

The rapidity of recovery depends upon the degree of pulmonary involvement. Resolution may take as long as 4 weeks.

PHOSPHATES, ORGANIC (Diazinon, Disyston, Malathion, Parathion, etc)

Many insecticides contain organic phosphates. Parathion is one of the most toxic examples. All inhibit cholinesterase, resulting in parasympathetic and central nervous system stimulation. Symptoms include headache, dizziness, blurred vision, diarrhea, abdominal pain, dyspnea, chest pain, bronchial constriction, pulmonary edema, respiratory failure, convulsions, cyanosis, coma, loss of reflexes and sphincter control, sweating, salivation, miosis, tearing, muscle fasciculations, and even generalized collapse.

Lowered red cell cholinesterase activity confirms the diagnosis.

Treatment

The patient *must* be decontaminated with soapy water or tincture of green soap as soon as possible to prevent further absorption.

Complete atropinization is mandatory. Begin with 50 μg/kg intravenously in a small child and 1–2 mg intravenously in an older child. Repeat every 15–30 minutes until dry mouth, mydriasis, and tachycardia appear. In addition, pralidoxime (2-PAM), 500 mg intravenously (injected slowly over a 5-minute period), should be given if symptoms are severe but may be delayed until confirmation of red cell cholinesterase depression has been made. Repeated administration of atropine may be necessary for 3–4 days following the onset of illness. 2-PAM should be continued in accordance with instructions.

Supportive measures include oxygen, artificial respiration, postural drainage of secretions, and measures to combat shock.

RAUWOLFIA DERIVATIVES

Rauwolfia derivatives produce parasympathetic effects: nasal congestion, salivation, sweating, bradycardia, abdominal cramps, and diarrhea. Parkinsonian symptoms occasionally develop.

Treatment

Give supportive treatment and remove the poison by emesis and lavage.

RIOT CONTROL DRUGS

Several riot control drugs are now available. In general they consist of a chemical in a hydrocarbon solvent (eg, kerosene) and, in some cases, a propellant (eg, Freon gas). The chemical agent typically causes lacrimation, photophobia, and, in some instances, nausea and vomiting. Skin sensitization and corneal scarring can occur, particularly when the chemical is released close to the victim's face or skin.

Treatment

The most effective treatment is prompt removal from the sprayed area and careful decontamination of the patient. After removing all clothes, the patient should shower carefully, using copious amounts of soap and water. An ophthalmologist should examine the eyes for possible corneal damage. Medical personnel involved in decontamination should wear surgical scrub suits and should also shower with copious amounts of soap and water when the decontamination is completed.

SALICYLATES

(See p 83.)

SCORPION STINGS

The toxin of the less venomous species of scorpions causes only local pain, redness, and swelling; that of the more venomous species causes generalized muscular pains, convulsions, nausea, vomiting, variable central nervous system involvement, and collapse.

Treatment

Keep the patient recumbent and quiet. Treatment of the wound is as for snake bite (see below). If absorption has occurred, give 5–20 mL of 10% calcium gluconate by slow intravenous infusion. Hot baths and 20 mL of 10% magnesium sulfate intravenously may be given for relief of pain. Provide adequate sedation and institute supportive measures. Hot compresses of sodium bicarbonate solution will relieve local pain if there is no systemic involvement. Corticotropin (ACTH) or the corticosteroids may be of value in severe cases. Antivenin is of value in cases involving the more venomous species of scorpions (eg, those found in the extreme southwestern USA).

SNAKE BITES

Snake venom may be neurotoxic or hemotoxic. Neurotoxin (cobra, coral snake) causes respiratory paralysis; hemotoxin (rattlesnake, copperhead, moccasin, pit viper) causes hemolysis, tissue destruction, and damage to the endothelial lining of the blood vessels. Manifestations consist of local pain, thirst, nausea and vomiting, profuse perspiration, local swelling and redness, abdominal cramps, urticaria, dilated pupils, stimulation followed by depression, extravasation of blood, respiratory difficulty, muscle weakness, hemorrhage, and circulatory collapse.

Note: Thirty to 70% of snake bites do not result in envenomation. Crotalid bites can be expected to show local hemorrhage if envenomation occurred.

Treatment

Keep the patient recumbent and quiet. Treat shock or respiratory failure with all available means. A tourniquet that occludes venous and lymphatic return should be applied, although its value is questionable. (If envenomation of the arterial tree is suspected or if prolonged delay in definitive treatment is unavoidable, the tourniquet should completely occlude arterial supply.) The tourniquet should be left on until antivenin is given. Release of the tourniquet prior to administration of the antivenin can cause shock and death. It is better to lose a limb than a life.

Immobilize the bitten part in a dependent position if possible. The value of ice packs is very dubious and, if prolonged, may cause frostbite. Incision for suction is probably useless unless done within the first 30 minutes. With compromise of circulation due to swelling of a limb, a joint-to-joint splitting fasciotomy may rarely be used.

Administer antivenin* as indicated. If the bite is major, give antivenin intravenously; be prepared to treat possible anaphylactic reactions. If use of antivenin is not certain, do *not* perform a skin test, as this will sensitize the patient. The first dose should be large; the smaller the victim, the larger the dose. In a child weighing 10–18 kg (20–40 lb), 3–5 vials (10 mL each) may be required; 7–10 have been given as the first dose. Inject the dose intramuscularly. If the patient is seen late, antivenin may be given intravenously diluted in 5% dextrose in water. An additional vial of antivenin should be given every 1–2 hours if swelling or pain continues to progress. Concurrent administration of corticosteroids may lessen the risks associated with administration of the antivenin. A dosage of 1 g of hydrocortisone sodium succinate (Solu-Cortef) initially is suggested. Cortisone, 50–100 mg every 6–8 hours, is helpful.

Give supportive measures (fluids, sedatives) and tetanus and gas gangrene prophylaxis as indicated. Transfusions may be necessary to counteract hemotoxic venom.

*The Oklahoma Poison Information Center maintains an index of antiserum availability; telephone (405) 271–5454.

SPIDER BITES

Black Widow Spider

The bite of a female black widow spider *(Latrodectus mactans)* causes pain at the site of injection. Clinical manifestations include generalized muscular pains with severe abdominal cramps, irritability, nausea and vomiting, variable central nervous system symptoms, profuse perspiration, labored breathing, and collapse. Convulsions may occur, especially in children. Examination reveals a small papule at the area of the bite, boardlike rigidity of the abdomen, restlessness, and hyperactive deep reflexes.

Keep the patient recumbent and quiet with adequate sedation. Antivenin *(Latrodectus mactans)*, 2.5 mL intramuscularly, repeated in 1 hour if symptoms have not markedly improved, although traditional, may not be of value and should be reserved for seriously symptomatic patients. Morphine or codeine may help control pain. A tetanus toxoid booster should be given to the previously immunized child (if a booster has not been given in 4 years), and tetanus immune globulin should be given to the nonimmunized child. Corticosteroids may relieve symptoms. To reduce muscle irritability, 10% calcium gluconate may be given intravenously and repeated as needed. Diazepam, 0.1 mg/kg, may decrease muscle spasm.

Brown Spider

The North American brown recluse spider (violin spider, *Loxosceles reclusa*) is most commonly seen in the central and midwestern areas of the USA. Its bite characteristically produces a localized reaction with progressively more severe pain within 8 hours. The initial bleb on an erythematous ischemic base is replaced by a black eschar within a week. Systemic signs include cyanosis, a morbilliform rash, fever, chills, malaise, weakness, nausea and vomiting, joint pains, and hemolytic reactions, with hemoglobinuria, jaundice, and delirium.

There is no specific antivenin. Hydrocortisone, 1 g given intravenously over a 24-hour period, is indicated for systemic complications. Hydroxyzine (Vistaril), 1 mg/kg/d orally, is reported to be useful for its muscle relaxant, antihistaminic, and tranquilizing effects. The advisability of total excision of the lesion at the fascial level to minimize necrosis is debatable but should not be delayed if circulatory compromise occurs as a result of swelling.

TRANQUILIZERS
(Phenothiazine Compounds)

Phenothiazine compounds produce extrapyramidal motor symptoms (opisthotonos, oculogyric crisis, torticollis, trismus, rigidity) and convulsions.

Treatment

Diphenhydramine, 10–25 mg intravenously or orally, or other antiparkinsonism drugs may dramatically reverse the extrapyramidal symptoms. This therapy is *not* helpful in cases where overdosage of phenothiazine produces central nervous system and respiratory depression. Only supportive measures are indicated in these situations, and emergency treatment (p 735) should be followed.

TRICYCLIC ANTIDEPRESSANTS
(Amitriptyline, Doxepin, Imipramine, Nortriptyline, etc)

Amitriptyline (Elavil), doxepin (Sinequan), imipramine (Tofranil), nortriptyline (Aventyl), and other tricyclic antidepressants characteristically cause cardiac arrhythmias, central nervous system abnormalities (agitation, hallucinations, seizures, and coma), and other signs of atropinism such as dilated pupils, malar flushing, dry mouth, hyperpyrexia, and urinary retention. Some of the newer cyclic antidepressants such as amoxapine are relatively free of cardiovascular toxicity but cause central nervous system toxicity, with subsequent convulsions.

Treatment

Give 0.5 mg of physostigmine salicylate intravenously over 1 minute. This dose may be repeated every 5 minutes until a total dose of 2 mg has been given. Repeated doses at 20- to 30-minute intervals may be necessary because the drug is rapidly metabolized. The lowest effective dose should be given, and the drug should only be used to control convulsions, severe coma, hypertension, hallucinations, and arrhythmias. Use of sodium bicarbonate is also helpful in correcting and preventing recurrence of cardiac arrhythmias. Relative contraindications to physostigmine include gangrene, urinary obstruction, bowel obstruction, asthma, and diabetes. If it is deemed necessary to use it in these circumstances, have available atropine in half the physostigmine dosage being given; atropine will reverse toxic findings of physostigmine. Arrhythmias may require the use of lidocaine or phenytoin.

Pediatric Procedures* | 32

RESTRAINT & POSITIONING

The optimal care of children logically includes an understanding of specific procedures often required in diagnosis and management. In most cases of failure to complete a procedure successfully, the fault lies in undue haste in preparing a struggling or crying patient. The physician should therefore become acquainted with various methods of restraining pediatric patients. Before starting any procedure, all items of equipment that may be needed should be set out for immediate use as required.

In using total body restraint, be certain that cardiorespiratory function is not impaired. When prolonged restraint is required, make certain that restraining devices remain secure, do not become excessively restricting, and are as comfortable as possible. After a procedure has been completed, the physician should personally observe the child long enough to be certain that no untoward reaction has developed.

VENIPUNCTURE

The antecubital and external jugular veins are the safest and most frequently used large vessels for venipuncture and withdrawal of blood. (The femoral vein should be employed only in emergencies.) Smaller vessels in the dorsa of the hands and feet and scalp veins may also be used for withdrawing blood samples. Applying negative pressure with a syringe attached to the needle may cause collapse of these vessels because of their small size. Therefore, for these vessels, a different technique should be employed to obtain blood (see below).

The skin should be cleansed thoroughly with alcohol, soap and water, or a disinfectant (eg, an iodinated organic compound of isopropyl alcohol). In an uncooperative patient, the use of a catheter between the needle and the syringe will facilitate entry into the vein and subsequent withdrawal of blood.

*Revised with the assistance of Jane C. Burns, MD.

Antecubital Vein Puncture

If accessible, the antecubital vein is the best vein for the purpose of venipuncture in larger infants and children and is often easily entered even in the neonate.

External Jugular Vein Puncture

A. Preparation: Wrap the child firmly so that the arms and legs are adequately restrained. The wraps should not extend higher than the shoulder girdle. Place the child on a flat, firm table so that both shoulders are touching the table; the head is rotated fully to one side and extended partly over the end of the table so as to stretch the vein (see Fig 32–1). Adequate immobilization is essential.

B. Technique: Use a 21- or 23-gauge pediatric scalp vein infusion set ("butterfly"; ie, a needle attached to plastic wings and tubing) for withdrawing blood. The child should be crying and the vein distended when entered. Thrust the needle under the skin and apply gentle, constant negative pressure with the syringe as the vein is entered. This will prevent air embolism resulting from air being drawn into the vein when the child inspires. After removing the needle, exert firm pressure over the vein for 3–5 minutes while the child is in a sitting position.

Femoral Vein Puncture

Caution: This is a hazardous procedure, particularly in the neonate, and should be employed only in emergencies. Septic arthritis of the hip may complicate femoral vein puncture as a result of accidental

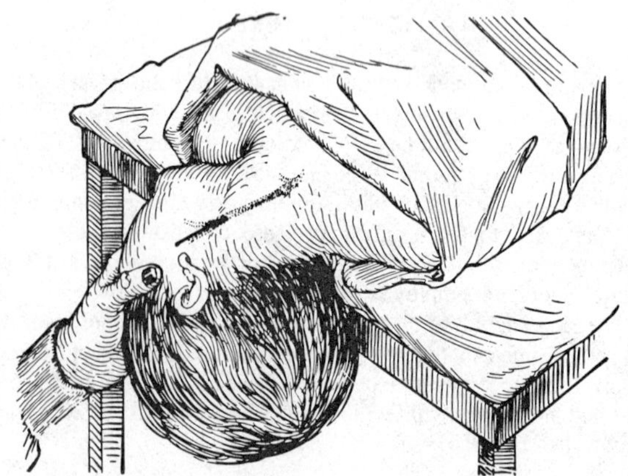

Figure 32–1. External jugular vein puncture.

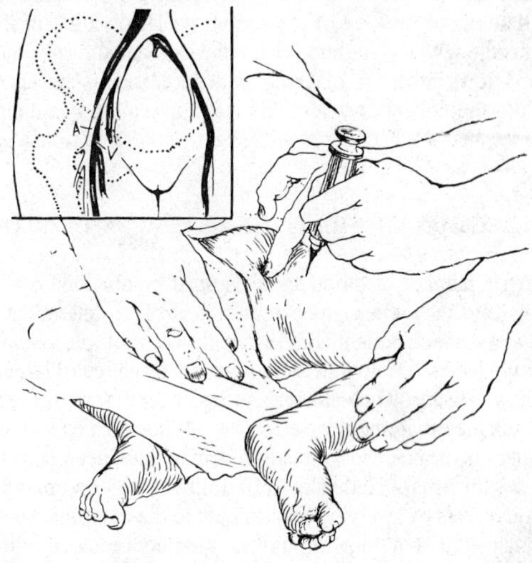

Figure 32–2. Femoral vein puncture.

penetration of the joint capsule. Arteriospasm with serious vascular compromise of the lower extremity may result from hematoma formation. Great care should be exercised in cleansing the skin prior to venipuncture so as to decrease the risk of infection.

A. Preparation: Place the child on a flat, firm table. Abduct the leg so as to expose the inguinal region. Use strict sterile precautions.

B. Technique: Locate the femoral artery by its pulsation. The left femoral vein is preferable because it lies medial to the artery throughout its course (see Fig 32–2). Be certain of the position of the femoral pulse at the time of puncture. Insert a short-beveled needle into the vein (perpendicularly to the skin) about 3 cm below the inguinal ligament; use the artery as a guide (see Fig 32–2). If blood does not enter the syringe immediately, withdraw the needle slowly, drawing gently on the barrel of the syringe; the needle sometimes passes through both walls of the vein, and blood is obtained only when the needle is being withdrawn. After removing the needle, exert firm, steady pressure over the vein for 3–5 minutes. If the artery has been entered, check the limb periodically during the next hour. If blanching of the extremity occurs, the application of heat may be of value.

Small Vein Puncture

After cleansing the skin, securely grasp the child's hand or foot in a manner that allows milking of the extremity. Using a 21- or 23-gauge straight needle with a clear hub, pierce the skin and advance the needle until blood flows into the hub. Gently milk the extremity and allow blood to drip into the collection vial. This technique allows sampling from small vessels that would collapse with negative pressure from a syringe.

COLLECTION OF MULTIPLE SPECIMENS OF BLOOD

When a number of blood samples must be obtained over a short period of time (eg, when glucose and electrolyte determinations are needed for a diabetic patient with ketoacidosis), multiple venipunctures may be avoided by employing an indwelling 22-gauge or larger Teflon intravenous catheter. The catheter and stylet are inserted in an arm or hand vein in the usual manner (see below). When the stylet is removed, the catheter hub is attached by means of a male Luer adapter to a buffalo cap filled with heparinized saline (10 units/mL). Blood may be withdrawn at intervals by applying a tourniquet to the extremity, inserting a needle attached to a syringe through the sterilely prepared rubber port, and drawing off and discarding the saline solution. A second needle and syringe are then used to collect the blood specimen. The tourniquet is removed, and the buffalo cap and catheter are subsequently cleared by injecting heparinized saline through the rubber port.

INTRAVENOUS THERAPY

A. Sites: For small infants, a scalp, wrist, hand, foot, or arm vein will usually be most convenient. Any accessible vein may be used in an older child. If the vein cannot be entered, fluids may be administered by hypodermoclysis, and blood may be given intraperitoneally in an emergency.

B. Equipment: A gravity apparatus is used with a closed-drip chamber in the tubing not far below the container; the tubing should hang perpendicularly. The chamber should be one-fourth to one-third full and the tubing below it free of air. Flow is regulated by a screw clamp on the tubing or the clamp that comes with special intravenous tubing. Use a pediatric scalp vein infusion set (butterfly) with a 25-gauge or larger needle or a Teflon intravenous catheter with removable stylet.

C. Technique:

1. Insertion of the butterfly–First flush the tubing with an isotonic solution. Insert the needle under the skin, and disconnect the syringe from the tubing so that blood return can occur when the needle tip enters the vein. Advance the needle until blood return is noted in the tubing. Holding the needle stationary, remove the tourniquet, reattach the syringe to the tubing, and attempt to flush solution into the vein. Watch carefully for evidence of fluid extravasation. Secure the needle and wings of the butterfly in place with plastic tape. Bolster the wings of the butterfly as needed with cotton to hold the needle at a proper angle. Coil the butterfly tubing and tape away from the needle entry site. Attach intravenous tubing.

2. Insertion of the catheter–The catheter/stylet apparatus consists of an intravenous catheter with removable stylet. Insert the apparatus under the skin, and advance it until blood drips from the catheter hub. Holding the stylet stationary, advance the catheter over the stylet into the vessel. Withdraw the stylet and attach intravenous tubing to the catheter hub. Secure the catheter in place carefully. Sandbags will be useful in holding the child's head. Sandbags or a padded board may be used for immobilizing the extremities.

D. Rate: Infusion sets are available in 2 different drip sizes, macrodrip and minidrip. The macrodrip set (for adults) delivers larger drops such that 10–15 drops usually equal 1 mL (depending on the manufacturer). The minidrip set, in which 60 drops equal 1 mL, is of value when small volumes are being given (drops/min = mL/h). Either of these gravity drip systems may be attached to a pump for more controlled administration of fluids.

E. Precautions: The rate of flow should be checked frequently. An accurate record must be kept of the amount and type of fluid added. For small infants (particularly if premature), a pump system is preferable for careful control of the volume of intravenous fluid infused. Phlebitis usually develops after a few days. It is best to remove the needle and change its location every 48–72 hours. If possible, avoid the use of hypertonic solutions. For the patient receiving fluids in an extremity, use foam rubber to maintain the limb in a position of greater comfort. Inspect the limb at regular intervals for evidence of undue pressure and circulatory embarrassment.

Venous Cutdown

Venous cutdown is indicated for small infants and for situations in which a seriously ill older child is in urgent need of fluids and difficulty is encountered in entering a vein. In these cases, expose a vein surgically and, under direct visualization, insert a Teflon catheter with an inner needle stylet.

A. Sites: The saphenous vein running anterior to the medial malleolus of the tibia will be found the most satisfactory. It can be entered at any point along its course. Hence, by starting at the ankle, the same vein can be used 2 or 3 times if necessary.

B. Equipment: An intravenous infusion set is prepared as for

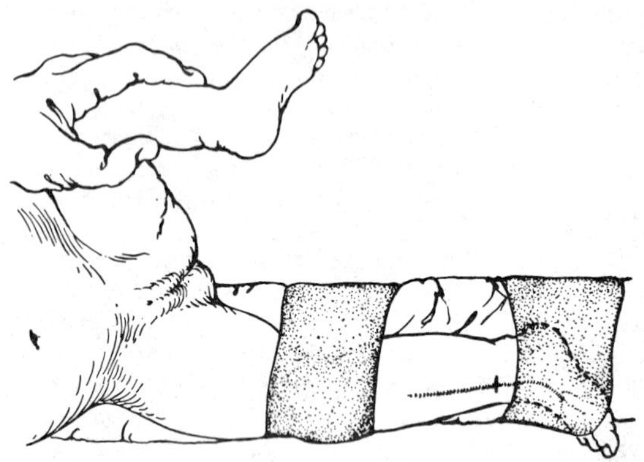

Figure 32–3. Position and taping of leg for venous cutdown.

continuous venoclysis (see above). A Teflon catheter with inner stylet is easiest to use. A pediatric cutdown tray containing scalpel, hemostats, forceps, and curved clamps should be available.

C. Preparation: Apply a tourniquet. Cleanse the skin and drape the leg as for a surgical procedure, using sterile precautions. The foot can be securely taped to a sandbag or board splint (see Fig 32–3). Make a large wheal with 1 or 2% lidocaine solution (without epinephrine) in the skin over the vein.

D. Technique:

1. Incision–With a scalpel, make an incision just through the skin. The incision should be about 1 cm long and at a right angle to the direction of the vein. Using a fine curved clamp, spread the incision widely, dissecting through the subcutaneous fat in a direction parallel to the vein.

2. Identification of the vein–Usually, the vein is seen lying on the fascia. Some dissection of subcutaneous fat may be necessary. Insert a curved clamp to the periosteum and bring the vein to the surface (see Fig 32–4). Be certain it is a vein, not a nerve or tendon, by noting the flow of blood. Pass 2 silk ties (No. 00) under the isolated vein (see Fig 32–5). Using a hemostat, dissect the vein free for a length of 1–2 cm. Apply gentle traction on proximal and distal ties to maximally expose the vessel. In small infants, the vein is small and fragile; great care must be taken in handling it.

3. Insertion of the catheter–Introduce the catheter with the stylet needle bevel-up. When the needle is in vessel lumen, hold the stylet stationary and gently advance the catheter. Withdraw the stylet and

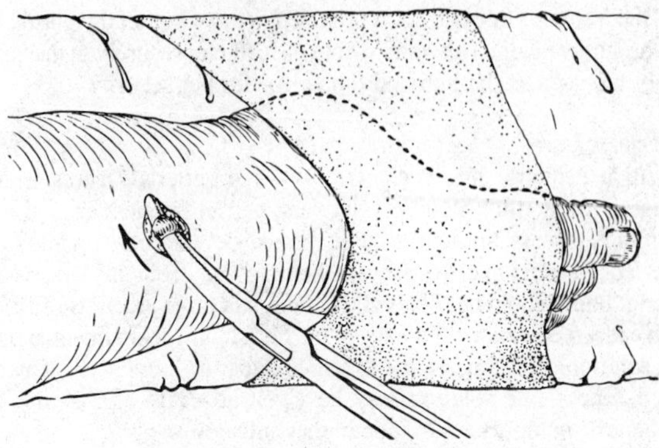

Figure 32–4. Isolation of vein for venous cutdown.

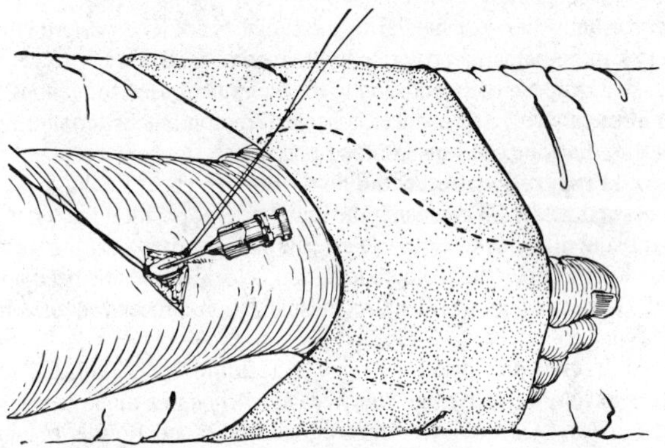

Figure 32–5. Venous cutdown with ligatures in place.

release tension on the proximal tie so that the catheter may be threaded and blood return ascertained. If there is no blood flow, remove the tourniquet and attempt to inject a small amount of intravenous solution into the vein. Watch for a wheal or extravasation of fluid, indicating that the catheter is not in the vessel. If the catheter flushes easily, remove the proximal and distal ligatures and suture the plastic wings of the catheter hub to the skin. This can most easily be accomplished by placing a skin closure suture on either side of the catheter hub. Tie the suture, and then pass the free ends through holes provided in the wings of the plastic hub. Tie the suture again. This should hold the catheter securely in the vessel. Apply tape across the hub and tubing for further security.

Arterial "Line"

In a pediatric intensive care unit, intra-arterial access is often necessary to monitor blood pressure and permit frequent arterial blood sampling. Access through a "line" must be carefully monitored by experienced personnel to prevent hemorrhage from the access site. Arterial lines should not be used to administer large amounts of fluid or to give any medications. Patency of the line should be maintained by use of a solution of normal saline to which heparin, 2 units/mL, has been added. The saline solution may be given at a rate of 2–4 mL/h by mechanical pump to ensure continuous infusion.

A. Sites: The radial artery and posterior tibial artery are the most appropriate vessels for cannulation because of the presence of collateral circulation. Use of more proximal arteries is dangerous because of the possibility of vessel thrombosis resulting in distal ischemia. The location of the vessel should be determined by palpating the pulse. The radial artery usually lies just medial to the radial head. The posterior tibial artery can be palpated posterior to the medial malleolus.

B. Equipment: In addition to the equipment used for venous cutdown (see above), a transducer is needed for continuous monitoring of systolic, diastolic, and mean blood pressures.

C. Preparation: Secure the child's limb on a board splint to expose the desired vessel. When using the radial artery, position the wrist in a slightly dorsiflexed position. Cleanse the skin and drape as for a surgical procedure. For percutaneous cannulation, a local anesthetic need not be used. (For cannulation under direct visualization, proceed as for venous cutdown.)

D. Technique: Insert a 22-gauge Teflon catheter with the stylet needle bevel-up (no syringe attached) at a 45-degree angle to the skin surface. Advance the stylet until the arterial blood flow is obtained. Adjust the position of the needle until blood return is maximal. Holding the stylet stationary, lower the catheter and stylet until they are flush with the skin and then advance the catheter. Remove the stylet and attach intravenous tubing to the hub of the catheter by use of a T-connector. Secure the catheter in place as for venous cutdown.

HYPODERMOCLYSIS

In an emergency when a vein cannot be entered, fluids may be placed under the skin.

A. Sites: For small infants, hypodermoclysis may be given by syringe, using the subcutaneous tissues of the axillae, upper back, thighs (preferred in older children), or lower abdomen. In most instances, the intravenous route is preferred, since hypodermoclysis may cause a marked shift in body fluids.

B. Equipment: A 20- or 50-mL syringe and a 20-gauge needle are used.

C. Preparation: Rigid aseptic precautions are necessary. The infant must be restrained to prevent bending or breaking the needle.

D. Technique: Use *only* isotonic solutions, injected slowly. If the center of the injected area becomes pale, change the position of the needle point. Gentle massage will diffuse fluid into the tissues. In infants, up to 50 mL can be injected in each site at one time. In children, give 30–40 mL/kg at one time. Larger amounts can be given over a longer period by means of a gravity apparatus with a Y-tube and 2 needles.

INTRAPERITONEAL THERAPY

Isotonic fluids and blood may be administered by the intraperitoneal route, but the intravenous route is preferred.

URINE COLLECTION

Voided Urine

A pediatric urine collector (a plastic bag with a round opening surrounded by an adhesive surface that binds to the skin) may be used. After application, the diaper may be reapplied. Urine may also be collected with a bird cup (for girls) or a test tube (for boys) fitted in a specimen band.

If a specimen is to be used for culture, the most reliable methods that decrease the chances of contamination of the specimen are catheterization and percutaneous bladder aspiration. Voided midstream collections are difficult to obtain from children and are subject to contamination.

Catheterization

A. Equipment: If the procedure is being performed to obtain a single specimen for culture, use an appropriately sized plastic feeding tube (No. 5 French feeding tube). If the catheter is to remain in place for continuous monitoring of urine output, use a Foley catheter with balloon and a closed sterile collection system. Have ready gloves and drapes, iodine solution, urine cup for specimen collection, normal saline solution to inflate the Foley balloon, and lubricant for the catheter; these should all be sterile.

B. Technique: Have adequate personnel available to restrain the patient during the procedure.

1. Female patients–Place the female patient in the frog-leg position to expose the urinary meatus. Separate the labia majora, and prepare and drape the patient as for a surgical procedure. Using sterile gloves, apply lubricant to the end of the catheter and pass the catheter through the urethral opening. Continue to thread the catheter gently until urine flow is obtained. Allow the first aliquot of urine to drain out of the catheter. Collect subsequent urine for culture. If a Foley catheter is used, inflate the balloon with the appropriate volume of normal saline solution (the volume is written on the catheter); inflation is through a one-way valve in the sidearm tubing. Pull back on the catheter to test that the balloon is in the bladder and that the catheter is secured. Tape the tubing to the thigh and attach the sterile collection unit and tubing.

2. Male patients–Hold the male patient's legs in extension. Prepare the glans as for a surgical procedure, retracting the foreskin if present. Proceed as above, taking special care to advance the catheter gently while applying gentle traction on the penis, with the meatus pointed cephalad. If resistance is encountered, retract the catheter slightly, change the angle of entry, and attempt to pass the catheter again.

C. Follow-Up Measures: To prevent phimosis in male patients, remember to return the foreskin to its normal position after catheter insertion. Some authorities recommend use of a single dose of a urinary tract antibiotic (eg, nitrofurantoin [Macrodantin], 2 mg/kg) following in-and-out catheterization in an attempt to prevent infection resulting from the possible introduction of bacteria into the bladder during the procedure.

Suprapubic Percutaneous Bladder Aspiration

Suprapubic percutaneous bladder aspiration is preferable to catheterization when a sterile urine specimen is required for culture and bacterial count.

A. Preparation: The bladder must be full before the procedure is attempted. Cooperative patients should be urged to drink liberal quantities of fluid without voiding. Local anesthesia may be used but is generally not necessary. Inadvertent perforation of a distended adjacent viscus may occur if the bladder is not sufficiently distended. Place the patient in a supine position, with the lower extremities held in the frog-leg position. Prepare the skin carefully as for a spinal puncture.

B. Technique: Introduce a 22-gauge straight needle (attached to a syringe) 1 cm above the pubis, with the needle perpendicular to the skin. With a quick, firm motion, advance the needle while applying gentle traction on the syringe. Stop when urine is aspirated. After urine has been obtained, withdraw the needle with a single, swift motion.

OBTAINING SPINAL FLUID BY LUMBAR PUNCTURE

Lumbar Puncture in Children & Older Infants

A. Preparation: Have a helper restrain the patient in the flexed lateral position on a firm, flat table. Scrub and wear sterile gloves. Draw an imaginary line between the 2 iliac crests and use the intervertebral space immediately above or below this line (L3-4 interspace). Prepare the skin surrounding this area as for a surgical procedure, with iodine and alcohol or other suitable antiseptic. Drape the area with sterile towels. Infiltrate the skin and subcutaneous tissues with 1–2% lidocaine (not necessary in infants and young children).

B. Technique: Use a short 21- to 23-gauge needle for infants; use a long 21-gauge needle for older children. Insert the lumbar puncture needle, with the stylet bevel-up, just below the vertebral spine in the midline (see Fig 32–6). Keep the needle perpendicular to both planes of

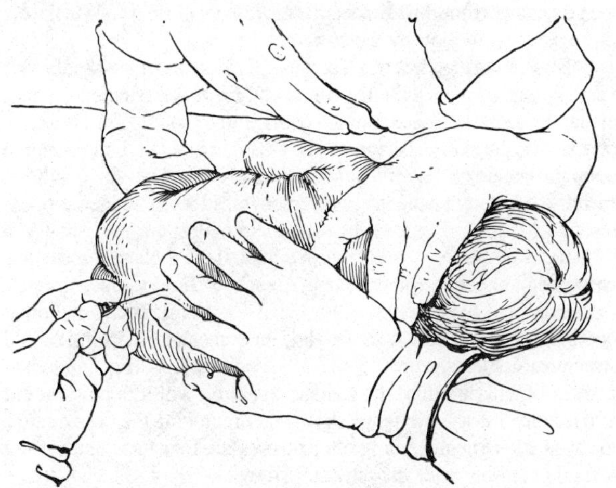

Figure 32–6. Lumbar puncture with assistance of nurse.

the back or pointing a little towards the head. A distinct "give" is usually felt when the dura is pierced; if in doubt, remove the stylet to watch for fluid. When fluid is obtained, a 3-way stopcock and manometer may be attached to measure opening pressure (at the beginning of collection) and closing pressure (at the end of collection). Cardiorespiratory function should be monitored throughout the procedure.

Lumbar Puncture in Small Infants

For small infants, lumbar puncture may be performed at the level of the superior iliac crests, with the patient in a sitting position and leaning forward. Cerebrospinal fluid may flow very slowly, and the "give" may not be felt in small infants. Gentle aspiration with a small syringe may be necessary.

BODY CAVITY PUNCTURES

Subdural Puncture

Caution: This procedure should be performed by a neurosurgeon when possible, because of the risks of bleeding and of damage to important underlying structures.

A. Preparation: Shave the scalp overlying the anterior fontanelle to a distance of at least 2 cm beyond the margin of the fontanelle. Use sterile precautions as for any surgical procedure. Restrain the child securely. The operator's hands should be braced against the skull during the procedure to minimize undesired movement of the needle in the event of unexpected motion by the patient.

B. Technique: Insert a 22-gauge lumbar puncture needle with a very short bevel at the extreme lateral margin of the fontanelle, at least 2 cm lateral to the midline, to avoid damage to major blood vessels. After penetrating the skin, pass the needle 2–3 mm parallel to the scalp; then point the needle tip perpendicular to the surface and advance cautiously. Piercing the tough dura is easily recognized by a sudden "popping through" feeling. Remove the stylet. Normally, not more than a few drops (up to 1 mL) of clear fluid is obtained. If the subdural fluid contains blood or pus, remove a sufficient amount of fluid to decompress the fontanelle, but never remove more than 10–15 mL at any one time on one side; removal of too much fluid may result in a shift of midline structures. Repeat the procedure on the opposite side. (For children over 2 years of age in whom the fontanelle has closed, a trephine opening ["bur hole"] is usually necessary.) After removing the needle, elevate the head 10–15 degrees and exert firm pressure for a few minutes. Apply a sterile dressing over the puncture sites.

Thoracentesis

Thoracentesis is used to remove pleural fluid or air for diagnosis or treatment.

Caution: Risks include introduction of a new infection; pneumothorax or hemothorax (or both) as a result of tearing of the lung; hemoptysis; syncope (pleuropulmonary reflex or air embolus); and pulmonary edema as a result of too rapid removal of large amounts of fluid. None of these are common if reasonable care is taken.

A. Sites: Locate the fluid or air by physical examination and by x-ray. If entering at the base, locate the bottom of the opposite uninvolved lung as a guide so the puncture will not be below the pleural cavity. Enter the dependent pleural cavity to remove fluid, or enter the superior chest (usually through the second interspace anteriorly, 1–2 cm lateral to the sternum when the patient is in a supine position) to relieve pneumothorax.

B. Equipment: For evacuation of a pneumothorax, use a 19-gauge needle (butterfly) with a 50-mL syringe attached to the tubing via a 3-way stopcock. For removal of pleural fluid, use an 18- to 19-gauge Teflon catheter (with inner removable stylet) attached to a 20-mL syringe via a 3-way stopcock. If a large amount of fluid is to be removed, it can be pumped through a rubber tube attached to the sidearm of the stopcock, thereby avoiding leakage of air into the pleural space.

C. Preparation: The patient should sit up, if possible, and lean forward against a bedstead or chair back. If too ill or too young to sit up, the patient should be held with the involved side (ie, lung with the effusion) in the most dependent position. Strict sterile precautions should be used. Scrub and wear sterile gloves. Prepare the skin surgically and use suitable drapes, preferably a large drape with a hole in the center. Use 1–2% lidocaine to infiltrate the skin and down to the pleura.

D. Technique: Insert the stylet and catheter in an interspace, passing just above the edge of the rib. The intercostal vessels lie immediately below each rib. Usually, it is not difficult to know when the pleura is pierced, but suction on the needle at any stage will show whether or not fluid has been reached. Remove the inner stylet, and quickly attach the stopcock and syringe to the hub of the catheter, thereby avoiding creation of a pneumothorax. In cases of long-standing infection, the pleura may be thick and the fluid loculated, necessitating more than one puncture site. If a large amount of fluid is present, it should be removed slowly at intervals, 100–500 mL each time, depending on the size of the patient. Pleural fluid is apt to coagulate unless it is frankly purulent; thus, to facilitate examination, an anticoagulant should be added to the fluid after it is removed.

Peritoneal Puncture

Peritoneal puncture can be used diagnostically to find evidence of blood, other body fluid, or pus and to obtain specimens for bacterial culture. Rarely, blood, albumin, or fluids may be administered by this route.

Caution: The procedure is dangerous if the intestines are distended or if the bladder is not empty. There is a risk of puncturing the distended bowel, which may be adherent to the abdominal wall.

Adhere to rigid surgical techniques. Use an 18- to 19-gauge catheter with inner stylet. Enter at a level about halfway between the symphysis and the umbilicus in the lower quadrant or in the midline. In infants, enter at the lateral edge of the rectus muscle to avoid penetrating the bladder. The needle should enter obliquely to avoid leakage afterward. As soon as the fluid is reached, remove the stylet and attach the syringe to the catheter to withdraw the fluid. Ascitic fluid will flow out readily. Pus can be aspirated with a sterile syringe.

BONE MARROW PUNCTURE

Bone marrow puncture is indicated for diagnosis of blood dyscrasias, neuroblastoma, lipidosis, and reticuloendotheliosis. It is also used to obtain specimens for culture. The procedure should be done with great caution when a defect of the clotting mechanism is suspected.

A. Sites: In children, the posterior iliac crest is the preferred site. When the child is restrained in a prone position, the iliac crest can be located and a spot can be marked approximately 1 cm below the crest. Puncture of the sternal marrow is rarely indicated in children. The site between the tibial tubercle and the medial condyle over the anteromedial aspect is recommended by some for bone marrow puncture in infants.

B. Preparation: Prepare the skin surrounding the area as for a surgical procedure. Scrub and wear sterile gloves. Use 1% lidocaine solution to infiltrate the skin and tissues down to the periosteum.

C. Technique: Use a 21-gauge lumbar puncture needle for infants; use an 18- or 19-gauge special marrow needle with a short bevel for older children. Insert the needle with stylet in place, perpendicular to the skin, through the skin and tissues, down to the periosteum. Push the needle through the cortex, using a screwing motion with firm, steady, and well-controlled pressure. Generally some "give" is felt as the needle enters the marrow; the needle will then be firmly in place. Immediately fit a dry syringe (20- to 50-mL) onto the needle and apply strong suction for a few seconds. A small amount of marrow will enter the syringe; this should be smeared on glass coverslips or slides for subsequent staining and counting. Remove the needle after withdrawing marrow, and exert local pressure for 3–5 minutes or until all evidence of bleeding has ceased. Apply a dry dressing.

EXCHANGE TRANSFUSION FOR ERYTHROBLASTOSIS FETALIS

A. Preparation: After adequate preparation of the infant (respirations and temperature stabilized and maintained, gastric contents removed, proper restraint, humidified oxygen being administered), drape the umbilical area. Cut off the cord about ½ inch or less from the skin. Control any bleeding.

B. Technique:

1. Identification of the vein–The 2 arteries are white and cordlike; the single vein is larger and thin-walled. If the vein cannot be visualized in the cord stump, make a small transverse incision above the umbilicus.

2. Cannulation and catheterization–Cannulate the vein gently (usually to a distance of 6–8 cm) with polyethylene tubing. Determine the position of the catheter by cross-table lateral x-ray. The catheter should be in the vena cava or sinus venosus and not in the portal vein or its branches. Secure the catheter with umbilical tape.

3. Transfusion–Employing sterile packaged equipment specifically prepared for this procedure, remove 10 mL of blood at a time (save the first blood withdrawn for laboratory studies) and replace it with an equivalent amount of blood preserved with citrate-phosphate-dextrose (CPD) less than 3 days old. Use type-specific or group O Rh-negative blood cross-matched with the mother. Give twice the blood volume (blood volume equals about 85–100 mL/kg) for a "complete" exchange. The time for a 2-volume exchange is optimally 1½–2 hours. When the infant is severely affected, a full exchange should not be attempted immediately after birth. Instead, small doses of sedimented erythrocytes should be given, alternating with slow withdrawal of the infant's blood until the venous pressure is less than 10 cm of water and the hematocrit is 45–50%.

C. Precautions: The infant should be monitored closely (blood pressure, venous pressure, blood gases, glucose) and homeostasis maintained with adjunctive therapy. If the infant becomes irritable, administer calcium gluconate, 1–2 mL of 10% solution, slowly through the polyethylene tubing (rinsing the tubing with saline solution before and after the drug is introduced). Do not give any further calcium if there is slowing of the pulse. Cardiac arrest rarely occurs and should be treated with tracheal intubation and the administration of oxygen by artificial ventilation; closed chest massage; intravenous or intracardiac sodium bicarbonate to correct acidosis; and supportive measures as indicated.

Appendix

DRUG THERAPY*

Precautions

Older children should never be given a dose greater than the adult dose. Adult dosages are given below to show limitations of dosages in older children when calculated on the basis of weight. All drugs should be used with caution in children, and dosages should be individualized. In general, the smaller the child, the greater the metabolic rate; this may increase the dose needed. Dosage may also have to be adjusted for body temperature (metabolic rate is increased about 10% for each degree centigrade); for obesity (adipose tissue is relatively inert metabolically); for edema (depending on whether the drug is distributed primarily in extracellular fluid); for the type of illness (kidney and liver disease may impair metabolism of certain substances); and for individual tolerance (idiosyncrasy). The dosage recommendations on the following pages should be regarded only as estimates; careful clinical observations and the use of pertinent laboratory aids are necessary. Established drugs should be used in preference to newer and less familiar drugs.

Drugs should be used in early infancy only for significant disorders. In both full-term and premature infants, detoxifying enzymes may be deficient or absent; renal function relatively inefficient; and the blood-brain barrier and protein binding altered. At any age, oliguria requires a reduction of dosage.

Dosages have not been determined as accurately for newborn infants as for older children.

Whenever possible, reference should also be made to the printed literature supplied by the manufacturer, particularly for drugs that are used infrequently.

Determination of Drug Dosage†

A. Surface Area: This is probably the most accurate method of estimating the dose for a child. (See Table 1 and Figs 1 and 2.)

$$\text{Child dose} = \frac{\text{Surface area of child in m}^2 \times \text{Adult dose}}{1.75}$$

or

$$\text{Surface area of child in m}^2 \times 60 = \text{Percentage of adult dose}$$

*Revised with the assistance of Robert Peterson, MD.

†To convert dose in g/kg to dose in gr/lb, multiply g dosage by 7.

Table 1. Determination of drug dosage from surface area.*

Weight (kg)	Weight (lb)	Approximate Age	Surface Area (m^2)	Percentage of Adult Dose
3	6.6	Newborn	0.2	12
6	13.2	3 mo	0.3	18
10	22	1 yr	0.45	28
20	44	5.5 yr	0.8	48
30	66	9 yr	1	60
40	88	12 yr	1.3	78
50	110	14 yr	1.5	90
65	143	Adult	1.7	102
70	154	Adult	1.76	103

*If adult dose is 1 mg/kg, dose for 3-month-old infant would be 2 mg/kg.

B. Weight: Use the following (adapted from Leach and Wood) to calculate the child dose in mg/kg if the adult dose is 1 mg/kg.

Patient Age	Multiply Adult Dose by
Adult	1
12 yr	1.25
1–7 yr	1.5
2 wk–1 yr	2

Administration of Drugs

A. Route of Administration:

1. Oral–Tablets may be crushed between spoons and given with chocolate, honey, jam, or maple or corn syrups. Powdered drugs should be mixed in the vehicle and held between 2 layers, not floated on the top. Many regularly prescribed drugs are commercially available in special pediatric preparations. Warn parents that the attractively flavored drug must be kept out of reach of children in the home. Avoid administering drugs with important foods. Attempt to administer the entire dose in one spoonful.

2. Parenteral–Parenteral administration of certain drugs may sometimes be necessary, especially in the hospital. Its use as a matter of convenience should be evaluated in the light of the psychic trauma that may result.

3. Rectal–Rectal administration is often very useful, especially for home use. (Rectal dosages are approximately twice the amount given orally.) The physician must make certain, however, that rectal absorption is adequate before depending upon this route for a specific drug. Drugs may be given rectally in corn starch solution (not more than 60 mL); they are best given through a tube, but an enema bulb may be used.

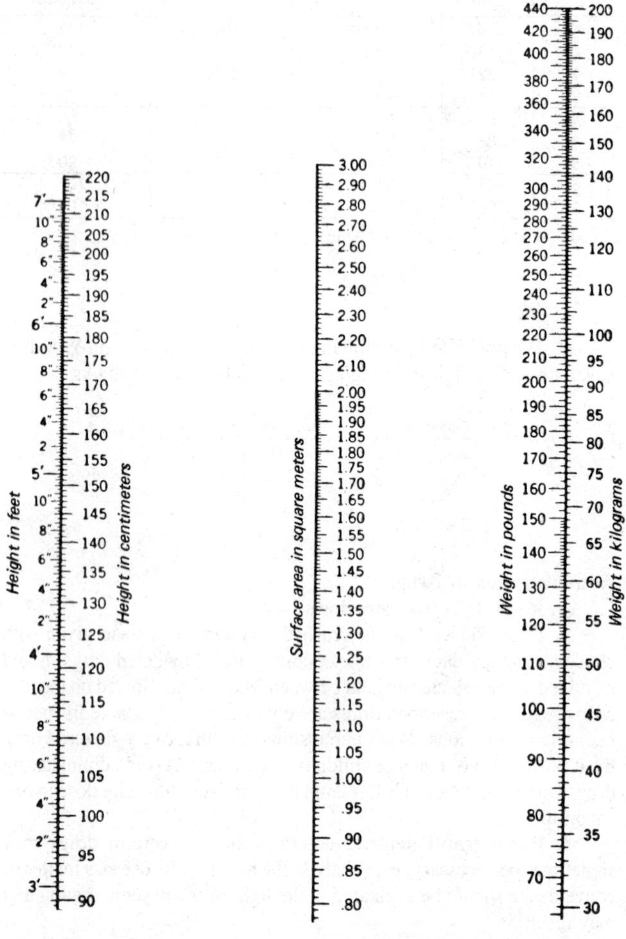

Figure 1. Nomogram for the determination of body surface area of children and adults. (Reproduced, with permission, from Boothby WM, Sandiford RB: Nomographic charts for the calculation of the metabolic rate by the gasometer method. *Boston MSJ* 1921;185:337.)

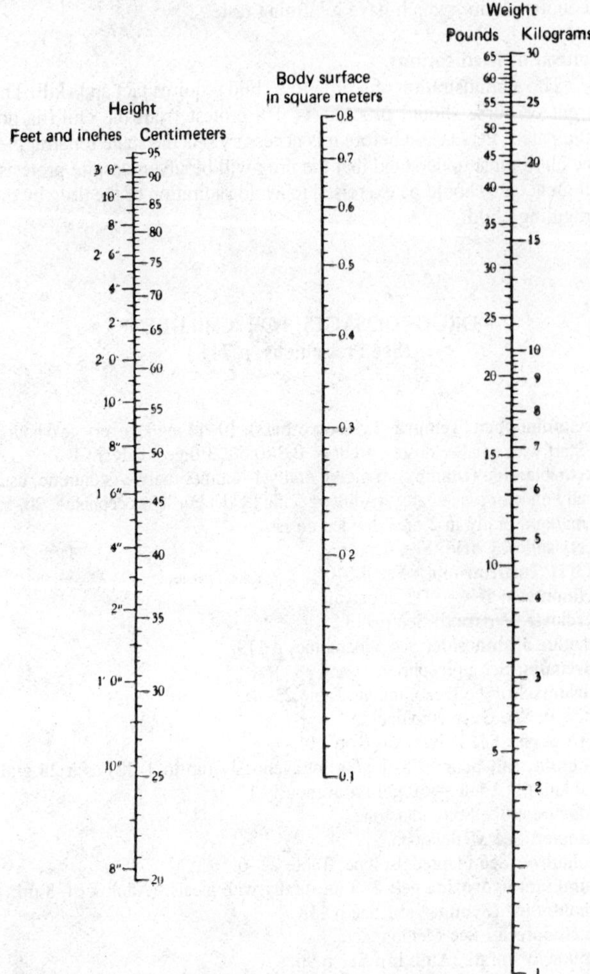

Figure 2. Nomogram for the determination of body surface area of children. (Reproduced, with permission, from Dubois EF: *Basal Metabolism in Health and Disease.* Lea & Febiger, 1936.)

B. Flavoring Agents for Drugs: Drugs for children should be attractive in flavor. Syrups are more useful as flavoring agents than are alcoholic elixirs, which have a burning taste.

Refusal of Medications

The administration of a drug to a child requires tact and skill. The parent or nurse should proceed as if a protest from the child is not anticipated. Persuasion before it is necessary sets the stage for struggle. The child must understand that the drug will be given despite protests, but great care should be exercised to avoid aspiration of the drug by the struggling child.

DRUG DOSAGES FOR CHILDREN*

(See Precautions, p 744.)

Acetaminophen (Tempra, Tylenol; others): 10–15 mg/kg every 4–6 hours. Start with smaller dose. (Adult = 0.3–0.6 g 3 times daily.)
Acetazolamide (Diamox): 5 mg/kg orally 1–4 times daily. As diuretic, usually once or twice daily. (Adult = 5 mg/kg/d.) For hydrocephalus, 20–55 mg/kg/d orally in 2 or 3 divided doses.
Acetylsalicylic acid: See Aspirin.
ACTH (corticotropin): See p 540.
Actinomycin D: See Dactinomycin.
Acyclovir (Zovirax): See p 118.
Adenine arabinoside: See Vidarabine, p 119.
Adrenalin: See Epinephrine.
Adriamycin: See Doxorubicin, Table 23–4.
Adroyd: See Oxymetholone.
Aerosporin: See Polymyxin B, p 114.
Albumin, salt-poor: 0.5–1 g/kg intravenously (up to 1 dL) as a 25 g/dL solution. (Adult = 50 g/d intravenously.)
Aldactone: See Spironolactone.
Aldomet: See Methyldopa.
Alphadrol: See Fluprednisolone, Table 22–6.
Aluminum hydroxide gel: 2–8 mL orally with meals. (Adult = 4–8 mL.)
Amantadine (Symmetrel): See p 118.
Amethopterin: See Methotrexate.
Amikacin sulfate (Amikin): See p 96.
Aminophylline: Orally, 4–6 mg/kg every 6 hours. (Adult = 0.25 g.) Intravenously, 4–6 mg/kg every 6 hours by continuous infusion of 0.9 mg/kg/h. Intramuscular and rectal administration not recommended. Caution in younger children.

*Revised with the assistance of Robert Peterson, MD.

Aminosalicylic acid (PAS): See p 99.
Ammonium chloride: 75 mg/kg/d orally in 4 divided doses. As single expectorant dose, 0.06–0.3 g orally. (Adult = 0.3 g.) As diuretic, 60–75 mg/kg/d orally. (Adult = 4 g/d.)
Amobarbital sodium (Amytal): As sedative, 1–2 mg/kg orally every 6–8 hours. As hypnotic, 5 mg/kg every 6 hours. Caution: Observe for respiratory depression and hypotension with hypnotic dosage.
Amoxicillin: See p 111.
Amphetamine sulfate (Benzedrine): 0.5 mg/kg/d orally in 3 divided doses (not over 15 mg/d). (Adult = 5–15 mg.) Caution.
Amphotericin B (Fungizone): 0.25 mg/kg/d intravenously slowly. Increase to 1–1.5 mg/kg/d diluted 1 mg in 10 mL. (Adult = 50–100 mg/d intravenously.) Caution: Toxic. (See p 99.)
Ampicillin: See p 110.
Amytal: See Amobarbital sodium.
Anadrol: See Oxymetholone.
Ancef: See Cefazolin, p 100.
Ancobon: See Flucytosine, p 105.
Ansolysen: See Pentolinium.
Antepar: See Piperazine, p 668.
Apomorphine: 0.06–0.1 mg/kg subcutaneously. Use with extreme caution. May cause depression and potentiate the depressant action of central nervous system depressant drugs. Note: Syrup of ipecac preferred for emesis.
Apresoline: See Hydralazine.
AquaMephyton: See Phytonadione.
Aralen: See Chloroquine.
Aramine: See Metaraminol bitartrate.
Arfonad: See Trimethaphan.
Aristocort: See Triamcinolone, Table 22–6.
Ascorbic acid (vitamin C): See Table 4–5 and p 64.
Asparaginase (Elspar): 5000–10,000 IU/m^2 intravenously daily to weekly. (See also Table 23–4.)
Aspirin: As analgesic, 65 mg (1 gr) per year of age for each dose. (Adult = 0.3–0.65 g.) For rheumatic fever, 65–130 mg (1–2 gr)/kg/d to maintain a blood level of 20–30 mg/dL. (Adult = 6–8 g.) As antipyretic, up to 30–65 mg/kg/d. Try smaller dose first. Obtain blood levels for higher doses.
Atarax: See Hydroxyzine.
Atropine sulfate: 0.01 mg/kg subcutaneously, intramuscularly, or intravenously, depending upon clinical setting. Repeat as necessary for desired therapeutic effect. For cardiac arrest, use intravenous route only. (Adult = 0.3–1 mg.) Caution.
Azathioprine (Imuran): 3–5 mg/kg/d orally.
Azlocillin: See p 113.
Azulfidine: See Sulfasalazine.
Bacitracin: See p 99.
Bactrim: See Trimethoprim with sulfamethoxazole, p 115.

See Precautions, p 774.

BAL: See Dimercaprol, pp 482, 740.
Banthine: See Methantheline.
BCNU (carmustine): See Table 23–4.
Belladonna tincture: 0.1 mL/kg/d orally in 3 divided doses. (Adult = 0.6 mL 3 times daily.) Do not give over 0.6 mL in a single dose or over 3.5 mL/d.
Benadryl: See Diphenhydramine.
Benemid: See Probenecid.
Bentyl: See Dicyclomine.
Benzathine penicillin G: See p 112.
Benzedrine: See Amphetamine sulfate.
Betamethasone (Celestone): See Table 22–6.
Bethanechol chloride (Urecholine; others): Orally, 0.6 mg/kg/d in 3 divided doses. (Adult = 10–30 mg 3–4 times daily.) Subcutaneously, 0.15–0.2 mg/kg/d. (Adult = 2.5–5 mg.) Caution: Have atropine available for bradycardia.
Bicillin C-R: See Penicillins, p 110.
Bisacodyl (Dulcolax; others): 0.3 mg/kg orally or rectally.
Blenoxane: See Bleomycin, Table 23–4.
Bleomycin (Blenoxane): See Table 23–4.
Blood fraction products: See pp 404–405.
Bonine: See Meclizine.
Brompheniramine (Dimetane; others): For children under 6 years of age, 0.5 mg/kg/d. For children over 6 years of age, 4 mg 3–4 times daily. (Adult = 4–8 mg 3–4 times daily.)
Busulfan (Myleran): 0.06 mg/kg/d orally. (Adult = 2 mg 1–3 times daily.)
Cafergot: See Ergotamine-caffeine.
Calciferol (vitamin D_2): 400 IU/d for maintenance. For hypo- and pseudohypoparathyroidism in children, 2000 IU (50 μg/kg/d). For renal osteodystrophy, 25–200 thousand units/d.
Calcium chloride (27% calcium): For newborns, 0.3 g/kg/d orally as a 2–5% solution. For infants, 1–2 g/d as a dilute solution. For children, 2–4 g/d. (Adult = 2–4 g 3 times daily.) Caution.
Calcium EDTA (calcium edathamil disodium; Versenate): 75 mg/kg/d intramuscularly in 3 or 4 divided doses. Caution: Inject slowly and stop if bradycardia occurs. (See also p 482.)
Calcium lactate (13% calcium): 0.5 g/kg/d in divided doses orally in dilute solution. (Adult = 4–8 g 3 times daily.)
Calcium mandelate: 2–8 g/d orally, depending on age. (Adult = 3 g 4 times daily.)
Carbenicillin: See p 111.
Carmustine (BCNU): See Table 23–4.
Castor oil: For infants, 1–5 mL orally. For children, 5–15 mL orally. (Adult = 15–60 mL orally.)
CCNU (lomustine): See Table 23–4.
Ceclor: See Cefaclor, p 100.
Cefaclor (Ceclor): See p 100.

Cefamandole (Mandol): See p 100.
Cefazolin (Ancef, Kefzol): See p 100.
Cefotaxime (Claforan): See p 100.
Cefoxitin (Mefoxin): See p 101.
Celestone: See Betamethasone, Table 22–6.
Celontin: See Methsuximide.
Cephalexin (Keflex): See p 101.
Cephalothin (Keflin): See p 101.
Charcoal, activated: 0.5–1 g/kg. (Adult = 30–50 g.)
Chloral hydrate (Noctec): Orally or rectally, 12.5–50 mg/kg as single hypnotic dose (adult = 0.5–2 g); or 4–20 mg/kg (not over 1 g) as single sedative dose (adult = 0.25–1 g). May repeat in 1 hour to obtain desired effect; then repeat every 6–8 hours (not over 50 mg/kg/d).
Chlorambucil (Leukeran): 0.1–0.2 mg/kg/d. (Adult = 0.2 mg/kg.)
Chloramphenicol (Chloromycetin): See p 102.
Chlordiazepoxide (Librium; others): For children over 6 years of age, 0.5 mg/kg/d orally in 3–4 divided doses.
Chloromycetin: See Chloramphenicol, p 102.
Chloroquine (Aralen): To treat active disease, 10 mg/kg as first dose and 5 mg/kg as second dose 6 hours later; on subsequent days, 5 mg/kg once daily. For prophylaxis, 5 mg/kg once daily, beginning 2 weeks prior to exposure; continue for 8 weeks after leaving endemic area.
Chlorothiazide (Diuril): For infants under 6 months of age, 30 mg/kg/d orally in 2 divided doses. For children, 20 mg/kg/d. (Adult = 0.5–1 g once or twice daily.)
Chlorpheniramine (Chlor-Trimeton, Teldrin; others): For children, 0.35 mg/kg/d orally in 4 divided doses. (Adult = 2–4 mg 3–4 times daily; long-acting, 8–12 mg 2–3 times daily.)
Chlorpromazine (Thorazine): Orally, 0.5 mg/kg every 4–6 hours. Intramuscularly, 0.5 mg/kg every 6–8 hours as needed but not over 40 mg/d for children up to 5 years of age and not over 75 mg/d for children 5–12 years of age. Rectally, 2 mg/kg. (Adult = 10–50 mg.)
Chlorpropamide: Initially, 8 mg/kg/d in 3 divided doses. (Adult = 250 mg/d.) Caution.
Chlor-Trimeton: See Chlorpheniramine.
Cholestyramine (Cuemid, Questran): For children over 6 years of age, 240 mg/kg/d orally in 3 divided doses. (Adult = 4 g 3–4 times daily.)
Citrovorum factor (leucovorin calcium): 1–6 mg/d orally. (Adult = 3–10 mg.)
Claforan: See Cefotaxime, p 100.
Cleocin: See Clindamycin, p 103.
Clindamycin (Cleocin): See p 103.
Clonazepam (Clonopin): See Table 21–4.
Clonopin: See Clonazepam, Table 21–4.
Cloxacillin: See p 113.

Codeine phosphate: As analgesic for children, 0.5 mg/kg every 4–6 hours. (Adult = 30–60 mg every 4–6 hours.) As antitussive for children, 1–1.5 mg/kg/d in 4–6 divided doses. (Adult = 10–20 mg every 4–6 hours as necessary.)
Colace: See Dioctyl sodium sulfosuccinate.
Compazine: See Prochlorperazine.
Co-Pyronil: See Pyrrobutamine.
Cortef: See Hydrocortisone, Table 22–6.
Corticosteroids: See Table 22–6.
Corticotropin (ACTH): See p 540.
Cortisone (Cortone): See Table 22–6.
Cortone: See Cortisone, Table 22–6.
Cortril: See Hydrocortisone, Table 22–6.
Cosmegen: See Dactinomycin.
Cotazym (pancreatic replacement): 0.3–0.6 g with each feeding. (Adult = 1–3 capsules with meals.)
Co-trimoxazole: See Trimethoprim with sulfamethoxazole, p 115.
Cuemid: See Cholestyramine.
Cuprimine: See Penicillamine.
Curare: See Tubocurarine.
Cyclizine (Marezine): For children 6–10 years of age, 3 mg/kg/d orally in 3 divided doses. For adolescents and adults, 50 mg every 4–6 hours as necessary.
Cyclophosphamide (Cytoxan): As a loading dose, 2–8 mg/kg/d orally or intravenously for 7 or more days or 15–50 mg/kg once a week. For maintenance, 2–5 mg twice weekly. (See also Table 23–4.)
Cycloserine (Seromycin): 10–20 mg/kg/d orally. (Adult = 250 mg twice daily.)
Cyproheptadine (Periactin): 0.25 mg/kg/d orally in 3 or 4 divided doses. Maximum for children 2–6 years of age, 12 mg/d; for those 7–14 years of age, 16 mg/d. (Adult = 12–16 mg/d.)
Cytarabine (cytosine arabinoside; Cytosar): 2 mg/kg/d by direct injection; 0.5–1 mg/kg/d by infusion. (See also Table 23–4.)
Cytomel: See Triiodothyronine.
Cytosar: See Cytarabine.
Cytosine arabinoside: See Cytarabine.
Cytoxan: See Cyclophosphamide.
Dactinomycin (actinomycin D; Cosmegen): 0.015 mg/kg/d intravenously for 5 days. (Same as adult dose.) (See also Table 23–4.)
Daraprim: See Pyrimethamine, pp 659, 664.
Darvon: See Propoxyphene.
Daunomycin: See Daunorubicin, Table 23–4.
Daunorubicin (daunomycin): See Table 23–4.
DDAVP: See Desmopressin.
Decadron: See Dexamethasone, Table 22–6.
Decapryn: See Doxylamine succinate.

See Precautions, p 774.

Deferoxamine mesylate (Desferal): 50 mg/kg intramuscularly every 6 hours or by intravenous infusion at a rate of 15 mg/kg/h. Caution: Hypotension occurs if intravenous infusion is too rapid.

Delalutin: See Progesterone-17-caproate.

Delatestryl: See Testosterone enanthate.

Delestrogen: See Estradiol valerate.

Delta-Cortef: See Prednisolone, Tablc 22–6.

Deltasone: See Prednisone, Tables 22–6 and 23–4.

Demerol: See Meperidine.

Dendrid: See Idoxuridine.

Depo-Provera: See Medroxyprogesterone acetate.

Desferal: See Deferoxamine mesylate.

Deslanoside: See Table 13–5.

Desmopressin (1-desamino-8-D-arginine vasopressin; DDAVP): 5–15 mg in the morning and 2.5–7.5 mg at night.

Desoxycorticosterone (Percorten): See Table 22–6.

Desoxycorticosterone acetate (Doca): See Table 22–6.

Desoxycorticosterone pivalate: See Table 22–6.

Dexamethasone (Decadron, Hexadrol): See Table 22–6.

Dexedrine: See Dextroamphetamine sulfate.

Dextroamphetamine sulfate (Dexedrine; others): 2–15 mg/d orally in 3 divided doses. For older children, start with smaller dose (not over 1 mg/kg/d). (Adult = 5–15 mg/d.) Caution.

Dextromethorphan hydrobromide (Romilar; others): 1 mg/kg/d in 3–4 divided doses. (Adult = 15–30 mg 3–4 times daily.)

Diamox: See Acetazolamide.

Dianabol: See Methandrostenolone.

Diazepam (Valium; others): Orally, 0.12–0.8 mg/kg/d in 3–4 divided doses. Intravenously, 0.1 mg/kg slowly. (Adult = 2–10 mg 2–4 times daily.) Caution: Respiratory depression and arrest.

Diazoxide (Hyperstat): 2.5–10 mg/kg intravenously.

Dicloxacillin: See p 113.

Dicodid: See Hydrocodone bitartrate.

Dicyclomine (Bentyl): For infants, 5 mg as syrup 3–4 times daily. For children, 10 mg 3–4 times daily. (Adult = 10–20 mg 3–4 times daily.)

Diethylstilbestrol: See Stilbestrol.

Digitalis preparations: See Table 13–5.

Dihydrocodeinone bitartrate: See Hydrocodone bitartrate.

Dihydrotachysterol: Initially, 1–4 mL/d (1.25 mg/mL) orally. As maintenance, 0.5–1 mL 3–5 times weekly. (Adult = 4–10 mL initially and then 1–2 mL.)

Dilantin: See Phenytoin.

Dimenhydrinate (Dramamine; others): 5 mg/kg/d orally in 4 divided doses. (Adult = 50–100 mg.)

Dimercaprol (BAL): See pp 482, 740.
Dimetane: See Brompheniramine.
Dioctyl sodium sulfosuccinate (Colace, Doxinate; others): 3–5 mg/kg/d orally in 3 divided doses. (Adult = 60–480 mg/d.)
Diodrast: See Iodopyracet.
Diphenhydramine (Benadryl; others): Orally, 4–6 mg/kg/d in 3–4 divided doses. Intravenously, 2 mg/kg infused over 5 minutes as an antidote for phenothiazine toxicity. (Adult = 100–200 mg/d orally.)
Diphenoxylate (in Lomotil; others): For older children, 2.5 mg 3–5 times daily. Decrease dose as relieved. (Adults = 5 mg 3–4 times daily and reduce.) Caution.
Diphenylhydantoin sodium: See Phenytoin.
Diuril: See Chlorothiazide.
Doca: See Desoxycorticosterone acetate, Table 22–6.
Dolophine: See Methadone.
Doxinate: See Dioctyl sodium sulfosuccinate.
Doxorubicin (Adriamycin): See Table 23–4.
Doxylamine succinate (Decapryn): 2 mg/kg/d orally.
Dramamine: See Dimenhydrinate.
Dulcolax: See Bisacodyl.
Durabolin: See Nandrolone.
Edathamil calcium disodium: See Calcium EDTA.
Edecrin: See Ethacrynic acid.
Edrophonium chloride (Tensilon): As test dose for infants, 0.2 mg/kg intravenously. Give only one-fifth of dose slowly initially; if tolerated, give remainder. (Adult = 5–10 mg intravenously.)
EDTA: See Calcium EDTA.
Efudex: See Fluorouracil.
Elspar: See Asparaginase.
Emetine hydrochloride: See p 661.
Ephedrine sulfate: Orally, 0.5–1 mg/kg. May repeat every 4–6 hours. (Adult = 25 mg.) Intramuscularly, 0.2 mg/kg every 6 hours. Intravenously, 50 mg/1000 mL. Adjust drip rate to patient's response.
Epinephrine (Sus-Phrine): For 1:1000 aqueous solution, 0.01–0.025 mL/kg (maximum dose, 0.5 mL) subcutaneously. (Adult = 0.5–1 mL.) For 1:200 aqueous solution, 0.05–0.1 mL subcutaneously, one dose only. Use smallest effective dose.
Equanil: See Meprobamate.
Ergotamine-caffeine (Cafergot; others): For children, one tablet at onset of attack; then one tablet every 30 minutes as necessary, but no more than 3 tablets per attack. (Adults = 2–4 tablets containing 1 mg of ergotamine and 100 mg of caffeine per tablet, but no more than 6 tablets per attack.) Rectal administration not recommended for children.
Erythrocin: See Erythromycin, p 104.

Erythromycin (Erythrocin, Ilosone, Ilotycin, Pediamycin; others): See p 104.

Esidrix: See Hydrochlorothiazide.

Estinyl: See Ethinyl estradiol.

Estradiol cypionate in oil: 1–2 mg/mo intramuscularly for teenage girls.

Estradiol valerate (Delestrogen; others): 10 mg/mo intramuscularly for teenage girls. (Adult = 10–20 mg intramuscularly every 2–3 weeks.)

Ethacrynic acid (Edecrin): For children, 1 mg/kg/d as one oral dose. (Adults = 50–100 mg initially.) As maintenance for children, 1 mg/kg intravenously. Caution: Ototoxic.

Ethambutol (Myambutol): See p 104.

Ethinyl estradiol (Estinyl; others): 0.02–0.05 mg orally 1–3 times daily for teenage girls. (Adult = 0.05 mg 1–3 times daily.)

Ethionamide (Trecator): See p 105.

Ethosuximide (Zarontin): For children under 6 years of age, 20 mg/kg/24 h orally as starting dose. For those over 6 years of age, 250–500 mg/d as starting dose. (See also Table 21–4.)

Ethotoin (Peganone): 25–75 mg/kg/d orally in divided doses. (Adult = 0.5 g orally 4–6 times daily.)

Ferrous salts: See p 389.

Flagyl: See Metronidazole, p 108.

Florinef: See Fludrocortisone, Table 22–6.

Flucytosine (Ancobon): See p 105.

Fludrocortisone (Florinef): See Table 22–6.

Fluorouracil (Efudex; others): For adults, 15 mg/kg/d for 4 days, not to exceed 1 g/d. If no toxicity occurs, give 7.5 mg/kg on sixth, eighth, tenth, and 12th days of treatment. Discontinue at end of 12th day even if no toxicity is apparent. May repeat in 6 weeks after last injection of previous course if no ty is noted. (See also Table 23–4.)

Fluoxymesterone (Halotestin; others): In prepubertal children, up to 0.15 mg/kg/d orally in 2 divided doses. In pubertal children, up to 0.1 mg/kg/d. (Adult = 2–10 mg/d.)

Fluprednisolone (Alphadrol): See Table 22–6.

Fulvicin: See Griseofulvin, p 106.

Fungicides: See pp 241–244.

Fungizone: See Amphotericin B.

Furadantin: See Nitrofurantoin, p 109.

Furazolidone (Furoxone): 5 mg/kg/d in 4 divided doses.

Furosemide (Lasix): For infants and children, 1 mg/kg intravenously; 2 mg/kg intramuscularly; or 2 mg/kg orally. Frequency usually once or twice daily. May need larger dose in older children.

Furoxone: See Furazolidone.

Gantanol: See Sulfamethoxazole, p 115.

Gantrisin: See Sulfisoxazole, p 115.

Garamycin: See Gentamicin, p 105.

Gemonil: See Metharbital.

See Precautions, p 774.

Gentamicin (Garamycin; others): See p 105.

Gentian violet (methylrosaniline chloride): 2 mg/kg/d orally in 3 divided doses, not to exceed 30 mg. (Adult = 65 mg.)

Glucagon: For newborns, 0.025–0.1 mg/kg as single intravenous dose. Try smaller dose first. May repeat in 30 minutes. For older children, 0.25–1 mg subcutaneously, intramuscularly, or intravenously as single dose.

Glucocorticoids: See Table 22–6.

Glycerin: 1–1.5 g/kg as single oral dose.

Gold sodium thiosulfate: 1 mg/kg weekly.

Gonadotropin, chorionic: 500–1000 units intramuscularly 2–3 times each week for 5–8 weeks.

Grifulvin: See Griseofulvin, p 106.

Grisactin: See Griseofulvin, p 106.

Griseofulvin (Fulvicin, Grifulvin, Grisactin): See p 106.

Guanethidine sulfate (Ismelin): 0.2 mg/kg/d orally as single dose. Increase dose at weekly intervals by same amount. (Adult = 10 mg/d.) Larger doses possible for hospitalized adults. Caution: Not recommended for infants.

Haldol: See Haloperidol.

Haldrone: See Paramethasone, Table 22–6.

Haloperidol (Haldol): Contraindicated in children under 3 years of age; safety is not yet established. For children 3–6 years of age, 0.01–0.03 mg/kg/d orally. For older children, 1–2 mg 2–3 times daily. (Adults = not more than 15 mg/kg/d. Initially, 1–2 mg 2 or 3 times daily. As maintenance, 1–2 mg 3–4 times daily.)

Halotestin: See Fluoxymesterone.

Heparin: Intravenously, 0.5 mg/kg. This may be repeated every hour. One mg/kg every 4 hours is recommended for intravascular clotting. Control with clotting time. (Adult = 50 mg.) Subcutaneously, 4 mg/kg. Will prolong clotting time for 20–24 hours.

Herplex: See Idoxuridine.

Hexadrol: See Dexamethasone, Table 22–6.

Hexylresorcinol: 0.1 g per year of age orally, not to exceed 1 g. (Adult = 1 g.)

Histamine: For provocative test, 0.02 mg/m^2 intravenously. Caution: Phentolamine should be available.

HN2: See Mechlorethamine.

Hyaluronidase (Wydase): 500 viscosity units or 150 turbidity-reducing units in 1 mL of sterile water or saline at site of fluid administration.

Hycodan: See Hydrocodone bitartrate.

Hydeltra: See Prednisolone, Table 22–6.

Hydralazine (Apresoline; others): Orally, 0.15 mg/kg 4 times daily. Increase to tolerance. Intramuscularly or intravenously with reserpine, 0.1–0.2 mg/kg every 6–24 hours. Intravenously or intramuscularly alone, 1.5–3.5 mg/kg/d in 4–6 divided doses. (Adults = initial parenteral dose of 10–20 mg; single oral dose of 100 mg.)

Hydriodic acid: 1–5 mL of 1.4% syrup every 4 hours in fruit juice.

Hydrochlorothiazide (Esidrix, HydroDiuril; others): For infants under 6 months of age, 2–3 mg/kg/d in 2 divided doses. For children, 2 mg/kg/d. (Adult = 25–200 mg/d.)

Hydrocodone bitartrate (Dicodid, Hycodan): 0.6 mg/kg/d orally. (Adult = 5–10 mg.) Caution.

Hydrocortisone (Cortef, Cortril, Hydrocortone, Solu-Cortef; others): See Table 22–6.

Hydrocortone: See Hydrocortisone, Table 22–6.

HydroDiuril: See Hydrochlorothiazide.

Hydroxyzine (Atarax; others): 1–2 mg/kg/d orally in 3 divided doses. Preoperatively, 1 mg/kg/d intramuscularly. (Adult = 25–50 mg 3 times daily.)

Hykinone: See Menadione sodium bisulfite.

Hyperstat: See Diazoxide.

Iodoquinol (Yodoxin): 40 mg/kg/d orally in 2–3 divided doses. (Adult = 0.2 g/7 kg/d.)

Idoxuridine (Dendrid, Herplex, Stoxil): See p 119.

Ilosone: See Erythromycin, p 104.

Ilotycin: See Erythromycin, p 104.

Imferon: See p 389.

Imipramine (Tofranil): Not generally recommended for children under 6 years of age. Initial dose for children, 25 mg/d; may increase to 50 mg/d for preadolescents and 75 mg/d for adolescents. (Adult = 75 mg initially, increased up to 150 mg/d.)

Immune globulin: See pp 404, 415.

Imuran: See Azathioprine.

Inderal: See Propranolol.

INH: See Isoniazid.

Insulin: See Table 22–7 and pp 546, 550.

Iodopyracet (Diodrast): 35% for intravenous urography and retrograde aortography; 70% for intravenous angiocardiography; or 7% in saline with hyaluronidase for subcutaneous injection.

Ipecac syrup: For children under 8 years of age, 15 mL orally. For those over 8 years of age, 30 mL. Give water. Ambulate. Repeat in 20 minutes as needed. Recover dose (lavage) if not vomited. (Adult = 30 mL.) Caution: Never use fluid extract of ipecac as emetic.

Iron: See Table 4–5 and p 389.

Iron dextran complex: See p 389.

Ismelin: See Guanethidine sulfate.

Isoniazid (INH; Nydrazid; others): 15–20 mg/kg/d (up to 30 mg if necessary). Maximum, 300 g/d. (See also pp 106, 334, 651.)

Isoproterenol hydrochloride (Isuprel, Norisodrine; others): Sublingually, 2–10 mg 3 times daily for older children (not oftener than every 3–4 hours). Oral inhalation, 5–15 breaths of 1:200 solution (not more than 0.5 mL). Intravenously, by dilute infusion only, 0.1 to 1 μg/kg/min. Monitor ECG and heart rate. (Adult = 15 mg sublingually 4 times daily.)

Isoproterenol sulfate (Norisodrine): 1–2 inhalations of 1:200 or 1:400 dilution.

Isuprel: See Isoproterenol hydrochloride.

Kanamycin (Kantrex): See p 107.

Kantrex: See Kanamycin, p 107.

Kayexalate: See Sodium polystyrene sulfonate.

Keflex: See Cephalexin, p 101.

Keflin: See Cephalothin, p 101.

Kefzol: See Cefazolin, p 100.

Ketoconazole (Nizoral): See p 107.

Kenacort: See Triamcinolone, Table 22–6.

Kenalog: See Triamcinolone, Table 22–6.

Konakion: See Phytonadione.

Lasix: See Furosemide.

Latrodectus mactans **antivenin:** See p 755.

Leucovorin calcium: See Citrovorum factor.

Leukeran: See Chlorambucil.

Levallorphan (Lorfan): For infants, 0.02–0.05 mg intravenously or intramuscularly; repeat if necessary. (Adult = 1–2 mg.) May give levallorphan tartrate 1 minute after vomiting begins as result of administration of apomorphine for treatment of poisoning.

Levarterenol: See Norepinephrine.

Levophed: See Norepinephrine.

Levothyroxine sodium (Synthroid; others): 0.1 mg is equivalent to 65 mg (1 gr) of Thyroid, USP, or 25–30 μg of triiodothyronine.

Librium: See Chlordiazepoxide.

Lidocaine (Xylocaine; others): 1 mg/kg intravenously slowly for arrhythmia. Repeat as needed. (Adult = 50–100 mg intravenously slowly.)

Lincocin: See Lincomycin, p 108.

Lincomycin (Lincocin): See p 108.

Liothyronine: See Triiodothyronine.

Liquid petrolatum, liquid paraffin: See Mineral oil.

Liver injection, crude: 2 mL/d intramuscularly. (Adult = 2 mL/d.)

Lomidine: See Pentamidine isethionate, p 666.

Lomotil: See Diphenoxylate.

Lomustine (CCNU): See Table 23–4.

Lorfan: See Levallorphan.

Lypressin (lysine-8 vasopressin; Syntopressin): 30–55 units/d as a nasal spray.

Magnesium hydroxide: See Milk of magnesia.

Magnesium sulfate: As anticonvulsant or for hypertension, 0.1–0.4 mL/kg of 50% solution intramuscularly every 4–6 hours if renal function is adequate. Intravenously, 10 mL (100 mg)/kg intravenously slowly as 1% solution. Caution: Check blood pressure carefully and have calcium available. As cathartic for children, 0.25 g/kg. (Adult = 10–30 g.)

Mandelamine: See Methenamine mandelate.

Mandol: See Cefamandole, p 100.

Mannitol (Osmitrol): As test dose for oliguria, 0.2 g/kg intravenously. For edema, 1–2.5 g/kg intravenously over 2–6 hours. For cerebral edema, 1–2.5 g/kg over ½–6 hours.

Marezine: See Cyclizine.

Matulane: See Procarbazine.

Mebendazole (Vermox): 100–200 mg/d as single oral dose for 3 consecutive days. (See also p 108.)

Mechlorethamine (nitrogen mustard, HN2; Mustargen): Inject slowly, diluted, 0.1 mg/kg/d for 4 days intravenously. (Adult = 0.1 mg/kg/d for 4 days.) (See also Table 23–4.)

Mecholyl: See Methacholine.

Meclizine (Bonine): 2 mg/kg orally every 6–12 hours. (Adult = 25–50 mg.)

Medrol: See Methylprednisolone, Table 22–6.

Medroxyprogesterone acetate (Depo-Provera): For children under 4 years of age, 100–150 mg per injection every 2 weeks. For those over 4 years of age, 150–200 mg per injection every 2 weeks.

Mefoxin: See Cefoxitin, p 101.

Mellaril: See Thioridazine.

Menadiol disodium diphosphate (vitamin K analog): For infants, 2.5–5 mg. Repeat every 12–24 hours as necessary. For children, 5–10 mg. Repeat every 12–24 hours as necessary.

Menadione sodium bisulfite (Hykinone): 1 mg intramuscularly. Not for infants. (Adult = 0.5–2 mg intramuscularly.)

Meperidine (Demerol): For children, 1–1.5 mg/kg every 3–4 hours as necessary. (Adult = 50–150 mg every 3–4 hours as necessary.)

Mephenesin (Tolserol): Orally, 40–130 mg/kg/d in 3–5 divided doses. Intravenously, 1–3 mg/kg as 2% solution slowly. (Adult = 1–3 g 3 times daily.)

Mephentermine sulfate (Wyamine): 0.4 mg/kg orally, intramuscularly, or slowly intravenously as single dose. (Adult = 15–20 mg intramuscularly.)

Mephenytoin (Mesantoin): 3–10 mg/kg/d orally. Start smaller dose and gradually increase. (Adult = 0.1–0.3 g 3 times daily.)

Mephobarbital (Mebaral): 6–12 mg/kg/d orally in 2–4 divided doses. (Adult = 200–600 mg/d in 2–4 divided doses.) (See also Table 21–4.)

Mephyton: See Phytonadione.

Meprobamate (Equanil, Miltown; others): For children over 3 years of age, 7–30 mg/kg/d orally in 2–3 divided doses. (Adult = 400–800 mg 3 times daily.)

Mercaptopurine (6-MP; Purinethol): 2.5–4 mg/kg/d orally in 3 divided doses. (Same as adult dose.) Caution. (See also Table 23–4.)

Mestinon: See Pyridostigmine.

Metandren: See Methyltestosterone.

Metaraminol bitartrate (Aramine): 0.04–0.2 mg/kg subcutaneously or intramuscularly; 0.3–2 mg/kg in 500 mL solution for intravenous infusion. (Titrate by effect or by blood pressure readings.) (Adult = 2–10 mg intramuscularly or 0.5–5 mg intravenously.)

Methacholine (Mecholyl): For arrhythmia in young children, 0.1–0.4 mg/kg subcutaneously or intramuscularly. May be increased by 25% every 30 minutes. Oral starting dose is approximately 18 times greater.
Methacycline (Rondomycin): See Tetracyclines, p 116.
Methadone (Dolophine): 0.7 mg/kg/d orally in 4–6 divided doses for analgesia.
Methandrostenolone (Dianabol): 0.04 mg/kg/d orally. (Adult = 2.5–5 mg/d.)
Methantheline (Banthine): 4–8 mg/kg/d orally or intramuscularly in 4 divided doses. (Adult = 50–100 mg 3 times daily.)
Methapyrilene hydrochloride: 0.2–0.3 mg/kg, up to 5 doses each day.
Metharbital (Gemonil): 5–12 mg/kg/d orally in divided doses. (Adult = 1.2 g orally 2–3 times daily.)
Methdilazine (Tacaryl): 0.3 mg/kg/d orally in 2 divided doses.
Methenamine mandelate (Mandelamine): 60 mg/kg/d orally in 4 divided doses. Maintain acid urine. (Adult = 1–1.5 g 4 times daily.)
Methicillin: See p 112.
Methimazole (Tapazole): 0.4 mg/kg/d in 3 divided doses. As maintenance, one-half of initial dose. (Adult = 15–60 mg.)
Methocarbamol (Robaxin): 40–65 mg/kg/d orally in 4–6 divided doses. (Adult = 1.5–2 g 3–4 times daily.)
Methotrexate (amethopterin): Orally or intramuscularly, 0.12 mg/d. (Adult = 5–10 mg/d.) Intrathecally, 0.25–0.5 mg/kg/d. Intravenously, 3–5 mg/kg as a single dose every other week. Caution: Toxic. (See also Table 23–4.)
Methoxamine hydrochloride (Vasoxyl): 0.25 mg/kg intramuscularly as single dose. (Adult = 15 mg intramuscularly.)
Methsuximide (Celontin): 20 mg/kg/d orally in divided doses. (Adult = 300 mg 1–3 times daily.) (See also Table 21–4.)
Methylatropine nitrate: 1:10,000 alcoholic solution. Initial dose, 0.05 mg subcutaneously. Increase to 0.3 mg as needed. (Adult = 1–2.5 mg every 3–4 hours.)
Methyldopa (Aldomet): For children, 5–10 mg/kg intravenously every 6–8 hours to a total dose of 20–40 mg/kg/d. Orally, initial dosage of 10 mg/kg/d in divided doses every 6–12 hours. Increase to 5–10 mg/kg/d at intervals of 2–7 days. Maximum, 40 mg/kg/d in divided doses every 6–12 hours. Caution. (Adult = 0.5–1 g/d initially; adjust at 2- to 7-day intervals.)
Methylene blue: 0.1–0.2 mL/kg of 1% solution intravenously. (Adult = 100–150 mg.)
Methylphenidate (Ritalin): For children over 6 years of age, initial dose of 5 mg with breakfast and lunch. May need larger dose subsequently. Orally, 0.25–0.75 mg/kg. Intramuscularly or slowly intravenously, 0.5 mg/kg. (Adult = 10 mg 3 times daily.) Caution.
Methylprednisolone (Medrol): See Table 22–6.
Methyltestosterone (Metandren, Oreton; others): 0.08–0.15 mg/kg/d sublingually. (As much as 10–20 mg/d has been used in preadolescents.) (Adult = 5–10 mg.)

Meticortelone: See Prednisolone, Table 22–6.
Meticorten: See Prednisone, Tables 22–6 and 23–4.
Metrazol: See Pentylenetetrazol.
Metronidazole (Flagyl): See p 108.
Mezlocillin: See p 113.
Milk of magnesia: 0.5 mL/kg orally. (Adult = 15–30 mL.)
Milontin: See Phensuximide.
Miltown: See Meprobamate.
Mineralocorticoids: See Table 22–6.
Mineral oil: For children over 6 years of age, 10–20 mL twice daily. (Adult = 15–30 mL.)
Mintezol: See Thiabendazole.
Morphine sulfate: 0.12–0.2 mg/kg intravenously or intramuscularly every 4 hours as needed to a maximum of 15 mg. (Adult = 10–15 mg.) Caution: Emesis, respiratory depression.
Moxalactam (Moxam): See p 108.
Moxam: See Moxalactam, p 108.
Mustargen: See Mechlorethamine.
Myambutol: See Ethambutol, p 104.
Mycifradin: See Neomycin, p 109.
Mycostatin: See Nystatin, p 109.
Myleran: See Busulfan.
Mysoline: See Primidone.
Nafcillin: See p 113.
Nalidixic acid (NegGram): See p 109.
Naloxone (Narcan): 0.01 mg/kg intravenously or intramuscularly. Higher doses (0.05 mg/kg) may be required to reverse propoxyphene overdoses.
Nandrolone (Durabolin): For infants, 12.5 mg intramuscularly every 2–4 weeks. For children, 25 mg intramuscularly every 2–4 weeks.
Narcan: See Naloxone.
Nebcin: See Tobramycin, p 116.
NegGram: See Nalidixic acid, p 109.
Nembutal: See Pentobarbital sodium.
Neobiotic: See Neomycin, p 109.
Neolin: See Penicillins, p 110.
Neomycin (Mycifradin, Neobiotic): See p 109.
Neostigmine (Prostigmin): Orally, 0.25 mg/kg. (Adult = 15 mg.) Intramuscularly, 0.025–0.045 mg/kg. (Adult = 0.25–1 mg.) For myasthenia test, 0.04 mg/kg intramuscularly. Caution: Atropine should be available.
Neo-Synephrine: See Phenylephrine.
Niacinamide (nicotinamide): See Table 4–5 and p 63.
Niclocide: See Niclosamide, p 671.
Niclosamide (Niclocide, Yomesan): See p 671.
Nicotinamide (niacinamide): See Table 4–5 and p 63.
Nitrofurantoin (Furadantin): See p 109.
Nitrogen mustard: See Mechlorethamine.

Nizoral: See Ketoconazole, p 107.
Noctec: See Chloral hydrate.
Norepinephrine (levarterenol; Levophed): Start at 0.05 μg/kg/min, and titrate rate by blood pressure.
Norethandrolone: 0.4–0.8 mg/kg/d orally. (Adult = 30–50 mg/d.)
Norisodrine: See Isoproterenol.
Nydrazid: See Isoniazid.
Nystatin (Mycostatin; others): See p 109.
Oleandomycin: See Erythromycin, p 104.
Omnipen: See Penicillins, p 110.
Oncovin: See Vincristine.
Opium tincture, camphorated: See Paregoric.
Oreton: See Methyltestosterone.
Osmitrol: See Mannitol.
Oxacillin: See p 113.
Oxandrolone: 0.05–0.25 mg/kg/d orally.
Oxymetholone (Adroyd, Anadrol): 0.1–0.3 mg/kg/d orally. For children weighing under 20 kg, 2.5 mg. For those over 20 kg, 3.75 mg.
Pancreatin (pancreatic enzymes): 0.3–0.6 g with each feeding. Increase as necessary. (Adult = 2–5 g.)
Papaverine: 1–6 mg/kg/d orally, intravenously, or intramuscularly in 4 divided doses. (Adult = 0.1 g.)
Paradione: See Paramethadione.
Paraldehyde: Orally, 0.1–0.15 mL/kg. (Adult = 4–16 mL.) Rectally, 0.3–0.6 mL/kg in 1 or 2 parts of vegetable oil. (Adult = 16–32 mL.) Intramuscularly, 0.1 mL/kg as single anticonvulsant dose (not over 10 mL). (Adult = 4–10 mL.) Intravenously, 0.02 mL/kg, very slowly. (Adult = 1–2 mL.) Caution: Intravenous administration may cause respiratory distress or pulmonary edema. Avoid plastic equipment.
Paramethadione (Paradione): Same dose as Trimethadione.
Paramethasone (Haldrone): See Table 22–6.
Parathyroid injection: 50–300 units subcutaneously or intramuscularly, and then 20–40 units every 12 hours. (Adult = 50–100 units 3–5 times daily.)
Paregoric (opium tincture, camphorated): Morphine content, 0.4 mg/mL. For infants up to 12 months of age, 0.06 mL per month of age; for those 5 years of age, 2 mL. May repeat every 3–4 hours if no drowsiness or respiratory depression. (Adult = 4 mL.) Caution: Respiratory arrest.
PAS: See Aminosalicylic acid, p 99.
PBZ: See Tripelennamine.
Pediamycin: See Erythromycin, p 104.
Peganone: See Ethotoin.
Penbritin: See Penicillins, p 110.
Penicillamine (Cuprimine): For infants over 6 months of age, 250 mg/d. For older children and adults, 1 g/d orally in 4 divided doses. Increase as indicated. Use D-penicillamine only.
Penicillin G: See p 111.

Penicillins: See p 110.
Pentamidine isethionate (Lomidine): See p 666.
Pentobarbital sodium (Nembutal): 1–1.5 mg/kg orally, up to 3–5 mg/kg as single sedative dose. (Adult = 100 mg.)
Pentobarbitone sodium: See Pentobarbital sodium.
Pentolinium (Ansolysen): Orally, 1 mg/kg/d. (Adult = 20–200 mg 3 times daily.) Intramuscularly or subcutaneously, 0.035–0.15 mg/kg. (Adult = 2.5–10 mg.) Start smaller dose and increase gradually.
Pentothal: See Thiopental sodium.
Pentylenetetrazol (Metrazol): 20 mg/kg diluted intravenously slowly. Caution.
Percorten: See Desoxycorticosterone, Table 22–6.
Periactin: See Cyproheptadine.
Permapen: See Penicillins, p 110.
Phenacemide (Phenurone): 20–30 mg/kg/d orally. For children 5–10 years of age, 0.25 g orally 3 times daily initially. (Adult = 0.5 g 2–4 times daily.)
Phenergan: See Promethazine.
Phenobarbital: As sedative, 0.5–2 mg/kg as single dose orally every 4–6 hours. As anticonvulsant, 3–5 mg/kg intramuscularly (intravenously only with extreme caution). (As much as 15–20 mg/kg intravenously has been recommended in neonates.) For epilepsy, starting doses as follows: for children under 3 years of age, 16 mg 3 times daily; 3–6 years, 32 mg 2 times daily; over 6 years, 32 mg 3 times daily. (Adult = 30 mg.) As hypnotic, 3–6 mg/kg orally. (Adult = 100–200 mg.) (See also Table 21–4.)
Phenobarbital sodium: Subcutaneously or intramuscularly, 4–10 mg/kg as anticonvulsant. Orally, 1–5 mg/kg as single sedative dose. (Adult = 15–100 mg.) Intramuscularly or rectally, 1 mg/kg as single sedative dose. (Adult = 30 mg.) Rectally, 3–5 mg/kg as anticonvulsant. Acts more rapidly than phenobarbital. (Adult = 0.3 g.)
Phenoxymethyl penicillin: See p 112.
Phensuximide (Milontin): 20–40 mg/kg/d orally in divided doses. (Adult = 0.5–1 g 2–3 times daily.)
Phentolamine (Regitine): 0.05–0.1 mg/kg intravenously. May repeat in 5 minutes and then as needed to control hypertension. Caution. Therapeutic dose, 5 mg/kg/d orally in 4 divided doses. (Adult = 5 mg intravenously.)
Phenurone: See Phenacemide.
Phenylephrine (Neo-Synephrine; others): Intramuscularly or subcutaneously, 0.1 mg/kg. Orally, 1 mg/kg/d in 6 divided doses. For nasal vasoconstriction, 3–10 mg orally. (Adult = 10–25 mg.)
Phenytoin (diphenylhydantoin sodium; Dilantin): Orally, 2–8 mg/kg/d in 3 divided doses. Try smaller dose first. Intramuscularly or intravenously, 1–5 mg/kg/d. (Larger doses have been recommended in neonates.) Rectally, 8–15 mg/kg/d. (Adult = 0.3–0.5 g/d.) (See also Table 21–4.)
Phytonadione (vitamin K_1; AquaMephyton, Mephyton, Konakion): Prophylactic dose, 0.5–5 mg intramuscularly. Therapeutic dose, 5–10 mg intramuscularly, intravenously, or orally.

See Precautions, p 774.

Pilocarpine hydrochloride: 0.5, 1, and 2% as eyedrops; 0.1 mg/kg as single intramuscular or subcutaneous dose.
Piperacillin: See p 113.
Piperazine citrate or phosphate (Antepar): See p 668.
Pitressin and Pitressin tannate: See Vasopressin.
Pituitary, posterior, powder: Small pinch (approximately 40–50 mg) nasally 4 times daily as needed. (Adult = 30–60 mg 2–3 times daily.)
Plasma: 10–15 mL/kg intravenously. (See also p 405.)
Polycillin: See Penicillins, p 110.
Polymyxin B (Aerosporin): See p 114.
Posterior pituitary: See Pituitary, posterior.
Potassium chloride: See pp 77, 87–88.
Povan: See Pyrvinium pamoate.
Pralidoxime (Protopam): 25–50 mg/kg as 5% solution intravenously.
Prednisolone (Delta-Cortef, Hydeltra, Meticortelone, Sterane): See Table 22–6.
Prednisone (Deltasone, Meticorten): See Tables 22–6 and 23–4.
Primidone (Mysoline): 12–24 mg/kg/d. For children under 8 years of age, start with 125 mg 2 times daily; for those over 8 years of age, 250 mg 2 times daily. Increase slowly as needed. (Adult = 250 mg as initial dose.) (See also Table 21–4.)
Priscoline: See Tolazoline.
Pro-Banthine: See Propantheline.
Probenecid (Benemid): Initial dose, 25 mg/kg; then 10 mg/kg orally every 6 hours. (Adult = 1–2 g initially; then 0.5 g every 6 hours.) Not recommended for children under 2 years of age.
Procainamide (Pronestyl): Orally, 8–15 mg/kg every 4–6 hours. Intramuscularly, 6 mg/kg every 4–6 hours. Intravenously (for emergency use only), 2 mg/kg at a rate not to exceed 0.5–1 mg/kg/min. Monitor by continuous ECG and blood pressure recording every minute.
Procaine penicillin G: See p 112.
Procarbazine (Matulane): 8 mg/kg orally as initial dose. Caution. (See also Table 23–4.)
Prochlorperazine (Compazine): Orally or rectally, 0.25–0.375 mg/kg/d in 2–3 divided doses. (Adult = 25 mg rectally 2 times daily or 5 mg orally 3–4 times daily.) Intramuscularly, 0.25 mg/kg/d; irritating to tissues. Toxicity: Parkinsonism and tetanuslike seizures. Avoid overdosage.
Progesterone-17-caproate (Delalutin; others): 125 mg intramuscularly for teenage girls.
Promethazine (Phenergan; others): As antihistaminic, 0.5 mg/kg orally at bedtime; 0.1 mg/kg orally 3 times daily. For nausea and vomiting, 0.25–0.5 mg/kg rectally or intramuscularly. For sedation, 0.5–1 mg/kg intramuscularly.
Pronestyl: See Procainamide.
Propantheline (Pro-Banthine): 1–2 mg/kg/d orally in 4 divided doses after meals. (Adult = 15–30 mg 3–4 times daily.)

Propoxyphene (Darvon; others): 3 mg/kg/d orally in divided doses every 4–6 hours. Not recommended for children under 12 years of age. (Adult = 32–65 mg 3–4 times daily.)

Propranolol (Inderal): Intravenously, 0.01–0.15 mg/kg. Orally, 0.5 to 2 mg/kg/d every 6 hours. Larger doses may be necessary in thyrotoxicosis.

Propylthiouracil: 6–7 mg/kg/d in 3 divided doses at intervals of 8 hours. As maintenance, one-third to one-half of initial dose. (See also p 526.)

Prostaphlin: See Penicillins, p 110.

Prostigmin: See Neostigmine.

Protamine sulfate: 2.5–5 mg/kg; then 1–2.5 mg/kg intravenously. (Adult = 50 mg intravenously every 4–6 hours.)

Protopam: See Pralidoxime.

Pseudoephedrine hydrochloride (Sudafed; others): 4 mg/kg/d in 4 divided doses.

Purinethol: See Mercaptopurine.

Pyridostigmine (Mestinon): 7 mg/kg/d in 5–6 divided doses. Increase as necessary. (Adult = 600 mg/d.)

Pyrimethamine (Daraprim): See pp 659, 664.

Pyrrobutamine (Co-Pyronil): 0.6 mg/kg/d. (Adult = 15 mg 3–4 times daily.)

Pyrvinium pamoate (Povan): 5 mg/kg/d. (Adult = 5 mg/kg.)

Questran: See Cholestyramine.

Quinidine sulfate: As test dose, 2 mg/kg orally. If tolerated, give 3–6 mg/kg every 2–3 hours. (Adult = 200 mg.) Therapeutic dose, 30 mg/kg/d in 4–5 divided doses.

Regitine: See Phentolamine.

Reserpine (Serpasil; others): Orally, 0.005–0.03 mg/kg/d in 4 divided doses. Intramuscularly, 0.02–0.07 mg/kg every 12–24 hours. Initially, try smaller dose (except in life-threatening situations) and double in 4–6 hours if response is inadequate. May give with hydralazine. (Adult = 0.1–0.5 mg/d.)

Rifampin: See p 114.

Ritalin: See Methylphenidate.

Robaxin: See Methocarbamol.

Romilar: See Dextromethorphan hydrobromide.

Rondomycin: See Tetracyclines, p 116.

Scopolamine: 0.006 mg/kg as single dose orally or subcutaneously.

Secobarbital sodium (Seconal): Orally, 2–6 mg/kg as a single sedative or light hypnotic dose. (Adult = 100 mg.) Rectally, 6 mg/kg as a minimal hypnotic dose. (Adult = 200 mg.)

Seconal: See Secobarbital sodium.

Septra: See Trimethoprim with sulfamethoxazole, p 115.

Seromycin: See Cycloserine.

Serpasil: See Reserpine.

Sodium nitrite: 10 mg/kg for every 12 g/100 mL of hemoglobin. May repeat one-half dose in 30 minutes.

Sodium phosphate: 150–200 mg/kg orally. (Adult = 4–8 g.)

See Precautions, p 774.

Sodium polystyrene sulfonate (Kayexalate): For children, 1 mEq of potassium per gram of resin. Calculate dose on basis of desired exchange. Instill rectally in 10% glucose. May be administered every 6 hours. (Adult = 15 g orally 1–4 times daily in small amount of water or syrup [3–4 mL/g of resin].)
Sodium sulfate: 150–200 mg/kg orally as a 50% solution. (Adult = 8–12 g.)
Solu-Cortef: See Hydrocortisone, Table 22–6.
Spectinomycin (Trobicin): See p 114.
Spironolactone (Aldactone): For children, 1–3 mg/kg orally 2–4 times daily. (Adults = 25–100 mg 2–4 times daily.) Start with smaller dose. Caution.
Stanozolol (Winstrol): 0.1 mg/kg/d.
Staphicillin: See Penicillins, p 110.
Sterane: See Prednisolone, Table 22–6.
Stilbestrol: 0.1–1 mg/d. (Adult = 0.5–1 mg.)
Stoxil: See Idoxuridine.
Streptomycin sulfate: See p 114.
Sudafed: See Pseudoephedrine hydrochloride.
Sulfadiazine: See p 115.
Sulfamethoxazole (Gantanol; others): See p 115.
Sulfasalazine (Azulfidine; others): 50–100 mg/kg/d at 4- to 6-hour intervals. (Adult = 1 g 4–6 times daily.)
Sulfisoxazole (Gantrisin): See p 115.
Sulfonamides: See p 115.
Sus-Phrine: See Epinephrine.
Symmetrel: See Amantadine, p 118.
Synthroid: See Levothyroxine sodium.
Syntopressin: See Lypressin.
Tacaryl: See Methdilazine.
Tapazole: See Methimazole.
Teldrin: See Chlorpheniramine.
Tempra: See Acetaminophen.
Tensilon: See Edrophonium chloride.
Testosterone: (1) Testosterone enanthate (Delatestryl): 200 mg intramuscularly every 4 weeks for teenage males. (2) Testosterone cypionate: 50–200 mg intramuscularly every 2–4 weeks for teenage males. (3) Testosterone propionate in oil: 10–50 mg intramuscularly 2–6 times a week for adults or teenage males. (4) Testosterone microcrystals in aqueous suspension: 100 mg intramuscularly every 2–3 weeks. (5) Testosterone pellets: 300 mg every 3 months.
Tetrachlorethylene: See p 669.
Tetracyclines: See p 116.
Tetraethylammonium chloride: As test dose, 250 mg/m² intravenously. Caution: Phentolamine should be available. (Adult = 10–15 mg/kg intravenously or intramuscularly.)
Theophylline: Bioavailable preparation, 10–20 mg/kg/d orally every 6 hours. As therapeutic agent for asthma in older children, use 100% bioavailable preparation, 12–28 mg/kg/d. (Adult = 5–20 mg/kg/d.)

See Precautions, p 774.

Thiabendazole (Mintezol): 44 mg/kg/d (maximum, 3 g) in divided doses.

Thiamine hydrochloride: See Table 4–5 and p 62.

Thiopental sodium (Pentothal): 10–20 mg/kg rectally slowly for basal anesthesia.

Thioridazine (Mellaril): For children 2–12 years of age, 0.5–3 mg/kg/d; increase until maximum therapeutic effect is obtained. For older children, 20–40 mg/d. Not for children under 2 years of age. (Adult = 20–200 mg/d; for psychoses, 200–800 mg/d.)

Thorazine: See Chlorpromazine.

Ticarcillin: See p 113.

Tigan: See Trimethobenzamide.

Tobramycin (Nebcin): See p 116.

Tofranil: See Imipramine.

Tolazoline (Priscoline): Intravenously, 1 mg/kg/bolus, followed by 1 mg/kg/h continuous infusion. Caution: Hypotension. For children up to 5 years of age, 2–10 mg orally. For those over 5 years of age, 5–15 mg orally or intramuscularly. Increase by 2–10 mg every 4 hours as needed until flush or "goose pimples" appear. (Adult = 12.5 mg 3 times daily.)

Tolonium chloride: Initial dose, 2.5–7.5 mg/kg/d intravenously. Subsequent dose, 2–5 mg/kg/d intravenously. (Adult = 6–8 mg/kg.)

Tolserol: See Mephenesin.

Toluidine blue: See Tolonium chloride.

Trecator: See Ethionamide, p 105.

Triamcinolone (Aristocort, Kenacort, Kenalog): See Table 22–6.

Tribromoethanol: 65–100 mg/kg rectally, not to exceed 8 g. (Adult = 60 mg/kg.)

Trichlormethiazide: 0.03–0.1 mg/kg/d orally. (Adult = 2–8 mg/d.)

Tridione: See Trimethadione.

Triethylenemelamine (TEM): Initial dose, 5 mg/d orally. Subsequent dose, 1 mg/d or 0.04 mg/kg orally. (Adult = 5 mg; then 2.5 mg.) Caution.

Triiodothyronine (liothyronine; Cytomel): 25–30 μg is equivalent to 65 mg of thyroid, USP, or 0.1 mg of levothyroxine sodium.

Trimethadione (Tridione): 15–50 mg/kg/d orally. Start with smaller dose and increase gradually. (Adult = 0.3–2 g.) (See also Table 21–4.)

Trimethaphan camsylate (Arfonad): Adult = 1–15 mg/min intravenously.

Trimethobenzamide (Tigan): 15 mg/kg/d in divided doses. For children weighing under 15 kg, one-half suppository (100 mg) 3 times daily. For children over 15 kg, 100 mg orally 3 times daily or 100–200 mg rectally 3 times daily.

Trimethoprim with sulfamethoxazole (co-trimoxazole; Bactrim, Septra): See p 115.

Tripelennamine (PBZ): 3–5 mg/kg/d orally in 3–6 divided doses, not to exceed 300 mg/d. (Adult = 50 mg 4 times daily.)

Trisulfapyrimidines: See Sulfonamides, p 115.

Trobicin: See Spectinomycin, p 114.

Tubocurarine (curare): 0.2–0.4 mg/kg/d intramuscularly or subcutaneously. Caution. (Adult = 6–9 mg.)
Tylenol: See Acetaminophen.
Unipen: See Penicillins, p 110.
Urea: Orally, 0.8 g/kg/d in 3 divided doses. (Adult = 8 g.) Intravenously, 0.5–1.5 g/kg over a period of 30–60 minutes. (Adult = 1–1.5 g/kg.)
Urecholine: See Bethanechol chloride.
Valium: See Diazepam.
Vancocin: See Vancomycin, p 116.
Vancomycin (Vancocin): See p 116.
Vasopressin injection (Pitressin): 0.125–0.5 mL (20 units/mL) intramuscularly. Short duration. (Adult = 0.25–0.5 mL.)
Vasopressin tannate injection (Pitressin): 0.2–2 mL (5 units/mL in oil) intramuscularly every 2–4 days as needed. Start with smaller doses and increase. Effective 1–3 days. (Adult = 0.3–1 mL.) (See also Desmopressin.)
Vasoxyl: See Methoxamine hydrochloride.
Velban: See Vinblastine.
Vermox: See Mebendazole, p 108.
Versenate: See Calcium EDTA, p 482.
Vidarabine (adenine arabinoside): See p 119.
Vinblastine (Velban): 0.1–0.2 mg/kg/wk as single intravenous dose. (Adult = 0.1–0.15 mg/kg intravenously weekly.)
Vincristine (Oncovin): 0.05–0.15 mg/kg/wk as single intravenous dose. (Same as adult.) (See also Table 23–4.)
Viokase (pancreatic replacement): 0.3–0.6 g with each feeding. (Same as adult dose.)
Vitamin A: See Table 4–5 and p 59.
Vitamin C: See Ascorbic acid, Table 4–5 and p 64.
Vitamin D: See Table 4–5 and p 64.
Vitamin D_2: See Calciferol.
Vitamin K_1: See Phytonadione.
Winstrol: See Stanozolol.
Wyamine: See Mephentermine sulfate.
Wydase: See Hyaluronidase.
Xylocaine: See Lidocaine.
Yodoxin: See Iodoquinol.
Yomesan: See Niclosamide, p 671.
Zarontin: See Ethosuximide.
Zovirax: See Acyclovir, p 118.

NORMAL BLOOD CHEMISTRY VALUES & MISCELLANEOUS OTHER HEMATOLOGIC VALUES*†

(Values may vary with the procedure employed.)

Determinations for:
(S) = Serum
(B) = Whole blood
(Hb) = Hemoglobin
(P) = Plasma
(RBC) = Red blood cells

Acid-Base Measurements (B)
pH: 7.38–7.42 from 14 minutes of age and older.
Pa_{O_2}: 65–76 mm Hg (8.66–10.13 kPa).
Pa_{CO_2}: 36–38 mm Hg (4.80–5.07 kPa).
Base excess: −2 to +2 mEq/L, except in newborns (range, −4 to −0).

Acid Phosphatase (S, P)
Values using *p*-nitrophenyl phosphate buffered with citrate (end-point determination).
Newborns: 7.4–19.4 IU/L at 37 °C.
2–13 years: 6.4–15.2 IU/L at 37 °C.
Adult males: 0.5–11 IU/L at 37 °C.
Adult females: 0.2–9.5 IU/L at 37 °C.

ACTH: See Corticotropin.

Adenosine Triphosphate (RBC)
Premature infants: 5.66 μmol/g of hemoglobin.
Adults: 3.86 μmol/g of hemoglobin.

Alanine Aminotransferase (ALT, SGPT) (S)
Newborns (1–3 days): 1–25 IU/L at 37 °C.
Adult males: 7–46 IU/L at 37 °C.
Adult females: 4–35 IU/L at 37 °C.

Aldolase (S)
Newborns: 17.5–47.8 IU/L at 37 °C.
Children: 8.8–23.9 IU/L at 37 °C.
Adults: 4.4–12 IU/L at 37 °C.

Aldosterone (P)
First year: 25–140 ng/dL.
Second year: 9–25 ng/dL.

Alkaline Phosphatase (S)
(See Table, below.)

Ammonia (P)
Newborns: 90–150 μg/dL (53–88 μmol/L); higher in premature and jaundiced infants.
Thereafter: 0–60 μg/dL (0–35 μmol/L).

Alkaline phosphatase in serum.

Values at 37 °C using *p*-nitrophenyl phosphate buffered with AMP (kinetic).

Group	Males (IU/L)	Females (IU/L)
Newborns (1–3 days)	95–368	95–368
2–24 months	115–460	115–460
2–5 years	115–391	115–391
6–7 years	115–460	115–460
8–9 years	115–345	115–345
10–11 years	115–336	115–437
12–13 years	127–403	93–336
14–15 years	79–446	78–212
16–18 years	58–331	35–124
Adults	41–137	39–118

*Adapted from Meites S (editor): *Pediatric Clinical Chemistry,* 2nd ed. American Association for Clinical Chemistry, 1982, and many other sources.
†Revised with the assistance of Keith B. Hammond, MS.

Amylase (S)
Neonates: Undetectable.
2–12 months: Levels increase slowly to adult levels.
Adults: 28–108 IU/L at 37 °C.

Androstenedione (P)
(See Table, below.)

Antihemophilic Globulin (Factor VIII) (P)
Children: 82–157 units/dL.

α_1-Antitrypsin (S)
1–8 weeks: 127–404 mg/dL.
3–12 weeks: 145–362 mg/dL.
1–2 years: 160–382 mg/dL.
2–15 years: 148–394 mg/dL.

Ascorbic Acid: See Vitamin C.

Aspartate Aminotransferase (AST, SGOT) (S)
Newborns (1–3 days): 16–74 IU/L at 37 °C.
Adult males: 8–46 IU/L at 37 °C.
Adult females: 7–34 IU/L at 37 °C.

Base Excess: See Acid-Base Measurements.

Bicarbonate, Actual (P)
Calculated from pH and Pa_{CO_2}.
Newborns: 17.2–23.6 mmol/L.
2 months–2 years: 19–24 mmol/L.
Children: 18–25 mmol/L.
Adult males: 20.1–28.9 mmol/L.
Adult females: 18.4–28.8 mmol/L.

Bilirubin (S)
Levels after 1 month are as follows:
Conjugated: 0–0.3 mg/dL (0–5 μmol/L).
Unconjugated: 0.1–0.7 mg/dL (2–12 μmol/L).
For peak newborn levels, see Table (below).

Bleeding Time
1–3 minutes.

Androstenedione in plasma.

Group	Males ng/dL (nmol/L)	Females ng/dL (nmol/L)
Cord blood	31–139 (1.1–4.9)	17–186 (0.6–6.5)
1–3 months	12–56 (0.1–2.0)	11–27 (0.4–0.9)
3–5 months	3–54 (0.1–1.9)	3–31 (0.1–1.1)
5–7 months	3–31 (0.1–1.1)	4–24 (0.1–0.8)
7–12 months	3–22 (0.1–0.8)	... ...
Adults	57–157 (2.0–5.5)	75–227 (2.6–7.9)

Bilirubin in serum.

Peak Newborn Level mg/dL (μmol/L)	Percentage of Newborns (Birth Weight) Exceeding Peak Level		
	(< 2001 g)	(2001–2500 g)	(> 2500 g)
20 (342)	8.2%	2.6%	0.8%
18 (308)	13.5%	4.6%	1.5%
16 (274)	20.3%	7.6%	2.6%
14 (239)	33.0%	12.0%	4.4%
11 (188)	53.8%	23.0%	9.3%
8 (137)	77.0%	45.4%	26.1%

Blood Volume
Premature infants: 98 mL/kg.
At 1 year: 86 mL/kg (range, 69–112 mL/kg).
Older children: 70 mL/kg (range, 51–86 mL/kg).

BUN: See Urea Nitrogen.

C Peptide (S)
5–15 years (8:00 AM fasting): 1–4 ng/mL.
Adults (8:00 AM fasting): < 4 ng/mL.
Adults (nonfasting): < 8 ng/mL.

Calcium (S)
Premature infants (first week): 3.5–4.5 mEq/L (1.7–2.3 mmol/L).
Full-term infants (first week): 4–5 mEq/L (2–2.5 mmol/L).
Thereafter: 4.4–5.3 mEq/L (2.2–2.7 mmol/L).

Carbon Dioxide, Total (S, P)
Cord blood: 15–20.2 mmol/L.
Children: 18–27 mmol/L.
Adults: 24–35 mmol/L.

Carotene (S, P)
0–6 months: 0–40 μg/dL (0–0.75 μmol/L).
Children: 50–100 μg/dL (0.93–1.9 μmol/L).
Adults: 100–150 μg/dL (1.9–2.8 μmol/L).

Cation-Anion Gap (S, P)
5–15 mmol/L.

Ceruloplasmin (Copper Oxidase) (S, P)
21–43 mg/dL (1.3–2.7 μmol/L).

Chloride (S, P)
Premature infants: 95–110 mmol/L.
Full-term infants: 96–116 mmol/L.
Children: 98–105 mmol/L.
Adults: 98–108 mmol/L.

Cholesterol (S, P)
Premature cord blood: 47–98 mg/dL (1.2–2.5 mmol/L).
Full-term cord blood: 45–98 mg/dL (1.1–2.5 mmol/L).
Full-term newborns: 45–167 mg/dL (1.2–4.3 mmol/L).
3 days–1 year: 69–174 mg/dL (1.8–4.5 mmol/L).
2–14 years: 120–205 mg/dL (3.1–5.3 mmol/L).
14–19 years: 120–210 mg/dL (3.1–5.4 mmol/L).
20–29 years: 120–240 mg/dL (3.1–6.2 mmol/L).
30–39 years: 140–270 mg/dL (3.6–7 mmol/L).
40–49 years: 150–310 mg/dL (3.9–8 mmol/L).
50–59 years: 160–330 mg/dL (4.1–8.5 mmol/L).

Cholinesterase (S, RBC)
2.5–5 μmol/min/mL of serum (pseudocholinesterase).
2.3–4 μmol/min/mL of red cells.

Christmas Factor (Factor IX) (P)
Children: 100 ± 22 units/dL.

Circulation Time, Decholin
3–6 years: 8–12 seconds.
6–12 years: 7.5–15 seconds.
12–15 years: 10–16 seconds.

Circulation Time, Fluorescein
Upper limit of normal, based on weight.
10 kg: 8 seconds.
20 kg: 8.4 seconds.
40 kg: 11.3 seconds.

Coagulation Time (Test Tube Method)
3–9 minutes.

Complement (S)
C3: 96–195 mg/dL.
C4: 15–20 mg/dL.

Copper (S)
Cord blood: 26–32 μg/dL (4.1–5.2 μmol/L).
Newborns: 26–32 μg/dL (4.1–5.2 μmol/L).
1 month: 73–93 μg/dL (11.5–14.6 μmol/L).
2 months: 59–69 μg/dL (9.3–10.9 μmol/L).
6 months–5 years: 27–153 μg/dL (4.2–24.1 μmol/L).
5–17 years: 94–234 μg/dL (14.8–36.8 μmol/L).
Adults: 70–118 μg/dL (11–18.6 μmol/L).

Copper Oxidase: See Ceruloplasmin.

Corticotropin (ACTH) (P)
Morning (8:00 AM): 20–100 pg/mL (4.4–22 pmol/L).

Cortisol (S, P)
Morning (8:00 AM): 5–25 μg/dL (0.14–0.68 μmol/L).
Evening: 5–15 μg/dL (0.14–0.41 μmol/L).

Creatine (S, P)
0.2–0.8 mg/dL (15.2–61 μmol/L).

Creatine Kinase (S, P)
Newborns (1–3 days): 40–474 IU/L at 37 °C.
Adult males: 30–210 IU/L at 37 °C.
Adult females: 20–128 IU/L at 37 °C.

Creatinine (S, P)
(See Table, below.)

Creatinine in serum and plasma.

Group	Males mg/dL (μmol/L)	Females mg/dL (μmol/L)
Newborns (1–3 days)*	0.2–1.0 (17.7–88.4)	0.2–1.0 (17.7–88.4)
1 year	0.2–0.6 (17.7–53.0)	0.2–0.5 (17.7–44.2)
2–3 years	0.2–0.7 (17.7–61.9)	0.3–0.6 (26.5–53.0)
4–7 years	0.2–0.8 (17.7–70.7)	0.2–0.7 (17.7–61.9)
8–10 years	0.3–0.9 (26.5–79.6)	0.3–0.8 (26.5–70.7)
11–12 years	0.3–1.0 (26.5–88.4)	0.3–0.9 (26.5–79.6)
13–17 years	0.3–1.2 (26.5–106.1)	0.3–1.1 (26.5–97.2)
18–20 years	0.5–1.3 (44.2–115.0)	0.3–1.1 (26.5–97.2)

*Values may be higher in premature newborns.

Dehydroepiandrosterone sulfate in serum.

Group	Males μg/dL (μmol/L)	Females μg/dL (μmol/L)
Premature infants	223–303 (5.8–7.9)	223–303 (5.8–7.9)
Full-term infants	54–64 (1.4–1.7)	54–64 (1.4–1.7)
1–8 years	12–23 (0.3–0.6)	18–36 (0.5–0.9)
8–10 years	49–69 (1.3–1.8)	... ...
8–12 years	... ...	75–155 (2.0–4.1)
10–14 years	105–155 (2.7–4.1)	... ...
12–14 years	... ...	150–188 (3.9–4.9)
14–20 years	203–325 (5.3–8.5)	198–288 (5.2–7.5)

Creatinine Clearance
Values show great variability and depend on specificity of analytical methods used.
Newborns (1 day):
5–50 mL/min/1.73 m^2
(mean, 18 mL/min/1.73 m^2).
Newborns (6 days):
15–90 mL/min/1.73 m^2
(mean, 36 mL/min/1.73 m^2).
Adult males: 85–125 mL/min/1.73 m^2.
Adult females: 75–115 mL/min/1.73 m^2.

Dehydroepiandrosterone Sulfate (S)
(See Table, p 802.)

17β-Estradiol (P)
(See Table, below.)

Estrone (P)
(See Table, below.)

Factor: See Antihemophilic Globulin, Christmas Factor, Proaccelerin, and Prothrombin.

Fatty Acids, "Free" (P)
Newborns: 435–1375 μEq/L.
4 months–10 years (14-hour fast): 500–900 μEq/L.
4 months–10 years (19-hour fast): 730–1200 μEq/L.
Adults (14-hour fast): 310–590 μEq/L.
Adults (19-hour fast): 405–720 μEq/L.

Fatty Acids, Total Esterified (P, RBC)
(See Table, below.)

17β-Estradiol and estrone in plasma.

Group	17β-Estradiol		Estrone	
	Males (pg/mL)	Females (pg/mL)	Males (pg/mL)	Females (pg/mL)
0–8 years	2–4	1–10	7–20	11–20
Tanner I	2–6	7–14	10–20	16–20
Tanner II and III	2–16	24–126	15–51	23–91
Tanner IV and V	11–29	41–270	23–50	41–177
Adults				
Follicular	...	40–150	...	...
Luteal	...	100–400	...	...

Total esterified fatty acids in plasma and red blood cells.

Fatty Acid*	Plasma mg/dL	Plasma (% of Total)	Erythrocytes mg/dL	Erythrocytes (% of Total)
16:0	29.4–55.8	(20.7–28.3)	24.8–49.0	(18.5–28.3)
16:1	1.4–6.8	(1.1–2.5)	0.0–9.4	(0.0–4.9)
18:0	11.2–28.6	(6.9–16.1)	13.7–47.3	(13.1–26.5)
18:1	21.9–51.1	(16.9–24.5)	11.6–46.8	(12.7–23.3)
18:2	24.5–78.5	(19.5–39.1)	0.7–47.9	(6.1–22.1)
20:3	0.0–8.0	(0.0–4.9)	0.8–7.6	(0.8–4.4)
20:4	5.5–26.9	(3.2–15.6)	14.2–46.2	(12.5–26.3)

*Ratio of number of carbons to number of unsaturated bonds.

Ferritin (S)
Newborns: 20–200 ng/mL (mean, 117 ng/mL).
1 month: 60–550 ng/mL (mean, 350 ng/mL).
1–15 years: 7–140 ng/mL (mean, 31 ng/mL).
Adult males: 50–225 ng/mL (mean, 140 ng/mL).
Adult females: 10–150 ng/mL (mean, 40 ng/mL).

Fibrinogen (P)
200–500 mg/dL (5.9–14.7 μmol/L).

Folate (S)
Prepubertal children: Mean folic acid values are reported to be slightly higher than mean adult values but remain within the normal range.
Adults: 3–21 ng/mL.

Follicle-Stimulating Hormone (FSH) (S)
(See Table, below.)

FSH: See Follicle-Stimulating Hormone.

Galactose (S, P)
1.1–2.1 mg/dL (0.06–0.12 mmol/L).

Galactose 1-Phosphate (RBC)
Normal: 1 mg/dL of packed erythrocyte lysate; slightly higher in cord blood.
Infants with congenital galactosemia on a milk-free diet: < 2 mg/dL.
Infants with congenital galactosemia taking milk: 9–20 mg/dL.

Galactose-1-Phosphate Uridyl Transferase (RBC)
Normal: 308–475 ImU/g of hemoglobin.
Heterozygous for Duarte variant: 225–308 ImU/g of hemoglobin.
Homozygous for Duarte variant: 142–225 ImU/g of hemoglobin.
Heterozygous for congenital galactosemia: 142–225 ImU/g of hemoglobin.
Homozygous for congenital galactosemia: < 8 ImU/g of hemoglobin.

Gastrin (S)
Newborns (1–7 days): 20–300 pg/mL.
Children (8- to 12-hour overnight fast): < 10–125 pg/mL.
Adults (8- to 12-hour overnight fast): < 10–100 pg/mL.

Follicle-stimulating hormone in serum.

Values based on World Health Organization Human Pituitary Standard 69/104.

Group	Males (mIU/mL)	Females (mIU/mL)
Newborns (1–7 days)	<1–2.4	<1–2.4
2 weeks–1 year	<1–20	<1–31
Prepubertal children	<1–3.2	<1–5
Tanner II	2–7	1–6
Tanner III	2–8	1.5–9
Tanner IV	2–8	2–9
Tanner V	2–8	1–9
Adults	1–8	...
Follicular	...	1–9
Midcycle	...	4–30
Luteal	...	<1–7
Postmenopausal	...	20–160

GH: See Growth Hormone.

Glomerular Filtration Rate
Newborns: About 50% of values for older children and adults.
Older children and adults: 75–165 mL/min/1.73 m^2 (levels reached by about 6 months).

Glucose (S, P)
Premature infants: 20–80 mg/dL (1.11–4.44 mmol/L).
Full-term infants: 30–100 mg/dL (1.67–5.56 mmol/L).
Children and adults (fasting): 60–105 mg/dL (3.33–5.88 mmol/L).

Glucose-6-Phosphate Dehydrogenase (RBC)
150–215 units/dL.

Glucose Tolerance Test (S)
(See Table, p 806.)

γ-Glutamyl Transpeptidase (S)
0–1 month: 12–271 IU/L at 37 °C (kinetic).
1–2 months: 9–159 IU/L at 37 °C (kinetic).
2–4 months: 7–98 IU/L at 37 °C (kinetic).
4–7 months: 5–45 IU/L at 37 °C (kinetic).
7–12 months: 4–27 IU/L at 37 °C (kinetic).
1–15 years: 3–30 IU/L at 37 °C (kinetic).
Adult males: 9–69 IU/L at 37 °C (kinetic).
Adult females: 3–33 IU/L at 37 °C (kinetic).

Glycogen (RBC)
Cord blood: 10–338 μg/g of hemoglobin.
4½–19 hours: 48–361 μg/g of hemoglobin.
2–12 months: 32–134 μg/g of hemoglobin.
1–12 years: 22–109 μg/g of hemoglobin.
Adults: 20–105 μg/g of hemoglobin.

Glycohemoglobin (Hemoglobin A_{1c}) (B)
Normal: 6.3–8.2% of total hemoglobin.
Diabetic patients in good control of their condition ordinarily have levels < 10%.
Values tend to be lower during pregnancy.

Growth Hormone (GH) (S)
After infancy (fasting specimen): 0–5 ng/mL.
In response to natural and artificial provocation (eg, sleep, arginine, insulin, hypoglycemia): > 8 ng/mL.
During the newborn period (fasting specimen): GH levels are high (15–40 ng/mL) and responses to provocation variable.

Haptoglobin (S)
50–150 mg/dL as hemoglobin-binding capacity.

Hematocrit (B)
At birth: 44–64%.
14–90 days: 35–49%.
6 months–1 year: 30–40%.
4–10 years: 31–43%.

Hemoglobin (P)
No more than 0.5 mg/dL (0.3 μmol/L).

Hemoglobin A_{1c}: See Glycohemoglobin.

Hemoglobin Electrophoresis (Hb)
A_1 hemoglobin: 96–98.5% of total hemoglobin.
A_2 hemoglobin: 1.5–4% of total hemoglobin.

Hemoglobin, Fetal (B)
At Birth: 50–85% of total hemoglobin.
At 1 year: < 15% of total hemoglobin.
Up to 2 years: Up to 5% of total hemoglobin.
Thereafter: <2% of total hemoglobin.

17-Hydroxyprogesterone: See Progesterone.

Immunoglobulins (S)
(See Table, below.)

Insulin: See Glucose Tolerance Test and Table (below).

Inulin Clearance
< 1 month: 29–88 mL/min/1.73 m^2.
1–6 months: 40–112 mL/min/1.73 m^2.
6–12 months: 62–121 mL/min/1.73 m^2.
1 year: 78–164 mL/min/1.73 m^2.

Iron (S, P)
Newborns: 20–157 μg/dL (3.6–28.1 μmol/L).
6 weeks–3 years: 20–115 μg/dL (3.6–20.6 μmol/L).

Iron (cont'd)
3–9 years: 20–141 μg/dL (3.6–25.2 μmol/L).
9–14 years: 21–151 μg/dL (3.8–27 μmol/L).
14–16 years: 20–181 μg/dL (3.6–32.4 μmol/L).
Adults: 40–175 μg/dL (7.2–31.3 μmol/L).

Iron-Binding Capacity (S, P)
Newborns: 59–175 μg/dL (10.6–31.3 μmol/L).
Children and adults: 250–400 μg/dL (45–72 μmol/L).

Immunoglobulins in serum.

Group	IgG (mg/dL)	IgA (mg/dL)	IgM (mg/dL)
Cord blood	766–1693	0.04–9	4–26
2 weeks–3 months	299–852	3–66	15–149
3–6 months	142–988	4–90	18–118
6–12 months	418–1142	14–95	43–223
1–2 years	356–1204	13–118	37–239
2–3 years	492–1269	23–137	49–204
3–6 years	564–1381	35–209	51–214
6–9 years	658–1535	29–384	50–228
9–12 years	625–1598	60–294	64–278
12–16 years	660–1548	81–252	45–256

Glucose tolerance test results in serum.

Normal levels based on results in 13 normal children given glucose, 1.75 g/kg orally in one dose, after 2 weeks on a high-carbohydrate diet.

Time	Glucose		Insulin		Phosphorus	
	mg/dL	(mmol/L)	μU/mL	(pmol/L)	mg/dL	(mmol/L)
Fasting	59–96	(3.11–5.33)	5–40	(36–287)	3.2–4.9	(1.03–1.58)
30 minutes	91–185	(5.05–10.27)	36–110	(258–789)	2.0–4.4	(0.64–1.42)
60 minutes	66–164	(3.66–9.10)	22–124	(158–890)	1.8–3.6	(0.58–1.16)
90 minutes	68–148	(3.77–8.22)	17–105	(122–753)	1.8–3.6	(0.58–1.16)
2 hours	66–122	(3.66–6.77)	6–84	(43–603)	1.8–4.2	(0.58–1.36)
3 hours	47–99	(2.61–5.49)	2–46	(14–330)	2.0–4.6	(0.64–1.48)
4 hours	61–93	(3.39–5.16)	3–32	(21–230)	2.7–4.3	(0.87–1.39)
5 hours	63–86	(3.50–4.77)	5–37	(36–265)	2.9–4.4	(0.94–1.42)

Lactate (B)
Venous blood: 5–18 mg/dL (0.5–2 mmol/L).
Arterial blood: 3–7 mg/dL (0.3–0.8 mmol/L).

Lactate Dehydrogenase (LDH) (S, P)
Values using lactate substrate (kinetic).
Newborns (1–3 days): 30–348 IU/L at 37 °C.
1 month–5 years: 150–360 IU/L at 37 °C.
5–8 years: 150–300 IU/L at 37 °C.
8–12 years: 130–300 IU/L at 37 °C.
12–14 years: 130–280 IU/L at 37 °C.
14–16 years: 130–230 IU/L at 37 °C.
Adult males: 70–178 IU/L at 37 °C.
Adult females: 42–166 IU/L at 37 °C.

LATS: See Long-Acting Thyroid Stimulator.

LDH: See Lactate Dehydrogenase.

Lead (B)
< 30 μg/dL (< 1.4 μmol/L).

Leucine Aminopeptidase (S, P)
Newborns: 29–59 IU/L.
1 month–adults: 15–50 IU/L.

LH: See Luteinizing Hormone.

Lipase (S, P)
20–136 IU/L based on 4-hour incubation.

Lipoprotein Cholesterol (P)
Fasting levels for lipoprotein cholesterol in children 4–17 years:
High-density lipoprotein (HDL) cholesterol: 37–73 mg/dL.
Low-density lipoprotein (LDL) cholesterol: 66–145 mg/dL.
Very low density lipoprotein (VLDL) cholesterol: 6–15 mg/dL.

Lipoprotein Cholesterol, High-Density (HDL) (S)
(See Table, below.)

Long-Acting Thyroid Stimulator (LATS) (S)
None detectable.

Luteinizing Hormone (LH) (S)
(See Table, p 808.)

Magnesium (RBC)
3.92–5.28 mEq/L (1.96–2.64 mmol/L).

Magnesium (S, P)
Newborns: 1.5–2.3 mEq/L (0.75–1.15 mmol/L).
Adults: 1.4–2 mEq/L (0.7–1 mmol/L).

Manganese (S)
Newborns: 2.4–9.6 μg/dL (2.44–1.75 μmol/L).
2–18 years: 0.8–2.1 μg/dL (0.15–0.38 μmol/L).

Methemoglobin (B)
0–0.3 g/dL (0–186 μmol/L).

High-density lipoprotein cholesterol in serum.

Group	Males mg/dL (mmol/L)	Females mg/dL (mmol/L)
6–7 years	24–78 (0.62–2.02)	31–67 (0.80–1.73)
8–9 years	36–76 (0.93–1.97)	31–75 (0.80–1.94)
10–11 years	36–76 (0.93–1.97)	31–71 (0.80–1.94)
12–13 years	25–85 (0.65–2.20)	38–78 (0.98–2.09)
14–15 years	28–68 (0.72–1.76)	30–70 (0.78–1.81)
16–17 years	28–68 (0.72–1.76)	31–79 (0.80–2.04)

Mucoprotein, Tyrosine (S)
2.5–3.5 mg/dL.

Osmolality (S, P)
270–290 mosm/kg.

Oxygen Capacity (B)
1.34 mL/g of hemoglobin.

Oxygen Saturation (B)
Newborns: 30–80% (0.3–0.8 mol/mol of venous blood).
Thereafter: 65–85% (0.65–0.85 mol/mol of venous blood).

Pa_{CO_2}: See Acid-Base Measurements.

Pa_{O_2}: See Acid-Base Measurements.

Partial Thromboplastin Time (P)
Children: 42–54 seconds.

pH: See Acid-Base Measurements.

Phenylalanine (S, P)
0.7–3.5 mg/dL (0.04–0.21 mmol/L).

Phosphatase: See Acid Phosphatase and Alkaline Phosphatase.

Phospholipid (S)
Cord blood: 48–160 mg/dL (0.62–2.07 mmol/L).
2–13 years: 166–247 mg/dL (2.14–3.19 mmol/L).
13–20 years: 193–338 mg/dL (2.49–4.37 mmol/L).

Phosphorus, Inorganic (S, P)
Premature infants:
At birth: 5.6–8 mg/dL (1.81–2.58 mmol/L).
6–10 days: 6.1–11.7 mg/dL (1.97–3.78 mmol/L).
20–25 days: 6.6–9.4 mg/dL (2.13–3.04 mmol/L).
Full-term infants:
At birth: 5–7.8 mg/dL (1.61–2.52 mmol/L).
3 days: 5.8–9 mg/dL (1.87–2.91 mmol/L).
6–12 days: 4.9–8.9 mg/dL (1.58–2.87 mmol/L).
Children:
1 year: 3.8–6.2 mg/dL (1.23–2 mmol/L).
10 years: 3.6–5.6 mg/dL (1.16–1.81 mmol/L).
Adults: 3.1–5.1 mg/dL (1–1.65 mmol/L).
(See also under Glucose Tolerance Test.)

Luteinizing hormone in serum.

Values based on World Health Organization Human Pituitary Standard 68/40.

Group	Males (mIU/mL)	Females (mIU/mL)
Newborns (1–7 days)	1.5–3	1.5–3
2 weeks–1 year	3.5–25	2.1–14
Prepubertal children	< 1–4	< 1–4
Tanner II	< 1–5	< 1–5
Tanner III	2–10	< 1–10
Tanner IV	2–10	3–11
Tanner V	4.5–11	2–12
Adults	3–10	...
Follicular	...	3–11
Midcycle	...	18–70
Luteal	...	2–11
Postmenopausal	...	25–70

Potassium (RBC)
87.2–97.6 mmol/L.

Potassium (S, P)
Premature infants: 4.5–7.2 mmol/L.
Full-term infants: 3.7–5.2 mmol/L.
Children: 3.5–5.8 mmol/L.
Adults: 3.5–5.5 mmol/L.

Proaccelerin (Factor V) (P)
Children: 61–127 units/dL.

Progesterone (S)
Cord blood: 8,000–56,000 ng/dL.
Newborns (1–7 days): Levels are markedly elevated in the neonate but fall rapidly to reach prepubertal levels by 7 days, where they remain until puberty.
For levels in children over 1 year of age and levels in adults, see Table (below).

Progesterone (17-Hydroxyprogesterone) (S)
Cord blood: 900–5,000 ng/dL.
Newborns (1–7 days): Levels decrease rapidly during the first week to reach 60–150 ng/dL by 7 days.
Males (1–12 months): Levels increase after the first week to peak values (120–200 ng/dL) between 30 and 60 days. Values then decline gradually to reach prepubertal levels by 1 year.

Progesterone (17-Hydroxyprogesterone) (cont'd)
Females (1–12 months): Levels gradually decrease during the first 12 months to reach prepubertal levels.
For levels in children over 1 year of age and levels in adults, see Table (below).

Prolactin (S)
Cord blood: 61–590 ng/mL.
Newborns (1–7 days): 30–495 ng/mL.
1–8 weeks: Levels decline during the first 2 months of life to levels observed in prepubertal and pubertal children and adults.
Male children and adults: 3–18 ng/mL.
Female children and adults: 3–24 ng/mL.

Prostaglandin E (P)
Newborns: 1000–1730 pg/mL.
2–3 days: 60–150 pg/mL.
1–6 years: 125–200 pg/mL.
6–14 years: 160–340 pg/mL.
Adults: 450–550 pg/mL.

Proteins (S)
(See Table, p 810.)

Prothrombin (Factor II) (P)
Children: 81–123 units/dL.

Prothrombin Time (P)
Children: 11–15 seconds.

Progesterone and 17-hydroxyprogesterone in serum.

Group	Progesterone		17-Hydroxyprogesterone	
	Males (ng/dL)	Females (ng/dL)	Males (ng/dL)	Females (ng/dL)
Prepubertal children (1–10 years)	7–33	7–33	3–90	3–82
Tanner II	< 10–33	< 10–55	5–115	11–98
Tanner III	< 10–48	10–450	10–138	11–155
Tanner IV	10–108	< 10–1300	29–180	18–230
Tanner V	21–82	< 10–950	24–175	20–265
Adults	13–97	...	27–199	...
Follicular	...	15–70	...	15–70
Luteal	...	200–2500	...	35–290

Protoporphyrin, "Free" (FEP, ZPP) (B)
Values for free erythrocyte protoporphyrin (FEP) and zinc protoporphyrin (ZPP) are 1.2–2.7 μg/g of hemoglobin.

Pseudocholinesterase (S)
2.5–5 μmol/min/mL.

Pyruvate (B)
Resting adult males (arterial blood): 50.5–60.1 μmol/L.
Adult (venous blood): 34–102 μmol/L.

Pyruvate Kinase (RBC)
7.4–15.7 units/g of hemoglobin.

Renin Activity (P)
3–6 days: 8–14 ng/mL/h.
0–3 years: 3–6 ng/mL/h.
Children: 1.3–2.6 ng/mL/h.

Sedimentation Rate (Micro) (B)
<2 years: 1–5 mm/h.
>2 years: 1–8 mm/h.

Serotonin (S, P)
Children: 127–187 ng/mL.
Adults: 119–171 ng/mL.

SGOT: See Aspartate Aminotransferase.

SGPT: See Alanine Aminotransferase.

Sodium (S, P)
Children and adults: 135–148 mmol/L.

Somatomedin C (S)
Newborns: 0.17–0.62 U/mL.
1–5 years: 0.14–0.94 U/mL.
6–12 years: 0.87–2.06 U/mL.
13–17 years: 1.35–3 U/mL.
Adults: 0.61–2.04 U/mL.

Sugar: See Glucose.

T_3: See Triiodothyronine.

T_4: See Thyroxine.

TBG: See Thyroxine-Binding Globulin.

Testosterone (S)
Males:
Newborns: 75–400 ng/dL.
1–7 months: Levels decrease rapidly the first week to 20–50 ng/dL and then increase to 60–400 ng/dL between 60 and 80 days. Levels then decline gradually to the prepubertal range by 7 months.
Females:
Newborns: 20–64 ng/dL.
1–7 months: Levels decrease during the first month to < 10 ng/dL and remain there until puberty.
For levels in children over 1 year of age and levels in adults, see Table (p 811).

Thrombin Time (P)
Children: 12–16 seconds.

Proteins in serum.

Values are for cellulose acetate electrophoresis and are in g/dL. SI conversion factor: g/dL × 10 = g/L.

Group	Total Protein	Albumin	α-Globulin	α_2-Globulin	β-Globulin	γ-Globulin
At birth	4.6–7.0	3.2–4.8	0.1–0.3	0.2–0.3	0.3–0.6	0.6–1.2
3 months	4.5–6.5	3.2–4.8	0.1–0.3	0.3–0.7	0.3–0.7	0.2–0.7
1 year	5.4–7.5	3.7–5.7	0.1–0.3	0.5–1.1	0.4–1.0	0.2–0.9
>4 years	5.9–8.0	3.8–5.4	0.1–0.3	0.4–0.8	0.5–1.0	0.4–1.3

Thyroid-Stimulating Hormone (TSH) (S)
Levels increase shortly after birth to levels as high as 30–40 μIU/mL. Levels return to the adult normal range (1.6–10.9 μIU/mL) by about 10–14 days.

Thyroxine (T_4) (S)
1–2 days: 11.4–25.5 μg/dL (147–328 nmol/L).
3–4 days: 9.8–25.2 μg/dL (126–324 nmol/L).
1–6 years: 5–15.2 μg/dL (64–196 nmol/L).
11–13 years: 4–13 μg/dL (51–167 nmol/L).
> 18 years: 4.7–11 μg/dL (60–142 nmol/L).

Thyroxine, "Free" (Free T_4) (S)
1–2.3 ng/dL.

Thyroxine-Binding Globulin (TBG) (S)
1–7 months: 2.9–6 mg/dL.
7–12 months: 2.1–5.9 mg/dL.
Prepubertal children: 2–5.3 mg/dL.
Pubertal children and adults: 1.8–4.2 mg/dL.

α-Tocopherol: See Vitamin E.

Transaminase: See Alanine Aminotransferase and Aspartate Aminotransferase.

Triglycerides (S, P)
< 19 years (12- to 14-hour fast): 10–130 mg/dL (0.11–1.47 mmol/L).
20–29 years (12- to 14-hour fast): 10–140 mg/dL (0.11–1.58 mmol/L).
30–39 years (12- to 14-hour fast): 10–150 mg/dL (0.11–1.69 mmol/L).
40–49 years (12- to 14-hour fast): 10–160 mg/dL (0.11–1.81 mmol/L).
50–59 years (12- to 14-hour fast): 10–190 mg/dL (0.11–2.14 mmol/L).

Triiodothyronine (T_3) (S)
1–3 days: 89–405 ng/dL.
1 week: 91–300 ng/dL.
1–12 months: 85–250 ng/dL.
Prepubertal children: 119–218 ng/dL.
Pubertal children and adults: 55–170 ng/dL.

Trypsinogen, Immunoreactive (S, P)
Newborns: 5–97 ng/mL.
99.5th percentile: 136 ng/mL.
99.8th percentile: 162 ng/mL.

TSH: See Thyroid-Stimulating Hormone.

Testosterone in serum.

Group	Males (ng/dL)	Females (ng/dL)
Prepubertal children	3–10	<3–10
Tanner II	18–150	7–28
Tanner III	100–320	15–35
Tanner IV	200–620	13–32
Tanner V	350–970	20–38
Adults	350–1030	10–55

Tyrosine (S, P)
Premature infants: 3–30.2 mg/dL (0.17–1.67 mmol/L).
Full-term infants: 1.7–4.7 mg/dL (0.09–0.26 mmol/L).
1–12 years: 1.4–3.4 mg/dL (0.08–0.19 mmol/L).
Adults: 0.6–1.6 mg/dL (0.03–0.09 mmol/L).

Tyrosine Mucoprotein: See Mucoprotein.

Urea Clearance
Premature infants: 3.5–17.3 mL/min/1.73 m^2.
Newborns: 8.7–33 mL/min/1.73 m^2.
2–12 months: 40–95 mL/min/1.73 m^2.
$\geqslant$2 years: > 52 mL/min/1.73 m^2.

Urea Nitrogen (S, P)
1–2 years: 5–15 mg/dL (1.8–5.4 mmol/L).
Thereafter: 10–20 mg/dL (3.5–7.1 mmol/L).

Uric Acid (S, P)
Males:
0–14 years: 2–7 mg/dL (119–416 μmol/L).
> 14 years: 3–8 mg/dL (178–476 μmol/L).
Females:
0–14 years: 2–7 mg/dL (119–416 μmol/L).
> 14 years: 2–7 mg/dL (119–416 μmol/L).

Vitamin A (S, P)
Values of < 20 μg/dL (0.7 μmol/L) should be considered abnormally low.

Vitamin B_{12} (S, P)
330–1025 pg/mL (243–756 pmol/L).

Vitamin C (Ascorbic Acid) (S, P)
Plasma: 0.2–2 mg/dL (11–114 μmol/L).

Vitamin D (S)
1,25-Dihydroxycholecalciferol: 25–49 pg/mL.
25-Hydroxycholecalciferol: 26–31 ng/mL.

Vitamin E (α-Tocopherol) (S, P)
Premature infants: 0.05–0.35 mg/dL (1.2–8.4 μmol/L).
Full-term infants: 0.10–0.35 mg/dL (2.4–8.4 μmol/L).
2–5 months: 0.2–0.6 mg/dL (4.8–14.4 μmol/L).
6–24 months: 0.35–0.8 mg/dL (8.4–19.2 μmol/L).
2–12 years: 0.55–0.9 mg/dL (13.2–21.6 μmol/L).
Breast-fed infants: 0.6–1.1 mg/dL (14.4–26.4 μmol/L).

Volume (B)
Premature infants: 98 mL/kg (mean).
Full-term infants: 75–100 mL/kg.
1 year: 69–112 mL/kg (mean, 86 mL/kg).
Older children: 51–86 mL/kg (mean, 70 mL/kg).

Volume (P)
Full-term neonates: 39–77 mL/kg.
Infants: 40–50 mL/kg.
Older children: 30–54 mL/kg.

Water (B, S, RBC)
Whole blood: 79–81 g/dL.
Serum: 91–92 g/dL.
Red blood cells: 64–65 g/dL.

Xylose Absorption Test (B)
Following a 5-g loading dose, the laboratory will report the D-xylose concentration of the baseline and 60-minute samples in mg/dL. The difference between these 2 values should be corrected to a constant surface area of 1.73 m^2 according to the formula shown below.

$$\text{Corrected blood value} = \frac{(\text{Value}_{60\ min} - \text{Value}_{baseline}) \times \text{Actual surface area}}{1.73}$$

Xylose Absorption Test (cont'd)
The actual surface area can be derived from a number of available nomograms using the patient's weight and height.
Normal corrected blood values: 9.8–20 mg/dL.
Effect of age and sex: No significant differences between males and females. No significant differences in ages 14–92.

Zinc (S)
Males: 83–88 μg/dL (12.7–13.5 μmol/L).
Females: 85–91 μg/dL (13–13.9 μmol/L).
Females taking oral contraceptives: 86–93 μg/dL (13.2–14.2 μmol/L).
At 16 weeks of gestation: 66–70 μg/dL (10.1–10.7 μmol/L).
At 38 weeks of gestation: 54–58 μg/dL (8.3–8.9 μmol/L).

NORMAL VALUES: URINE, BONE MARROW, DUODENAL FLUID, FECES, SWEAT, & MISCELLANEOUS*†

URINE

Acidity, Titratable
20–50 mEq/d.

Addis Count
Red cells (12-hour specimen): < 1 million.
White cells (12-hour specimen): < 2 million.
Casts (12-hour specimen): < 10,000.
Protein (12-hour specimen): < 55 mg.

Albumin
First month: 1–100 mg/L.
Second month: 0.2–34 mg/L.
2–12 months: 0.5–19 mg/L.

Aldosterone
Newborns: 0.5–5 μg/24 h (20–140 μg/g of creatinine).
Prepubertal children: 1–8 μg/24 h (4–22 μg/g of creatinine).
Adults: 3–19 μg/24 h (1.5–20 μg/g of creatinine).

δ-Aminolevulinic Acid: See Porphyrins.

Ammonia
2–12 months: 4–20 μEq/min/m².
6–16 years: 4–16 μEq/min/m².

Calcium
4–12 years: 4–8 mEq/L (2–4 mmol/L).

Catecholamines (Norepinephrine, Epinephrine)
(See Table, p 814.)

Chloride
Infants: 1.7–8.5 mmol/24 h.
Children: 17–34 mmol/24 h.
Adults: 140–240 mmol/24 h.

Copper
0–30 μg/24 h.

Coproporphyrin: See Porphyrins.

*Adapted from Meites S (editor): *Pediatric Clinical Chemistry,* 2nd ed. American Association for Clinical Chemistry, 1982, and many other sources.
†Revised with the assistance of Keith B. Hammond, MS.

Corticosteroids (17-Hydroxycorticosteroids)
0–2 years: 2–4 mg/24 h (5.5–11 μmol).
2–6 years: 3–6 mg/24 h (8.3–16.6 μmol).
6–10 years: 6–8 mg/24 h (16.6–22.1 μmol).
10–14 years: 8–10 mg/24 h (22.1–27.6 μmol).

Creatine
18–58 mg/L (1.37–4.42 mmol/L).

Creatinine
Newborns: 7–10 mg/kg/24 h.
Children: 20–30 mg/kg/24 h.
Adult males: 21–26 mg/kg/24 h.
Adult females: 16–22 mg/kg/24 h.

Epinephrine: See Catecholamines.

Follicle-Stimulating Hormone (FSH)
(See Table, below.)

FSH: See Follicle-Stimulating Hormone.

Homovanillic Acid
Children: 3–16 μg/mg of creatinine.
Adults: 2–4 μg/mg of creatinine.

17-Hydroxycorticosteroids: See Corticosteroids.

5-Hydroxyindoleacetic Acid
0.11–0.61 μmol/kg/7 h, based on results in 15 well-nourished, apparently healthy, mentally defective children on a tryptophan load.

Hydroxyproline, Total
5–14 years: 38–126 mg/24 h (290–961 μmol/24 h).

17-Ketosteroids
(See Table, p 815.)

Luteinizing Hormone (LH)
(See Table, below.)

Catecholamines in urine.

Group	Total Catecholamines μg/24 h	Norepinephrine μg/24 h (nmol/24 h)	Epinephrine μg/24 h (nmol/24 h)
< 1 year	20	5.4–15.9 (32–94)	0.1–4.3 (0.5–23.5)
1–5 years	40	8.1–30.8 (48–182)	0.8–9.1 (4.4–49.7)
6–15 years	80	19.0–71.1 (112–421)	1.3–10.5 (7.1–57.3)
> 15 years	100	34.4–87.0 (203–514)	3.5–13.2 (19.1–72.1)

Follicle-stimulating hormone and luteinizing hormone in urine.

Group	Follicle-Stimulating Hormone		Luteinizing Hormone	
	Males (IU/24 h)	Females (IU/24 h)	Males (IU/24 h)	Females (IU/24 h)
Prepubertal children	< 1–3.3	< 1–3.4	< 1–5.6	1.4–4.9
Tanner II	1–7	2–6	1.5–11	3–10
Tanner III	2–9	3–8	2.5–13	5–18
Tanner IV	2–10	3–9	5–16	6–21
Tanner V	3–12	2–11	4–28	5–24
Adults	3–11	2–15	9–23	4–30

Mercury
< 50 μg/24 h (249 nmol/24 h).

Metanephrine & Normetanephrine
< 2 years: < 4.6 μg/mg of creatinine (23.3 nmol).
2–10 years: < 3 μg/mg of creatinine (15.2 nmol).
10–15 years: < 2 μg/mg of creatinine (10.3 nmol).
> 15 years: < 1 μg/mg of creatinine (5.1 nmol).

Mucopolysaccharides
Acid mucopolysaccharide screen should yield negative results. Positive results after dialysis of the urine should be followed up with a thin-layer chromatogram for evaluation of the acid mucopolysaccharide excretion pattern.

Norepinephrine: See Catecholamines.

Normetanephrine: See Metanephrine and Normetanephrine.

Osmolality
Infants: 50–600 mosm/kg.
Older children: 50–1400 mosm/kg.

Phosphorus, Tubular Reabsorption
78–97%.

Porphobilinogen: See Porphyrins.

Porphyrins
δ-Aminolevulinic acid: 0–7 mg/24 h (0–53.4 μmol/24 h).
Porphobilinogen: 0–2 mg/24 h (0–8.8 μmol/24 h).
Coproporphyrin: 0–160 μg/24 h (0–244 nmol/24 h).
Uroporphyrin: 0–26 μg/24 h (0–31 nmol/24 h).

Potassium
26–123 mmol/L.

Pregnanetriol
2 weeks–2 years: 0–0.2 mg/24 h (0–0.59 μmol/24 h).
2–16 years: 0.3–1.1 mg/24 h (0.89–3.27 μmol/24 h).

Sodium
Infants: 0.3–3.5 mmol/24 h (6–10 mmol/m^2).
Children and adults: 5.6–17 mmol/24 h.

Testosterone
Prepubertal children: 0.2–2.3 μg/24 h (0.3–5 μg/g of creatinine).
Adult males: 40–130 μg/24 h.
Adult females: 2–11 μg/24 h.

Urobilinogen
< 3 mg/24 h (< 5.1 μmol/24 h).

Uroporphyrin: See Porphyrins.

17-Ketosteroids in urine.

Group	Males mg/24 h (μmol/24 h)	Females mg/24 h (μmol/24 h)
0–14 days	0.5–2.5 (1.7–8.7)	0.5–2.5 (1.7–8.7)
2 weeks–2 years	0.0–0.5 (0.0–1.7)	0.0–0.5 (0.0–1.7)
2–6 years	0.0–2.0 (0.0–6.9)	0.0–2.0 (0.0–6.9)
6–8 years	0.0–2.5 (0.0–8.7)	0.0–2.5 (0.0–8.7)
8–10 years	0.7–4.0 (2.4–13.9)	0.7–4.0 (2.4–13.9)

Vanilmandelic Acid (VMA)

Because of the difficulty in obtaining an accurately timed 24-hour collection, values based on microgram per milligram of creatinine are the most reliable indications of VMA excretion in young children.

1–12 months: 1–35 μg/mg of creatinine (31–135 μg/kg/24 h).

1–2 years: 1–30 μg/mg of creatinine.

2–5 years: 1–15 μg/mg of creatinine.

5–10 years: 1–14 μg/mg of creatinine.

10–15 years: 1–10 μg/mg of creatinine.

Adults: 1–7 μg/mg of creatinine (1–7 mg/24 h; 5–35 μmol/24 h).

VMA: See Vanilmandelic Acid.

Xylose Absorption Test

Mean 5-hour excretion expressed as percentage of ingested load.

<6 months: 11–30%.

6–12 months: 20–32%.

1–3 years: 20–42%.

3–10 years: 25–45%.

>10 years: 25–50%.

Or: % excretion >(0.2 × age in months) + 12.

BONE MARROW CYTOLOGY

Eosinophils (all stages): 1–10%.

Lymphocytes: 5–45%.

Metamyelocytes: 7–30%.

Monocytes: 0–7%.

Myeloblasts: 0–4%.

Myelocytes: 7–25%.

Normoblasts: 4–35%.

Polymorphonuclear leukocytes (PMNs): 5–30%.

Promyelocytes: 0–6%.

Pronormoblasts: 0–8%.

Other cells: Occasionally seen.

DUODENAL FLUID VALUES

Enzymes

Amylase: (Anderson).

0–2 months: 0–10 units/mL.

2–6 months: 10–20 units/mL.

6–12 months: 40–150 units/mL.

1–2 years: 100–225 units/mL.

2–5 years:125–275 units/mL.

Carboxypeptidase:

0.4–1 unit (Ravin).

Chymotrypsin:

11–65 units (Ravin).

Protease:

18–70 units (Free-Meyers).

Trypsin: (Anderson or as noted).

0–2 months: 110–160 units/mL.

2–6 months: 115–160 units/mL.

6–12 months: 120–290 units/mL; 3–10 units (Nothman et al).

1–2 years: 200–300 units/mL.

2–5 years: 200–275 units/mL.

pH

6–8.4

Viscosity

<3 minutes (Shwachman).

FECES

Chymotrypsin

3–14 mg/72 h/kg.

Fat, Percentage of Dry Weight

2–6 months: 5–43%.

6 months–6 years: 6–26%.

Fat, Total

2–6 months: 0.3–1.3 g/d.

<1 year: <4 g/d.

Children: <3 g/d.

Adolescents: <5 g/d.

Adults: <7 g/d.

Lipids, Split Fat

Adults: >40% of total lipids.

Lipids, Total

Adults: Up to 7 g/d on normal diet, 10–27% of dry weight.

Nitrogen
Infants: < 1 g/d.
Children: < 1.2 g/d.
Adults: < 3 g/d.

Urobilinogen
2–12 months: 0.03–14 mg/d.
5–10 years: 2.7–39 mg/d.
10–14 years: 7.3–99 mg/d.

SWEAT

Electrolytes
Values for sodium or chloride or both. Elevated values in the presence of a family history or clinical findings of cystic fibrosis are diagnostic of cystic fibrosis.
Normal: < 55 mmol/L.
Borderline: 55–70 mmol/L.
Elevated: > 70 mmol/L.

MISCELLANEOUS

Amylo-1,6-Glucosidase Debrancher (Liver)
> 1 μmol/min/g of wet tissue.

Chloride
Breast milk: 2.5–30 mmol/L.
Cow's milk: 20–80 mmol/L.
Muscle: 20–26 mmol/kg of wet fat-free tissue.
Spinal fluid: 120–128 mmol/L.

Copper (Liver)
< 20 μg/g of wet tissue.

Glucose-6-Phosphatase (Liver)
> 5 μmol/min/g of wet tissue.

Lactate Dehydrogenase (LDH) (CSF)
17–59 IU/L at 37 °C.

Potassium
Breast milk: 12–17 mmol/L.
Cow's milk: 20–45 mmol/L.
Muscle: 160–180 mmol/L of wet fat-free tissue.

Proteins (CSF)
Total proteins:
Newborn: 40–120 mg/dL (0.4–1.2 g/L).
1 month: 20–70 mg/dL (0.2–0.7 g/L).
Thereafter: 15–40 mg/dL (0.15–0.4 g/L).
Gamma globulin:
Children: Up to 9% of total.
Adults: Up to 14% of total.

Sodium
Breast milk: 4.7–8.3 mmol/L.
Cow's milk: 22–26 mmol/L.
Muscle: 33–43 mmol/kg of wet fat-free tissue.

THERAPEUTIC DRUG LEVELS*†

(Values are for serum or plasma.)

Amikacin
15–25 μg/mL.

Aminophylline: See Theophylline.

Aspirin
Antipyretic or analgesic:
20–100 μg/mL.
Anti-inflammatory: 100–250 μg/mL.

Carbamazepine
8–12 μg/mL.

Chloramphenicol
10–20 μg/mL; levels in excess of 25 μg/mL may be dangerous in the newborn infant.

Digoxin
0.8–2 ng/mL.

Diphenylhydantoin: See Phenytoin.

Ethosuximide
40–100 μg/mL.

Gentamicin
5–10 μg/mL.

Phenobarbital
15–40 μg/mL (65–172 μmol/L).

Phenytoin
10–20 μg/mL (0.4–0.8 μmol/L).

Primidone
5–12 μg/mL.

Theophylline
10–20 μg/mL; great patient variability seen within the therapeutic range.

Tobramycin
5–10 μg/mL.

Valproic Acid
50–100 μg/mL.

*Adapted from Meites S (editor): *Pediatric Clinical Chemistry*, 2nd ed. American Association for Clinical Chemistry, 1982, and many other sources.

†Revised with the assistance of Keith B. Hammond, MS.

Table 2. Normal peripheral blood values at various age levels.

Value	1st d	2nd d	6th d	2 wk	1 mo	2 mo
Red blood cells* (million/μL)	5.9 (4.1–7.5)	6 (4.0–7.3)	5.4 (3.9–6.8)	5 (4.5–5.5)	4.7 (4.2–5.2)	4.1 (3.6–4.6)
Hemoglobin (g/dL)	19 (14–24)	19 (15–23)	18 (13–23)	16.5 (15–20)	14 (11–17)	12 (11–14)
White blood cells* (per μL)	17,000 (8–38)		13,500 (6–17)	12,000	11,500	11,000
PMNs (%)	57	55	50	34	34	33
Eosinophils* (total) (per μL)	20–1,000				150–1,150	
Lymphocytes (%)	20	20	37	55	56	56
Monocytes (%)	10	15	9	8	7	7
Immature white blood cells (%)	10	5	0–1	0	0	0
Platelets (per μL)	350,000		325,000	300,000		
Nucleated red blood cells/100 white blood cells*	0–10		0.0–0.3	0	0	0
Reticulocytes (%)	3 (2–8)	3 (2–10)	1 (0.5–5.0)	0.4 (0.0–2.0)	0.2 (0.0–0.5)	0.5 (0.2–2.0)
Mean diameter of red blood cells (μm)	8.6				8.1	
MCV† (fl)	85–125		89–101	94–102	90	
MCHC† (%)	36		35	34		
MCH† (pg)	35–40		36	31	30	
Hematocrit (%)	54 ± 10		51	50	35–50	

*Total nucleated red blood cells: first day, $< 1000/\mu L$.

†MCV = mean corpuscular volume. MCHC = mean corpuscular hemoglobin concentration. MCH = mean corpuscular hemoglobin.

Table 2 (cont'd). Normal peripheral blood values at various age levels.

Value	3 mo	6 mo	1 yr	2 yr	5 yr	8–12 yr	Adults	
							Males	Females
Red blood cells* (million/μL)	4 (3.5–4.5)	4.5 (4–5)	4.6 (4.1–5.1)	4.7 (4.2–5.2)	4.7 (4.2–5.2)	5 (4.5–5.4)	5.4 (4.6–6.2)	4.8 (4.2–5.4)
Hemoglobin (g/dL)	11 (10–13)	11.5 (10.5–14.5)	12 (11–15)	13 (12–15)	13.5 (12.5–15.0)	14 (13.0–15.5)	16 (13–18)	14 (11–16)
White blood cells* (per μL)	10,500	10,500	10,000	9,500	8,000	8,000	7,000 (5–10)	
PMNs (%)	33	36	39	42	55	60	57–68	
Eosinophils* (total) (per μL)	70–550	70–550					100–400	
Lymphocytes (%)	57	55	53	49	36	31	25–33	
Monocytes (%)	7	6	6	7	7	7	3–7	
Immature white blood cells (%)	0	0	0	0	0	0	0	
Platelets (per μL)	260,000			260,000		260,000	260,000	
Nucleated red blood cells/100 white blood cells*	0	0	0	0	0	0	0	
Reticulocytes (%)	2 (0.5–4.0)	0.8 (0.2–1.5)	1 (0.4–1.8)	1 (0.4–1.8)	1 (0.4–1.8)	1 (0.4–1.8)	1 (0.5–2.0)	
Mean diameter of red blood cells (μm)	7.7		7.4		7.4		7.5	
MCV† (fl)	80	78	78	80	80	82	82–92	
MCHC† (%)		33		32	34	34	34	
MCH† (pg)	27	26	25	26	27	28	27–31	
Hematocrit (%)	35	30–40	36	37	31–43	40	40–54	37–47

*Total nucleated red blood cells: first day, $< 1000/\mu L$.

†MCV = mean corpuscular volume. MCHC = mean corpuscular hemoglobin concentration. MCH = mean corpuscular hemoglobin.

LABORATORY TESTS*

TESTS OF LIVER FUNCTION

Alkaline Phosphatase (ALP) Test

A. Specimen: Serum.

B. Normal Values: See p 799. Serum ALP activity during childhood varies according to age; thus, values in children are difficult to interpret. The measurement of serum ALP isoenzymes, which theoretically would help to establish the tissue origin of the enzymes, presents significant technical problems and also renders interpretation difficult. This test, and the measurement of heat-labile (bone) ALP, cannot be recommended at this time.

C. Interpretation: ALP activity is increased in diseases of liver and bone. In hepatic disease, an increased serum ALP level is generally accepted as an indication of biliary obstruction. Levels are also increased in primary hyperparathyroidism, in secondary hyperparathyroidism due to renal disease, in various forms of rickets, in osteitis deformans juvenilia, in malabsorption, and with renal tubular dystrophies. Levels may also be increased in Recklinghausen's disease of bone and in idiopathic hypophosphatasia; the latter disease is associated with rickets and the excretion of excess phosphoethanolamine in the urine.

γ-Glutamyl Transpeptidase (GGTP) Test

A. Specimen: Serum.

B. Normal Values: See p 805.

C. Interpretation: The serum GGTP test is sensitive for liver disease, particularly that due to biliary obstruction, and is particularly useful in screening for liver disease. In the nonjaundiced patient, the GGTP test is superior to tests for alkaline phosphatase, 5′-nucleotidase, and transaminases. Elevated GGTP levels are not confined to a single category of liver disease and may be found in the majority of liver disorders. Liver disease is unlikely to be present if the serum GGTP level is completely normal; however, because of the lack of specificity for hepatic tissue, the converse may not be true.

Serum Protein (Chromatography) Electrophoresis

A. Specimen: Serum.

B. Normal Values: See p 810.

C. Interpretation:

1. Acute hepatitis–Levels of α_2-globulin are increased; γ-globulin levels are markedly increased by the second week. These

*Revised with the assistance of Keith B. Hammond, MS.

changes become marked in chronic cases where the albumin level also is decreased.

2. Massive hepatic necrosis–There is a marked decrease in α-globulin levels and sometimes in β-globulin levels.

3. Cirrhosis–Levels of α-globulin sometimes are increased, but, characteristically, there is a large diffuse increase of γ-globulin levels.

4. Nephrosis–See Chapter 18.

TESTS OF CARBOHYDRATE METABOLISM

Disaccharide (Lactose, Sucrose) Tolerance Tests

These tests are performed in the same manner as the one-dose (oral) glucose tolerance test (see below), except that the loading dose of disaccharide should be twice the dose of glucose.

Epinephrine Tolerance Test

A. Specimen and Test Material: Fasting blood and blood are drawn 15, 30, 60, and 120 minutes after injection of epinephrine (1:1000 solution), 0.1 mL subcutaneously. Collect urine an hour before injection and at 4 consecutive 2-hour periods after injection.

B. Normal Values: Blood glucose levels rise 30–75 mg/dL in 1 hour.

C. Interpretation: The rise in glucose levels is subnormal in organic liver disease, glycogen storage disease, and malnutrition states.

Glucagon Tolerance Test

A. Specimen and Test Material: Fasting blood and specimens are taken at 20, 40, and 60 minutes after glucagon, 20–40 μg/kg, is given intramuscularly.

B. Normal Values: There is an abrupt increase of 40–60% or more in the fasting blood glucose level by 20 minutes.

C. Interpretation: Flat curves are found in cases of glycogen storage disease, in severe liver disease, during the hypoglycemic period in ketotic hypoglycemia, and in small-for-dates neonates.

Glucose Tolerance Test (Intravenous)

A. Specimen and Test Material: Fasting blood and specimens are taken at 5, 15, 30, 45, and 60 minutes after glucose, 0.5 g/kg in a 20–50% solution, is given over a period of 2–4 minutes.

B. Normal Values: The peak value is reached at 5 or 10 minutes, and normal is reached at 45–60 minutes.

C. Interpretation: Elevated values indicate carbohydrate intolerance.

Glucose Tolerance Test (One-Dose, Oral)

A. Specimen and Test Material: Fasting blood and blood specimens are drawn 30, 60, 90, 120, and 180 minutes after glucose is given; in suspected cases of carbohydrate reactive hypoglycemia, samples should also be taken at 4 and 5 hours. Give glucose as an approximate 20% aqueous solution, with flavoring added, in the following dosages: up to 18 months, 2.5 g/kg; 1½–3 years, 2 g/kg; and over 12 years, 1.75 g/kg. Collect urine prior to the test and after 1 and 2 hours, and test for glycosuria. The child should have been on a diet of average carbohydrate intake for 2 weeks prior to the test.

B. Normal Values: There is a rise of 30–80 mg, a peak in 30–60 minutes after ingestion, and a return to fasting level in 120–180 minutes. Levels in capillary blood may be slightly higher than those in venous blood. See also p 806.

C. Interpretation: Abnormal responses consist of (1) fasting sample of greater than 110 mg/dL; (2) elevation of greater than 170 mg/dL; (3) 3-hour sample of greater than 110 mg/dL or above baseline level. A combination of the above results suggests carbohydrate intolerance. The response is the same in newborns, but the fasting point is lower than in older infants. High, prolonged curves are found in hepatic disorders, septicemia, pneumonia, tuberculous meningitis, acute nutritional disturbances, diabetes mellitus, exogenous obesity, and glycogen storage disease. Flat curves are found in encephalitis, in hypothyroidism, in celiac disease, and with delayed gastric emptying. In hyperinsulinism, the immediate response may be normal, but an abrupt fall to hypoglycemic levels may occur.

Insulin-Glucose Tolerance Test

A. Specimen and Test Material: Fasting blood and specimens are taken at 10, 20, 30, 60, 90, 120, and 180 minutes after administration of insulin, 0.1 unit/kg intravenously. At 30 minutes, give glucose, 0.8 g/kg orally. ***Caution:*** In children with potential insulin sensitivity, be ready to terminate the test at any time by giving glucagon or intravenous glucose.

B. Normal Values: There is a fall to 20% of the fasting level of blood glucose in 30 minutes, a prompt rise to 100–200 mg/dL at 90 minutes, and a subsequent fall to normal by 180 minutes.

C. Interpretation: In idiopathic hypoglycemia, adrenal deficiency, and hypopituitarism, there is a normal response to insulin and a diminished response to glucose.

Insulin Tolerance Test

A. Specimen and Test Material: Fasting blood and blood are drawn 10, 30, 45, 60, 90, and 120 minutes after injection of insulin, 0.1 unit/kg intravenously (preferred) or 0.25 unit/kg subcutaneously. Use only one-half to one-third of the calculated dose in children with potentially enhanced insulin sensitivity. ***Caution:*** Safety precautions are as for the insulin-glucose tolerance test, which is preferred.

B. Normal Values: After intravenous administration, the blood glucose level drops to 50% of the fasting level in 15–30 minutes. A fall of the blood glucose value to greater than 50% of the fasting level and a delay of over 90 minutes in the return to fasting levels are considered abnormal by some.

C. Interpretation: Normal newborns have a low tolerance. There is slow or blunted insulin responsiveness with exogenous obesity, some stages of diabetes mellitus, and excessive production of hyperglycemic hormones. A rapid drop is found in adrenal or pituitary insufficiency, starvation, organic intracranial lesions, and in cases with inadequate epinephrine response.

Laevo-Leucine Tolerance Test

A. Specimen and Test Material: Fasting blood and specimens are taken at 15, 30, 45, and 60 minutes after ingestion of laevo-leucine, 150 mg/kg orally or 75–100 mg/kg intravenously, or after ingestion of casein. Casein is given as an approximate 20% aqueous solution in the following dosages: up to 18 months, 2.5 g/kg; 1½–3 years, 2 g/kg; 3–12 years, 1.75 g/kg; and over 12 years, 1.25 g/kg (minimum, 10 g; maximum, 50 g).

B. Normal Values: There is no significant fall in the blood glucose level.

C. Interpretation: A fall in the blood glucose level to 50% of control levels occurs in 30–45 minutes in cases of sensitivity to leucine.

Tolbutamide Tolerance Test

A. Specimen and Test Material: Fasting blood and specimens are taken at 15, 30, 60, 90, 120, and 180 minutes after intravenous administration of sodium tolbutamide, 25 mg/kg (maximum, 1 g) in 10 mL distilled water, infused over a period of 2 minutes. The patient should have been on a high-carbohydrate diet for at least 3 days. ***Caution:*** Terminate the test with 50% glucose if severe hypoglycemic symptoms develop.

B. Normal Values: There is a 25–40% decrease in blood glucose levels in 30 minutes. The return of blood sugar to fasting levels is slow in children. False-positive results are relatively common in children.

C. Interpretation: In hyperinsulin states, there may be a rapid decrease in blood glucose to levels below 40 mg/dL from 30–120 minutes after administration of tolbutamide, and there may be failure to return to normal levels in 3 hours.

TESTS OF RENAL FUNCTION

Addis Sediment Count

A. Specimen: All urine passed from 7:00 PM to 7:00 AM is collected. No fluids are given after 4:00 PM.

B. Normal Values: See p 813.

C. Interpretation: It has not been definitely established whether abnormal Addis counts in children are evidence of anatomic pathology only or of functional impairment as well.

Creatinine Clearance Test

A. Specimen: The timed collection of urine is made between 7:00 PM and 7:00 AM and assayed for creatinine. Blood specimens are drawn at the beginning and end of the period.

$$Ccr = \frac{UV}{P} \times \frac{1.73}{SA}$$

where Ccr = creatinine clearance; U = urinary concentration of creatinine; V = total volume of urine divided by number of minutes in the collection period; P = average of the 2 plasma creatinine levels; and SA = surface area in square meters.

B. Normal Values: See pp 803, 814.

C. Interpretation: Creatinine clearance is a reflection of glomerular filtration rate and declines with the advance of renal insufficiency.

TESTS OF ENDOCRINE FUNCTION

Corticotropin (ACTH) 17-Hydroxycorticosteroid Test

A. Specimen and Test Material: A 24-hour urine specimen is drawn before injection, on the last day of injection, and on the day after injection of corticotropin (ACTH), 0.5 unit/kg intravenously in isotonic saline or glucose solution, infused over a period of 8 hours on 2 or more successive days.

B. Normal Values: There is an increase in output of 17-hydroxycorticosteroids to 2–3 times that of baseline value. A 2-fold or greater rise of urinary 17-hydroxycorticosteroids following use of corticotropin gel, 20 units intramuscularly every 12 hours for a 3-day period, is a normal response. See also p 814.

C. Interpretation: A normal response rules out primary hypoadrenocorticism; a normal response occurs with hypoadrenocorticism secondary to hypopituitarism except in some cases of long-standing ACTH deficiency.

Corticotropin (ACTH) Test (Thorn Test)

A. Specimen and Test Material: Fasting blood and blood are drawn after 4 hours. Corticotropin (ACTH), 5–25 mg, is given subcutaneously or intramuscularly.

B. Normal Values: There is a fall in the eosinophil count of greater than 50% in 4 hours. The normal fall in eosinophil count indicates normal function of the adrenal cortex. See also p 802.

C. Interpretation: Failure to cause a fall in eosinophil count indicates adrenal insufficiency. This test is most reliable in nonallergic patients.

Growth Hormone Test

A. Specimen and Test Material: Fasting blood and specimens are taken at 15 minutes (for glucose concentration) and at 30 and 60 minutes (for glucose concentration and assay of human growth hormone) after administration of crystalline insulin, 0.1 unit/kg intravenously. ***Caution:*** Be ready to terminate the test at any time by giving glucose orally or intravenously or by giving glucagon orally.

B. Normal Values: The 30- or 60-minute sample will reflect a rise in serum growth hormone level (> 7 pg/mL rise from fasting level) in children whose blood glucose level falls below 55 mg/dL or below 66% of the fasting concentration. See also p 805.

C. Interpretation: The fasting sample may have undetectable amounts of human growth hormone. In the presence of a fall in blood glucose of one-third to one-half below fasting level, an increase of less than 7 pg/mL suggests an impaired growth hormone response to hypoglycemia and a possible deficiency of growth hormone. Further clinical evaluation of growth hormone and repeat testing should be carried out before a definitive diagnosis is made. Response is decreased in hypothyroidism and may be abnormal in deprivation dwarfism.

The administration of arginine monohydrochloride, 0.5 g/kg as a 5–10% solution over a 30-minute interval (adult dose, 30 g), will provide a significant rise in plasma concentration of human growth hormone 30–90 minutes postinfusion. Growth hormone levels also rise without artificial stimulation 60–90 minutes after the onset of natural sleep.

Metyrapone (Metopirone; SU-4885) Test

A. Specimen and Test Material: A 24-hour urine specimen for 17-hydroxycorticosteroids is drawn on the day before and the day after giving metyrapone, 300 mg/m^2 orally (never < 250 or > 750 mg) every 4 hours for 6 doses.

B. Normal Values: A 2- to 4-fold rise in levels of 17-hydroxycorticosteroid over control values usually occurs on the day following administration of the drug. Metyrapone inhibits 11β-hydroxylation and blocks the conversion of 11-deoxycortisol to cortisol. Lowered serum cortisol produces compensatory increased secretion of ACTH from the normal pituitary gland, with resultant elevated production of 11-deoxycortisol and raised urinary levels of 17-hydroxycorticosteroid or 17-ketosteroid (or both).

C. Interpretation: Failure to respond occurs with primary adrenocortical failure and in conditions characterized by decreased ACTH production.

Triiodothyronine (T_3) Suppression Test

A. Specimen and Test Material: Radioactive iodine uptake determination is made before and on the seventh day after the administration of 75–125 μg of triiodothyronine daily for 8 days.

B. Normal Values: There is suppression of uptake to 60% or less of the initial amount.

C. Interpretation: Lack of normal suppression occurs with hyperthyroidism.

Water Deprivation Test for Diabetes Insipidus (See p 515.)

Water Load Test of Adrenal Function

A. Specimen and Test Material: Nothing is given by mouth after 6:00 PM. At 10:30 PM, the patient voids and discards urine. Collect and measure urine at 7:30 AM. At 7:30 AM, give water (20 mL/kg) orally within 30 minutes. Collect and measure urine at 9:00 AM, 10:00 AM, 11:00 AM, and 12:00 noon.

B. Normal Values: A normal individual excretes over 70% of the water load within 4 hours, with the greatest volume being excreted during the second hour (9:00 AM–10:00 AM). One of the hourly volumes should exceed the night volume.

C. Interpretation: With adrenal insufficiency, less than 65% of the water load is excreted. The test may not be valid in diabetes insipidus, renal disease, and liver disease.

TESTS OF PANCREATIC & ENTERIC FUNCTION

Sweat Electrolyte Test

A. Specimen: At least 50 mg (0.05 mL) of sweat is collected by pilocarpine iontophoresis. A collection of less than 50 mg should be considered inadequate and the test repeated. Because of the late development of the sweat glands, it is sometimes difficult to obtain sufficient amounts of sweat in the newborn period, and testing may have to be delayed until after the patient is 6 weeks of age.

B. Normal Values: See p 817.

C. Interpretation: A positive sweat test result is an important parameter in the diagnosis of cystic fibrosis. Unfortunately, the test is performed poorly in many clinical laboratories, particularly those where sweat analysis is infrequently requested. A properly performed sweat test should involve pilocarpine iontophoresis, measurement of the volume and weight of sweat collected, and measurement of sodium and chloride concentrations. The sodium and chloride concentrations in sweat are consistently and markedly elevated in almost all cases of cystic fibrosis. Elevated sweat electrolyte levels may be found in a number of other conditions, ie, untreated adrenal insufficiency, nephrogenic diabetes insipidus, and certain forms of ectodermal dysplasia.

Xylose Absorption Test

A. Specimen and Test Material: The test is performed after an overnight fast, but a free fluid intake is actively encouraged before and during the test. A baseline blood sample is drawn into a fluorideoxalate tube. Five grams of D-xylose are freshly dissolved in 250 mL of water and quickly swallowed by the patient. A second blood sample is drawn exactly 60 minutes after the xylose dose. Since micromethods are available for the determination of xylose, capillary blood may be used. The difference between the 2 values should be corrected to a constant surface area of 1.73 m^2 according to the following formula:

$$\text{Corrected blood value} = \frac{(\text{Value}_{60\ min} - \text{Value}_{baseline}) \times \text{Actual surface area}}{1.73}$$

The actual surface area can be derived from a number of available nomograms using the patient's weight and height.

B. Normal Values: The normal corrected blood value is 9.8–20 mg/dL. See also p 812.

C. Interpretation: Xylose absorption is a technically simple, reliable, and informative gauge of upper bowel absorption. Xylose absorption is normal in colitis, liver disease, and primary pancreatic deficiencies. In children, it is abnormal in cystic fibrosis, indicating that the malabsorption in this state is not solely a reflection of deficient pancreatic enzymes.

FLUORESCEIN STRING TEST IN UPPER GASTROINTESTINAL HEMORRHAGE

A white string or umbilical tape 4–5 feet long, weighted at the end with lead shot, is marked lengthwise with radiopaque thread taken from surgical sponges. Interval markers of similar thread are placed horizontally at 1-inch intervals. The string is swallowed and allowed to progress through the gastrointestinal tract overnight while feedings are withheld. An x-ray of the abdomen is obtained to determine whether the string has passed through the pylorus. While the patient is on the x-ray table, fluorescein sodium (Fluorescite) processed with sodium bicarbonate is given intravenously (infants, 1–2 mL; children, 5 mL; adults, 20 mL). After 4 minutes, the string is removed and promptly examined for gross blood and under Wood's light or ultraviolet light for fluorescence.

The presence of blood and fluorescence indicates an actively bleeding site. The presence of blood without fluorescence indicates that there is a bleeding point that was not active at the time of the test. By comparing a measured bloody or fluorescent segment of the string with its location on the x-ray, the site of bleeding can be determined.

Note: Because fluorescein is not stable, the string must be examined promptly. Fluorescein is excreted by the biliary system and ultimately enters the duodenum.

Table 3. Schedule and checklist for performance of pediatric screening procedures.*

Factor to Be Assessed	Age of Child: 3–7 d	2–6 wk	4–5 mo	6–7 mo	8–10 mo	11–14 mo	16–19 mo	22–25 mo	3–4 yr	5–7 yr	8–10 yr	11–12 yr	13–15 yr	16–21 yr
Medical status (by general and developmental history)														
Physical status (by physical examination)			■											
Immunization status†	■	■						■	■		■	■		■
Dental care status‡	■	■	■	■	■	■	■	■						
Visual acuity (by observation and report)		■	■		■		■		■	■	■	■	■	■
Visual acuity (by test)	■	■	■	■	■	■	■	■						
Hearing acuity (by observation and report)		■	■		■				■	■	■	■	■	■

Hearing acuity (by audiometry)§														
Height, weight, and head circumference														
Psychomotor development (by screening test)//														
School progress														
Tuberculin sensitivity¶														
Bacteriuria (girls only)														
Anemia														
Sickle cell disease														

See footnotes on last page of table.

Key: Empty boxes mean that the procedure should be done at the age indicated at the top of the column. The procedure should be done at the next scheduled visit if not done at the recommended time.

Table 3 (cont'd). Schedule and checklist for performance of pediatric screening procedures.*

	Age of Child													
Factor to Be Assessed	**3–7 d**	**2–6 wk**	**4–5 mo**	**6–7 mo**	**8–10 mo**	**11–14 mo**	**16–19 mo**	**22–25 mo**	**3–4 yr**	**5–7 yr**	**8–10 yr**	**11–12 yr**	**13–15 yr**	**16–21 yr**
Sickle cell and hemoglobin C traits														
Lead absorption#														
Phenylketonuria and galactosemia**														

*Adapted from Frankenberg WK, North AF: *A Guide to Screening.* US Department of Health, Education, and Welfare Publication No. SRS 74-24516. US Government Printing Office, 1974.

†A visit at approximately 2 mo of age is necessary to begin the normal immunization schedule.

‡Visual inspection of the mouth and teeth is part of the medical examination at all ages.

§Test hearing yearly from age 3–6 yr.

//Test development earlier and more frequently in known high-risk groups.

¶Test tuberculin less frequently or omit in known low-risk groups.

#Test only exposed children. Test every 6 mo from age 1–3 yr.

**Preferably test at 4–7 d.

Key: Empty boxes mean that the procedure should be done at the age indicated at the top of the column. The procedure should be done at the next scheduled visit if not done at the recommended time.

DIFFERENTIAL DIAGNOSIS OF CERTAIN COMMON SYMPTOMS & SIGNS*

(See p 773 for contents.)

ABDOMINAL ENLARGEMENT

Abdominal Wall Disorders
- Hernia, inguinal
- Hernia, umbilical
- Musculature, absent
- Neoplasms
- Omphalocele

Ascites
- Cardiac failure, congestive
- Chylous ascites
- Cirrhosis, biliary or portal
- Glomerulonephritis
- Hepatitis, viral
- Hypoproteinemia
- Nephrotic syndrome
- Obstruction, hepatic vein
- Obstruction, vena cava
- Pericarditis, constrictive
- Peritonitis
- Polyserositis, idiopathic

Neoplasms & Cysts
- Adrenal tumor
- Bowel, duplication of
- Choledochal cyst
- Dermoid cyst
- Hepatic cyst
- Mesenteric cyst or tumor
- Neuroblastoma
- Omental cyst
- Ovarian cyst or tumor
- Pancreatic cyst
- Polycystic kidney
- Sarcoma, retroperitoneal
- Teratoma, retroperitoneal
- Urachal cyst
- Vitelline duct cyst
- Wilms' tumor
- Other intra-abdominal tumors

Tympanites (Meteorism)
- Adynamic ileus
- Air swallowing
- Colitis, ulcerative
- Cystic fibrosis
- Fecal impaction
- Gastroenteritis
- Malabsorption syndrome
- Megacolon
- Obstruction, intestinal
- Peritonitis
- Pneumoperitoneum
- Septicemia
- Tracheoesophageal fistula

Miscellaneous
- Abscess, peritoneal
- Bladder distention
- Enteritis, regional
- Fecal impaction
- Gastric dilatation
- Hemorrhage, adrenal
- Hepatomegaly
- Hydrocolpos
- Hydronephrosis
- Hydrops of gallbladder
- Intussusception
- Megacolon
- Obstruction, intestinal
- Pregnancy
- Splenomegaly
- Volvulus

CONVULSIONS OR COMA (OR BOTH)

Brain Trauma
- Concussion or contusion
- Hematoma, epidural
- Hematoma, parenchymal
- Hematoma, subdural

*Adapted from Green and Richmond, Berkowitz, Douthwaite, MacBryde, Matousek, Nellhaus, and other sources.

Central Nervous System Disorders
- Degenerative diseases, cerebromacular
- Degenerative diseases, spinocerebellar (Friedreich's ataxia, etc)
- Encephalopathies, demyelinizing
- Gaucher's disease, infantile
- Leukodystrophy (Krabbe's)
- Leukodystrophy, metachromatic
- Niemann-Pick disease
- Schilder's disease
- Sclerosis, diffuse
- Tay-Sachs disease

Central Nervous System Tumors

Cerebrovascular Disorders
- Aneurysm, ruptured cerebral artery
- Embolus, cerebral
- Embolus, fat
- Encephalopathy, hypertensive
- Glomerulonephritis with encephalopathy
- Hematoma, extradural
- Hematoma, subdural
- Hemiplegia, acute infantile
- Hemorrhage with intracranial tumor
- Hemorrhage, other intracranial
- Hemorrhage, parenchymal
- Hemorrhage with pertussis
- Hemorrhage, subarachnoid
- Occlusion, venous, with severe dehydration
- Thrombosis of cerebral vessels
  - Anemia, sickle cell
  - Heart disease, congenital
  - Occlusion, cerebral vein
- Thrombosis, platelet
- Thrombus, cerebral
- Vasospasm

Epilepsy
- Akinetic (drop) seizure
- Cataplexy
- Convulsive equivalent
- Focal seizure
- Grand mal seizure
- Infantile spasm
- Motor and sensory seizure
- Myoclonic seizure
- Narcolepsy
- Petit mal seizure
- Psychomotor seizure

Hyperpyrexia
- Febrile convulsion
- Heat stroke
- (See Fever, Chapter 2.)

Hypoxia
- Anesthesia
- Asphyxia
- Breath-holding spells
- Cardiac diseases
- Hypertension, pulmonary
- Respiratory diseases
- Respiratory failure

Infectious Diseases
- Abscess, intracranial
- Botulism
- Encephalitis
- Encephalopathy, pertussis
- Infectious mononucleosis
- Meningitis
- Panencephalitis, subacute sclerosing
- Pertussis
- Poliomyelitis
- Rabies
- Shigellosis
- Syphilis
- Tetanus
- Toxoplasmosis
- Other acute infectious diseases

Metabolic & Storage Diseases
- Acidosis
- Adrenal insufficiency
- Aminoacidurias
- Histidinemia
- Homocystinuria
- Hypercalcemia
- Hypernatremia
- Hyperosmolarity
- Hyperuricemia
- Hyperventilation
- Hypocalcemia
  - Hypoparathyroidism
  - Rickets
  - Steatorrhea, chronic
  - Tetany of newborn
  - Tetany, postacidotic
- Hypoglycemia
- Hypomagnesemia
- Hyponatremia
- Ketoacidosis, diabetic

Metabolic & Storage Diseases (cont'd)
- Liver insufficiency
- Maple syrup urine disease
- Phenylketonuria
- Pyridoxine deficiency and dependency
- Renal insufficiency
- Water intoxication

Narcolepsy

Poisonings & Drug Reactions
- Alcohol
- Anticonvulsants
- Antidiuretics
- Antihistamines
- Boric acid
- Camphor
- Carbon monoxide
- Carbon tetrachloride and other hydrocarbons
- Diamthazole (Asterol)
- Drug addiction
- Drug withdrawal
- Encephalopathy, toxic
- Ether anesthesia
- Gasoline
- Glue sniffing
- Insecticides
- Kerosene
- Metals, heavy (arsenic, lead, mercury, thallium)
- Plants, poisonous
- Pyrethrum
- Renal insufficiency
- Salicylates
- Sedatives
- Sodium fluoride
- Strychnine
- Sympathomimetic drugs
- Tranquilizers
- Water intoxication

Postinfectious Disorders & Immunization Reactions
- Ataxia, acute cerebellar
- Encephalopathy after pertussis vaccine
- Encephalopathy after smallpox vaccine
- Myelitis, postinfection

Miscellaneous
- Anaphylaxis
- Ataxia-telangiectasia
- Bloch-Sulzberger syndrome
- Cerebral palsy
- Cyst, intracranial
- Effusions, subdural
- Encephalopathy, hemorrhagic
- Encephalopathy, toxic, with systemic disease
- Hemiplegia, acute infantile
- Hydrocephalus
- Kernicterus
- Landry-Guillain-Barré syndrome
- Lupus erythematosus
- Myelitis, transverse
- Shock
- Sturge-Weber syndrome
- Von Recklinghausen's disease

DIARRHEA OF INFANCY (SEVERE)

Allergy & Intolerance Disorders
- Celiac disease
- Cystic fibrosis
- Disaccharide intolerance
- Galactose intolerance
- Glucose intolerance
- Milk protein sensitivity

Anatomic Disorders
- Blind loops
- Fistula
- Hirschsprung's disease
- Stenosis of bowel
- Vagotomy

Deficiency Diseases
- Abetalipoproteinemia
- Agammaglobulinemia
- Copper deficiency
- Kwashiorkor
- Magnesium deficiency
- Vitamin deficiencies

Endocrine Disorders
- Addison's disease
- Adrenogenital syndrome
- Thyrotoxicosis
- Tumors, neural crest

Infectious Diseases
- Bacterial infections
- Enteric infestations
- Enteritis, candidal
- Enteritis, staphylococcal
- Infections adjacent to intestine
- Viral infections

Miscellaneous
- Acrodermatitis enteropathica
- Altered intestinal flora
- Colitis, ulcerative
- Darrow-Gamble syndrome
- Enteropathy, exudative
- Hyperacidity
- Sprue

FAILURE TO THRIVE OR SHORT STATURE (OR BOTH)

Central Nervous System Disorders
- Cerebral abnormalities
- Cerebral damage
- Diencephalic syndrome
- Down's syndrome
- Hematoma, subdural
- Hydranencephaly
- Hypothalamic lesions
- Laurence-Moon-Biedl syndrome
- Schilder's disease

Endocrine Disorders
- Adrenal insufficiency
- Cushing's syndrome
- Diabetes mellitus
- Gonadal dysgenesis
- Hypopituitarism
- Hypothalamic lesions
- Hypothyroidism
- Pseudohypoparathyroidism

Metabolic & Storage Diseases
- Acidosis, renal tubular
- Aminoacidurias
- De Toni-Fanconi-Debré syndrome
- Galactosemia
- Gaucher's disease, infantile
- Glycogen storage disease
- Hypercalcemia, idiopathic
- Hypophosphatasia
- Poisonings (vitamin A; acrodynia)

Nutritional Disturbances
- Anorexia, psychologic
- Diabetes, poorly controlled
- Disaccharidase deficiency
- Fructose intolerance
- Gastrointestinal disease, chronic (regional enteritis, megacolon, etc)
- Malabsorption syndrome
- Malnutrition, intrauterine
- Malnutrition, postnatal
- Zinc deficiency

Skeletal Disorders
- Chondrodystrophia calcificans congenita
- Chondrodystrophy
- Diaphyseal dysplasia
- Hunter's syndrome
- Hurler's syndrome
- Morquio's syndrome
- Osteochondritis
- Osteogenesis imperfecta
- Osteopetrosis
- Rickets, all types
- Spinal diseases
- Other congenital defects

Variations From Normal
- Delayed growth, normal
- Dwarfism, familial
- Dwarfism, racial
- Genetic ("primordial") disorders
- Prematurity
- Prenatal disorders (intrauterine disorders; low-birth-weight infant)

Other Unclassified Types of Dwarfism
- "Bird-headed dwarf"
- Bloom's syndrome
- Cornelia de Lange syndrome
- Leprechaunism
- Progeria
- Progeroid syndrome
- Rubinstein-Taybi syndrome
- Silver's syndrome
- Trisomy 13-15 syndrome
- Trisomy 18 syndrome

Miscellaneous
- Acidosis, chronic
- Allergies, chronic
- Anemia, chronic
- Circulatory disorders
- Deprivation dwarfism
- Hepatic and biliary tract disease
- Infection or infestation, chronic
- Malignant disease
- Parental neglect
- Pulmonary disease, chronic
- Renal disease, chronic
- Reticuloendotheliosis

FEVER OF OBSCURE ORIGIN

Blood Disorders & Neoplastic Diseases
- Agranulocytosis
- Anemia, hemolytic
- Anemia, sickle cell
- Hodgkin's disease
- Leukemia
- Transfusion reaction
- Tumor of cervical cord
- Tumor, Ewing's
- Other tumors

Central Nervous System Disorders
- Convulsive states
- Hemorrhage, intracranial
- Hypothalamic lesions
- Medullary lesions
- Third ventricle lesions
- Tumors of brain

Dehydration

Drug Reactions

Hemorrhage, External & Internal

High Environmental Temperature

"Hypersensitization" Diseases
- Dermatomyositis
- Lupus erythematosus
- Polyarteritis nodosa
- Rheumatic fever
- Rheumatoid arthritis
- Serum sickness

Immunization Reactions

Infectious Diseases

Bacterial, mycotic, parasitic, spirochetal, and viral infections of various tissues, organs, and systems, including:

- Abscess
  - Alveolar
  - Appendiceal
  - Intracranial
  - Perinephritic
  - Pulmonary
  - Retropharyngeal
  - Subphrenic
- Amebiasis
- Appendicitis
- Ascariasis
- Bronchiectasis
- Brucellosis
- Cat-scratch fever
- Cholangitis
- Coccidioidomycosis
- Empyema
- Encephalitis
- Endocarditis, bacterial
- Exanthems
- Hepatitis
- Histoplasmosis
- Infectious mononucleosis
- Influenza
- Leptospirosis
- Lymphocytosis, acute
- Malaria
- Mastoiditis
- Mediastinitis
- Meningitis
- Myalgia, epidemic
- Myocarditis
- Osteomyelitis
- Otitis media
- Pancreatitis
- Poliomyelitis
- Psittacosis
- Rat-bite fever
- Salmonellosis
- Septicemia
- Shigellosis
- Sinusitis
- Spinal epidural infections
- Streptococcal disease
- Syphilis

Infectious Diseases (cont'd)
Torulosis
Toxoplasmosis
Trichinosis
Tuberculosis
Tularemia
Urinary tract infections
Yellow atrophy, acute

Miscellaneous
Agammaglobulinemia
Bacterial product reaction
Cardiac failure, congestive
Colitis, ulcerative
Degenerative diseases
Dysautonomia, familial
Ectodermal dysplasia
Enteritis, regional
Fever, etiocholanolone
Fever, factitious
Fever, psychogenic
Hyperostosis, infantile cortical
Hyperthyroidism
Myeloproliferative disorders
Periodic disease
Sarcoidosis
Tachycardia, paroxysmal atrial
Thyroiditis
Yellow atrophy of liver, acute

HEPATOMEGALY

Blood Disorders & Neoplastic Diseases
Anemia, hemolytic
Anemia, sickle cell
Erythroblastosis fetalis
Leukemia
Lymphomas
Myelofibrosis
Neuroblastoma
Tumors, hepatic (malignant and benign; primary and metastatic)
Other tumors

Infectious Diseases
Abscess, pyogenic hepatic
Amebiasis or amebic abscess
Ascariasis
Brucellosis
Cholangitis due to various organisms

Infectious Diseases (cont'd)
Coxsackievirus infection
Cytomegalic inclusion disease
Echinococcosis
Hepatitis, viral (infectious and serum type)
Histoplasmosis
Infectious mononucleosis
Leptospirosis
Rubella syndrome
Septicemia
Syphilis
Toxoplasmosis
Tuberculosis
Visceral larva migrans

Metabolic & Storage Diseases
Amyloidosis
Cirrhosis of liver
Cystic fibrosis of pancreas
Cystinosis
Diabetes, poorly controlled
Galactosemia
Gaucher's disease
Glycogen storage disease
Hemochromatosis
Hemosiderosis
Hurler's syndrome
Hyperlipidemia, idiopathic
Infiltration (fatty) due to malnutrition
Letterer-Siwe disease
Lipogranulomatosis
Niemann-Pick disease
Osteoporosis
Porphyria
Vitamin A poisoning
Xanthomatosis

Vascular Disorders
Cardiac failure, congestive
Pericarditis, constrictive
Thrombosis of hepatic vein (Chiari's disease)

Miscellaneous
Atresia, biliary duct
Cirrhosis, biliary
Cirrhosis, portal
Cyst, choledochal
Cysts, congenital
Diabetic mothers' offspring
Drugs and toxins

Miscellaneous (cont'd)
Hemangioma
Hemorrhage
Hepatoma, traumatic
Lupus erythematosus
Macroglobulinemia
Sarcoidosis
Wilson's disease

HYPERTENSION

Cardiovascular Disorders
Aortic insufficiency
Arteriosclerosis
Coarctation of aorta
Ductus arteriosus
Polycythemia vera
Stenosis, mitral

Central Nervous System Disorders
Diencephalic disorders
Encephalitis
Increased intracranial pressure
Poliomyelitis, bulbar
Tumors, hypothalamic or pontine

Endocrine Disorders
Adrenogenital syndrome
Cushing's syndrome
Diabetes mellitus
Gonadal dysgenesis
Hyperaldosteronism
Hyperthyroidism
Neuroblastoma
Pheochromocytoma
Tumors, adrenal

Poisonings & Drug Reactions
Acrodynia
Adrenocorticosteroids
Arachnidism
Carbon monoxide
Corticosteroids
Hypercalcemia, idiopathic
Lead poisoning, chronic
Licorice ingestion
Mercury poisoning
Sodium chloride
Sympathomimetic drugs
Thallium
Vitamin D

Renal Disorders
Aneurysm, renal artery
Congenital abnormality
Glomerulonephritis, acute and chronic
Hemolytic-uremic syndrome
Horseshoe kidney
Hydronephrosis
Hypoplastic kidney
Nephrosis, lower nephron
Obstruction, renal artery
Perinephritis
Polycystic kidney
Pyelonephritis
Tuberculosis
Tumors (eg, Wilms' tumor)

Miscellaneous
Angiitis
Dysautonomia
Emotional stress
"Hypersensitization" diseases
Hypertension, essential or idiopathic
Polyarteritis nodosa
Porphyria
Trauma

JAUNDICE

Biliary Obstruction
Atresia, biliary*
Cholangitis*
Cholelithiasis
Cyst, choledochal*
Cystic disease of liver*
Extrinsic pressure
Inspissated bile syndrome*
Peritoneal adhesions
Stenosis, pyloric*
Tumors of bile ducts
Tumors of liver

Deficiency Diseases
Glucose-6-phosphate dehydrogenase deficiency*
Glucuronyl transferase deficiency
- Cretinism*
- Crigler-Najjar disease*
- Gilbert's disease*
- "Physiologic" disease of newborn*

*Items that should be considered in infants with jaundice.

Deficiency Diseases (cont'd)

Uridine diphosphopyridine deficiency*
Wilson's disease

Hemolysis Excess

Anemia, acquired hemolytic*
Anemia, congenital hemolytic*
Erythroblastosis fetalis*
Hemoglobinopathy (Bart's, Zurich, etc)*

Hepatocellular Damage

Infectious Diseases
- Amebiasis
- Ascaris
- Cholangitis
- Cytomegalic inclusion disease*
- Echinococcosis
- Hepatitis, congenital*
- Hepatitis, plasma cell
- Hepatitis, serum
- Herpes simplex*
- Infectious mononucleosis
- Leptospirosis
- Sepsis*
- Syphilis*
- Toxoplasmosis
- Tuberculosis
- Yellow fever

Poisonings and drug reactions
- Hydrocarbons (carbon tetrachloride, chloroform, etc)

Metals, heavy
Novobiocin*
Vegetable toxins
Other drugs competing for albumin
- Heme pigments
- Intravenous fat
- Salicylates
- Sodium glucuronate
- Sulfonamides

*Items that should be considered in infants with jaundice.

Hepatocellular Damage (cont'd)

Poisonings and drug reactions (cont'd)
- Other drugs competing for conjugating mechanisms
  - Caffeine with sodium benzoate*
  - Chloramphenicol*
  - Corticosteroids*
  - Salicylates*
  - Sulfonamides*
  - Vitamin K, water-soluble*
- Other drugs with increased hemolysis
  - Vitamin K, synthetic*

Neoplasms & Cysts

Hemangiomas
Hodgkin's disease
Neoplasms, metastatic
Tumors of bile ducts
Tumors of liver

Miscellaneous

Breast feeding*
Cirrhosis (Laennec's biliary)
Cretinism*
Cystic fibrosis of pancreas
Dubin-Johnson syndrome
Galactosemia*
Hypoxia in neonates*
Leukemia, congenital*
Tyrosinosis

LYMPHADENOPATHY

Blood Disorders

Anemia, hemolytic
Anemia, Mediterranean
Anemia, sickle cell

Infectious Diseases

Bacterial mycotic, parasitic, spirochetal, and viral infections including:
- Brucellosis
- Candidiasis
- Cat-scratch fever
- Chickenpox
- Coccidioidomycosis

Infectious Diseases (cont'd)
- Granulomas
- Histoplasmosis
- Infectious mononucleosis
- Leptotrichosis
- Measles
- Mumps
- Mycobacteria, atypical, infections
- Rubella
- Salmonellosis
- Scarlet fever
- Septicemia
- Toxoplasmosis
- Tuberculosis
- Tularemia
- Vaccinia

Metabolic & Storage Diseases
- Cystinosis
- Gaucher's disease
- Lipidosis, secondary
- Niemann-Pick disease
- Reticuloendothelioses

Neoplastic Diseases
- Hodgkin's disease
- Leukemia
- Lymphosarcoma
- Metastases
- Neuroblastoma
- Other tumors

Poisonings & Drug Reactions
- Antithyroids
- Hydantoins
- Iodides
- Mercurials
- PAS
- Sulfonamides

Miscellaneous
- Eczema
- Oculoglandular syndrome
- Sarcoidosis
- Silicosis

PURPURA

Fibrinogen Deficiency

Plasma Coagulation Defects
- Acquired defect
- Congenital hereditary defect
- (See Table 17–1.)

Qualitative Platelet Abnormalities

Thrombocytopenia
- Aldrich's syndrome
- Allergy
- Anemia, aplastic
- Coagulation, intravascular*
- Cytomegalic inclusion disease*
- Drug reactions*
- Exchange transfusion reaction
- Gaucher's disease
- Hemangiomatosis*
- Hypersplenism
- Infections*
- Irradiation
- Isoimmunization of newborn*
- Leukemia
- Lipid storage disease
- Neonatal thrombocytopenia*
- Neuroblastoma
- Niemann-Pick disease
- Poisons and toxins*
- Postinfection disease
- Systemic disease
- Thrombocytopenic purpura, congenital*
- Thrombocytopenic purpura, idiopathic
- Thrombotic thrombocytopenic purpura
- Tumors
- Xanthomatosis

Vascular Disorders
- Anaphylactoid purpura
- Ehlers-Danlos syndrome
- Infections
    - Cytomegalic inclusion disease*
    - Diphtheria
    - Exanthems
    - Meningococcosis
    - Rickettsial disease
    - Sepsis*
    - Syphilis, congenital*
    - Toxoplasmosis*
    - Typhoid fever

*Items that should be considered in neonates with purpura.

Vascular Disorders (cont'd)
- Letterer-Siwe disease
- Metabolic disease
  - Cushing's disease
  - Diabetes
  - Uremia
- Osteogenesis imperfecta
- Poisonings and drug reactions*
- Scurvy
- Steroids
- Telangiectasia, hereditary*
- Trauma
- Von Willebrand's syndrome

SEXUAL PRECOCITY

Complete ("True") Precocious Puberty
- Constitutional (functional or idiopathic) disorders
- Cerebral disorders
  - Cystic arachnoiditis
  - Encephalopathy, degenerative
  - Hydrocephalus, internal
  - Hypothalamic lesions (hamartomas, hyperplasia, congenital malformations, tumors)
  - McCune-Albright syndrome
  - Pineal or corpora quadrigemina tumors
  - Postencephalitis disorder
  - Postmeningitis disorder
  - Toxoplasmosis
  - Tuberculoma of central nervous system
  - Tuberous sclerosis
  - Tumors near third ventricle
  - Von Recklinghausen's disease
- Drug reactions

*Items that should be considered in neonates with purpura.

Incomplete ("Pseudo") Precocious Puberty
- Adrenogenital syndrome
  - Hyperplasia, adrenocortical
  - Tumors, adrenocortical
- Drug-induced sexual precocity (heterosexual and isosexual)
- Premature pubarche (premature adrenarche)
- Premature thelarche (premature gynarche)
- Tumors, gonadal
  - Tumors of ovaries
    - Choriocarcinoma
    - Dysgerminoma
    - Follicle cysts
    - Granulosa cell tumor
    - Luteoma
    - Teratoma
    - Theca cell tumor
  - Tumors of testes
    - Ectopic adrenal tissue tumor
    - Interstitial cell tumor
    - Teratoma

Miscellaneous
- Down's syndrome (rare)
- Hypothyroidism
- Laurence-Moon-Biedl syndrome
- Silver's syndrome
- Teratoma, presacral
- Tumors, primary liver cell
  - With disturbed androgen metabolism
  - With elevated gonadotropin levels

SPLENOMEGALY

Blood Disorders & Neoplastic Diseases
- Anemia, hemolytic (congenital and acquired)
- Anemia, iron deficiency
- Anemia, Mediterranean
- Anemia, sickle cell
- Erythroblastosis fetalis
- Hemoglobinopathies
- Hodgkin's disease
- Hypersplenism
- Leukemia
- Lymphosarcoma
- Myeloproliferative disorders
- Thrombocytopenic purpura

Infectious Diseases
- Brucellosis
- Common communicable diseases
- Coxsackievirus infection
- Cytomegalic inclusion disease
- Hepatitis
- Histoplasmosis
- Infectious mononucleosis
- Rubella syndrome
- Salmonellosis
- Syphilis
- Toxoplasmosis, congenital
- Tuberculosis
- Tularemia

Metabolic & Storage Diseases
- Amyloidosis
- Cystinosis
- Galactosemia
- Gaucher's disease
- Hemosiderosis
- Hurler's syndrome
- Hyperlipidemia, idiopathic familial
- Letterer-Siwe disease
- Niemann-Pick disease
- Porphyria
- Xanthomatosis

Vascular Disorders
- Cardiac failure, congestive
- Cirrhosis of liver
- Pericarditis, constrictive
- Thrombosis, hepatic vein (Chiari's disease)
- Thrombosis, splenic or portal vein

Miscellaneous
- Abscess, splenic
- Cystic fibrosis
- Cysts
- Hemangioma
- Hemorrhage, subcapsular
- Lupus erythematosus
- Osteopetrosis
- Rheumatoid arthritis
- Sarcoidosis
- Serum sickness
- Waldenström's macroglobulinemia

VOMITING

Central Nervous System Disorders
- Abscess, intracranial
- Concussion
- Edema, cerebral
- Effusion, subdural
- Encephalitis
- Epilepsy
- Hematoma, subdural
- Hemorrhage, intracranial
- Hydrocephalus
- Meningitis
- Migraine
- Pseudotumor cerebri
- Tumors, intracranial

Gastrointestinal Disorders (Obstructive Mechanical)
- Adhesive bands
- Atresia, esophageal
- Atresia, intestinal
- Bowel, duplication of
- Bowel, malrotation of
- Hernia, diaphragmatic
- Hernia, incarcerated or strangulated
- Hirschsprung's disease
- Imperforate anus
- Intussusception
- Meconium ileus
- Meconium plug
- Pancreas, annular
- Stenosis, intestinal
- Stenosis, pyloric
- Volvulus

Infectious Diseases
- Gastrointestinal infections
- Bacterial, fungal, granulomatous, parasitic, and viral infections
- Systemic infections

Metabolic Disorders
- Acidosis
- Hypercalcemia
- Hypoadrenalism
- Hypocalcemia
- Hypoglycemia
- Hypokalemia
- Renal insufficiency

Poisonings & Drug Reactions

Ammonia
Bleaches
Boric acid
Digitalis
Iron
Lead poisoning
Lye
Petroleum distillates
Salicylates
Theophylline

Miscellaneous

Allergy, gastrointestinal
Celiac disease
Cyclic vomiting
Equilibrium disturbances
Foreign bodies
Hemorrhagic diseases
Hyperpyrexia
Motion sickness
Occlusion, mesenteric vascular
Rumination
Shock
Vomiting, psychogenic

Table 4. Cerebrospinal fluid in pathologic conditions.*

Condition	Pressure (mm of H_2O)	Appearance	White Blood Cells (per μL)		Pandy	Protein (mg/dL)	Glucose (mg/dL)	Chloride† (mEq/L)
			Number	Type				
Normal (adult)‡	40–200	Clear.	0–5§	Mono.	0	15–40	40–80	110–128
Newborn	N	Clear or xanthochromic.	0–30 (variable)	PMN 60% (rbc 0–700).		20–170	Average, 80	N
Infant (1 mo)	N	Clear.	0–15	Mostly PMN.		20–70		
"Bloody tap"	N	Pink or red; clearer in successive tubes.	Negative benzidine on supernatant.	rbc and wbc as in peripheral blood.	0 to +	N to slightly incr.	N	N
Brain abscess, unruptured	Incr.	Clear.	10–60	Mono.	0 to +	20–80	N	N
Brain tumor	Usually incr; may be N.	Clear.	Occasionally up to 500.	PMN or lymphocytes.	0 to ++	N to slightly to markedly incr.	N	N
Carcinomatosis, intracranial	Incr.	Clear.	Up to 1000.	Mono.	0 to ++	60–100	Decr.	N
Choriomeningitis, lymphocytic	Incr to greatly incr.	Clear or opalescent.	100–2000	Lymphocytes; early PMN.	++ to ++++	60–200	N	N
Diabetic coma	N	Clear.	N		0	N	High.	N
Encephalitis, lead	N to very high.	Clear.	Up to 100.	Mono.	0 to ++++	100–600 or more.	N	N
Encephalitis, *Toxoplasma*	N to incr.	Clear or opalescent.	30–2000	Mono.	0 to +++	N to greatly incr.	N	N
Encephalomyelitis, equine and St. Louis	Usually incr; may be N.	Clear or opalescent.	Up to 1000.	Early PMN; later mono.	0 to +++	Early N; later 60–200.	N to slightly incr.	N
Guillain-Barré syndrome	Incr.	Clear.	N	Mono.	+ to ++++	Slightly to markedly incr.	N	N
Hematoma, subdural	N to incr.	Clear or xanthochromic.	N to 20.	May have PMN.	0 to ++	N to moderately incr.	N	N
Hemorrhage, subarachnoid	Incr.	Grossly bloody; supernatant xanthochromic.	See // below.	rbc and wbc as in peripheral blood.	0 to ++	N to slightly incr.	N to slightly incr.	N to slightly incr.

Meningismus	Incr.	Clear.	N	Mono.	0 to ±	N	N	N
Meningitis, acute purulent bacterial¶	Up to 300 or more.	Turbid.	500–15,000	PMN.	++ to +++	Up to 500 or more.	Low or absent.	103–116
Meningitis, tuberculous	Up to 300 or more.	Clear or opalescent.	30–500	Early mixed; later mono.	++ to +++	Up to 300 or more.	0–45	Early N; later 94–100.
Mumps	Usually incr; may be N.	Clear or opalescent.	150–2000 (average, 400)	Mono.	0 to +++	Early N; later 60–200.	N	N
Neurosyphilis#	N to incr.	Clear or opalescent.	N to 200.	Mono.	0 to ++	N to 200.	N	N
Poliomyelitis	N to incr.	Clear or opalescent.	15–400 (average, 90)	Early PMN; later mono.	0 to +	30–60; later 100–600.	N	N
Rabies	N to incr.	Clear or opalescent.	30–1000	PMN.	0 to ++	N to incr.	N	N
Uremia	Incr.	Clear.	N	N	+ to ++	N to slightly incr.	N	N to slightly incr.
Other encephalitides (rubeola, varicella)	Usually incr; may be N.	Clear or opalescent.	15–1000	Early PMN; later mono.	0 to +	60–200	Usually N; may be decr.	N

*Cerebrospinal fluid lactate dehydrogenase activity is 50 units (range, 22–73) in infants < 1 wk of age and 14 units (range, 0–40) in older children. The range is 50–2000 units in children with bacterial meningitis and 3–48 units in those with aseptic meningoencephalitis.

†Reported as NaCl in mg/dL and as Cl^- in mEq/L.

‡Additional normal findings: Calcium, 4–6 mg/dL; magnesium, 2.5–3.3 mEq/L; potassium, 2.8–4.2 mEq/L; sodium, 130–165 mEq/L; phosphorus, 1.5–3.0 mg/dL; specific gravity, 1.005–1.009; pH, 7.33–7.42; carbon dioxide combining power, 18–31 mEq/L.

§Up to 10 cells/μL in infants and up to 8 cells/μL in children < 5 yr of age.

//Many rbc for 8–12 d. Crenated after 12 h.

¶Lactic acid content (normal, 9–20 mg/dL) elevated and pH (normal, 7.28–7.35) reduced in bacterial meningitis.

#If a patient has a positive result in the serologic test for syphilis, even small amounts of blood in the spinal fluid may give a false-positive test result on the fluid. If a traumatic bloody tap is obtained, it should be repeated in 2–3 wk.

N = Normal	Decr = Decreased	PMN = Polymorphonuclear neutrophils	rbc = Red blood cells
Mono = Mononuclear cells	Incr = Increased		wbc = White blood cells

Table 5. Chromosomal disorders.*

Chromosomal Disorder	Chromosome		Possible Mechanism	Usual Age of Mother	Prominent Characteristics
	Number	Abnormality			
I. Autosomal anomalies					
1. Down's syndrome (mongolism; trisomy 21 syndrome)					See Chapter 21. Other findings include abnormal dermatoglyphics with high axial triradius, arch tibial on foot, ulnar loops on all fingers and simian creases, abnormal tryptophan metabolism. Parents may have increased incidence of taste abnormalities (insensitivity to quinine and certain thiourea type compounds). Translocation type may be familial; standard and mosaic types usually are not. Parents of translocation type may have 45 chromosomes including translocation with a normal phenotype. Abnormalities may be less severe in the mosaic type.
a. Standard or regular type (1:900 births)	47	Trisomy 21.	Meiotic nondisjunction.	Older mother in one-third of cases.	
b. Translocation type (5% of patients with Down's syndrome; 50% of these are familial)	46	Trisomy 21 with one 21 attached to chromosome 13, 21, or 22.	Translocation.	No relation to maternal age.	
c. Mosaic type (2.7% of all cases)	46 and 47	One set normal; other with trisomy 21.	Error in early mitotic division.		
2. Trisomy 18 syndrome (E_1 group trisomy) (1:8000 births; sex ratio = 4 males: 1 female)	47	Trisomy 18.	Meiotic nondisjunction.	More frequent with advanced maternal age.	Flexion deformity of fingers with index finger over third finger, "rocker bottom" deformity of feet, prominent occiput, retrognathia, mental retardation, intrauterine growth retardation, failure to thrive, short sternum, small pelvis, dorsiflexed ("hammer") big toe, renal or skeletal anomalies, early death.
3. Partial deletion of short arm of 18 (18p monosomy; $18p^-$)	46	Partial deletion of short arm of 18.	Chromosomal break.	Unknown.	Microcephaly, epicanthic folds, rounded facies, hypotonia, severe psychomotor retardation, short stature.

4. Partial deletion of long arm of 18 (18q monosomy; $18q^-$)	46	Partial deletion of long arm of 18.	Chromosomal break.	Unknown.	Atresia of ear canals, high-arched palate, microcephaly, retraction of mid face, receding chin, prominent anthelix, spindle-shaped fingers, psychomotor retardation, short stature. Absence of IgA immunoglobulin has been noted in one-third of cases.
5. Trisomy 13 syndrome (D group trisomy; D_1 group trisomy) (1:5000–1:10,000 births)	47	Trisomy 13.	Meiotic nondisjunction.	More frequent with advanced maternal age.	Cleft lip and palate; hyperconvex narrow fingernails, overriding index finger, retroflexible thumbs; simian line; posterior prominence of heels; abnormal scrotum; cryptorchidism; polydactyly; apparent deafness; cardiac anomalies; large fleshy nose; arhinencephaly; hypoplasia of frontal lobes; microphthalmos; colobomas; failure to thrive; mental retardation; early death.
6. Cat's cry syndrome (cri du chat syndrome)	46	Deletion of part of arm of 5.	Deletion.		"Catlike" cry, deformed larynx, microcephaly, micro-retrognathia, "moonlike" facies, failure to thrive, hypotonia, severe mental retardation. Chromosome abnormalities in some relatives. Abnormal dermatoglyphics.
7. Syndrome of congenital asymmetry and short stature (Silver's syndrome)	46 or 46/69	Most with normal karyotype; mosaicism (46/69) in small percentage.			Asymmetry, short stature, variations in sexual development (including precocity), intrauterine growth retardation, downturned mouth, incurved fifth fingers, elevated gonadotropins in some.
8. Chronic myelogenous leukemia	46	Abnormally small acrocentric chromosome 22 (Ph^1).	Balanced translocation: long arm of 22 to long arm of 9.		Chronic myelogenous leukemia. Low phosphatase of neutrophils. Chromosomal abnormality in bone marrow (90% of cases) and sometimes in peripheral blood.

*Revised with the assistance of Arthur Robinson, MD.

Table 5 (cont'd). Chromosomal disorders.*

Chromosomal Disorder	Chromosome Number	Chromosome Abnormality	Possible Mechanism	Usual Age of Mother	Prominent Characteristics
I. Autosomal anomalies (cont'd)					
9. Bloom's dwarfism	46	Multiple chromosome breaks, quadriradial figures; occasionally "pulverization."			Dwarfism, chronic erythematous rash, tendency toward malignant diseases (especially leukemia). Probably single gene autosomal recessive. Increased chromosomal breaks occasionally in close relatives.
10. Congenital aplastic anemia (Fanconi's anemia)	46	Increased number of chromosomal breaks.	Autosomal recessive.		Skeletal (especially thumbs and upper extremity), renal, and hematopoietic abnormalities. Skin pigmentation, gonad hypoplasia.
11. Trisomy 8 mosaicism	46 and 47	One set normal; other with trisomy 8.	Error in early mitotic division.	No relation to maternal age.	Short stature, unusual facies, abnormal pinnas, absent patellas, genitourinary anomalies, mental retardation.
12. $4p^-$ syndrome	46	Partial deletion of short arm of 4.	Chromosomal break.		Severe mental retardation, microcephaly, coloboma, prominent epicanthi, beaked nose, cleft palate, micrognathia, inguinal hernia.
13. $13q^-$ syndrome	46	Partial deletion of long arm of 13.	Chromosomal break.		Mental retardation, failure to thrive, microcephaly, coloboma, microphthalmia, hypoplastic or absent thumbs, congenital heart disease, genitourinary abnormalities. Occasionally, retinoblastoma.
14. $21q^-$ syndrome	46	Partial deletion of long arm of 21.	Chromosomal break.		Mental retardation, motor retardation, antimongoloid slant of eyes, cleft palate, hypospadias.
15. Cat-eye syndrome	47	Trisomy 22 or partial trisomy 22.	Chromosomal break.		Coloboma, anal atresia, mental retardation, antimongoloid slant of eyes, genitourinary and heart anomalies, micrognathia, low-set nipples.

16. Trisomy 9p syndrome (sex ratio = 1 male:2 females)	46	9p usually translocated to another chromosome.	Breakage or malsegregation of a reciprocal translocation.		Relatively frequent syndrome. Brachycephaly, bulbous nose, small deep-set eyes, brachymesophalangy, mental retardation.
II. Sex chromosome abnormalities†					
1. Klinefelter's syndrome (1:700 births)	47	Usually XXY. Also XXYY, XXXY, XXXYY, XXXXY, and mosaicism.	Nondisjunction.		See Chapter 21. Rarely fertile. Increased risk of mental retardation and of behavioral and emotional problems.
2. XX male	46	XX.	Interchange of X and Y chromosome during meiosis or loss of Y in mitosis. May be due to an autosomal gene for "sex reversal."		Normal phenotype, phenotype similar to Klinefelter's syndrome, or partial feminization. Not as tall as in Klinefelter's syndrome.
3. XYY sex chromosome anomaly (1:1000 births)	47	XYY.	Meiotic nondisjunction.		Tall stature, impulsivity or sociopathology in some adults.
4. XXXXY sex chromosome anomaly	49	XXXXY; sometimes XXXXY/XXXY.	Nondisjunction.		Mental retardation; synostosis of proximal radius and ulna; microcephaly, short stature, long legs, incurved phalanges, elongation of the radii, abnormal ossification centers, scoliosis, and hypertelorism; nuclear chromatin with 3 Barr bodies.

*Revised with the assistance of Arthur Robinson, MD.

†A few cases with other karyotypes, including several types of mosaicism, have also been described. Sterility is common to most.

Table 5 (cont'd). Chromosomal disorders.*

Chromosomal Disorder	Chromosome		Possible Mechanism	Prominent Characteristics
	Number	Abnormality		
II. Sex chromosome abnormalities (cont'd)†				
5. Turner's syndrome (Bonnevie-Ullrich-Turner syndrome; gonadal dysgenesis) (1:3000 births)	45 or 46	Usually 45,X; often mosaicism; may have 45,X, fragment X; or 46,Xi(Xq)—isochromosome of long arm.	Meiotic or mitotic nondisjunction; chromosome lag or breakage.	See Chapter 20.
6. Male pseudohermaphrodite; mixed gonadal dysgenesis	45 and 46	Missing Y chromosome in some cells. Mosaicism. 45,X/46,XY.	Mitotic nondisjunction or chromosome lag.	Some of findings present in Turner's syndrome, with infantile female secondary sexual characteristics but with a variable degree of masculinization of the genitalia. Tendency to develop gonadoblastomas.
7. Male pseudohermaphrodite; testicular feminizing syndrome	46	46,XY.		Tall, well-feminized, sterile female with testes. Probably a single gene defect that inhibits end-organ response to testosterone. Tendency to develop gonadoblastomas.
8. True hermaphrodite	46	46,XX; 46,XY; 46,XX/46,XY.	46,XX/46,XY: ovum fertilized by 2 sperms.	Ovum on one side and testis on other or ovotestis on one or both sides. Varying degrees of abnormal phenotypic sexual determinacy.
9. Triple-X sex chromosome anomaly (1:1000 births)	47	47,XXX; rarely, XXXX or XXXXX.	Nondisjunction.	Increased risk of intellectual and emotional disturbances reported in adults. Tendency toward tall stature.
10. Fragile X syndrome	46	46,fra(X)(q28)Y.	Break of long arm of Xq28 (inhibited by folic acid and thymidine). Heritable "marker X."	Mental retardation; large testes, head, and ears; prognathic jaw; jocular and repetitive speech.

*Revised with the assistance of Arthur Robinson, MD.

†A few cases with other karyotypes, including several types of mosaicism, have also been described. Sterility is common to most.

Index*

*See Appendix (p 778) for alphabetical listing of drugs (with dosages) not listed in the Index. See Appendix (p 833) for lists of differential diagnoses of certain common symptoms and signs. Only the major categories are listed in the Index.

JA (bact 4+)

RBC 30-35

WBC 2-4 HPF

1.013

pH 5.0

2+

Granucast Many/HPF

ANA pos

LE prep (-)

Kaye + Osky
Core Text of PEDS

T ≥ 106° = pyelonephritis
- meningitis
- pneumonia

Bulging Fontanelle

- ↑ intracranial pressure - f/ mass, meningitis
- Hyper/hypo Vit. A → (pseudotumor cerebri)
- Tetracycline (old)
  pt newly off steroid
- Roseola - classically → happy babies c̄ bulging fontanelle c̄ fever
  ↳ erythema subitum, 6 mo - 15 mo's
  emerges after fever breaks
  ↳ can → seizures